Harkness and Wagner's

Biology and Medicine of Rabbits and Rodents

FIFTH EDITION

Harkness and Wagner's

Biology and Medicine of Rabbits and Rodents

FIFTH EDITION

John E. Harkness, DVM, MS, MEd, DACLAM
College of Veterinary Medicine
(Professor Emeritus)
Mississippi State University
Mississippi State, Mississippi, USA

Patricia V. Turner, MS, DVM, DVSc, DACLAM
Ontario Veterinary College
University of Guelph
Guelph, Ontario, Canada

Susan VandeWoude, DVM, DACLAM
Colorado State University
Fort Collins, Colorado, USA

Colette L. Wheler, DVM, MVetSc
University of Saskatchewan
Saskatoon, Saskatchewan, Canada

Illustrations by Gianni A. Chiappetta

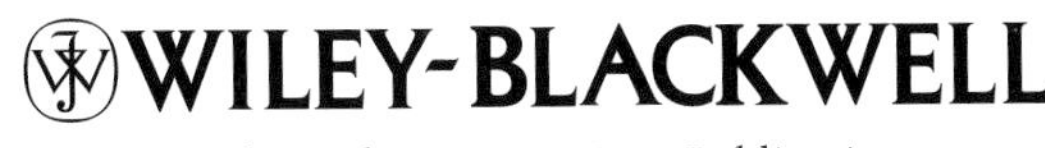

A John Wiley & Sons, Inc., Publication

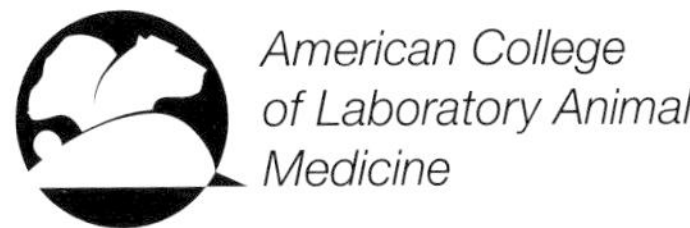

First edition first published 1977, Williams & Wilkins
Second edition first published 1983, Williams & Wilkins
Third edition first published 1989, Williams & Wilkins
Fourth edition first published 1995, Williams & Wilkins
Fifth edition first published 2010

Blackwell Publishing was acquired by John Wiley & Sons in February 2007. Blackwell's publishing program has been merged with Wiley's global Scientific, Technical, and Medical business to form Wiley-Blackwell.

Editorial Office
2121 State Avenue, Ames, Iowa 50014-8300, USA

For details of our global editorial offices, for customer services, and for information about how to apply for permission to reuse the copyright material in this book, please see our website at www.wiley.com/wiley-blackwell.

Library of Congress Cataloging-in-Publication Data

Harkness and Wagner's biology and medicine of rabbits and rodents / John E. Harkness ... [et al.]. – 5th ed.
p. ; cm.
Rev. ed. of: The biology and medicine of rabbits and rodents / John E. Harkness, Joseph E. Wagner. 4th ed. 1995.
Includes bibliographical references and index.
ISBN-13: 978-0-8138-1531-2 (alk. paper)
ISBN-10: 0-8138-1531-2 (alk. paper)
1. Laboratory animals–Diseases. 2. Rodents–Diseases. 3. Rabbits–Diseases. 4. Rodents as laboratory animals. 5. Rabbits as laboratory animals. I. Harkness, John E. II. Harkness, John E. Biology and medicine of rabbits and rodents. III. American College of Laboratory Animal Medicine. IV. Title: Biology and medicine of rabbits and rodents.
[DNLM: 1. Rodentia–physiology. 2. Animals, Laboratory. 3. Rabbits–physiology. 4. Veterinary Medicine. SF 996.5 H2825 2010]
SF996.5.H37 2010
636.932′2–dc22

2009027945

A catalog record for this book is available from the U.S. Library of Congress.

Set in 10 on 12 pt Times by Toppan Best-set Premedia Limited
Printed in Singapore by Markono Print Media Pte Ltd

1 2010

This edition is dedicated to a devoted teacher, colleague, and friend,
Dr. Joseph E. Wagner, 1938–2007.

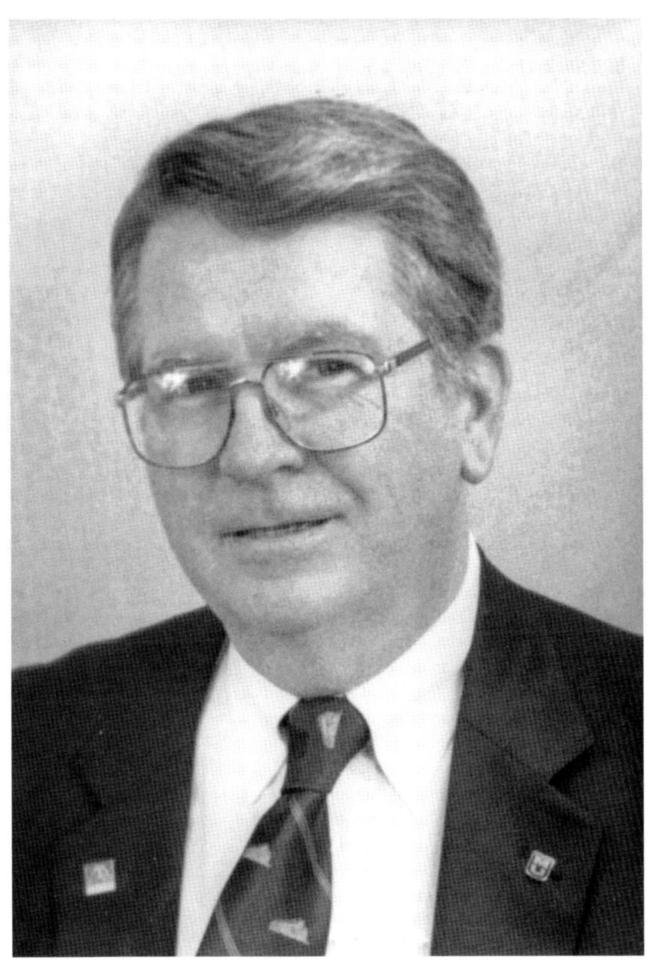

CONTENTS

PREFACE

The *Biology and Medicine of Rabbits and Rodents* provides concise, up-to-date, reasonably comprehensive information to anyone concerned with the health, care, and management of rabbits and rodents. The book is intended for veterinarians, students, technicians, scientists, breeders, and those with a background in the biological sciences. A basic knowledge of biology and an interest in rabbits and rodents as pets, production animals, or laboratory animals are assumed. Beyond this, the emphasis throughout is on the practical aspects of rabbit and rodent care and health, and substantial detail is provided about many aspects of biology and husbandry, clinical signs and procedures, and specific diseases and their diagnoses. Distinctions between animals used as production, laboratory, or pet animals are provided when relevant.

This book is intended to bridge the gap between the extremely comprehensive hardcover reference works on various species of laboratory animals and a variety of class notes, handbooks, proceedings, autotutorial materials, and other publications used as references in practice or for teaching. The care and use of rabbits and rodents has changed considerably since the last edition of this text. The goal when writing this edition was to retain the easy-to-read practical style characteristic of previous editions, but to expand discussion of management and diseases that have evolved significantly since 1995.

This edition was produced under the expert oversight of Dr. John Harkness, one of the original authors, to preserve the flavor and accessibility of previous editions. Every effort was made to correct errors and ommissions from previous editions, and we welcome suggestions for improving and updating the next edition. Undoubtedly, despite our best intentions, errors will be discovered, and for these we apologize. We hope the new material added to this text will be helpful to new and seasoned readers of previous editions.

The major changes in this edition include updating previously described conditions; reorganizing certain disease descriptions under common headings; adding descriptions of new diseases, refined techniques such as medical imaging, and husbandry practices; and adding information on chinchillas. The following diseases and conditions have been given new or expanded coverage: anorexia and dental disease, various dermatopathies and enteropathies of rabbits and rodents, hematuria and pigmented urine, *Helicobacter* spp infections of mice, listeriosis, murine norovirus infections, rabies virus infections, and viral hemorrhagic disease in rabbits. In chapter 6, some case reports have been deleted, others modified, and new ones added. Many references have been eliminated or updated and some web-based resources have been included. Finally, over 200 images have been added to this edition, some of which replace the line drawings present in previous editions, and several new tables have been included.

We are humbled to have had the pleasure of working on the new edition of this classic text that has enjoyed such a loyal following over the decades. We can only hope that readers will be satisfied with our efforts, and that the information contained on the following pages will be used to improve the welfare of these interesting species that have contributed to human lives in countless positive ways.

Patricia V. Turner
Guelph, Ontario

Susan VandeWoude
Fort Collins, Colorado

Colette L. Wheler
Saskatoon, Saskatchewan

ACKNOWLEDGMENTS

Many portions of this fifth edition of *Biology and Medicine of Rabbits and Rodents* have been rewritten and updated, and we are grateful to our colleagues in veterinary practice and animal care facilities for advancing the knowledge underlying many of these changes. We feel very fortunate to have had the opportunity to work together during the preparation of this material, and we learned a tremendous amount from each other. We gained a true appreciation of the depth and variety of knowledge that we all acquire during our diverse experiences working with these species in different environments, and would encourage all readers to take advantage of their peers and colleagues when seeking answers to small mammal cases. We recognize that in spite of our best efforts, errors may be present in the text, and we invite your comments for future editions.

We especially wish to recognize the support given by our families and thank them for their unfailing patience throughout this project. We thank Erica Judisch at Wiley-Blackwell for her excellent comments and suggestions throughout the preparation of this edition. Special thanks are also due to Jutta Hammermueller and Margaret Chiappetta for document searches and editorial assistance.

This project was undertaken by the American College of Laboratory Animal Medicine (ACLAM), and all proceeds from book sales will be used to support the educational mission of the ACLAM Foundation. We thank Dr. James Fox, Chair of the ACLAM Publications Committee, for his support and helpful guidance throughout this project.

PHOTOGRAPHY CREDITS

Every effort has been made to attribute photographs to their rightful owners, and we apologize in advance if we have inadvertently missed any contributor. We are deeply grateful to the following individuals and companies for providing permissions to use photographs in this book and for assisting with photography:

- Calgary, AB: Irene Phillips, Avenida All-Pet Clinic
- Centennial, CO: Animal Care Systems, Inc.
- Charles River Laboratories, Wilmington, MA: Katherine Pritchett-Corning
- Colorado State University, Fort Collins, CO: Matthew Johnston, with assistance by Hillary Lucero, Elisa French, Richard Heimbichner, Charles Kerlee, and Denise Ostmeyer
- Guelph, ON: Kendra A. Keels, Ontario Rabbit Industry Development Manager, and Robert Wright, Ontario Ministry of Agriculture and Food Rural Affairs
- McMaster University, Hamilton, ON: Shawn Petrik
- Oakville, ON: Catherine L. Havlicek
- Oregon Health and Science University, Portland, OR: Anne Bower and Manfred Baetscher
- Saskatoon, SK: Glen and Rebecca Grambo—Grambo Photography and Design, Inc., and Petland, Confederation Park Plaza
- Scarborough, ON: Kresimir Pucaj, Nucrotechnics
- State University of New York, Buffalo, NY: Lisa B. Martin
- University of Guelph, Guelph, ON: Marina Brash, David Hobson, Emily Martin, Amanda Martyn, Dean H. Percy, Dale Smith, and W. Michael Taylor, with assistance by Murray Hazlett, Amanda Healy, Annette Morrison, Jelena Ovari, Tim Sullivan, and Ashley Whiteman
- University of Saskatchewan, Saskatoon, SK: L. Dean Chapman, Leah Frei, Ernest D. Olfert, Dennilyn Parker, and Phyllis Paterson, with assistance by Peggy Nelles, Tania Liboiron, Monique Mayer, Michele Moroz, Lorilee Sereda, and Colleen Zielke
- University of Toronto: Karen Parisien and A.J. Wang

Harkness and Wagner's

Biology and Medicine of Rabbits and Rodents

FIFTH EDITION

Chapter 1

Introduction, General Husbandry, and Disease Prevention

INTRODUCTION

Populations of rabbits, rodents, and other small mammals used as pets are difficult to establish; however, a 2007 study conducted by the American Veterinary Medicine Association (AVMA) estimated that U.S. families own 6.2 million rabbits, 1.2 million hamsters, and just over one million guinea pigs. Only a small percentage of these owners obtain annual veterinary care for their small mammal pets.

Numbers of animals used in research are also difficult to determine because of the limitations of applicable surveys and estimates where fixed data does not exist. Based on United States Department of Agriculture Animal and Plant Health Inspection Service (USDA-APHIS) data, approximately 170,000 hamsters, 220,000 guinea pigs, and 240,000 rabbits have been used annually in the United States in research, testing, and teaching in recent years, while fewer numbers of gerbils and chinchillas have been used. The numbers of rats and mice used is significantly more difficult to estimate since these data are not collected or reported by U.S. federal agencies. Approximately one million mice were used in Canada in 2007, and this accounted for 47% of animals used in research (www.ccac.ca). Estimates of mice used in the United States in biomedical research range from six to one hundred million mice per year. It is even more difficult to find accurate references for numbers of rats used annually in research, though estimates of four million have been previously cited. Mice and rats are typically noted to account for 95–98% of all animals used in research in the United States. Availability of genetically characterized strains and stocks with increased relevance to the diseases being studied, sequencing of the mouse and rat genomes (completed in 2002 and 2005, respectively), development of transgenic technology, and ease and economy of housing in large numbers have significantly contributed to the popularity of these animals as models for many aspects of biomedical research.

Numbers of rabbits produced as a food source varies by region; in 2006, the European Union accounted for 63% of world production of rabbit meat with approximately 26,309 tons (53 million lb) produced annually, followed by China at 25% of the world production (faostat.fao.org). The United States and Canada accounted for approximately 2% and 0.2% of world rabbit meat production, respectively. Production is by-and-large proportional to per capita consumption, as rabbit meat is rarely exported from North America. Italy leads the world in terms of rabbit meat consumption with more than 5 kg (11 lb) per person annually; however, Greece, Belgium, and a number of Mediterranean countries also have significant per capita consumption.

With the exception of China, the number of rabbits used for fur and pelt production is much lower than the number raised for human consumption. Rabbit pelts harvested at slaughter for meat are typically of poor quality, as breed, age at harvest, and husbandry conditions differ significantly for optimal production of meat compared with pelts. Rex rabbits are the primary breed used for pelt harvest, whereas Angora rabbits are shorn regularly for use of their hair in thread production and weaving. France has historically lead world production of both quality skins and angora fiber, and significant industrial growth of fur farming has occurred in China during the last 2 decades. Hong Kong, Beijing, Milan, and Montreal are now the dominant sites for sale of rabbit furs to be used for textile processing.

Chinchillas have been used by humans as a source of pelts for clothing for centuries, a practice that drove them to near extinction in the wild in the early twentieth century. In 1983, it was estimated that the United States led production of chinchilla pelts (200,000 annually), but by the late twentieth century, South American and Eastern European suppliers significantly outpaced U.S. and Canadian production. Public perception about the use of animal pelts for fur has lead to development of specific industry husbandry guidelines. For example, commercial chinchilla ranching standards have been developed in Canada, and a U.S. chinchilla breed association (Empress Chinchilla Breeders) runs a humane care certification program for ranchers.

While veterinary care is relevant for all the aforementioned reasons, the subjects of this book—rabbits, guinea pigs, chinchillas, hamsters, gerbils, mice, and rats—do not constitute a large part of the typical small animal practice population, even if the practice specializes in exotic animals.*

Nevertheless, the human-animal bond applies regardless of animal size, and the client who has a rabbit or rodent as a pet may be as devoted to that pet as is the owner of a more traditional species, such as a dog or cat. These owners are often frustrated in their attempts to find veterinarians who are knowledgeable about their small mammal pet. Problems of management and husbandry are often at the root of disease issues and can often be ameliorated by appropriate client education. Small mammal practice does require a modicum of special knowledge; however, careful extrapolation of experiences with other small animals (dogs and cats) to rabbits and rodents is often useful and appropriate. Small animal clinicians usually are very competent with most small mammal problems and practitioners inclined to develop a client base in this area should not be deterred because of a perceived lack of specialized veterinary training.

Veterinary clinicians are likely to encounter rabbits and rodents in a wide spectrum of situations, presenting a significant challenge when compiling literature regarding management of health and diseases of these species. For example, rabbits and rodents may be produced by commercial breeders for the purposes of research and testing. Most animals raised in this manner are reared in specific pathogen-free barriers that preclude introduction of disease agents, and they are sold to research establishments that maintain highly controlled environments to house research animals. Because of the sophisticated nature of the research in which these animals are used, they are usually defined physiologically, genetically, and microbiologically. Rodents and rabbits in the retail pet trade have less certain genetic identification and health histories, and are often managed in ways that do not limit disease transmission among species and conspecifics. Commercial breeding operations for food and fiber production are intermediate between these two scenarios, emphasizing production as a goal, and employing management schemes that result in yet a third spectrum of disease issues. Therefore, medical challenges for private practitioners evaluating small mammal pets are substantially different from those seen by institutional laboratory animal veterinarians and veterinarians treating animals at commercial rabbit and rodent breeding operations.

Early literature describing the attributes of these species originated from the laboratory animal and commercial breeder industry; however, more recent texts have been developed with the private practitioner in mind, adopting an individual animal approach versus a herd health approach to treatment. Although the biology, physiology, and disease susceptibility of animals reared and kept for research production or as pets are similar, differences in purpose and management requirements should be kept in mind when reviewing the available literature on these animals. For example, housing requirements for mice held in a laboratory animal facility emphasize environmental and microbiological controls for the sake of experimental uniformity. These standards may exceed practical recommendations for owners rearing fancy mice for show or feeder prey for reptiles. Diseases described in the laboratory animal literature are typically those seen in specific strains and ages most commonly used for research (i.e., specific pathogen free [SPF] genetically defined stocks of rodents and New Zealand white rabbits) and

*Exotic animal practice typically refers to veterinary practices that treat avian, reptile, amphibian, and small mammal species.

are likely to differ substantially from common conditions of rodents purchased at the local pet store, chinchillas managed in a production setting, or neutered house rabbits approaching geriatric age. Treatment of animals reared for food or fur production may be limited due to the impact of drug residues or damage to pelts. Thus, it is important to use professional judgment when evaluating the literature and to consider the differences in management and purpose when formulating an appropriate diagnostic and therapeutic plan.

SOURCES OF INFORMATION

References for veterinarians who see rabbits and rodents in private practice are much more readily available today than a decade ago. Web resources abound, but should be regarded with some caution if unreferenced. Wikipedia (en.wikipedia.org), an online, free, collaborative encyclopedia, generally provides informative articles with specific references, or indicates where references are lacking. Wikipedia also provides links to other websites that are typically general in nature, informative, and well written. General references related to the practice of rabbit and rodent medicine are listed at the end of this chapter. Species-specific references are listed in chapters 2, 4, and 5. This text emphasizes general references and indices of current literature rather than exhaustive literature reviews.

Knowledge about rabbits and rodents among veterinarians varies considerably. Even among the most knowledgeable and successful practitioners, recommendations for treatment vary, depending on experience with what has worked and what has not. The Veterinary Information Network (VIN, www.vin.com) is a subscription-only online network that supports dialogue among veterinary practitioners, including specialists in rabbit and rodent medicine. Membership in VIN also provides ready access to a searchable literature and case database that includes exotic species. Laboratory animal veterinarians have extensive training in these species, particularly in matters relating to biology, husbandry, and diseases. Diagnostic laboratories specializing in rodent and rabbit diseases can also be helpful in suggesting appropriate work-ups or providing necropsy and specialized diagnostic services. Because many therapeutic recommendations are unpublished and empirically based, they should be accepted and used with caution. Despite these admonitions, skilled small animal practitioners with little specific knowledge about rabbits and rodents often do extremely well by applying general medical knowledge and by consulting with colleagues for suggestions. This is particularly true since many disease issues in these species are related to easily recognizable lapses in appropriate husbandry.

TAXONOMY, HISTORY, AND BEHAVIOR

Detailed taxonomy and history of domestication of rabbits and rodents can be found in chapter 2. Until the early 1900s, rabbits and rodents were classified similarly; however, anatomical and physiological studies indicated significant differences leading to reclassification of rabbits in a distinct order. Rabbits are members of the family Leporidae in the order Lagomorpha, whereas rodents are members of the order Rodentia. Rats, mice, gerbils, and hamsters are in the suborder Myomorpha ("rat-like"), while guinea pigs and chinchillas are classified in the suborder Hystricomorpha ("porcupine-like"). Differences in classification of rabbits and rodents relate to the dental anatomy and physiology, as well as to differences in nutrition, gastrointestinal function, and reproduction.

Rabbits and guinea pigs have been used for food (and domesticated to the extent of captive production for this purpose) for centuries; however, during the last century, breeding of these species, as well as of chinchillas, commenced for other purposes, including use of pelts (rabbits, chinchillas), use in biomedical research (primarily rabbits and guinea pigs), and as fancy show animals. While mention is made of domestication of mice in Asia as long ago as 1100 B.C., modern "fancy" rats and mice were first domesticated in the late nineteenth century. Though rats were occasionally used for food in times of famine, their initial domestication was for the once-popular sport of "rat-baiting," in which several rats were placed in a pit and bets taken on how long it would take a terrier to decimate the captives. Fancy rats and mice are relatively popular, and are judged in shows based upon color and behavior. As discussed, rats and mice are the predominant animals used in biomedical research; development of inbred and outbred stocks in the early twentieth century preceded the current explosion of genetically engineered strains (see later). Hamsters and gerbils were more recently domesticated and introduced as pets and as research animals in the 1950s. All of these species became popular as small mammal pets starting in the 1960s, concurrent with their availability in pet stores and from private breeders, and with growth of urban and suburban communities.

An understanding of the natural behavior of these animals is essential if provision of appropriate husbandry and veterinary care is to be made. All of the species described in this text are prey species, and as such, they are generally stressed in the presence of a perceived predator, such as a cat or dog, and have developed adaptive behaviors to avoid predation. One of the most prevalent of these is the propensity for active behaviors to be concentrated either during the dark phase of the daily cycle (nocturnal activity), or during dawn and dusk (crepuscular activity). This is most apparent in hamsters, which exhibit significant resistance to arousal during the light cycle, and is least apparent in guinea pigs, which scatter their activities over a 24-hour period. This fact may limit the ability of a clinician or owner to evaluate normal activity, in that the typical physical exam and evaluation will occur when the animal is less likely to be active, and may not be exhibiting evidence of pain. Behavioral evaluations are further complicated in that the "fight or flight" response initiated during an exam may override behaviors less conducive to overall survival. For this reason, evaluation during the dark phase and in the home cage can be beneficial for detecting subtle abnormalities. Evaluation in the home environment is often possible in a laboratory situation, and may be feasible when evaluating a colony-wide problem at a commercial breeding establishment. If animals must be moved from their normal area to an examination area, it is helpful to have a small, darkened secure transport cage and to minimize sudden and loud noises in the area of the cage. Many practices have developed procedures for specifically accommodating these small mammal pets; for example, restricting appointments to evening hours when no predator species will be present.

Rabbits and rodents also have highly developed senses of smell and hearing to aid in detection of predators. Therefore, it is likely less stressful to examine and house these animals outside the sight and smell of perceived predators. Prey species are often approached from above by predators, thus when picking up an animal, a slow, steady approach from the side will allow orientation to the movement. Rabbits and rodents are often calmed by a confident and encircling grasp, and by covering the eyes. This can be achieved by use of a towel or sleeve during the examination process.

In general, the amount of stress that may be induced by even minimally invasive clinical procedures should always be weighed against the benefit of intervention in rabbits and rodents to a far greater degree than is typically considered for dogs and cats. Stress can be minimized by thoughtful consideration of their natural behaviors, and by calm manipulations that take these behaviors into consideration.

REGULATORY CONSIDERATIONS

Rabbits and rodents used in biomedical research are subject to significant regulatory oversight. In the United States, the Animal Welfare Act (AWA), a federal law promulgated by the Animal Care Division of USDA-APHIS, outlines provisions and standards for rabbits, guinea pigs, chinchillas, hamsters, and gerbils, as well as other mammals used in biomedical research. Rats of the genus *Rattus* and mice of the genus *Mus* specifically bred for use in research are exempt. In 1998, USDA-APHIS issued a regulatory update advising that any retail pet store selling small mammals be licensed as a dealer subject to AWA regulations.

The Health Research Extension Act (HREA) provides standards for all vertebrate animals used in biomedical research funded by the United States Public Health Service (including the National Institutes of Health, Centers for Disease Control, and Food and Drug Administration). Specific measures of the HREA are outlined in a document published by the National Academies Press (NAP) under the auspices of the Institute for Laboratory Animal Research (ILAR), a division of the National Research Council (NRC), entitled *The Guide for the Care and Use of Laboratory Animals,* and often referred to as "The Guide." Laboratory animal veterinarians, and those acting as consultants to facilities using animals in biomedical research, should be well versed in this document. This and other guidelines for use of animals in biomedical research are referenced at the end of this chapter.

Regulations regarding the use of laboratory animals also exist in many other countries. In Canada, the Canadian Council on Animal Care (CCAC) has developed guidelines for the care and use of animals used in research, teaching, testing, and production. All vertebrate species, as well as cephalopods, are covered by these guidelines (www.ccac.ca). Any research institution holding animals and receiving Canadian federal funds for research must comply with CCAC guidelines and participate in regular on-site assessments of their facilities and operations. Participation is optional for private institutions not receiving federal money, but many organizations choose to comply with the CCAC guidelines to demonstrate a high level of commitment to humane animal care and use.

Regardless of the national framework of regulatory oversight, many countries around the world, including the United States and Canada, have a system of local ethical oversight in place in the form of an Animal Care Committee or Animal Ethical Review Board, whose purpose is to review the care and to safeguard the use of all animals housed in a facility for research, production, teaching, and testing.

GENETICALLY MODIFIED MICE

Animals have been selectively bred for centuries to develop genetic characteristics desired by humans. Since the 1980s, advances in recombinant DNA technology have greatly accelerated the capacity to manipulate the genome of domesticated species. This has been especially prominent in mice, which have blastocysts (early embryo stages) that are readily manipulated, and robust stem cells. In 1982, the first report of a genetically engineered mouse ("transgenic mouse") was demonstrated by inserting a growth hormone gene into the germline of an inbred mouse, resulting in an altered phenotype. Animals with the gene inserts weighed two to four times more than their nonmanipulated inbred siblings, providing a dramatic example of the utility of this technique. Further developments of this technology, and subsequent refinement of more sophisticated methods for specific gene targeting such as activation, deactivation, or replacement with an experimental gene, have resulted in propagation of many thousands of strains of mice used in laboratory studies for investigations in such varied fields as infectious and congenital diseases, development and differentiation, toxicology, cancer, immunology, and neurobiology. Animals altered by one of these several methodologies are collectively known as genetically modified mice (GMM) (see Table 1.1 for examples).

The first widely used technique developed for insertion of foreign DNA into the germline of an animal was microinjection. With microinjection, early embryos (blastocysts) are removed from the female mouse and then, using a specialized microscope, a fine glass pipette is used to pierce the cell membrane and inject prepared DNA into one of the embryonic nuclei (Figure 1.1).

The injected embryos are then surgically implanted into another recipient female and pups are delivered at term and reared by the mother. Offspring are typically tested at or about weaning for evidence of incorporated microinjected DNA sequences. An experienced laboratory produces pups from 30% to 60% of injected embryos; 10–40% of these will be transgenic. This technique results in random insertion of multiple copies of DNA sequences (1–200 copies) into the mouse genome. Multiple rounds of breeding ensue onto an inbred strain to develop stable homozygous lines, which are then used for further experimental manipulations.

More sophisticated knock-out technologies were later developed using methods that specifically impair or insert new genes into a designated site within the genome. Two important discoveries preceded this technology: (1) the ability to grow mouse embryonic stem (ES) cells in culture, and (2) understanding the process of homologous recombination during DNA replication. Undifferentiated ES cells

Table 1.1. Examples of genetically modified mice (GMM) and their uses in biomedical research.

Type of Modification	Procedure for Creation	Phenotype/Example
Oncogene expression, e.g., myc or ras	Microinjection	Expression evaluated in tissues for studies of tumorigenesis
Immune system alterations	Knockout	Interferon, cytokine, interleukin or specific immunocyte knockouts with specific immunodeficiencies
Regulation of gene expression	Microinjection or knockout	Regulatory element mutations used to study fetoprotein expression
Creation of animal models of single-gene mutations	Knockout	Cystic fibrosis resulting from disabling cystic fibrosis transmembrane regulator gene in mice
Creation of models for study of HIV-AIDS	Microinjection	Mutated HIV transgene develops Kaposi's sarcoma skin lesions in mice
Development of sensitive tests for toxicologic screening	Microinjection or knockout	Mice expressing a marker gene with a disabled promoter region; reversion of the promoter to an active form following exposure to potential toxicants can be screened in vitro following tissue harvest

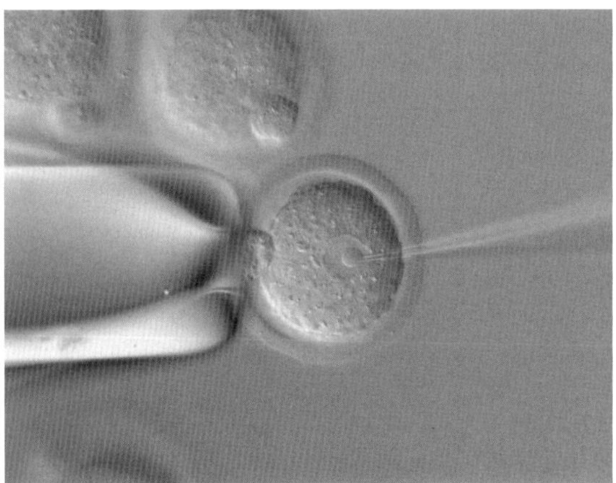

FIGURE 1.1. DNA being injected into an embryonic nucleus by microinjection. Courtesy of Anne Bower and Manfred Baetscher.

have the capacity to develop into any cell of the body when provided with appropriate cues; in the case of knock-out development, this includes mixing the stem cells with an early stage embryo (blastocyst). Commonly, segments of DNA with the altered gene of interest are mixed in a culture with mouse ES cells. Cells are subjected to an electrical field that opens pores in the cell membrane (electroporation). Some of the electroporated ES cells take up foreign DNA; following cell division, homologous recombination occurs between the ES genome and foreign DNA in a small fraction of cells, resulting in inactivation of the gene of interest. Cells that have undergone recombination are selected, microinjected into blastocysts, and implanted into recipient female mice. A percentage of offspring will be born as chimeras, that is, with cells of both the wild-type embryo and the altered ES cells, and these can be detected visually if the ES cells and blastocysts are each generated from mice of different coat colors (Figure 1.2).

Genetic testing and breeding will eventually result in genetically characterized stable mouse lines. Experienced laboratories will produce approximately two lines per DNA targeting sequence attempted; it takes a year or more for this success. Even more sophisticated GMMs are being produced that condi-

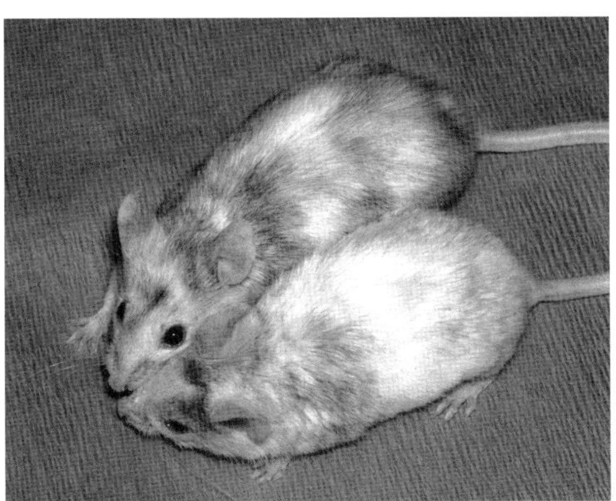

FIGURE 1.2. Two chimeric mice produced by knockout technology. Courtesy of Katherine Pritchett-Corning.

tionally express certain genes, allowing studies of the effects of "turning-on" or "turning-off" a gene in a specific tissue or at a specific developmental stage, for example.

The effects of genetic modification are unpredictable and may result in subtle phenotypic alterations that may not be clinically obvious. Veterinarians and veterinary pathologists have played an important role in developing, standardizing, and cataloguing mutant phenotypes, which in combination with complete genome sequences results in understanding of molecular and genetic contributions to physiology, behavior, and many disease processes.

As noted, these molecular and cellular manipulations have generated thousands of GMMs that either need to be propagated at low levels to keep the line viable, or preserved via cryopreservation of sperm, embryos, or ova for future use. In addition to the greatly expanded mouse populations, GMMs may be immunocompromised, have reduced fertility, or have increased morbidity or mortality, resulting in the need for more sophisticated monitoring and veterinary intervention for these animals. Veterinarians play an important role in developing management practices that consider the special needs of these animals and as advocates for their welfare and appropriate care.

Genetic engineering of rats has been much more difficult to master, though recent advances in embryonic stem cell technology hold promise for solving some of the technical difficulties that have hampered development of these animals. The unique physiology and behavior of rats compared to mice will make them very useful for certain studies, particularly in cardiovascular disease, neurobiology, and behavior. Development of genetically engineered rat strains would likely result in increased use of these animals in research.

EQUIPMENT NEEDS

Drugs and equipment available in a small animal practice can often be adapted for use in rabbits and rodents. Rabbits and cats, being approximately equal sizes, share some equipment requirements. Drugs, including anesthetics, and their dosages are discussed in other sections. Drugs must be used cautiously because virtually all use is extralabel in small mammal pets and small volumes are often administered, sometimes necessitating dilution of the stock drug. It is especially critical to be aware of labeling of drugs for potential use in meat rabbits to ensure that appropriate withdrawal times are followed prior to slaughter for human consumption.

Rodents weigh between 20 g (2/3 oz) for a mouse to approximately 1 kg (2.2 lb) for obese or pregnant guinea pigs. Scales with up to a 1–2 kg capacity with sensitivity to 5 g are essential, as is a weighing container for the animal. Obtaining an accurate body weight is extremely important, not only for correct dosing of small rabbits and rodents but also for monitoring changes in body weight, which are often the only objective data available for monitoring these small mammals over time. Other specialized considerations include (1) the need to perform oral examinations and tooth trimming in a small and narrow oral cavity; (2) specialized requirements for administration of volatile anesthetics to small animals with high metabolic rates; (3) maintenance of core body temperature during anesthesia; (4) anesthetic monitoring of rapid heart and respiratory rate in a small patient; and (5) dilution of stock drugs to avoid inaccuracies and overdosing. Some specialized items include those listed in Table 1.2 (adapted from Shoenberger, 1987).

Table 1.2. Equipment needs.

A. Physical Examination/Blood Collection/Drug Administration Needs

Scales able to accurately weigh animals 20 g to 10 kg
Towels/baskets/restraint devices (preferably dedicated to rabbits/rodents)
Small needles (22–27 gauge) and butterfly IV catheters
24 g IV catheters
Ball-tipped dosing needles—straight and curved (flexible plastic or stainless steel)
0.5 mL, 1 mL, 3 mL, and various straight- and curved-tip syringes
Microtainer tubes for blood samples (gel-separator, heparin, EDTA)
Microtip swabs for microbiology culture
Otoscope with several sets of plastic cones
Small bivalve vaginal or nasal speculum with light
Penlight
Gavage and feeding tubes
Sharp clippers (consider portable moustache clippers)
Pediatric stethoscope
Nebulization or oxygenation chamber
Bubblewrap, tubular gauze, or stockinette for draping small rodents
Small nail trimmer

B. Hospital In-Patient Needs

Caging with appropriate bedding material and environmental controls (preferably in a ward separate from other species)
Food crocks that are difficult to tip over and have low sides for easy access
Water bottles with operational valves or lixits
Herbivore critical care diet and/or species-specific appropriate diet
Food blender
Litter pans and litter appropriate for rabbits
Hide boxes, especially for guinea pigs

C. Anesthetic and Surgery Needs

Water-circulating heating pad
Incandescent heatlamp (also useful for vasodilation prior to blood collection) or other heating device (e.g., microwavable heating pads such as Safe-Warm® disks)
Ophthalmic surgical or microsurgical instruments
Small metal wound clips (8 mm) and wound clip applicator
Small gauge (3-0 to 5-0) suture materials with cutting/reverse cutting needles
Small surgical instruments
Inhalant gas vaporizer with nonrebreathing assembly and small face masks
Face masks (can be fashioned from syringe cases)
Small induction chambers (can be made from appropriately sized plastic containers with rubber gasket seals)
Surgical restraint blocks
Small cuffed and uncuffed endotracheal tubes (2-0 and larger)
Transparent or light-weight paper surgical drapes
Sterile cotton-tipped applicators
Dental equipment appropriate for rabbits and rodents (cheek dilator/spreader, rodent dental speculum, molar cutters, molar rongeur, rotating dental burr with extra-long shaft)

D. 'Bells and Whistles'

Radiologic and ultrasound equipment
Pediatric pulse oximeter
Dental x-ray unit or mammogram unit for radiology
Stereoscope for microvascular surgery
CT unit for dental radiographs
Oral specula and cheek dilators for dental surgeries
Rabbit/rodent table retractor/restrainer for dental procedures
Surgical retractor device
Radiosurgery equipment

MAJOR CONCERNS IN HUSBANDRY

A major consideration in preventive management is maintaining husbandry standards that reduce or eliminate factors that predispose to injury, disease, or development of abnormal behaviors and stereotypies. This includes establishing satisfactory methods for sanitation and providing escape-free and well-constructed caging. These concerns extend to animal housing for pets, as well as to research and commercial settings.

Behavioral Well-Being and Environmental Enrichment

Housing should be designed to provide for the behavioral well-being and physical comfort of the animals. It should take into consideration the normal behaviors, postures, and typical movements of each species. Regardless of their end purpose, whether as a companion animal, research subject, or for commercial production, these species will typically spend the majority of their life in close contact with the caged environment, and it is important to ensure that this environment is optimized. Animals housed in a suboptimal environment often develop abnormal behaviors detrimental to their health and purpose of use. With the exceptions of female hamsters and male rabbits, which often fight when pair- or group-housed, rabbits and rodents are highly social species. Housing social species in pair or group settings, whenever possible, is an important consideration for maintaining good behavioral health. Most of these animals naturally dig tunnels and live in burrows in the wild, and because of this are more appropriately housed on solid flooring with substrate and nesting material. Expanding an animal's options for species-specific behavior can positively affect both physiological and behavioral well-being. Environmental enrichment strategies for laboratory rabbits and rodents can be classified as structure and substrate, which include objects or parameters associated with the enclosure; manipulanda, which encourage fine motor activity; novel foods, which provide opportunities for variation in diet; and other enrichments that stimulate senses other than touch or taste. Examples of species-specific environmental enrichment are provided in chapter 2.

Housing

Primary enclosures (cages and pens) should be structurally sound, appropriate for the species housed, in good repair, free of sharp or abrasive surfaces, built for easy cleaning, constructed to prevent escape and intrusion, and large enough to provide freedom of movement and normal postural adjustments, such as eating, mating, and exercising. Unpainted wood, untreated metal, and other porous materials that are difficult to sanitize should not be used for long-term housing of rabbits or rodents. Flooring and nesting materials that prevent escape, provide the capacity to burrow and maintain thermoneutrality, and allow for adequate sanitation should be considered.

Physical Comfort

Animal caging should be dry, clean, well ventilated but protected from drafts, and kept away from excessive noise and direct sunlight. Regulatory guidelines for institutional temperature and humidity ranges are provided by the U.S. Animal Welfare Act, the ILAR guide, and the CCAC guidelines, volume 1 (Table 1.3). In general, the thermoneutral zone of rodents is 26–28 °C (79–82 °F), and these animals are comfortable in warm but not hot ambient temperatures. Rabbits prefer cooler temperatures because of their dense coat and may be more comfortable in 16–20 °C (61–68 °F) temperatures. Rabbits can tolerate much cooler ambient temperatures provided they are protected from drafts and are given dry bedding. Cages should never be placed in direct sunlight to prevent overheating of these animals, none of which have efficient cooling mechanisms.

Hairless and smaller rodents, such as mice, require higher ambient temperatures. Relative humidity in the cage should be maintained between 30% and 70%. Temperature or humidity extremes and variations can significantly contribute to disease susceptibility and should be closely monitored.

Room air changes in institutional animal facilities, using fresh or filtered air, are required to be at least 10–15 complete air changes per hour. This rate of exchange is recommended to reduce waste gasses, airborne particulates, and allergen load associated with a large number of animals housed at high

Table 1.3. Temperature and humidity guidelines.

Species	USDA AWA	ILAR Guide	CCAC Guidelines
Rabbits	40–90 °F	30–70% RH, 61–72 °F (16–22 °C)	40–70% RH, 16–22 °C
Guinea Pigs	60–85 °F	30–70% RH, 64–79 °F (18–26 °C)	40–70% RH, 18–22 °C
Hamsters	60–85 °F	30–70% RH, 64–79 °F (18–26 °C)	40–70% RH, 21–24 °C
Gerbils	Not specified	30–70% RH, 64–79 °F (18–26 °C)	40–70% RH, 15–24 °C
Chinchillas	Not specified	Not specified	Not specified
Mice	Not covered	30–70% RH, 64–79 °F (18–26 °C)	40–70% RH, 22–25 °C
Rats	Not covered	30–70% RH, 64–79 °F (18–26 °C)	40–70% RH, 20–25 °C

density. Fewer air exchanges are certainly adequate for small numbers of pet rodents in private homes. The size of the room, strain and sex of animal, number of animals present, number of animals per cage, and sanitization interval affect ventilation requirements. For pets, enclosed cages such as covered aquaria should be avoided, as these may result in poor air circulation and a build-up of potentially toxic levels of ammonia and carbon dioxide. Aquaria left in direct sunlight can also result in hyperthermia and rapid death. Drafts should also be avoided. A light intensity of 30 foot candles (323 lumens/m^2) at 1 meter above floor level (approximately equivalent to a dimly lit office) is adequate for routine care and recommended by the ILAR guide. Less light is needed to maintain circadian rhythms, and excessive illumination intensity may induce retinal degeneration in albino rats and mice. Animals in continuous light or dark may become infertile.

Housing for small rodents, particularly mice in laboratory animal facilities, has generated a unique industry, as methods to house large numbers of animals efficiently while limiting spread of adventitious pathogens have become increasingly important. Filter top caging was initially demonstrated to provide effective cage-level barriers to the spread of disease in the 1960s; however, modern caging systems now used widely were first introduced in the 1980s. The most economical microisolation system is "static," that is, air circulation between the room and cage is passive. This leads to a rapid build-up of high levels of ammonia and CO_2, necessitating frequent (typically semi-weekly) cage changes. Individually ventilated caging (IVC, also known as ventilated caging systems [VCS]) is now widely available commercially, and has replaced static cages in facilities with resources to purchase such units. Several companies produce IVC with different specifications. These may have high efficiency particulate air (HEPA) filtration for incoming or outgoing air, or both. The benefits of IVC, besides providing a significant barrier to spread of diseases between cages, that is, provision of biosecurity, include (1) very low accumulation of ammonia and CO_2 within cages, allowing for a longer interval between cage changes of up to 2 weeks; (2) a decrease in rodent allergens in the macroenvironment, with concomitant benefits to staff; and (3) provision of protection of staff and other animals from pathogens, that is, biosafety improvements (Figure 1.3).

IVC has also permitted the use of rodents that are immunodeficient because of genetics or experimental manipulations, providing a protected environment for animals that could otherwise succumb to opportunistic infections.

Health Maintenance

Facilities and caging should be cleaned and sanitized when necessary, usually one to three bedding changes per week for mice, rats, guinea pigs, chinchillas, and rabbits, and longer intervals (biweekly) for hamsters and gerbils. Ammonia gas, which reduces the disease resistance capabilities of the respiratory tract, is reduced by decreasing population density, use of IVC, and by providing good sanitation and frequent bedding changes. Vermin must be excluded from animal housing areas, as feral rats and mice are often a source of parasitic, viral, and bacterial pathogens. Different species and animals with unknown or non-SPF disease status should be housed separately, pref-

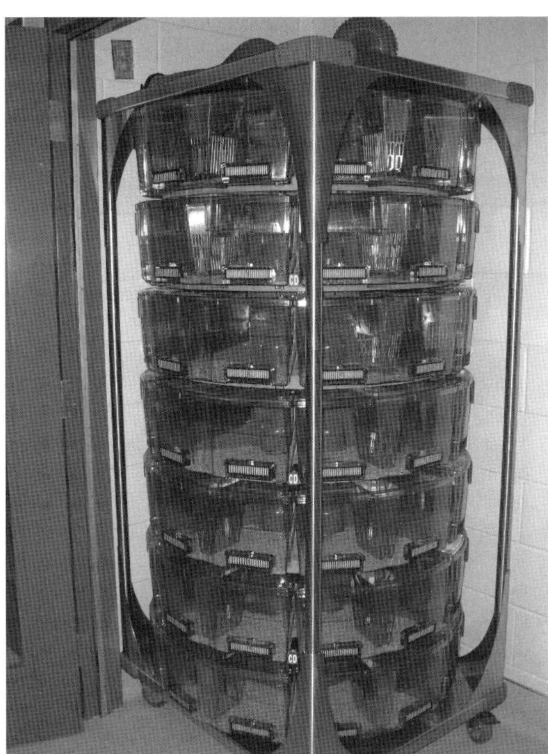

FIGURE 1.3. Example of OptiMICE® high-density mouse housing system, which provides individual cage ventilation.

erably in different rooms or in IVC. Professional and technical personnel or pet owners should examine animals at least daily for evidence of injury and disease. Stock and replacement animals should be obtained from reputable dealers or pet animal suppliers. Many animals in the pet trade are infected with one or more pathogenic organisms, and the stress and consequences of transport, marginal nutrition, mixing of species and sources of animals, inbreeding, and suboptimal environmental conditions may exacerbate existing disease conditions.

Nutrition

Food should be stored in closed containers, kept at room temperature or below, and observed regularly for mold or vermin. Feeding and watering devices should be kept clean, be designed or placed so as to prevent fecal and urine contamination, be appropriate for the species and age of animal housed, and be accessible and functional. Water should be fresh, clean, and available ad libitum. Specially designed watering bags with disposible valves or "lixits" have recently been manufactured for use in laboratory animal facilities, and may provide ergonomic and labor benefits in certain circumstances while still providing continuous access to potable water.

Rabbits and rodents should be fed a fresh, clean, nutritious, palatable feed on a regular basis and in an adequate quantity. Diets milled for laboratory animals typically include a milling date and should be used within 6 months of manufacture. Diets available for pets are highly variable, and seed-based diets should be avoided in lieu of a pelleted chow manufactured by a reputable company for the specific species being fed. Discounted, outdated, or improperly formulated feeds, supplements, and vitamin formulations should be avoided. Colorful, attractive displays of rodent and rabbit feeds in pet stores should be scrutinized closely. The most common deficiencies encountered in pet store rabbit and rodent feeds are low protein content (under 16% crude protein), excessively long storage with subsequent nutrient decomposition, and inappropriate species use, particularly for guinea pigs, which require vitamin C in the diet. Smaller-sized bags of food purchased more frequently are likely to provide more nutrients and vitamins to pets than large quantities of food that will take months to consume. Supplementation with grains, salt blocks, vitamins, and antibiotics is typically unnecessary if the diet is properly formulated. Treats such as fruit and vegetables should be fed sparingly and should never consist of more than 5–10% of the daily diet. Clean grass hay should be provided ad libitum for pet rabbits, guinea pigs, and chinchillas.

Although the nutritional requirements of rabbits and rodents have been investigated and reported, optimal nutrient levels for most species remain uncertain. Requirements known at present are available from feed company publications or from the publications of the National Academy of Sciences' National Research Council. With the important exception of ascorbic acid deficiency in guinea pigs and caloric, water, and protein deficiencies in all species, malnutrition is uncommon in rabbits and rodents. Primary nutritional imbalances may be manifested as weight loss or failure to gain, increased susceptibility to disease, hair loss, poor hair coat, prenatal mortality, agalactia, infertility, anemia, deformed bones, central nervous system abnormalities, or a reluctance to move. Subclinical nutritional deficiencies, excesses, or imbalances may be obscured by secondary bacterial infections or metabolic disorders. The importance of nutritional imbalances lies more in the predisposing role than in the causation of primary deficiency disease. The most prevalent nutritional problems in pet rabbit and rodents, and in laboratory animals in long-term studies, tend to be obesity associated with ad libitum feeding of high-calorie foodstuffs, including treats, and insufficient dietary fiber. More specific information about nutritional requirements and nutritional-related diseases for each species, and for pet versus laboratory animals, is provided in chapter 2.

Identification

Animals used in research or testing should be identified properly and clearly. Animals may be identified by cage cards, individual coat pattern, ear punch or notch (mice, rats, and hamsters), ear tag or stud, dye staining on light-colored fur, or tattooing, for example, ear, tail, footpad, or shaved flank (Figures 1.4–1.6).

Microchip devices that store animal identification information in association with physical parameters such as weight are used in some laboratory facilities and for pets. An example of an ear notch/punch code is shown in Figure 1.7. This method can be used for individually identifying the animal as well as for collection of tissue for DNA genotyping.

Cage cards with information specific to the animal and protocol are required in research settings. Permanent individual animal identification is often used together with cage cards since cards can be inadvertently mixed during cage cleaning and experimental manipulations.

FACTORS PREDISPOSING TO DISEASE

Certain organic or environmental factors increase the exposure or reduce the resistance of animals to disease. These factors must be considered by animal owners and caregivers in disease prevention efforts. Factors that influence disease susceptibility include environmental, genetic, metabolic, experimental, and dietary variables. Attention to these factors is extremely important in rabbit and rodent husbandry and disease prevention and control. Many aspects of husbandry procedures are mandated or discussed in detail in regulations governing the care and use of laboratory animals, and provide suitable guidelines for pet and production animals.

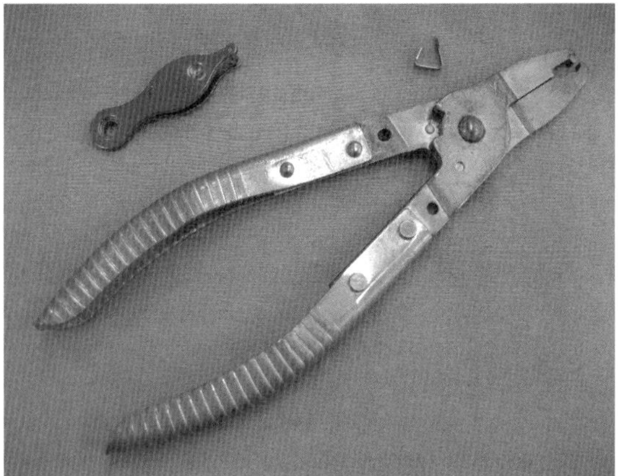

FIGURE 1.4. Example of instruments used for ear notching of mice (upper left) and ear tagging of rodents and rabbits (lower right).

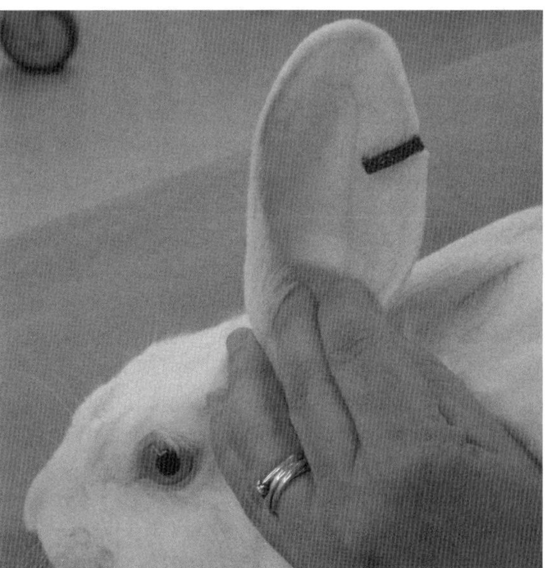

FIGURE 1.5. Ear tag in a rabbit.

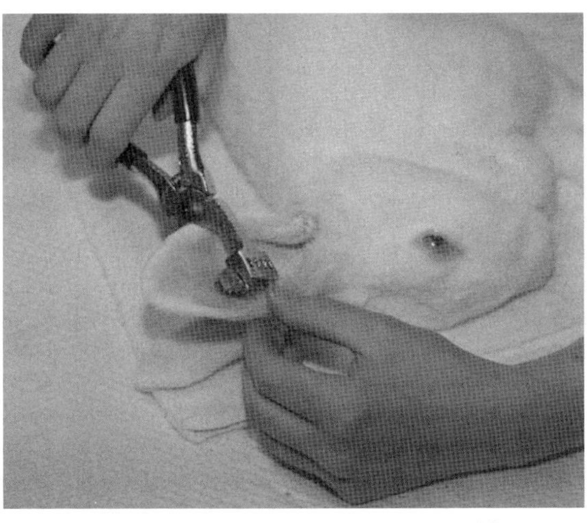

FIGURE 1.6a. Rabbit sedated and positioned for ear tattoo identification. Courtesy of Ernest Olfert.

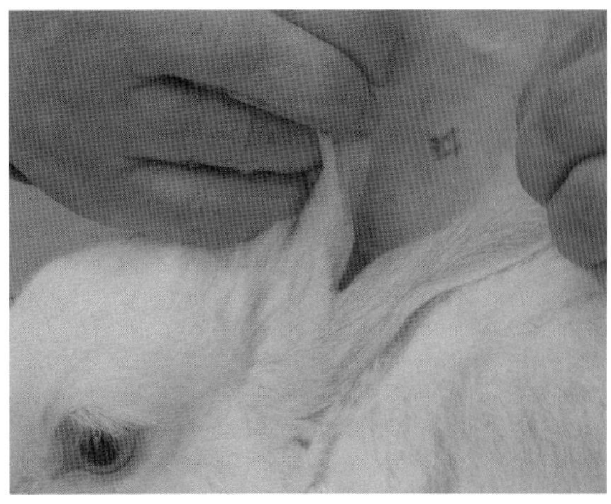

FIGURE 1.6b. Ear tattoo in a rabbit.

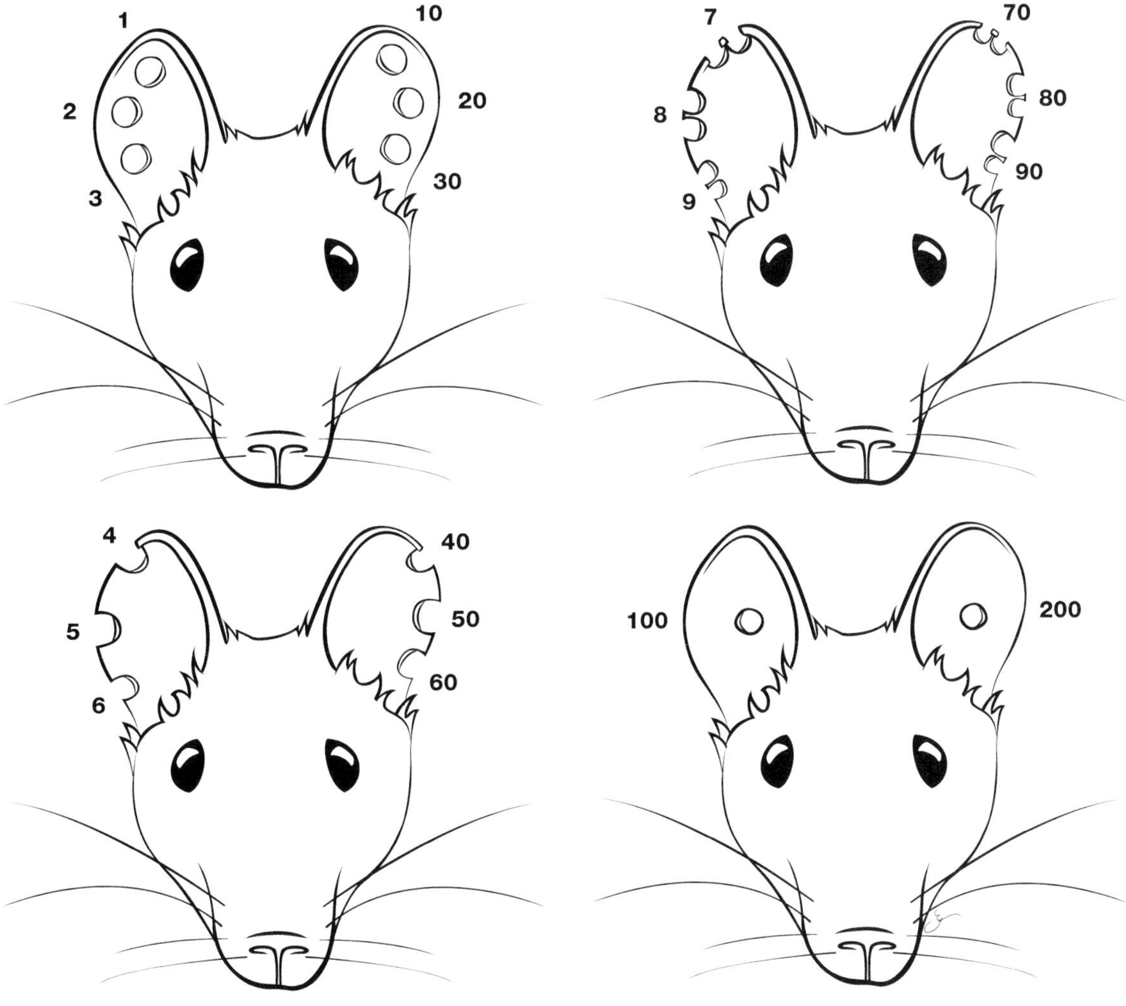

FIGURE 1.7. Standard ear notch punch codes for identification of rodents. The punches are combined to achieve the desired final number. Illustrations by Gianni A. Chiappetta.

Facility Cleaning, Disinfection, and Fumigation

Sanitation is a key process in rabbit and rodent maintenance. The high levels of sanitation dictated in an SPF research colony that may contain animals with immunodeficiencies or infected with certain pathogens on an experimental basis may not be necessary for pet and production facilities, but can be used as a basis for animal care. Clean cages are particularly important during pregnancy, lactation, and weaning; after the removal of sick animals; and preceding the introduction of new animals into the household or colony. Some species (including hamsters, some strains of mice, and primiparous animals of all species) are better left undisturbed immediately following parturition, as disturbances may affect maternal care.

Cages can be disinfected by washing with 82 °C (180 °F) water after removal of organic matter, or by applying a disinfectant solution to all surfaces. Disinfectant solutions, for example, phenolic, quaternary ammonium, or halogen compounds, including hypochlorites or dilute bleach solutions, are available in farm supply or feed stores or from specialty manufacturers. Instructions for use are on the labels of bottled concentrates. Clients are more likely to follow advice about disinfection if common household products, such as bleach and vinegar, are recommended. Detergents and disinfectants must be rinsed thoroughly from cleaned cages and feeders as residues may cause health effects or may alter experimental data. Laboratory settings typically use cage wash equipment designed specifically for this purpose as this greatly facilitates sterilization of caging on a consistent basis. Animal food bowls and water bottles can often be sanitized in home dishwashers, but kitchen dishcloths should never be shared between human and animal dishes, if items are hand washed, to prevent transmission of potential zoonotic bacteria and protozoa between animals and their human caregivers.

Disinfectants should be selected for broad spectrum activity, rapid kill effect, cleaning capacity, solubility, stability, residual activity, and lack of odor and toxicity. Disinfectants should be effective in the presence of organic materials, detergents, hard water, at varying pH levels, and on porous, rough, or cracked surfaces. Some disinfectant preparations should be avoided because they cloud clear plastic cages or cage accessories. Unfortunately, no single disinfectant meets all these criteria, and selection must be based on specific requirements. The effects of disinfectants vary with time of exposure, temperature and concentration of solution, and ionic content of the diluent. Important categories of microorganisms that are weakly or unaffected by standard disinfectant solutions are bacterial spores, coccidial oocysts, parasite ova, and nonenveloped viruses. *Pseudomonas* spp can be more resistant to disinfection than other bacteria and frequently contaminates watering devices, necessitating careful disinfection of these implements. Use of acidified water to decrease *Pseudomonas* spp is described in the mouse husbandry section of chapter 2.

Halogen-containing disinfectants, including hypochlorites and iodophores, are effective in acidic solutions, but they may stain or damage fabrics and have reduced activity in the presence of organic matter, soap, or detergent residues. A good, practical, and safe disinfectant for pet or food animal cages is a solution of 30 mL of a 5% sodium hypochlorite solution (laundry bleach) in one liter of water (1 oz per quart). A fresh mixture should be prepared just prior to use and used on clean cages only.

Phenol derivative compounds, the disinfectants least affected by environmental influences, kill the vegetative forms of both Gram-positive and Gram-negative bacteria except *Pseudomonas* spp, which require longer exposures and higher concentrations, after approximately 30 minutes of contact time. Germicidal activity is increased with increased concentration and temperature of the solution. Phenolic compounds, emulsified at 1–5% in weakly acidic, soapy water, have some antifungal, sporicidal, and virucidal activity. Because of a residual odor and toxicity, phenolic derivatives are not used to disinfect feeders and waterers.

Quaternary ammonium compounds are effective against Gram-positive bacteria but are considerably less effective in the presence of organic matter, soaps, and an acidic pH. These compounds are useful for general purpose disinfection and for cleaning feeders and waterers, though as mentioned previously, devices should be thoroughly rinsed afterward. Residues of these compounds on the nest box have been implicated as a cause of death among suckling rabbits. Other disinfecting substances used less often and for resistant organisms such as bacterial spores, parvoviruses, parasitic ova, and coccidial oocysts include 2% lye solution, formalin, ethylene oxide gas, and 10% ammonia solution.

The alkaline urine of rabbits, guinea pigs, and hamsters (above pH 8.0) contains phosphate and carbonate crystals that result in scale residues on caging. Acidic products, for example, dilute inorganic acids including white vinegar, can be used to dislodge the crystal accumulation. Some plastics are affected by alkaline detergents, which cause the transparent plastic cages to become cloudy and brittle. Acid detergent preparations are less destructive, but they will discolor aluminum.

Gas fumigation is an effective method for room and cage sanitization and for eliminating parasites and vegetative bacterial forms following removal of organic matter. Before gas fumigation is attempted, the room must be free of animals, airtight, warmed to at least 21 °C (70 °F), and wetted to raise the relative humidity to 80% or more. Formaldehyde gas is generated by heating paraformaldehyde crystals in an alkaline solution on a hot plate. Chlorine dioxide gas can also be used for fumigation. Because of the potential for severe toxicity, provisions must be made for exhausting fumes from the room without the entry of personnel, and stainless steel and other equipment that may be corroded by fumigants should be removed prior to fumigation.

New methods of sterilization and newer chemical sterilants have been developed in response to emergence of antibiotic-resistant organisms present in hospital settings. These include new aldehydes, acids, and surfactant agents. Many laboratory animal facilities have begun to use hydrogen peroxide plasma–generating systems to sterilize equipment and rooms that are temperature and corrosion sensitive with reasonable success.

ALLERGIES TO RABBITS AND RODENTS

The high prevalence of allergies to laboratory animals (laboratory animal allergy [LAA]) has been recognized for decades, and has been reported in 11–44% of people with repeated unprotected exposures to rabbits and rodents. It is likely that exposure in a laboratory animal setting under circumstances of repeated and frequent exposures to large numbers of animals, their dander, and their excreta contributes to the high prevalence of this syndrome. The allergic reactions among people in frequent contact with animals involve both contact (dermal and ocular allergic dermatitis and conjunctivitis) and inhalant (respiratory allergic rhinitis, bronchial hypersensitivity) syndromes. LAA may progress to asthma in up to 22% of affected persons, and can result in anaphylaxis in severely allergic persons. The generation of immunoglobulin E (IgE) against antigens produced by laboratory animals is a prerequisite for diagnosis of LAA. Specific clinical signs include runny and itchy eyes and nose, a persistent cough, asthma or shortness of breath, or various skin manifestations, including wheal and flare reactions, hives, and pruritic rashes (urticaria). Reactions may occur immediately, 15–20 minutes after exposure, or many hours later. It is difficult to be in contact with animals without having contact with allergens, as even very small quantities of allergens can trigger a reaction. Allergens have also been detected on clothing and in the cars and offices of people who have had animal contact in other areas.

Predisposing factors to development of allergies to animal allergens unrelated to occupational exposures include atopy (clinical hypersensitivity of hereditary predisposition) and smoking. The intensity, frequency, and directness of contact are the most important associations related to development of LAA. Allergies are usually species-specific, that is, particular to one species of animal or another, but not strain-specific. Development of one allergy increases the probability that allergies to additional antigens may occur. Development of LAA has been recorded in association with exposures to rats, guinea pigs, rabbits, mice, hamsters, and gerbils; virtually any laboratory animal can induce allergies in exposed and predisposed individuals. The most difficult allergies to manage are those to rats and mice, but this likely reflects the fact that the numbers of these animals are greatest in most laboratory animal facilities. Many mouse and rat urinary proteins belong to a family called lipocalins. These proteins resemble antigens of schistosomes, which are human trematodes (flukes). These proteins are highly prone to triggering IgE production, which likely accounts in part for the high proportion of the population susceptible to LAA. Three distinct mouse allergens and two allergens of rats have been described and are found in hair, dander, urine, and serum. Allergens have not been as well characterized in other species, though at least two lipocalin-like proteins have been identified in rabbits and guinea pigs and are present in urine, saliva, and dander.

Various animal factors influence the risk of exposure to laboratory animal allergens and examples of these follow. Female mice generate far fewer airborne allergens than do males. Airborne prealbumin and albumin are reduced when corncob bedding is used in place of wood shavings. Rabbit saliva is deposited on the fur during grooming. After drying, the allergens become airborne and serve as an important source of exposure to rabbit allergens. Allergens in aerosolized rat urine can be carried with ammonia gas. These exposures may be particularly dangerous because they can be associated with severe pulmonary congestion. Symptoms develop rapidly after sensitized persons enter rat facilities that have poor ventilation and infrequent cage cleaning. Proteinuria in rats increases with age; consequently, exposure to these animals puts people at higher risk for allergy development.

This discussion clearly illustrates that laboratory animal facilities should have occupational health programs in place that consider development of LAA as a risk of employment, and employees with predisposing factors should be identified and monitored as part of the program. The need for occupational health awareness is well described in the ILAR guide, and ILAR has also published a volume entitled *Occupational Health and Safety in the Care and Use of Research Animals* to provide additional information on this topic. Veterinarians, or owners with pets or production animals, should be aware of the possibility of development of LAA, and should seek the advice of a physician if they have reason to believe they have an allergy to rabbits or rodents.

Prevention

Rabbit and rodent airborne allergens can be measured, allowing for association between environmental exposures and development of LAA. This technology has also allowed evaluation of husbandry methods that decrease ambient concentrations of airborne allergens. These studies are the basis for recommendations for reduced occupational exposures. Because nonoccupational risks can increase the risk of development of LAA, many laboratory animal facilities include a preemployment risk assessment as part of their occupational health program.

An effective LAA prevention program includes education and training; implementation of personal protective equipment (PPE), including gloves, designated work clothes or laboratory coats, and respiratory protection; modification of work practices; and use of various engineering controls to reduce the level of allergen exposures. Use of ventilated cages that are pressurized negative to the room and that are opened only in ventilated changing stations reduces mouse allergens 10-fold relative to nonventilated caging handled on conventional change tables. Increasing room ventilation rates and humidity, use of low-dust bedding, wetting bedding prior to dumping, use of ventilated dump stations, and using room-level air filtration are all measures that decrease allergen exposures.

Persons experiencing allergic symptoms with exposure to laboratory animals should be evaluated by a physician with experience in allergy diagnosis and management. Diagnostic tests that may be performed include skin tests or in vitro assays that detect IgE reacting to laboratory animal allergens. Pulmonary function measurements may be used to assess asthmatic symptoms. Possible management for sensitized individuals includes reduction of exposure, pharmacologic treatment, or immunotherapy. Early intervention is essential, as prognosis for control of symptoms and overall outcome is highly dependent upon disease severity at the time of diagnosis.

Small mammal pet owners can minimize allergen exposure by keeping the animals in well-ventilated areas, providing regular sanitation of cages and the surrounding environment to reduce allergen levels, using dust-free bedding, and ensuring appropriate hand and clothing hygiene after handling these pets.

REFERENCES

Websites

http://www.afrma.org/—American Fancy Rat and Mouse Association. Information for owners of pet and show rats and mice.

http://www.ncbi.nlm.nih.gov/Genomes/—rat and mouse genome organization. Accessed March 6, 2009.

http://www.rabbit.org/—House Rabbit Society. Information for owners of companion animal rabbits.

Veterinary Information Network (VIN, www.vin.com) is a subscription online network that supports dialogue among veterinary practitioners, including specialists in rabbit and rodent medicine.

Wikipedia (en.wikipedia.org, an online, free, collaborative encyclopedia) generally provides informative articles with specific references or indicates where references are lacking. Specific entries include Chinchilla, Fancy Mouse, Fancy Rat, Fur Farming, Gerbil, Hamster, and Rabbit.

Journals

Exotic DVM is a journal providing "a practical resource for clinicians" and is published approximately four times per year by the Zoological Education Network (http://www.exoticdvm.com/).

The Journal of Exotic Pet Medicine (a continuation from Seminars in Avian and Exotic Pet Medicine) is published by Elsevier four times per year, and each issue includes a comprehensive, current overview of a special topic on exotic pet medicine.

Veterinary Clinics of North America: Exotic Animal Practice, published by Elsevier three times a year, offers the most current information on exotic animal treatment, updates on the latest advances, and a sound basis for choosing treatment options. Each issue focuses on a single topic in exotic animal practice. http://www.vetexotic.theclinics.com/.

General Texts

Fox JG, Anderson LC, Loew FM, Quimby FW (eds.). Laboratory Animal Medicine, 2nd ed. San Diego: Academic Press, 2002. The American College of Laboratory Animal Medicine has also sponsored textbooks and references on specific species, including Laboratory Hamsters (out of print), The Laboratory Rat, The Mouse in Biomedical Research, Anesthesia and Analgesia in Laboratory Animals, The Biology of the Guinea Pig (out of print), and The Biology of the Laboratory Rabbit (out of print). A CD-ROM including training materials is also available; for updates see www.aclam.org/education/products.html.

Hau J, Van Hoosier GL (eds.). Handbook of Laboratory Animal Science, 2nd ed., vols. I–III. Boca Raton, FL: CRC Press, Inc. 2002–2004. Note: CRC Press publishes a wide variety of texts related to laboratory animals and laboratory animal science, including individual species, animal models, and management of research issues. See: www.crcpress.com/. Accessed March 6, 2009.

Hrapkiewicz K, Medina L. Clinical Laboratory Animal Medicine: An Introduction, 3rd Ed. Ames, IA: Blackwell, 2004.

Laber-Laird K, Swindle MM, Flecknell PA. Handbook of Rodent and Rabbit Medicine. Tarrytown, NY: Elsevier Science, 1996.

Mitchell M, Tully T. Manual of Exotic Pet Practice. St Louis: Saunders Elsevier, 2009.

Poole TB (ed.). The UFAW Handbook of the Care and Management of Laboratory Animals, 7th ed. Oxford: Blackwell Science, 1999.

Quesenberry K, Carpenter J (eds.). Ferrets, Rabbits, and Rodents: Clinical Medicine and Surgery, 2nd ed. St Louis: Saunders, 2004.

Rowsell HC, et al. (eds.). The Guide to the Care and Use of Experimental Animals, vol 2. Ottawa, ON: Canadian Council on Animal Care, 1984. See: www.ccac.ca.

Special Emphasis Textbooks

Bays T, Lightfoot T, Mayer J. Exotic Pet Behavior. St Louis: Saunders Elsevier, 2006.

Carbone L. What Animals Want. New York: Oxford University Press, 2004.

Committee on Animal Nutrition. Nutrient Requirements of Rabbits, 7th ed. Washington, DC: National Academy Press, 1977.

Feldman DB, Seely JC (eds.). Necropsy Guide: Rodents and the Rabbit. Boca Raton, FL: CRC Press, 1988.

Oglesbee B. The 5-Minute Veterinary Consultant: Ferret and Rabbit. Ames, IA: Blackwell, 2006.

Paterson S (ed.). Skin Diseases of Exotic Pets. Oxford: Blackwell Science, 2006.

Percy DH, Barthold SW. Pathology of Laboratory Rodents and Rabbits, 3rd ed. Ames, IA: Blackwell, 2007.

Silverman S, Tell T. Radiology of Rodents, Rabbits, and Ferrets. St Louis: Elsevier Saunders, 2005.

Regulations and Guidelines

Canadian Council on Animal Care Guidelines. All are available in English and French through the home website, www.ccac.ca.

Institute for Laboratory Animal Research. Guide for the Care and Use of Laboratory Animals. Washington, DC: National Research Council, National Academies Press, 1996.

Regulation of Pocket Pets. Animal Welfare Information Center Bulletin, Fall 1998, vol. 9, no. 1–2.

United States Department of Agriculture (USDA)—Animal and Plant Health Inspection Service (APHIS). The Animal Welfare Act: An overview. http://www.aphis.usda.gov/publications/animal_welfare/content/printable_version/animal_welfare4-06.pdf. Note: Animal care reports and other relevant documents can be found on the APHIS website as well.

Willems RA. Animals in veterinary medical teaching: compliance and regulatory issues, the U.S. perspective. J Vet Med Educ. 2007, 34(5):615–619.

Genetically Modified Mice

AALAS. Laboratory Mouse Handbook. Memphis TN: American Association for Laboratory Animal Science, 2006.

Capecchi MR. Targeted gene replacement. Sci Amer. 1994, 270(3):52–59.

Houdebine LM. Transgenic Animals, Generation and Use. Amsterdam: Harwood Academic Publishers, 1997.

Jaenisch R. Transgenic animals. Science. 1998, 240(4858):1468–1474.

Merlino G. Transgenic animals in biomedical research. FASEB J. 1991, 5:2996–3001.

Pinkert CA. Transgenic Animal Technology, a Laboratory Handbook. London: Academic Press, 1998.

Ristevski S. Making better transgenic models. Mol Biotechnol. 2005, 29:153–163.

Sundberg JP, Tsutomu I. Genetically Engineered Mice Handbook. Boca Raton, FL: CRC Press, 2006.

Laboratory Animal Allergies

Bush R, Stave G. Laboratory animal allergy: an update. ILAR J. 2003, 44(1):28–55.

Elliott L, Heederik J, Marshall S, et al. Incidence of allergy and allergy symptoms among workers exposed to laboratory animals. Occup Environ Med. 2005, 62:766–771.

Reeb-Whitaker C, Harrison DJ, Jones R, et al. Control strategies for aeroallergens in an animal facility. J Allergy Clin Immunol. 1999, 103(1):139–146.

Schweitzer IB, Smith E, Harrison DJ. Reducing exposure to laboratory animal allergens. Comp Med. 2003, 53(5):487–492.

Numbers of Animals Used in Research

Abbott A. The renaissance rat. Nature. 2004, 428:464–466.

http://www.ccac.ca/en/Publications/New_Facts_Figures/analysis/analysis_index.htm.

http://www.minnesotamedicine.com/PastIssues/April2007/tabid/1578/Default.aspx.

http://www.vetmed.ucdavis.edu/Animal_Alternatives/whymice.htm.

Knight J, Abbott A. Full house. Nature. 2002, 417: 785–786.

Lazar J, Moreno C, Jacob HJ, et al. Impact of genomics on research in the rat. Genome Res. 2005, 15:1717–1728.

www.the-aps.org/pa/resources/bionews/animalNumber.htm. What Do USDA "Animal Use" Numbers Mean? Accessed March 6, 2009.

Meat and Fur Production

Empress Chinchilla. www.empresschinchilla.com. Accessed March 6, 2009

Endangered Species Handbook, Animal Welfare Institute. www.endangeredspecieshandbook.org/trade_chinchillas.php.

Lebas F, Coudert P, de Rochambeau H, Thebault RG. The Rabbit: Husbandry, Health and Production. FAO Animal Production and Health Series, no. 21, FAO—Food and Agricultural Organization of the United Nations, Rome 1997, FAO Corporate Document Repository.

Poley WG. Chinchilla Industry Council Market Report. www.chinchillaindustrycouncil.com/engl/markrep/markrep.htm.

Rabbits. Ontario Ministry of Agriculture, Food and Rural Affairs. www.omafra.gov.on.ca/english/livestock/alternat/rabbits.htm.

Standard Guidelines for the Operation of Chinchilla Ranches, www.omafra.gov.on.ca/english/livestock/alternat/facts/chinguid.htm.

Other References

Animal Welfare Information Center Bulletin, Fall 1998, vol. 9, nos. 1–2; www.nal.usda.gov/awic/newsletters/v9n1/9n1aphis.htm.

Baker DG (ed.). Parasites of Laboratory Animals, 2nd ed. Hoboken, NJ: Wiley-Blackwell, 2007.

Biosafety in Microbiological and Biomedical Laboratories, 5th ed. Washington, DC: U.S. Government Printing Office, 2007.

Committee on Occupational Safety and Health in Research Animal Facilities, Institute of Laboratory Animal Resources, Commission on Life Sciences. Occupational Health and Safety in the Care and Use of Research Animals. Washington, DC: National Research Council, National Academies Press, 1997.

Fisher PG. Equipping the exotic mammal practice. Vet Clin Exot Anim. 2005, 8:405–426.

Hafez ESE (ed.). Reproduction and Breeding Techniques for Laboratory Animals. Ann Arbor, MI: Books on Demand, 1970.

Hunskaar S, Fosse RT. Allergy to laboratory mice and rats: a review of its prevention, management, and treatment. Lab Anim. 1993, 27:206–221.

Hutchinson E, Avery A, VandeWoude, S. Environmental enrichment for laboratory rodents. ILAR J. 2005, 46(2):148–161.

Lennox AM. Equipment for exotic mammal and reptile diagnostics and surgery. J Exot Pet Med. 2006, 15:98–105.

McDonnell G, Russell AD. Antiseptics and disinfectants: activity, action, and resistance. Clin Microbiol Rev. 1999, 12(1):147–179.

Roughan JV, Flecknell PA. Behaviour-based assessment of the duration of laparotomy-induced abdominal pain and the analgesic effects of carprofen and buprenorphine in rats. Behav Pharmacol. 2004, 15(7):461–467.

Rowan AN. Of Mice, Models, and Men: A Critical Evaluation of Animal Research. Albany, NY: State University of New York Press, 1984.

Rutala WA, Weber DJ. New disinfection and sterilization methods. Emerg Infect Dis. 2001, 7(2):348–353.

Shek R. Role of housing modalities on management and surveillance strategies for adventitious agents of rodents. ILAR J. 2008, 49(3):316–325.

Shoenberger, D. Economic Considerations of Establishing an Exotic Pet Practice. In: Veterinary Clinics of North America—Small Animal Practice, vol. 17(5). Harkness JE (ed.). Philadelphia: Saunders, 1987; 981–1017.

Singer P. Animal Liberation. New York: Avon Books, 1977.

Chapter 2

Biology and Husbandry

Chapter 2 covers selected topics on the biology and husbandry of rabbits, guinea pigs, chinchillas, hamsters, gerbils, mice, and rats. The sections are divided into eleven categories: origin and description, anatomic and physiologic characteristics, the animal as a pet, housing, feeding and watering, reproduction, disease prevention, public health concerns, uses in research, biodata, and sources of information. The references listed in each section may be found in university and public libraries or ordered from bookstores or publishers. Relevant websites deemed to have reliable and current information as of this edition (2009) are also listed. Further information about the seven species included in this chapter is given, often in considerable detail, in the general reference works listed in chapter 1.

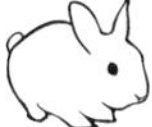

THE RABBIT

The domestic or European rabbit housed indoors or outdoors can be a pet, a show animal, a producer of meat, wool, or byproducts, or a research subject. Pet rabbit popularity has significantly increased in recent years, and consequently, so has the body of knowledge contributing to our understanding of individual rabbit husbandry and disease. If rabbits are raised in appropriate enclosures; receive adequate water and an appropriate diet; and are protected from predators, drafts and temperature extremes, obesity, and subclinical infections, they will grow rapidly, reproduce well, and live healthy lives.

Origin and Description

The domestic rabbit, *Oryctolagus cuniculus*, is a lagomorph of the family Leporidae. The other lagomorph family, Ochitonidae, consists of a few typically high-altitude-dwelling species known as pika. Domestic rabbits are descended from the wild rabbits of Europe and northwestern Africa, where wild *Oryctolagus* still exist. Rabbits have been at least semi-domesticated for nearly 200 years. Domestic rabbits have become feral in other areas of the world, most notably Australia. Wild rabbits are gregarious, burrowing, herbivorous, crepuscular animals related distantly to rodents and diverging from them in the Paleocene epoch (55–65 million years ago). Size, shape, and color variations, derived from centuries of selective breeding, define over 50 breeds that are recognized by the American Rabbit Breeders' Association (ARBA). Representatives of the large breeds (6.4–7.3 kg or 14–16 lb) are the giant chinchilla and the Flemish giant. Among the medium-sized breeds (1.8–6.4 kg or 4–14 lb) are the California and New Zealand white rabbits. Small breeds (0.9–1.8 kg or 2–4 lb) include the Dutch and Polish breeds (see Figure 2.1 for breed examples).

The albino New Zealand white is popular for meat production and research, rex and angora breeds are used for their fine hair and pelts, and the smaller breeds are typically found as pets, show, and research animals. Pet or house rabbits are often crosses of different breeds. Optimal husbandry and medical practices may vary among breeds, sources, sizes, and environments, and recommendations appropriate for colonies of New Zealand white rabbits, for example, may not be suitable for home-raised, individual pet rabbits that are litter box trained. Production rabbits require yet other considerations unique to their purpose.

Oryctolagus cuniculus is the only genus of European or domestic rabbit. Hares (*Lepus*) and cottontails (*Sylvilagus*) are in different genera. Hares and rabbits are named inconsistently, for example, the jackrabbit is really a hare and the Belgian hare is a rabbit. Rabbits are born naked and helpless (altricial), whereas hares are born furred and with their eyes open (precocious). Fertile, cross-genera matings do not occur due to different chromosome numbers (*Oryctolagus* spp has 44 chromosomes while *Lepus*

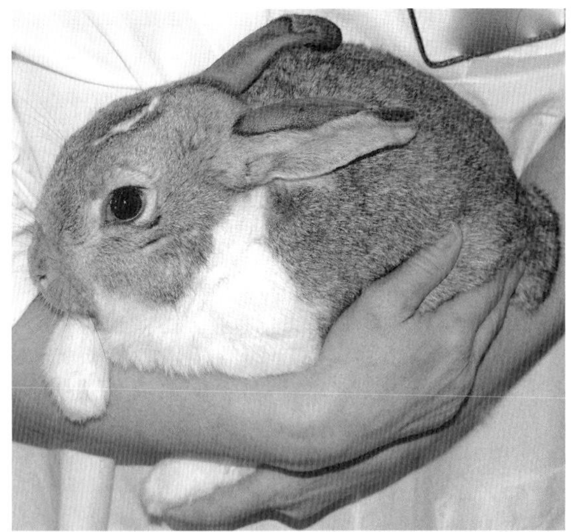

A

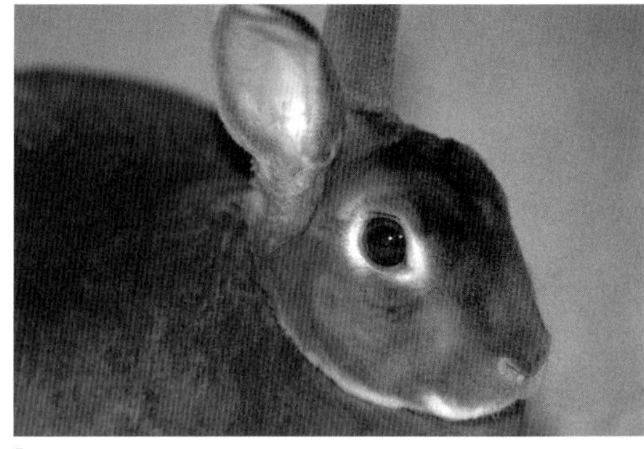

B

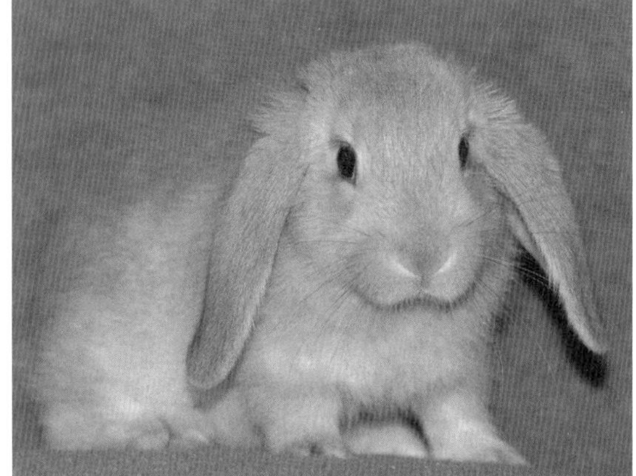

C

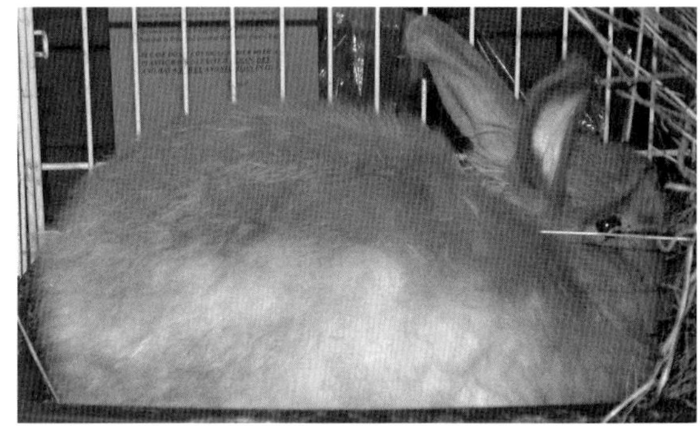

D

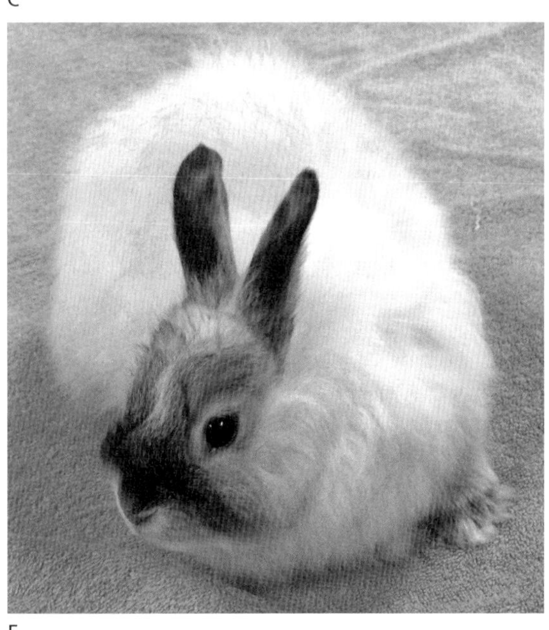

E

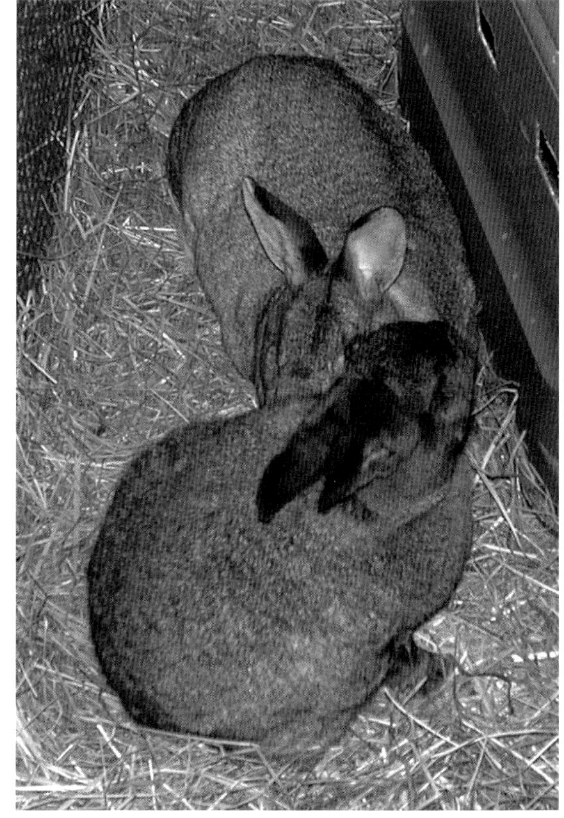

F

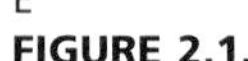

FIGURE 2.1.

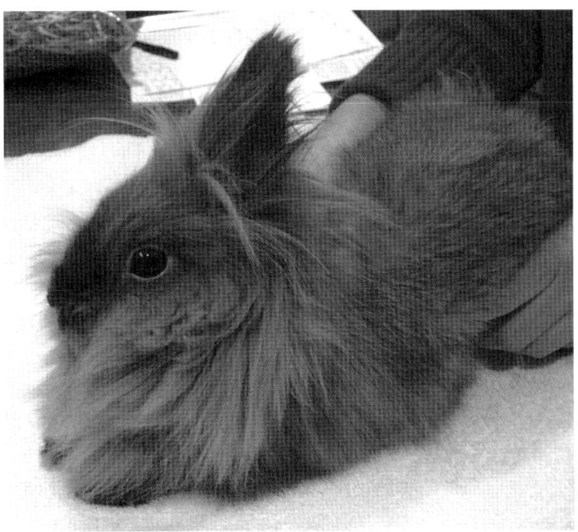
G

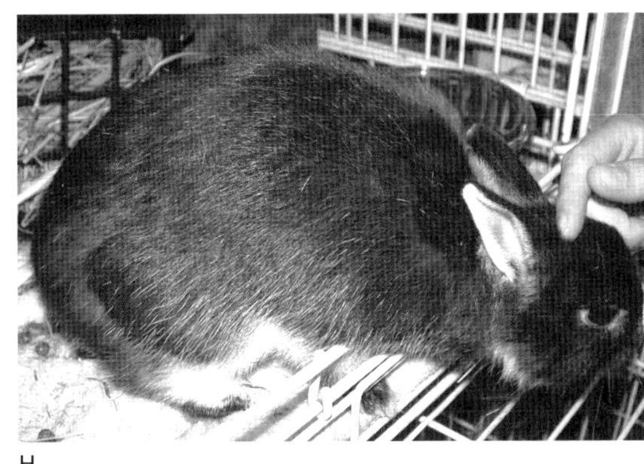
H

FIGURE 2.1. Typical appearance of several rabbit breeds. A: Dutch, B: Rex (courtesy of Glen and Rebecca Grambo), C: French lop (courtesy of Glen and Rebecca Grambo), D: Angora (courtesy of Matthew Johnston), E: Jersey wooly (courtesy of Matthew Johnston), F: Chinchilla (courtesy of Matthew Johnston), G: Lion head (courtesy of Matthew Johnston), and H: Netherland dwarf (courtesy of Matthew Johnston).

spp has 48 chromosomes). Orphaned young hares and cottontails are kept occasionally as pets, but inhalation pneumonia, injury, and death are common consequences of captivity. There are a few successfully maintained nondomesticated lagomorphs colonies used in research settings.

Anatomic and Physiologic Characteristics

Rabbits have a well-developed nictitating membrane or third eyelid. During sleep or anesthesia this membrane moves from the medial canthus across the cornea. Rabbits have a wide field of vision that reaches 190° for each eyeball. The wide pupillary dilation that they are capable of results in a light sensitivity approximately eight times that of humans. Rabbits possess a double retinal system of rods and cones and their eyes readily detect motion and apparently are very sensitive to the blues and greens present at twilight. These ocular characteristics facilitate recognition of predators via visual cues. Rabbits cannot visualize below the horizon, however, and use their sensitive vibrissae and lips to find forage. Rabbit ears are highly vascular organs that function in heat regulation, sound gathering, and as convenient sites for intravenous injections and blood sampling. This site might not be advisable for all breeds nor all materials to be injected, as perivascular injections of irritating substances may result in sloughing of the ear tips. The ears are fragile and sensitive and should not be used for restraint.

Rabbit teeth are open rooted (continuously growing). On each side of the mouth there are 2/1 incisors, 0/0 canines, 3/2 premolars, and 3/3 molars. Lagomorphs have a second pair of incisors ('peg teeth') in the upper jaw, one feature that classifies them into *Lagomorpha* versus *Rodentia* (Figures 2.2 and 2.3). Peg teeth protect the palate from trauma from lower incisors (Figure 2.4).

Malocclusion and dental overgrowth occur most often with incisors, which grow an average of 10–12 cm (4–4.8 in) per year throughout the rabbit's life. Peg teeth may overgrow also, as can the premolars and molars (cheek teeth). Malocclusion may result from either or both congenital anomalies in jaw and tooth formation and inadequate fiber and roughage in the diet.

The thoracic cavity is small compared with the capacious abdominal cavity, and this is important to remember when rabbits are positioned on their backs for surgery, as the intestinal weight on the diaphragm may interfere with normal chest excursions during breathing. The intestine is approximately 10 times the body length and includes a large cecum and glandular stomach. The vermiform appendix at the free end of the cecum and sacculus rotundus (the pale

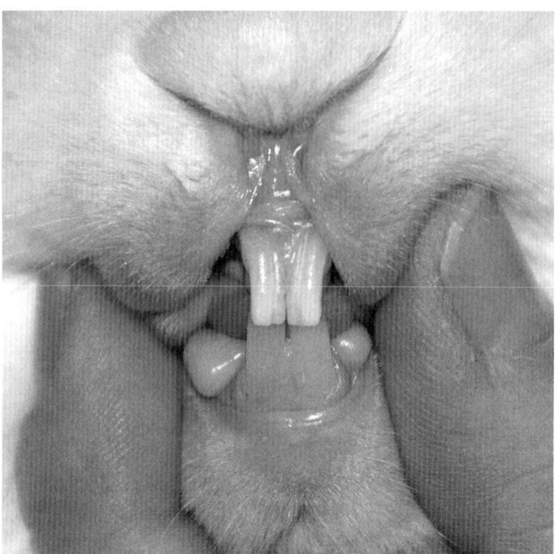

FIGURE 2.2. Normal rabbit incisors. Note the relative lengths of the maxillary and mandibular incisors.

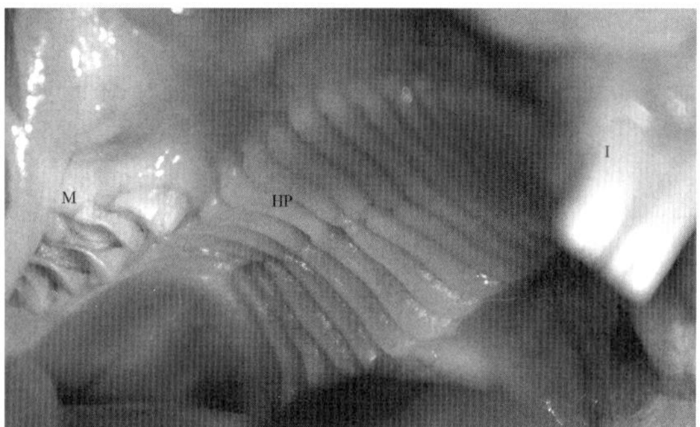

FIGURE 2.3. Lateral view of rabbit maxillary molar arcade taken from a postmortem specimen. The molars are difficult to visualize in a conscious animal without sedation. I: incisors, HP: hard palate, M: molars.

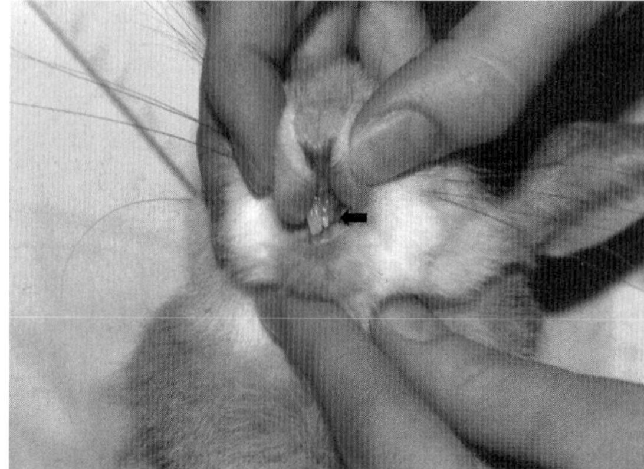

FIGURE 2.4. Dwarf rabbit missing left rostralmost maxillary incisor, revealing typical caudally located peg tooth (arrow).

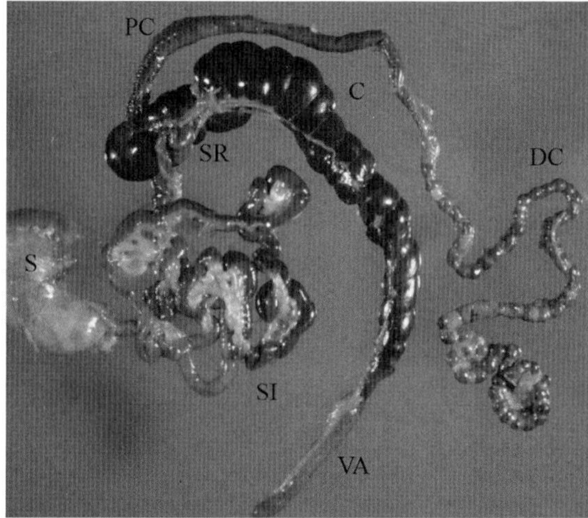

FIGURE 2.5. Normal gastrointestinal anatomy of the rabbit (S: stomach, SI: small intestine, SR: sacculus rotundus, C: cecum, VA: vermiform appendix, PC: proximal colon, DC: distal colon). Courtesy of Dean H. Percy. Reprinted with permission from Blackwell Publishing.

fleshy tissue at the ileocecal junction) are prominent lymphoid organs associated with the rabbit's intestine (Figure 2.5). The fragile skeleton comprises only 8% of the animal's body weight, compared to the cat's skeleton, which comprises 13% of its body weight. The long bones and lumbar spine, encased in relatively large muscle masses, are susceptible to fracture, particularly in young animals with incomplete growth plate calcification.

The rabbit has a comparatively small heart, and the right atrioventricular valve is bicuspid instead of tricuspid. Rabbits have delicate, thin-walled veins that tear easily, and they have a very narrow linea alba. The inguinal canals, leading to the inguinal pouches (scrotal sacs), remain open for the life of the rabbit. The testes descend at 12 weeks but are capable of abdominal retraction. Rabbits have 8–10 mammary glands, arranged in broad bands from the throat to the groin that are only visible in the mature female. Rabbit milk is high in fat and protein compared with other mammals. A separate cervix is present for each uterine horn.

Rabbits have a soft dense undercoat and thin skin, making clipping fur difficult but contributing to the versatility of the pelt. Rabbits do not have footpads but instead have coarse fur on the plantar and palmar surface of the tarsus and carpus, respectively, where they contact the ground. Cage surfaces should be solid or a polished wire to avoid damage to the feet, otherwise severe pododermatitis can develop.

The rabbit neutrophil, especially when observed in suppurative lesions, resembles an eosinophil because of the numerous intracytoplasmic eosinophilic granules. These cells are more appropriately termed heterophils because of their staining characteristics, but they have the same functions as neutrophils in other species. Heterophils and lymphocytes are present in an approximate ratio of 1 : 1 to 3 : 7, respectively, except during certain infections, when the ratio may reverse. Basophils are more common in rabbits (2–7% or more in differential white blood cell counts) than in other mammals. The composition of proteolytic and mucolytic enzymes in heterophils of the rabbit results in production of viscous suppurative exudates characteristically observed during bacterial infections.

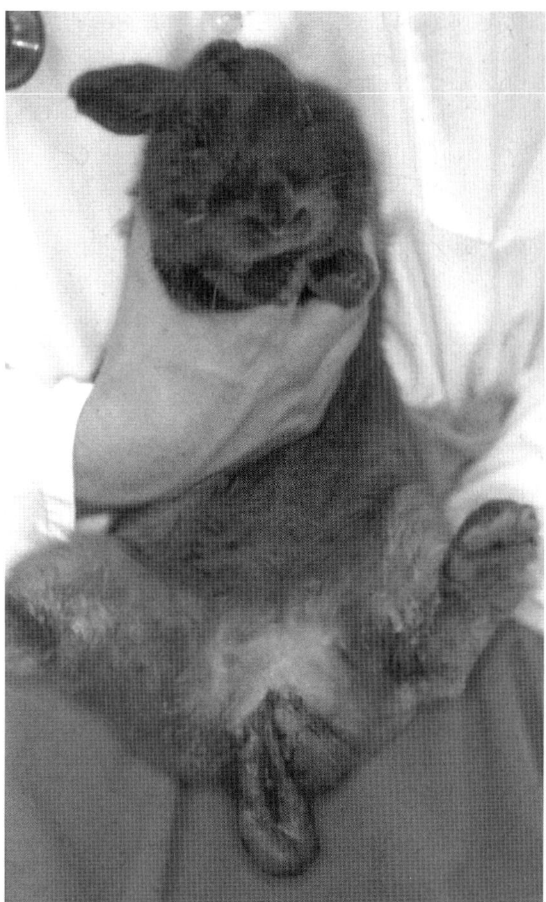

FIGURE 2.6. Male rabbit with scrotal wound and exposure of testis following fight with another male rabbit.

Rabbits as Pets

Behavior

Rabbits make good pets and can be litter box trained, particularly if they are neutered. Older bucks and primiparous does with strong territorial instincts may bite people, but such biting is uncommon unless a protruding finger is mistaken by the rabbit as a piece of carrot or other piece of food. Rabbits can, if improperly restrained or if naturally aggressive, inflict substantial scratches with their powerful rear limbs. Rabbits protect themselves through acute senses, burrowing, agonistic displays, and thumping of the rear limbs in response to perceived aggression. Otherwise, agonistic behavior is confined to the breeding cage, where pursuit, tail flagging, urination, squealing, and combat are exhibited. Aggressive behavior varies among breeds, with Dutch belted being more aggressive than New Zealand whites and lops, in that order. Rabbits thump as an isolated response to aversive (fearful or painful) situations. Sexually maturing rabbits (older than 3 months) often attack one another and may need to be housed separately. Wounding, pseudopregnancy, and infertility may occur in group-housed rabbits, unless groups are established before sexual activity begins or animals are neutered as juveniles and gradually introduced to one another (Figure 2.6). Introductions of new animals should be gradual and supervised. Mature rabbits of the opposite sex should be paired only at mating and separated afterward. It is recommended that house rabbits be neutered to decrease aggression, increase compatibility, and improve litter box behavior.

Life Span

A medium-sized rabbit has a breeding life from approximately 4.5 months to 3–4 years of age, an average life span of 5–6 years, and a possible longevity of 15 years. In general, dwarf breeds will live longer and reach sexual maturity earlier than larger breeds.

The breeding life of a doe may consist of 7–25 litters before the number of young per litter (7–8 for medium breeds) declines. This onset of senescence may be caused by progressive endometrial fibrosis and consequent failure of ova to be implanted.

Restraint

To carry a rabbit a short distance, the neck skin is grasped with one hand and the rear quarters supported with the other ("football" hold) (Figure 2.7); alternatively, a small rabbit can be grasped over the back. Grasping the rabbit under the thorax and supporting the rump so that the rabbit assumes a "C" shape position ("cradle" hold) has been suggested as a method that allows examination of the ventrum. Another method involves stretching the rabbit and holding against the body (upright hold). To carry longer distances, the rabbit should be placed on the bearer's forearm with its head concealed in the bend of the elbow. Commercial plastic restrainer devices are also available (Figure 2.8).

Covering the animal's eyes with a towel may help to allay fear and struggling. When rabbits are handled improperly, they may struggle vigorously and break their backs or scratch the handler. Wrapping a rabbit snugly in a towel or blanket ("towel wrap"; see Figure 2.9) may help to alleviate anxiety, prevent struggling, and facilitate examination or transportation of the animal for short distances.

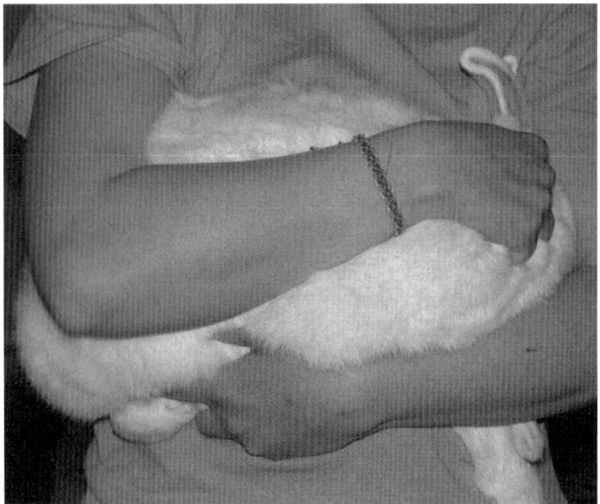

FIGURE 2.7. Football hold used for carrying rabbits short distances. The rabbit's face is tucked under the handler's elbow to minimize visual stimulation, and the rabbit's hind end is controlled by the handler's opposite forearm and elbow.

When rabbits must be carried long distances, a box or carrier is recommended. Rabbits should never be lifted or restrained by their ears.

Housing

Plans for rabbit hutches are freely available online or from libraries and feed companies. Assembled wire cages, with ancillary equipment, are available from farm-supply stores, pet stores, or mail-order houses that advertise in publications of rabbit breeder associations or at conventions. Caging is also advertised in professional and trade publications in animal science, laboratory animal science, and rabbit husbandry. Critical considerations in rabbit housing include the use of the animal (i.e., pet, laboratory, or production), structural strength, absence of sharp edges and rough surfaces, adequate size, wire construction [1×2.5 cm (0.4×1 in) mesh on floor and on lower walls if neonates are present and 2.5×5 cm (1×2 in) on sides], ease of cleaning, protection from climatic extremes, corrosion resistance, portability, and provision of self-feeding "J" hoppers and sipper-tube or dewdrop water valves. Pet and research rabbits are frequently housed in large pens, crates, or cages made of stainless steel or plastic with solid bottoms and litter substrate, such as wood shavings or straw (Figures 2.10 through 2.14). In breeding operations, male rabbits are typically separated at weaning, whereas does are housed individually from approximately 12 weeks of age.

Rabbits should be housed in areas that are commensurate with the animal's use, size, and weight, and in accordance with current regulations or guidelines (Table 2.1). Recommendations for pet animals vary, but have been suggested as enough floor space for three hops and tall enough to accommodate an animal standing on its hind legs. It is also suggested that house rabbits might be confined to a hutch during the day, but be provided supervised exercise on a daily basis.

Intact, young to mature, sibling does or neutered bucks may be housed together to enhance social enrichment and increased exercise. Animals should

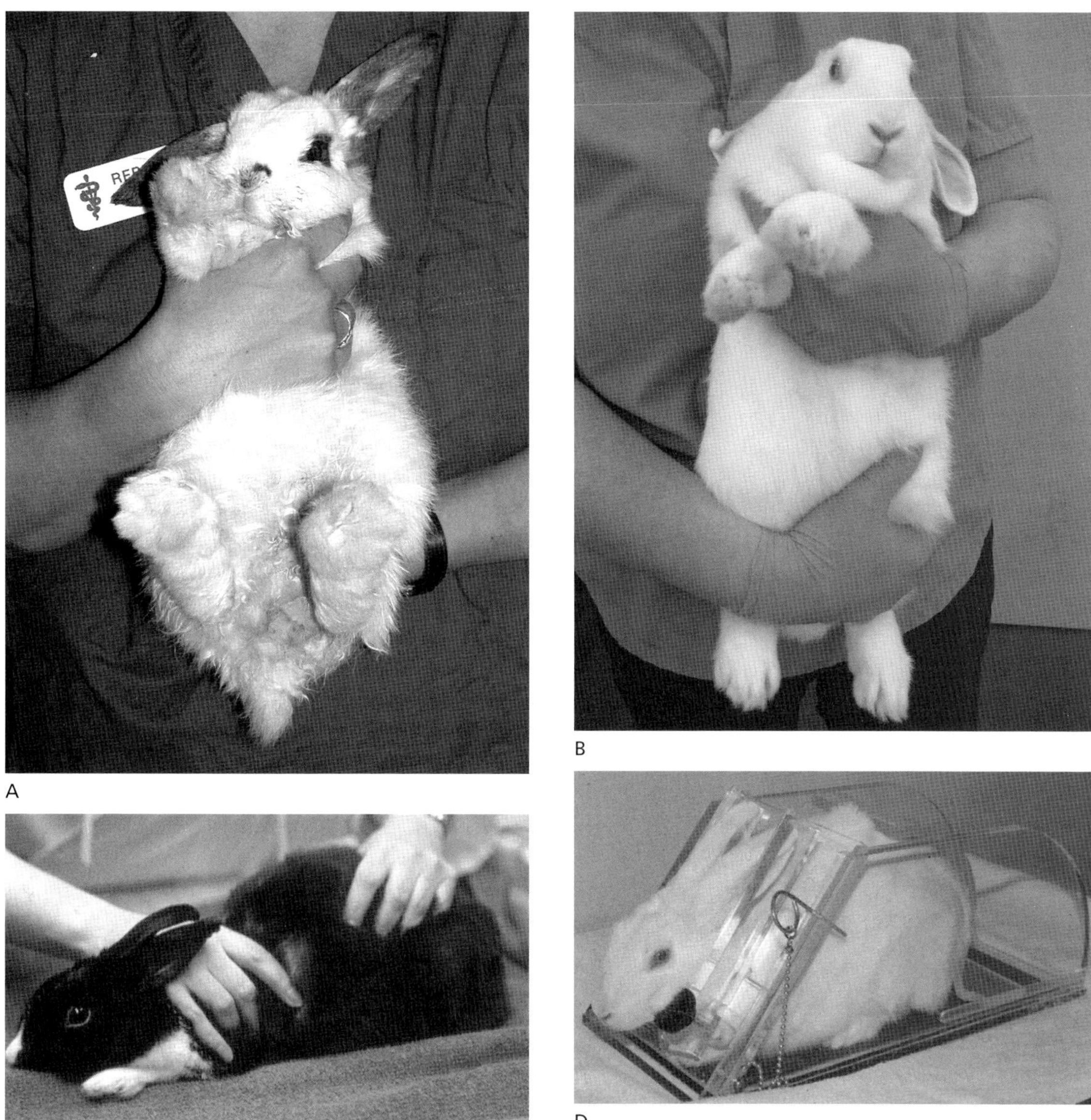

FIGURE 2.8. Alternate methods for rabbit restraint. A: cradle hold for small rabbits (courtesy of Matthew Johnston), B: upright body hold, C: table hold for injection, with hands pressing over the pelvic and pectoral limbs to prevent bolting, and D: plastic commercial rabbit restrainer (courtesy of Ernest D. Olfert).

be supervised closely to disrupt fighting during group establishment. Once dominance hierarchies are established, aggression will usually diminish.

Rabbits are generally housed indoors at temperatures between 4 °C and 29 °C (40–85 °F), with a recommended average between 16 °C and 21 °C (61–70 °F). Rabbit cages should not be placed in direct sunlight, to avoid overheating of animals. Lower environmental temperatures are tolerated well, and rabbits may be housed safely outside provided they are sheltered from wind and drafts, protected from predation and insect vermin, and kept

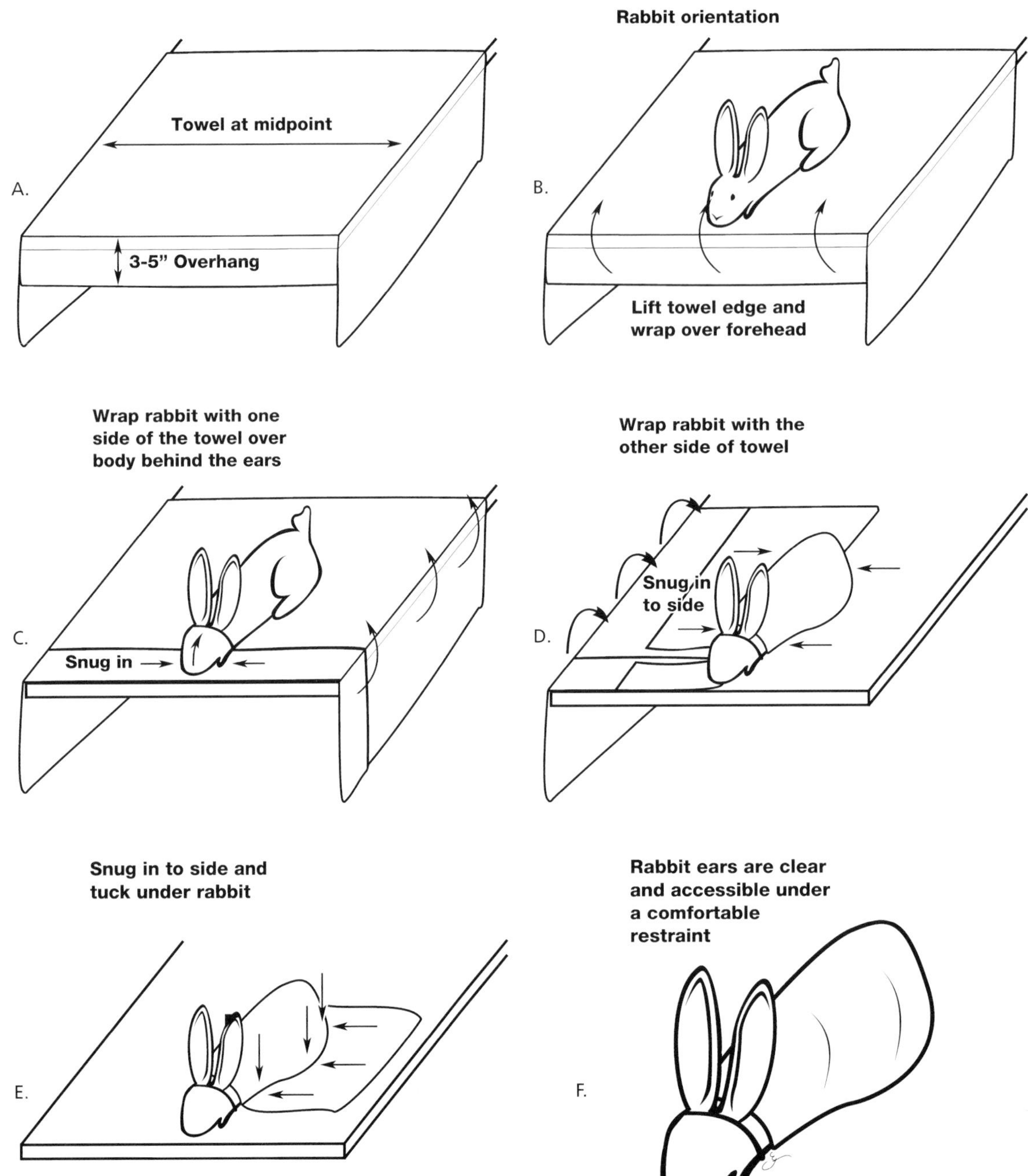

FIGURE 2.9. Visual instructions for performing the rabbit towel wrap. Start with a large towel placed on a flat surface or table, as illustrated (top left). Place the rabbit in the middle of the towel (top right) and wrap as indicated. The final photo (see next page) shows a snugly wrapped animal. The towel can be folded down from the face to make the animal more comfortable for longer periods of restraint or for face mask induction for anesthesia. Illustrations by Gianni A. Chiappetta.

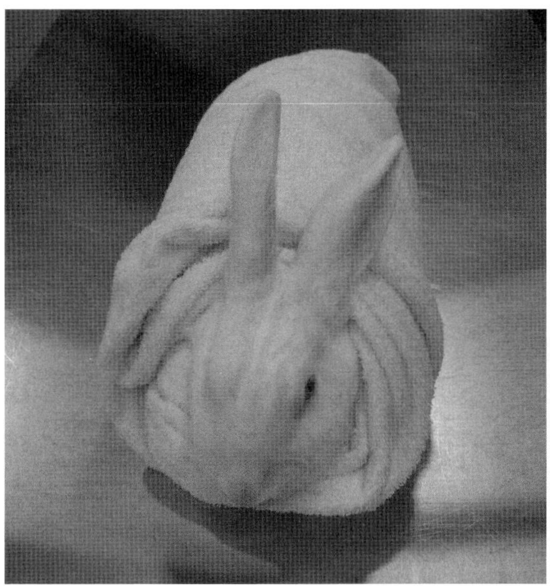

FIGURE 2.9. *(continued)*

warm and dry. In hot weather (above 29 °C or 85 °F), outdoor cages should be cooled by ventilation, shade, evaporator pads, or overhead sprinklers (care must be taken to prevent excessive wetting of rabbits).

Other characteristics of the rabbit's environment should include a moderate humidity (30–70%), adequate draft-free ventilation, regular removal of droppings, and a daily cycle of 14–16 hours light for females, 8–10 hours light for males, often compromised as 12h:12h light-dark cycles. Shortening of daylight hours may depress sexual activity, as may occur in the shortening days of autumn. Although hanging wire cages may remain superficially clean for weeks, hair and matted feces accumulate, requiring regular sanitation.

Rabbits use a preferred latrine area in their cage for defecation and urination, which makes house training possible. Litter trained rabbits may still soil outside the litter box on occasion. Pans for droppings should be emptied, and enclosed hutches should be cleaned weekly or more often, as needed. Flies are attracted to rabbit droppings, and hatched fly larvae or maggots may give the false impression that the rabbits have "worms" on their back quarters. Such a flystrike can have serious consequences for rabbit health and is an indication of a need for improved husbandry. Properly ventilated and dried manure troughs in production facilities can be left undisturbed for months. However, cleaning of rabbit cages to remove infectious agents is particularly important before parturition, during weaning, before installing new stock, and after removing a sick animal. Laboratory rabbit cages are sanitized with chemicals, steam, or a combination of these methods every 2 weeks per USDA Animal Welfare Act guidelines in the United States.

Due to their herbivorous diet, rabbit urine has a pH of approximately 8.2, which results in crystalli-

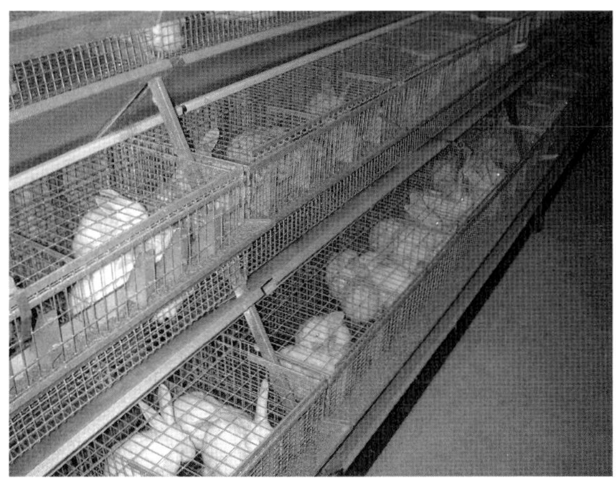

A

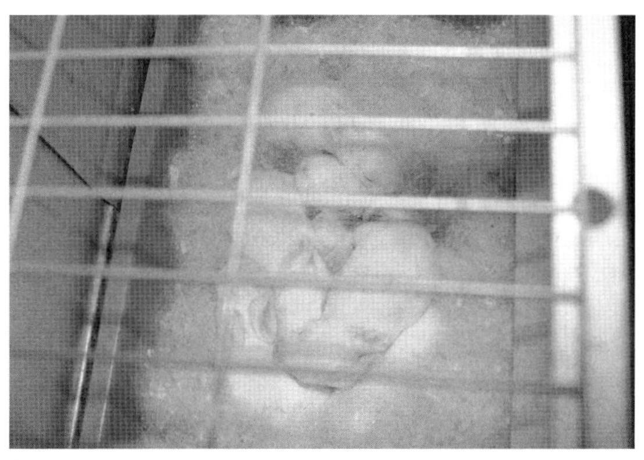

B

FIGURE 2.10. A. Typical double-row suspended wire housing used for commercial rabbit operations. Courtesy of Kendra Keels. B. Nest box with kits in commercial operation. Courtesy of Robert Wright.

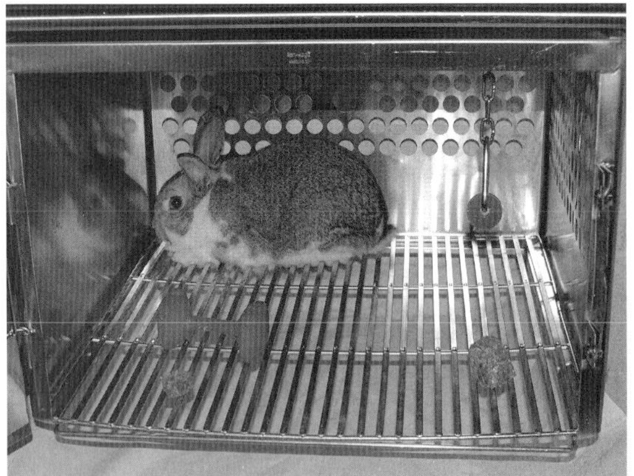

FIGURE 2.11. Stainless steel cage used for laboratory rabbit housing. Note the enrichment items in the cage, including the suspended chain and plastic chew toys. An alfalfa cube has been given as a treat.

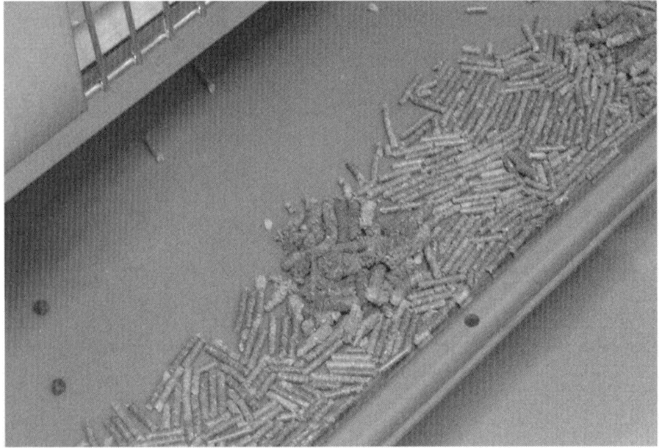

FIGURE 2.12. The pan under the rabbit cage may be filled with commercially available recycled paper pellets to absorb urine and control odors.

zation of minerals and turbid crystalluria. Rabbit urine varies in color from light yellow to deep orange or red brown because of porphyrin accumulation, and color is enhanced by dehydration and alkalinity. This may be mistaken for hematuria by owners. The carbonate and phosphate salt scale that accumulates on cage surfaces is difficult to remove, and requires soaking in acids prior to washing for adequate descaling.

Detergents, disinfectants, and lime-scale removers can be applied with a stiff brush in routine cage cleaning. Acidic solutions damage floors and metals and should be used cautiously. Sodium hypochlorite

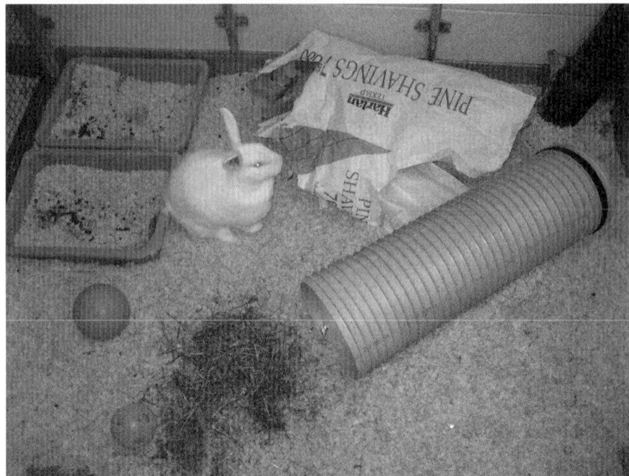

FIGURE 2.13. Loose pen housing for a laboratory rabbit. Pen contains two litter boxes filled with shavings plus a number of enrichment items including a paper bag to chew on, a tube for hiding, and balls for rolling or nibbling. Free-choice hay is available.

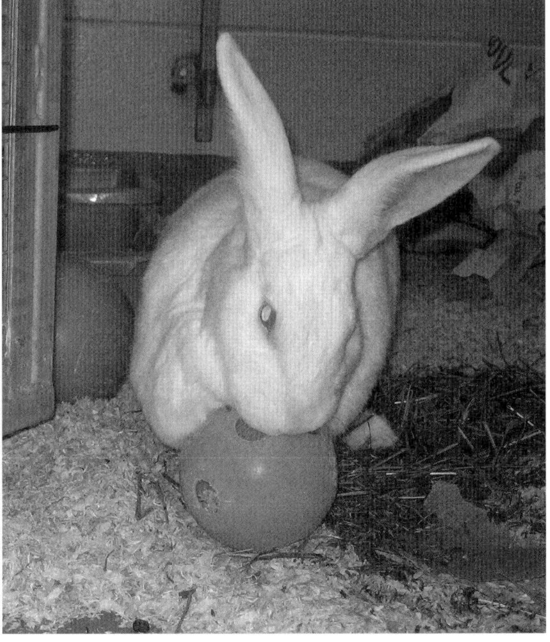

FIGURE 2.14. Rabbit chewing on whiffle ball used for enrichment.

(5%) or household bleach mixed at 30 mL per liter of water (1 oz per quart) is an excellent disinfectant for small animal caging but should be left in contact for at least 10 minutes before rinsing. Flaming may be necessary to remove hair and kill coccidial oocysts

Table 2.1. Cage size requirements for rabbits used in biomedical research in the United States and Canada.

Rabbit Size	Floor Space/Animal* ILAR Guide[a]	CCAC Guide[b]
Up to 2 kg (4.4 lb)	0.14 m^2 (1.5 ft^2)	
2–4 kg (4.4–8.8 lb)	0.28 m^2 (3 ft^2)	0.37 m^2
4–5.4 kg (8.8–11.9 lb)	0.37 m^2 (4 ft^2)	0.47 m^2
>5.4 kg (>11.9 lb)	0.46 m^2 (5 ft^2)	
Doe with litter	Additional 0.19 m^2 (2 ft^2)	0.93 m^2

* Based on current ILAR Guide for the Care and Use of Laboratory Animals (1996) and the CCAC's Guide to the Care and Use of Experimental Animals, vol. 1 (1993).
[a] Minimum cage height 0.35 m (13.7 in).
[b] Minimum cage height 0.4 m (15.6 in) for animals up to 4 kg and 0.45 m (17.6 in) for animals >4 kg.

and may be used for disinfection of production facilities. Absorbent compressed paper or wood chip is recommended as a substrate to line a house rabbit litter box, and the box is best spot cleaned on a daily basis with a complete change once every 1–2 weeks, depending on the type of litter used. Dilute vinegar can be used to remove scale. Clay or clumping litters should not be used in a rabbit litter box.

Breeding bucks should be sheltered from high temperatures to avoid periods of sterility. At temperatures of 29 °C (85 °F) and above, especially in heavily furred older rabbits in high humidity, heat stress may lead to death or infertility. Does may experience embryonic mortality under similar conditions. High temperatures lower feed intake and increase water consumption, whereas cold increases both, if the water remains unfrozen.

Feeding and Watering

Rabbits are monogastric, hindgut fermenting herbivores. They prefer low-fiber, high-protein, high-carbohydrate portions of plants, which are usually the tender, succulent portions. Some microbial digestion of cellulose occurs in the rabbit large intestine. The microflora also ferments ingesta, producing digestion products essential to nutrition, including amino acids, volatile fatty acids, B complex vitamins, and vitamin K. The rabbit utilizes these end-products by direct absorption across the mucosa or following cecotrophy (= coprophagia), in which cecal contents are re-ingested as cecotropes. Rabbits eat various forages, including leaves, grass, weeds, and byproducts. They digest 70–80% of forage protein, which makes them among the most efficient users of plant protein.

Consequences of good nutrition in the medium-sized production rabbit are gains of 30–40 g (1–1.4 oz)/day to a weight of 1.8–2.3 kg (4–5 lb) by 8–10 weeks; up to 11 litters of 7–8 young annually; and an absence of diet-related disease. Adult male rabbits eat 110–175 g (4–6 oz) of pellets/day; pregnant does eat 175–225 g (6–8 oz)/day; lactating does eat 225–450 g (8–16 oz)/day; rabbits 3–6 weeks of age eat 50–75 g (1.7–2.5 oz)/day; and rabbits 6–8 weeks of age eat 125–150 g (4–5 oz)/day. Rabbits begin eating dry feed at 16–18 days of age. Consumption varies with ambient temperature, water availability, and other factors. Diets high in starch and carbohydrates lead to a multitude of gastrointestinal and systemic diseases. Progressive production rabbit facilities provide high-fiber, low-energy diets to growing fryers, and a higher energy ration to breeding animals. Because of the capacity of rabbits to convert low-quality feed efficiently, they are an important food source not only for wild predator species but also for human populations. The meat is also low in cholesterol and fat, compared to other more common forms of meat, such as chicken, beef, or pork.

Rabbits naturally exhibit coprophagy, usually in the early morning, and ingest large quantities of

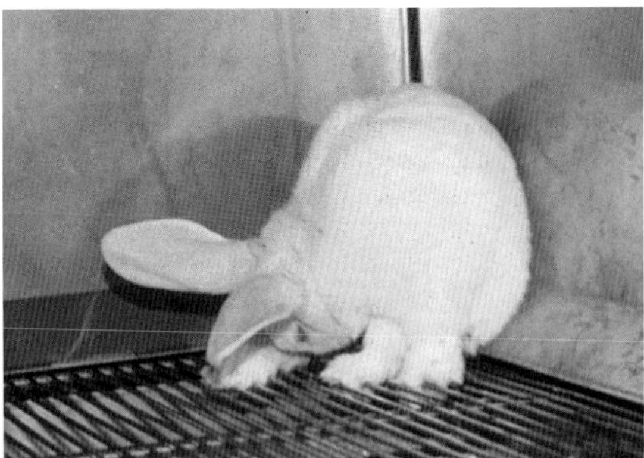

FIGURE 2.15. Coprophagy is a normal activity of a rabbit in which cecotropes are ingested directly from the anus. Housing animals on wire or slatted floors does not prevent coprophagy from occurring. Courtesy of Dean H. Percy.

protein- and vitamin-rich mucin-covered feces ("cecotropes") directly from the anus (Figure 2.15). This soft, moist, mucus-covered "night stool" is swallowed whole and may be seen in the stomachs of dead rabbits. Wire floors do not inhibit coprophagy.

Consumption

Rabbits are fastidious eaters and may reject otherwise acceptable foods because of odor, texture, form, or method of presentation. Rabbits eat to satisfy a specific caloric requirement. Under conditions of lower ambient temperatures, food consumption increases, which may lead to excessive protein consumption and secondary renal problems. Lower protein diets may be considered for winter feeding if rabbits are housed outside. At higher ambient temperatures, consumption decreases. In cold weather, dwarf rabbit breeds and does of any breed at peak lactation may not consume adequate calories and may develop a negative energy balance. Does with litters of more than 5 may require more rations, while does with smaller litters should be limit fed.

Rabbits prefer sweet foods, but despite this preference, high-calorie foods should be avoided. High-fiber, low-energy diets transit the gut rapidly, allowing increased intake both to satisfy caloric requirements and to fill the digestive tract. Cecotrope production is also reduced with low-fiber diets because of hindgut hypomotility. Hypomotility may lead to both diarrhea and cecal impaction.

Rabbits prefer pelleted diets of medium diameter (around 5 mm × 12 mm, or 0.2 × 0.5 in) with bentonite clay as a binder. Food intake peaks at mid-pregnancy and 2–3 weeks into lactation; intake decreases around kindling and around weaning (30 days postpartum). Restricting feed of growing fryers may improve food energy conversion without impairing weight gain. Restricting intake of energy-rich food to the doe postpartum (then gradually increasing) and to young animals postweaning may reduce undigested starch reaching the cecum and potential carbohydrate fermentation with secondary gut dysbiosis and diarrhea. Restricting intake also reduces abdominal fat deposits and rate of hair growth cycle, both characteristics that improve pelt quality and ease of removal.

Supplementation of a small daily amount (2–3 oz, 60–90 g) of pelleted high-fiber diet composed of timothy or prairie grasses, with ad libitum feeding of quality grass hay (high fiber, low calcium, for example, timothy or brome grass hay) is common. This type of diet has had noted success in reducing obesity, gastric stasis, urolithiasis, enteropathies, dental disorders, and hair chewing. Provision of salt, table scraps, vitamins, antimicrobials, and herbs without provision for a balanced diet is not advised. Rabbits can be given small quantities of fruits, carrots, and green leafy vegetables as treats, but these should never exceed 5–10% of the animal's daily intake and should not be fed to overweight animals. Acclimating rabbits to these "special foods" may be useful in young pet rabbits as they will be more inclined to eat them later in life as appetite stimulants, if they become sick.

Alfalfa, spinach, kale, and dandelion greens are all foods that are high in calcium and should only be fed in small amounts, on an intermittent basis, to minimize the potential for renal disease. Homemade nonpelleted diets are possible for neutered nonproduction rabbits, but the composition should be considered thoughtfully to avoid over-feeding of calcium-rich foods and to ensure that the diet is well balanced with sufficient levels of daily fiber, protein, and energy. Animals reared for meat production, or in the laboratory, are typically fed a pelleted diet balanced for fiber and protein, and supplemented with grass hay or small quantities of other food enrichment.

Because the rabbit's intestinal microflora is sensitive to the intestinal milieu (e.g., osmolarity, pH, starch content), changes in diet, especially in the 4- to 12-week-old rabbit that is transitioning from a fat- and protein-rich milk-based diet to a diet high in fiber, should be gradually made over a 4- to 5-day, period to allow adjustments in the balance of normal flora. Old and new feeds can be combined during this conversion period.

Intestinal Flora

The neonatal rabbit stomach has a pH of 5.0–6.5, which does not kill food microbes, but until 3 weeks of age, octanoic and decanoic fatty acids within the stomach keep microbial populations low. The higher stomach pH allows weanlings to acquire their adult gastrointestinal bacterial flora. Gastric acidity from weaning into adulthood has a pH of 1.0–2.0, which keeps the stomach and small intestine essentially free from resident bacteria. Facultative anaerobes (e.g., enterococci) colonize the large intestine early, followed by strict anaerobes, primarily Gram-negative *Bacterioides* spp. Spore-forming bacteria are present in smaller numbers, including low levels of several clostridial species. *Escherichia coli* may be present in low numbers. Lactobacilli are usually not present because of the lethal effects of low gastric acidity and bile acids and because of nonadhesion to the intestinal mucosa. If the cecal substrate contains increased amounts of highly soluble carbohydrate, clostridial and coliform bacteria may proliferate or produce enterotoxins, dysbiosis, diarrhea, and death.

Gastrointestinal Function

The rabbit's intestine eliminates fiber rapidly as hard, dry pellets and efficiently breaks down nonfiber components. Eighty percent of ingesta reaches the cecum by 12 hours postingestion. Rabbits chew thoroughly (120 times per minute) and reduce pelleted feed to powder, although mucin-wrapped cecotropes are swallowed whole.

Twenty-four hours after beginning a fast, the stomach may still be half full, partly because of coprophagy, and some content is still present 11 days into a fast. The small intestine functions as in other mammals. In the cecum and proximal colon, muscular, mechanical activity separates large particle insoluble fiber from soluble small particle carbohydrates and proteins. The insoluble fiber is passed through the haustrated colon and forms the familiar hard fecal pellets. During chyme separation, an aldosterone-mediated, active uptake of fluid occurs into the lumen of the upper colon, the fusus coli. The fluid then passes with small fiber and other solutes by retrograde motion into the cecum. Materials in this fluid undergo fermentation in the cecum and are packaged eventually by cecal and colonic action as soft or night feces, for consumption directly from the anus. Cecotropes have 26–29% protein and 14–18% fiber content, whereas dry fecal pellets have 9–15% protein and 28–30% fiber. Hard feces are passed for approximately 4 hours postfeeding and cecotropes for the next 4 hours. Rabbits usually eat at dusk. Bacterial action (mostly by *Bacterioides* spp) in the cecum produces volatile fatty acids (mostly butyric acid), B complex and K vitamins, and bacterial protein. Fatty acids are absorbed directly and are the major energy source for the hindgut, whereas vitamins and proteins are reprocessed after coprophagy. Heat treatment of feeds may alter starch and facilitate digestion. The lymphoid cecal appendix is rich in bicarbonate and may buffer cecal acids, or it may affect microbial fermentation in other ways.

Nutrient Requirements

Energy

The nutrient requirements of rabbits fed ad libitum are approximately 2,500 kilocalories/kg of diet during growth, gestation, or lactation, whereas maintenance requirements are 2,100 kcal/kg of diet. Growing and lactating rabbits, dwarf breeds, and rabbits in cold climates have higher caloric requirements. A once-daily feeding (limit feeding) of approximately 90–120 g (3–4 oz or 2/3 cup) of pellets will maintain an adult medium-sized rabbit at a constant weight.

Water

A 2 kg (4.4 lb) rabbit drinks as much water as a 10 kg (22 lb) dog. Rabbits consume twice as much water as food (weight basis) and the average daily water consumption is 120 mL/kg body weight (BW)/day. Consumption increases dramatically with higher ambient temperatures, with 335 mL consumed daily at 5 °C (41 °F) and 450 mL at 30 °C (86 °F). Food consumption over the same temperature change decreases from 184 g to 125 g per day. Rabbits on high-fiber or high-protein diets drink more water to moisten and move food and to remove the urea load, respectively. Food deprivation and lactation requirements also increase consumption; lactation by as much as 10-fold. The 24-hour urine volume is approximately 130 mL/kg BW/day at pH 8.

Fiber

Large-particle insoluble or lignin-containing fiber is not digested efficiently by rabbits and serves more to provide the bulk (i.e., pressure and irritation) needed for stimulating intestinal motility. Promotion of motility decreases diarrhea, which, in the rabbit, is typically associated with hypomotility. In addition to the well-established protection against enteritis, fiber dilutes the energy content of a diet, prevents obesity, reduces hair accumulation in the stomach, improves dental health, and reduces hair chewing. Rabbit growth rate is optimal at 10–15% crude fiber, and diarrhea may result if the level decreases below 10%. A 15–17% dietary fiber level is adequate, and levels greater than 17% may retard weight gain, which may be desirable in sedentary adult rabbits. High-fiber (22.5%) diets are fed to reduce obesity and hair accumulation in the stomach. Roughages include timothy or other grass-based meal, hay, rice hulls, grasses, and leaves.

Protein

Rabbits efficiently digest plant protein, and most protein in meat or research production diets is derived from alfalfa or other quality legumes, though the high calcium content of alfalfa can result in overfeeding of this nutrient. Rabbits obtain their amino acid requirements from simple forage and grain diets, and 10% of amino acids come from cecotropes, which buffer most deficiencies. Lysine and methionine are most likely to be marginal in rabbit feed. The optimal level of protein is 15–19%. Too high protein levels lead to increased dietary costs, high urea levels and ammonia formation, increased urine production and subsequent microenvironmental humidity, and because of increased gastrointestinal pH, increased enteritis problems. Protein sources include legumes (alfalfa, clover, peas, beans, peanuts), soybean and cottonseed meal, rapeseed meal, canola, sunflowers, fish, and milk. Soybean meal is highly palatable and highly digestible by rabbits, but is an expensive diet for production facilities.

Fermentable Carbohydrates

Carbohydrates (grain starch) provide much of the energy needed by the rabbit. High-energy diets contain approximately 3,200 kcal of metabolizable energy (ME)/kg feed, and lower energy diets contain approximately 2,500 kcal ME/kg feed. A 1 kg production rabbit (6 weeks of age) requires 290 kcal/day, a 1.5 kg rabbit (7.5 weeks of age) needs 348 kcal/day, and a 2.0 kg rabbit (9 weeks of age) requires 423 kcal/day. At peak lactation, a doe needs three to four times maintenance levels, or 1,092 kcal/day, which cannot be met by ingesting conventional diets at maximum practical levels, especially diets high in added hay. A postpartum estrus 1–7 days after kindling is associated with a positive energy balance; from 10 to 28 days postpartum, does are energy deficient. Higher energy lactation diets may be indicated (25% protein) in intensive breeding schemes. Low-fiber, high-energy, high-protein concentrates include cereal grains (corn, wheat, barley) and various milling byproducts: brans, middlings, mill runs, pulps, and tubers.

Minerals

The mineral needs of rabbits are met and exceeded easily because alfalfa and grain are often combined with limestone/calcium and a 0.5% trace mineral mix. Absorption of calcium from the gut is poorly regulated in rabbits compared with other species and appears to be independent of metabolic need or vitamin D level. Blood calcium levels are regulated homeostatically, and the relatively high plasma levels (12–16 mg/dL), efficient renal excretion and reabsorption, and bone reabsorption of calcium are characteristics of domesticated rabbits. Alfalfa, the primary constituent of commercial rabbit pellets, is high in calcium and may underlie the high levels of serum calcium seen in many rabbits. The alkaline turbid (pH 8) urine is the primary route of calcium excretion, whereas in other species, calcium is primarily eliminated in bile. High calcium levels together with other physiologic or pathologic processes may result in urolithiasis, red urine, or metastatic calcification and chronic renal disease, especially if excessive vitamin D is provided. As mentioned, dilution or replacement of higher calcium-containing alfalfa hay or alfalfa-based pellets with grass hay and pellets is advisable for pet rabbits that are not being bred intensively.

Vitamins

Vitamin supplementation in rabbits is usually unnecessary because alfalfa and recycling of nutrients via coprophagy supply most vitamins. Rabbits convert 100% of beta-carotene in the diet to vitamin A and the provisional requirement is met by a diet of 10,000 IU/kg. Sun-cured alfalfa has 50,000–150,000 IU/kg of vitamin A, and feed with 190,000 IU/kg of vitamin A can result in toxicity, including abortion, fetal resorption, small litters, hydrocephalus, and low survivability. Vitamin A deficiency produces similar signs. Low fetal uptake of vitamin A somewhat protects the fetus against overdose effects. The requirement for vitamin D is low because intestinal calcium absorption is efficient in the absence of vitamin D. Vitamin D toxicity does occur with levels higher than 2,300 IU/kg. Evidence of vitamin D intoxication includes emaciation, weakness, urolithiasis, renal disease, and widespread metastatic calcification. Vitamin E deficiency leads to infertility, abortions, still births, neonatal deaths, and muscular weakness. Vitamin E can be added to the diet, as required.

Reproduction

Sexing

Neonatal rabbits can be very difficult to sex; anogenital distance is the most reliable indicator (males being longer than females), but this may not be evident until animals are 10–20 days of age, and can be a problematic way to identify gender in a single-sex litter. The best policy for identifying the sex of a young rabbit is to recheck at 1 month of age if one is unsure. Males have a rounded, protruding penile sheath and os penis (baculum) with a rounded urethral opening, whereas females have an elongated vulva with a slit opening.

Stretching the perineum by lifting the tail (with the rabbit in sternal recumbency) provides a clear view of the anogenital structures and everts the penis from its sheath. The penis can be extruded at approximately 2 months of age. Paired blind, perineal, or inguinal pouches containing scent glands lie immediately lateral to the genital openings. These scent glands are used to mark kits and cage surfaces and may contain dried yellow-brown sebaceous material. In mature males, the hairless scrotal sacs are evident lateral and anterior to the penis. In immature males, the scrotal sacs are not readily apparent (Figures 2.16–2.18).

Other dimorphic sexual characteristics, some more certain indicators than are others, include the male's larger head size, the heavy dewlap or fold of skin at the throat of many large females and of some males, and the presence of hairless nipples in the mature female.

Breeding Stock Criteria

Many rabbit breeds exist, and obviously these breeds have specific phenotypic and genotypic criteria and breeding specifications, but the most popular rabbit breeds for meat and laboratory use are the New Zealand white and California breeds. Breeding stock may be selected for several criteria, but good health (*Pasteurella* and enteritis free) is essential. *Pasteurella*-free animals are available from SPF commercial rabbit breeders and are highly recommended for laboratory studies. SPF colonies are typically also free of hepatic coccidiosis, encephalitozoonosis, and *Bordetella* spp. Currently SPF New Zealand white and Dutch breeds are available from vendors. New Zealand white laboratory rabbits have been shown to suffer myriad health effects associated with *P. multocida* infection. The impact of pasteurellosis infection on other breeds of rabbits is less clear, and in most instances these animals are not selected as *Pasturella* free or SPF. Pasteurellosis contributes significantly to moribundity of production rabbits, and sneezing animals with nasal discharge should be culled regularly.

Moderately to highly heritable breeding characteristics of production rabbits include litter weight at 28 days and other characteristics related to growth and body weight. Traits of fertility and disease resistance have low heritability.

Other criteria for selection are consistent production of litters of 7–9 kits, a 570 g (19 oz) rabbit at 4 weeks and 1.8 kg (60 oz) rabbit at 8 weeks, dressing percentage of 57% or more, 10 teats, good mother-

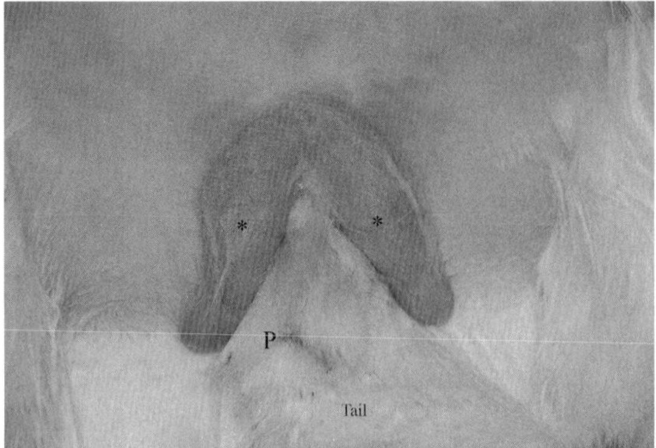

FIGURE 2.16a. External genitalia of the male rabbit (*: denotes paired scrotal sacs, P: penis).

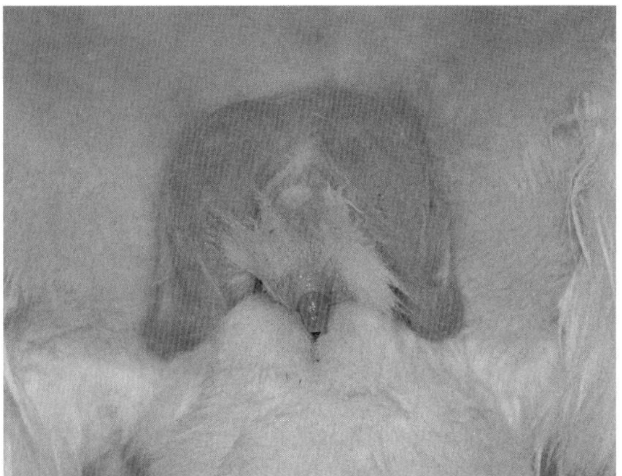

FIGURE 2.16b. External genitalia of the male rabbit with the penis extruded. The penis overlies the anus.

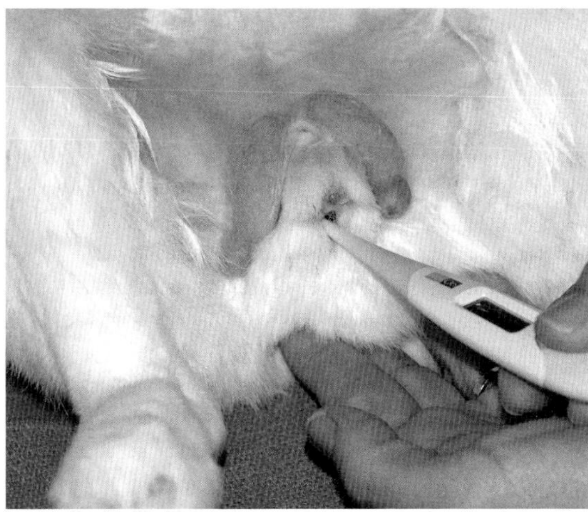

FIGURE 2.16c. Anus exposed during insertion of thermometer for rectal temperature collection.

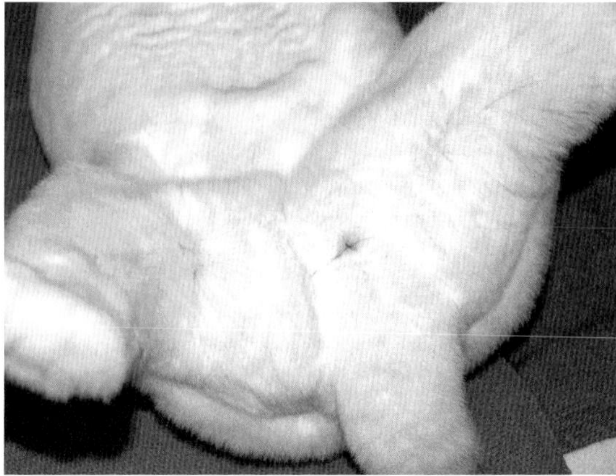

FIGURE 2.17. External genitalia of the female rabbit. Only the urogenital orifices are visible, as the tail must be retracted to visualize the anus.

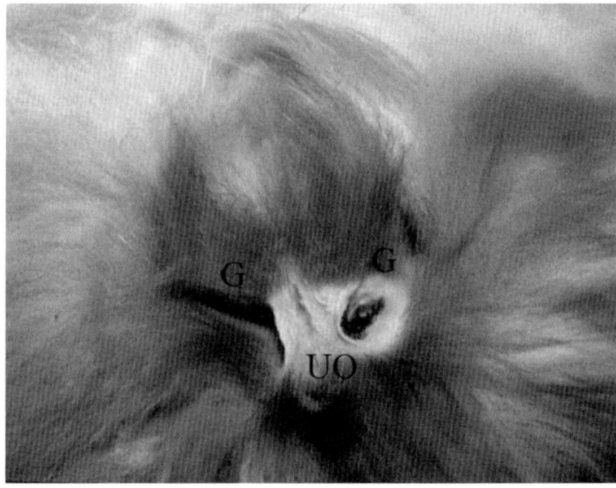

FIGURE 2.18. Paired inguinal glands in a female rabbit (UO: urogenital orifice, G: inguinal gland). The tail is at the bottom of the picture. Note the close proximity of the anus and urogenital orifice. Care must be taken to insert the thermometer into the correct orifice when obtaining a rectal temperature.

ing instincts, high food conversion efficiencies, good coat condition, and good body conformation. Milk production in does is best determined by litter weight at 21 days. An important criterion for meat rabbits is total litter weight at market age (8–10 weeks), which should be approximately 12.5–15 kg. Criteria for culling from a production herd are two consecutive litters (not counting the first litter) with less than 7 kits or exceeding 12, high nest box mortality, poor maternal behavior, poor survival (under 60%) to weaning and marketing, aggression, fur chewing, excitement, and reluctance to mate (conception rate should be 70–85%). Criteria for selection of breeders for laboratory rabbits would also include screening for congenital defects, such as buphthalmia or bradygnathism; breed selection characteristics would include parameters such as coat quality and color.

Buck Criteria

Buck quality is extremely important in intensive production systems, as each buck may service up to two dozen does or more if artificial insemination (AI) breeding systems are used. Bucks should be selected to minimize inbreeding and should be kept lean and active during their breeding lives of 2–3 years. If used weekly or twice weekly, bucks should be limit fed to control obesity. Selection of replacement bucks can be made as early as 21 days of age because, for males, weights at 21 days correlate well with weights at 56 days. Young bucks (5–6 months) should be placed with gentler does, because aggressive does may attack and permanently frighten the buck, ruining the animal as a breeder. Young bucks can be used two to three times per week, whereas mature bucks can be used once daily. Breeding bucks should be housed singly in cooler areas (less than 29 °C; 85 °F) of the facility but located conveniently near the does. For breeding, does are brought to the buck's cage and removed immediately after breeding (usually within 30 seconds of pairing) to minimize opportunities for buck aggression. When conception rate and litter size decrease in a group of does, the buck should be culled. The buck should be free from disease because disease may be transmitted by direct contact.

Doe Criteria

Does are bred by age (4–6 months), by weight (3–4 kg), and by observation of congestion of the vulva, which indicates receptivity. Age at breeding depends upon size and breed and ranges from 4 to 5 months of age for small breeds to up to 9 months for large breeds. Healthy production does produce between 20 and 25 litters before litter size decreases, and in intensive breeding systems these litters can be produced in 2–3 years. One replacement doe and buck should be planned per month for every 12 does and 5 bucks in production.

Mating

Rabbits release ova 9–13 hours after copulation. Does do not have an estrous cycle, but they do have a 7- to 10-day period of receptivity followed by 1–2 days of inactivity during which a new wave of follicles replaces the atretic precursors. Receptivity is indicated variably by a swollen, reddened vulva, restlessness, chin rubbing, and standing and allowing mounting. Rabbits may be receptive during periods of pregnancy and lactation with libido peaks approximately 26 and 39 days postpartum. Ovarian activity, reflecting hypothalamic changes, is diminished as days shorten. The use of a 16:8 or 14:10 hour light:dark cycle, adequate caloric intake, and a slightly increased ambient temperature may prevent or reduce this suppressive seasonal and environmental effect.

Does are carried to the buck's cage; if mating is to occur, it will be evident usually within 30 seconds. The pair together should be observed, at least two intromissions should occur, and the doe should not be left unsupervised with the buck more than 30 minutes to decrease opportunities for aggressive behavior.

Artificial Insemination

Artificial insemination can be an economic and efficient method of breeding large numbers of does; however, skill and labor are required that may negate other advantages of the procedure. Semen from a single buck may be extended to fertilize 500 does. Semen is collected from a trained and experienced buck using an artificial vagina in the presence of a receptive teaser doe. Such collections may occur two to three times each week. After obtaining the 0.3–1.0 mL ejaculate, the gel plug is removed, and the semen is kept at 37 °C and used within 12 hours or diluted in egg yolk sodium-citrate extender.

To induce ovulation, gonadotropin-releasing hormone (GnRH; 10 ug) or luteinizing hormone (LH or hCG; 1.25 mg in physiologic saline) is injected intramuscularly immediately following insemination. GnRH is preferable, as this short-chain peptide does not elicit an immune response. A vasectomized buck can also be used for copulation and ovulatory stimulus but is less desirable. A doe is restrained on her back or held between the thighs of the operator sitting on a stool; insemination is effected through a smooth 15 cm × 0.6 cm plastic or glass pipette inserted almost full length into the anterior vagina.

Breeding Schedules

The schedule or number of litters produced per year is determined by goal of production, that is, meat, show, or pet animal, breed characteristics, disease status, and feed selection. Intensive breeding (7–8 litters of 7–9 young per year) requires healthy, selected stock, high-energy diets, and no evidence of enterotoxemia. Five and six breeding cycles per year can be produced on a maintenance diet such as 14% protein and 20% fiber. Seven and eight cycles per year require a different composition, that is, 17% protein and 17% fiber. Implicit in higher protein rations are higher grain and higher starch (high energy), which predispose to enterotoxemia if the rabbit carries potentially enteropathogenic bacteria or is not managed properly.

Postpartum estrus occurs in most does 2–9 days after kindling and mating may occur at this time in production facilities. Postkindling days 14–28 are heavy lactation days, and conception is often unsuccessful during this period. In the five cycles/year schedule, each breeding cycle is 73 days. Thirty to 40 young are produced annually. In the eight cycles/year schedule, each breeding cycle is 45 days with 40–50 young produced yearly. Approximately 40 fryers per doe per year are needed to break even financially, but many commercial operations aim to produce 56 fryers per doe per year to increase profitability. Success of postpartum conception depends upon the doe condition, nutrition and disease status, and size of the litter being suckled.

Group Housing Production

Postpartum mating often occurs in animals reared in harem groups. Successive litters sometimes live together, though risk of maternal neglect is high for the youngest litter. Rabbits of different ages and litters may share nests, but stronger young survive at the expense of the smaller members. Disease is typically more common among group-housed rabbits. Thus there are several significant limitations to successfully using this breeding method compared to other production schemes previously described.

Pregnancy Detection

Abdominal palpation 10–14 days postbreeding will usually detect pregnancy. Ultrasound diagnosis and radiographic evaluation can also be used. Breeding failure detected at 10–14 days usually indicates a problem with individual rabbit fertility, whereas resorption detected at 28 days after initial pregnancy diagnosis is usually a husbandry problem.

A suggested method for palpation to detect pregnancy is to (1) hold the nape of neck with one hand; (2) place the other hand under the body between the hind legs and slightly in front of the pelvis; (3) place thumb on one side and fingers on the other side of the horns of the uterus (embryos will be marble-sized, and ventral in the abdominal cavity); and (4) gently rub the thumb and fingers against the doe's abdomen to distinguish the embryos from fecal pellets. Alternatively, the rabbit can be cradled in dorsal recumbency for palpation (Figure 2.19). Tense abdominal muscles will make detection of the uterus difficult.

Pregnancy

The rabbit's gestation period lasts 29–35 days, with an average of 32 days. Litters retained longer than 34 days are usually stillborn or contain large or abnormal fetuses. Pregnant rabbits are particularly sensitive to fetal loss at 13 days, when placentation

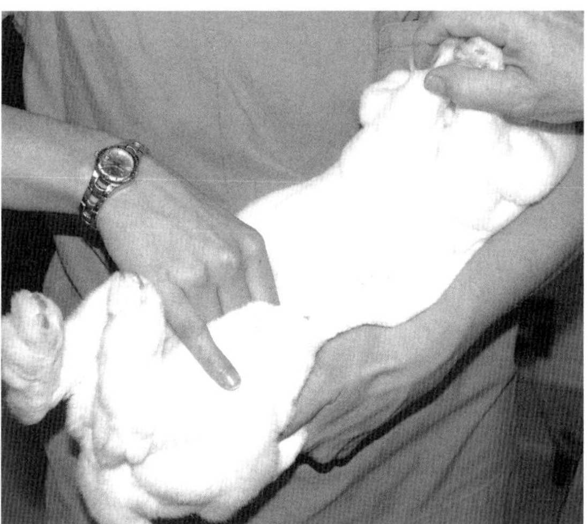

FIGURE 2.19. Palpating the female rabbit for pregnancy. Rabbits are palpated for pregnancy between 10 and 14 days of gestation and again at 26–28 days to detect possible resorption.

changes from the yolk sac to the hemochorial type, and at 23 days, when fetuses are more readily dislodged. Within 1 week of becoming pregnant, estrogen levels increase with respect to progesterone, the hair follicles relax, and the doe constructs a hair and material nest in a suitable box. Nest construction improves with successive litters. Because litter survival significantly improves with appropriately prepared nests, provision of nesting materials is recommended, particularly in summer when less hair is shed, and winter when more insulation is required. Straw, wood chips, sawdust, shredded paper, or leaves have been used to supplement nest building. Strong-smelling beddings, such as aromatic softwood chips, should be avoided because of the potential for respiratory irritation. Nests that become wet should be replaced.

The nest box itself is a substitute for the underground burrow found in the wild and provides protection of both doe and young from predators. Boxes should be protected from damp weather, should not allow kits to escape because does will not retrieve their young, and should be sanitized easily. Boxes may have a solid floor, but the surface should not be completely smooth, as a higher incidence of splayleg has been noted to occur when inadequate traction can be achieved by the developing neonate (Figure 2.20). Boxes may sit on the hutch floor, be attached to the front of the cage, or be subterranean and attached to the cage's floor. The subterranean box mimics the natural burrow, stops escape, and aids retrieval but may not be possible to install in multilayer caging systems. Boxes 41 cm (length) × 30 cm (width) × 30 cm (height) or larger are preferred. The box should be present for at least 10 days, and is usually removed at 2–3 weeks postpartum. A doe may not use the nest box and may scatter newborn young on the wire if the bedding in the box is damp, contaminated with urine and feces, or has an odor of disinfectants or predators. This typically results in rejection and death of the litter.

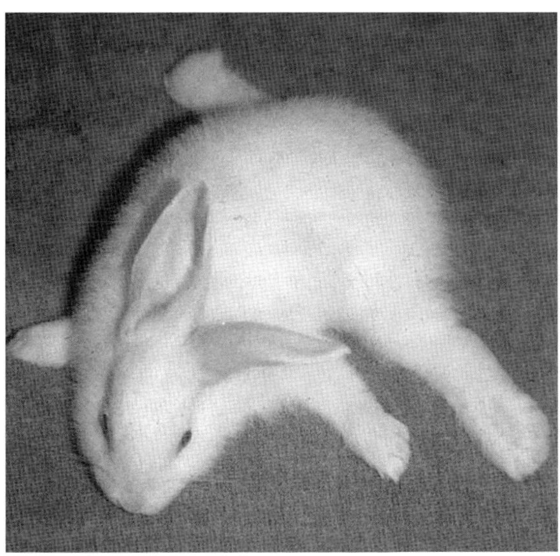

FIGURE 2.20. Young rabbit with splayleg. Courtesy of Ernest D. Olfert.

Parturition (Kindling)

Young are usually born at night. Oxytocin (0.2–3.0 units/kg IM) may be used in cases of dystocia or disruptions in labor. During delivery, the doe should not be disturbed. Optimal litter size is 8–10, and stronger, larger members of overly large litters should be fostered onto lactating does with young approximately the same age and size. Scent transfer is not a concern while fostering. Cannibalism is rare in rabbits. When it occurs, it may be associated with dead or deformed young, a hyperexcitable, primiparous doe, placentophagy, environmental disturbances, or a low-energy diet.

Metritis and retained fetuses or placentas may alter maternal behavior and cause the doe to scatter and neglect young. Maternal neglect has been associated with inadequate nest boxes, chilling or escape of offspring from the nest, disturbance of the doe (particularly when primiparous), and agalactia or mastitis.

Neonatal Period

Domestic rabbits at birth are virtually hairless, have sealed eyelids and ear canals, little crawling ability, and a body weight somewhere between 40 and 80 grams, depending on breed and litter size. Because of this, neonates are unable to maintain a stable body temperature if unfed or if the ambient temperature changes dramatically. Adequacy of ambient temperature can be assessed by observing the position of the kits. In warm environments (37 °C or 98 °F), the young disperse and assume an extended posture. At 25 °C (77 °F) neonates group, curl up, and move toward areas of higher temperature. Although neonatal rabbits increase heat production during cold stress through brown fat catabolism, shivering, and huddling with nest mates, body temperatures may decrease rapidly if the ambient temperature decreases to less than the critical temperature of 35 °C (95 °F) on day 1, 32 °C on day 5, or 29 °C on day 9. Nest box floors heated to 27 °C (81 °F) minimize chilling and reduce perinatal mortality.

The principal organ of thermogenesis in these neonates is brown fat. This triglyceride-rich tissue is found in the young of many species.

Nursing

The doe produces colostrum for 2–3 days postpartum, and then milk quantity increases and composition changes (protein 10%, fat 12%, sugar 2%) to a maximum production of 200–250 mL/day by 3 weeks. Quantity then decreases dramatically at 4 weeks, when most young are weaned. Young rabbits require only seconds to attach to a nipple after the doe's arrival in the nest. Location of the nipples by neonates is dependent on odor cues from the milk in the nipple areas. This dependence on odor (and certain tactile) cues for nursing may explain why newborn rabbits are difficult to bottle feed and hand raise. The environmental temperature and the suckling activity are linked to the onset of urinary and alimentary activity in the neonate. Rabbits require little maternal care to develop normally. Nursing time, except for the first day, is between 2.3 and 2.9 minutes. Several investigators have reported no significant differences between young rabbits with continuous access to the doe and young allowed access for only a few minutes in the morning or evening. The doe's time in the nest box is not related to milk production or to kit satiation. These observations are consistent with wild lagomorph behavior, in which the dam only visits the young once or twice daily. In the wild, this brief suckling period may decrease the risk of exposure of the young to predators.

The young begin eating maternal feces at 8 days, and wetting kits with milk stimulates urination. A primiparous mother has less milk than in subsequent litters, and litters of more than 10 may be too large for the number of nipples. In both cases, litter sizes may be reduced by fostering the strongest kits onto another doe. Orphaned or abandoned young may be fed a milk substitute with an eye dropper, doll's nursing bottle, or syringe without needle. Orphaned puppy or kitten milk or a replacer formula of 1/2 cup evaporated milk, 1/2 cup water, 1 egg yolk, and 1 tablespoon corn syrup may be used. At 2 weeks, young will begin eating fresh greens, and they will drink water from a bowl at 15–18 days. Overfeeding should be avoided.

A wild doe's acceptance of a litter and rejection and destruction of a strange litter are dependent primarily on olfactory cues. Unless characteristic odors are masked by perfume or the caretaker's distribution of a new scent to a fostered litter, strange young may be attacked and killed by the offended doe. This may occur even if the young are from the same territorial or social grouping as the host doe. However, this rejection is rarely a problem in domestic rabbits; young kits can be fostered readily with no special handling precautions. If a buck is present when a strange litter is introduced into a foster doe's cage, that buck may mark or chin the young and thereby protect them from doe aggression. In an established doe and litter group, the doe's odor guides and groups the young. Scent glands produce a secretion containing hydrocarbons, proteins, carbohydrates, esters and waxes, fatty acids (acetic and isovaleric), triglycerides, and steroids. The submandibular (or submental) and anal secretions, along with piles of feces and urine spray, are used to mark territories and individuals, whereas the inguinal scent is used to mark young rabbits and sexual partners. Chin-marking of does by bucks is a common behavior, especially after coitus and in new surroundings.

Weaning

Weaning naturally occurs 4–5 weeks postpartum. Weaning is stressful, and the young may decrease food consumption for 3 days, which may be related to a learning curve for operation of feeders and waterers. A dripping water valve attracts the young, and observation of other rabbits assists with learning. Growth is affected minimally if weanlings are moved to a clean new cage, or if the doe is removed and the litter left in the familiar environment of the nest box and maternal cage. This procedure may reduce the stress that accompanies weaning.

Several experiments have been conducted to determine the effects of handling young rabbits on subsequent behaviors; specifically exploratory, approach, sleep, and sexual behaviors. In these studies, the young were usually of the Dutch belted breed and were handled in various ways between days 1 and 20. Handling was restricted to 3 minutes daily, during which time the young were removed from the nest box, placed into a container with bedding, and then returned into the maternal nest. Although the experimental protocol varied, handled rabbits became more active, were more often awake and more exploratory, approached novel stimuli more often, and reached sexual maturity at an earlier age. This was more closely associated with stimulation occurring between days 11 and 20 than days 1 and 10.

Disease Prevention

The general recommendations for husbandry and disease prevention listed in chapter 1 should be observed, especially the removal of ammonia gas from the rabbit's environment. Common management practices with rabbits include periodic trimming of toenails and the exclusion of dogs, cats, and other animals, including insects, from the rabbitry. Wire flooring must be selected to minimize injury to limbs. Vaccination is not routinely practiced in rabbits, although vaccines for the poxvirus disease, myxomatosis, have been used during outbreaks outside of North America.

Special consideration should be given to neonatal and weanling rabbits in terms of minimizing disease. The nest box should be sanitized before use and kept clean and dry during use. Special provisions may be necessary to provide accessible food and water to young and to facilitate training to use feeders and waterers during the weaning period.

Public Health Concerns

Diseases of major public health importance in domestic rabbits are relatively rare. Salmonellosis, tularemia, rabies, ringworm (dermatophytosis), tuberculosis, and toxoplasmosis have been reported in domestic rabbits. Rabies vaccinations are not licensed for use in rabbits and are not given except in cases of high exposure probability, such as after a rabies outbreak in local skunks. Wounds caused by rabbit scratches may become infected with *Pasteurella multocida* or other bacteria, but this is rare.

Table 2.2. Biodata: rabbits.

Adult body weight: male (buck)	2–5 kg
Adult body weight: female (doe)	2–6 kg
Birth weight	30–80 g
Body surface area (cm^2)	$9.5 \times$ (weight in grams)$^{2/3}$
Rectal temperature	38.5–40.0 °C (101.3–104 °F)
Diploid number	44
Life span	5–6 yr or more
Food consumption	5 g/100 g/day
Water consumption	5–12 ml/100 g/day
GI transit time	4–5 hr
Breeding onset: male	6–10 mo
Breeding onset: female	4–9 mo
Cycle length	induced ovulator
Gestation period	29–35 days
Postpartum estrus	48 hours
Litter size	4–10
Weaning age	4–6 wk
Breeding duration	1–3 yr
Commercial	7–25 litters
Young production	2–4/mo
Milk composition	12.2% fat, 10.4% protein, 1.8% lactose

Uses in Research

Approximately 250,000 rabbits were used annually in research in the United States from 2000 to 2006 and approximately 9,000 were used annually in the same period in Canada. Rabbits are used most frequently as sources of hyperimmune sera and antibody. Other uses of rabbits in biomedical investigations include ocular research, dermal and reproductive toxicology, oncology, and infectious diseases.

Biodata

The values listed in Table 2.2 are approximations and may not represent the normal range in a given rabbit population.

References

Exotic DVM is a journal providing "a practical resource for clinicians" and is published approximately four times per year by the Zoological Education Network, 2324 S. Congress Avenue, Suite 2A, West Palm Beach, FL. The American Association of Laboratory Animal Science, 91910 Crestwyn Hills Dr., Memphis, TN, publishes several periodicals on species commonly used in laboratory animal medicine, including rabbits. The Talk Origins Archive gives useful information about the evolution of various animal species, http://www.talkorigins.org/faqs/faq-transitional.html.

Comprehensive works on rabbits, grouped by general emphasis, are:

Laboratory Rabbits

Manning P, Ringler D, Newcomer C (eds.). The Biology of the Laboratory Rabbit, 2nd ed. Orlando: Academic Press, 1994.

Poole TB (ed.). Uthe FAW Handbook of the Care and Management of Laboratory Animals, 7th ed. Oxford: Blackwell Science, 1999.

Rabbits and Rodents in Laboratory Animal Science. Proceedings 142, September 1990, Australian Society for Laboratory Animal Science (Post Graduate Committee in Veterinary Science, University of Sydney, Suite 93, Lincoln House, Sydney, South, NSW Australia, 2000).

Rowsell HC, et al. (eds.). The Guide to the Care and Use of Experimental Animals, vol. 2. Ottawa, ON: Canadian Council on Animal Care, 1984.

Smith C (ed.). Information Resources on the Care and Welfare of Rabbits. Beltville, MD: Animal Welfare Information Center, 2005. Also available online at www.nal.usda.gov/awic/pubs/Rabbits/rabbits.htm

Production Rabbits

Arrington L, Kelley K. Domestic Rabbit Biology and Production. Gainesville, FL: University Presses of Florida, 1986.

Cheeke PR (ed.). Rabbit Feeding and Nutrition. San Diego: Academic Press, 1987.

Cheeke PR, Patton NM, Lukefahr, DS, McNitt JI. Rabbit Production, 8th ed. Danville, IL: Interstate Printers and Publishers, 2000.

Patton N, Hagen K, Gorham J, Flatt R. Domestic Rabbits: Diseases and Parasites. Revised by J. Harkness in 2008, Pacific Northwest Extension Publication, PNW 310-E (update of 1976 publication, available online at http://extension.oregonstate.edu/catalog/pdf/pnw/pnw310-e.pdf).

Pet/House Rabbits

Flecknell P (ed.). BSAVA Manual of Rabbit Medicine and Surgery. Gloucester, UK: BSAVA, 2000.

Harcourt-Brown F. Textbook of Rabbit Medicine. Oxford: Elsevier Science, 2002.

Mitchell M, Tully T. Manual of Exotic Pet Practice. St Louis: Saunders Elsevier, 2009.

Quesenberry K, Carpenter J (eds.). Ferrets, Rabbits, and Rodents: Clinical Medicine and Surgery, 2nd ed. St Louis: Saunders, 2004.

Richardson V. Rabbits: Health, Husbandry and Diseases. Oxford: Blackwell Science, 2000.

Saunders R, Rees-Davies R. Notes on Rabbit Internal Medicine. Oxford: Blackwell, 2005.

Special Emphasis

Arvy L, More J. Atlas d'histologie du lapin (Histological Atlas of the Rabbit. Oryctolagus cuniculus). Paris: Librairie Maloine, 1975.

Barone R, Pavaux C, Bun PC. Atlas d'anatomie du lapin. (Atlas of Rabbit Anatomy). Paris: Masson, 1973.

Bays T, Lightfoot T, Mayer J. Exotic Pet Behavior: Birds, Reptiles and Small Mammals. St Louis: Saunders Elsevier, 2006.

Committee on Animal Nutrition: Nutrient Requirements of Rabbits, 7th ed. Washington, DC: National Academy Press, 1977.

DeBlas C, Wiseman J (eds.). The Nutrition of the Rabbit. New York: CABI, 1998.

Longo VG. Electroencephalographic Atlas for Pharmacological Research (Rabbit Brain Research, vol. 2). New York: Elsevier-North Holland, 1962.

Oglesbee B. The 5-Minute Veterinary Consultant: Ferret and Rabbit. Ames, IA: Blackwell, 2006.

Paterson S (ed.). Skin Diseases of Exotic Pets. Oxford: Blackwell Science, 2006.

Silverman S, Tell L. Radiology of Rodents, Rabbits, and Ferrets. St Louis: Elsevier Saunders, 2005.

Urban I, Richard P. A Stereotaxic Atlas of the New Zealand Rabbit's Brain. Springfield, IL: Charles C Thomas, 1972.

Other References on Rabbits

Bennett B. Storey's Guide to Raising Rabbits, 3rd ed. Pownal, VT: Storey, 2000.

Chapin RE, Smith SE. The calcium tolerance of growing and reproductive rabbits. Cornell Vet. 1967, 57:480–491.

Cheeke PR (ed.). Rabbit Feeding and Nutrition. San Diego: Academic Press, 1987.

Collewijn H. The Oculomotor System of the Rabbit and Its Plasticity (Studies of Brain Function Series, vol. 5). New York: Springer-Verlag, 1981.

Feldman DB, Seely JC (eds.). Necropsy Guide: Rodents and the Rabbit. Boca Raton, FL: CRC Press, 1988.

Foote RH, Simkin ME. Use of gonadotropic releasing hormone for ovulating the rabbit model. Lab Anim Sci. 1993, 43:383–385.

Gendron K. The Rabbit Handbook. Hauppauge, NY: Barron, 2000.

Girgis M. Stereotaxic Atlas of the Rabbit Brain. Saint Louis: Green, 1987.

Hrapkiewicz K, Medina L. Clinical Laboratory Animal Medicine: An Introduction, 3rd ed. Ames, IA: Blackwell, 2004.

Hunter S. Hop to It: A Guide to Training Your Pet Rabbit. Hauppauge, NY: Barron, 1991.

Jilge B. The rabbit: a diurnal or nocturnal animal? J Exp Anim Sci. 1991, 34:170–183.

Laber-Laird K, Swindle MM, Flecknell P. Handbook of Rodent and Rabbit Medicine. Tarrytown, NY: Elsevier Science, 1996.

Lebas F, et al. The Rabbit: Husbandry, Health & Production. Lanham, MD: UNIPUB, 1986.

Morton DB, et al. Refinements in rabbit husbandry. Lab Anim. 1993, 27:301–329.

Pavia A. Rabbits for Dummies. New York: Wiley, 2003.

Sandford JC. The Domestic Rabbit, 4th ed. Dobbs Ferry, NY: Collins UK, 1986.

Shek J, et al. Atlas of the Rabbit Brain and Spinal Cord. New York: S. Karger, 1985.

Veeramachaneni R, et al. Disruption of sexual function, FSH secretion, and spermatogenesis in rabbits following developmental exposure to vinclozolin, a fungicide. Reproduct. 2006, 131:805–816.

Wegler M. Rabbits: A Complete Pet Owner's Manual. Hauppange, NY: Barron, 1999.

Wingerd BD. Human Anatomy and Rabbit Dissection. Baltimore: Johns Hopkins, 1985.

Yu B, Tsen HY. Lactobacillus cells in the rabbit digestive tract and the factors affecting their distribution. J Appl Bacteriol. 1993, 75:269–275.

Websites for Rabbits

http://www.poultry.msstate.edu/extension/pdf/rabbit_production.pdf—commercial rabbit production.

http://www.ontariorabbit.ca/—Ontario Commercial Rabbit Growers Association.

http://www.omafra.gov.on.ca/english/livestock/alternat/rabbits.htm—production rabbit care and health.

http://www.rabbit.org/—American House Rabbit Society website.

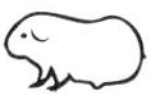

THE GUINEA PIG

The guinea pig or cavy is a docile caviomorph encountered often as a pet, show, or research animal or, in its native Andes Mountains, as a culinary delicacy. Guinea pigs are notable for their fastidious eating habits, absolute dependence on dietary vitamin C, relatively long gestation period, large and precocious young, and messy living habits.

Origin and Description

The guinea pig, *Cavia porcellus*, is a New World hystricognath related to the wild and semi-domesticated caviae (*Cavia aperea*) still found in the mountains and grasslands of Peru, Argentina, Brazil, and Uruguay. Andean Indians use *C. aperea* as a special food much as North Americans use the turkey. Other New World hystricognaths include agoutis, degus, and chinchillas. Guinea pigs are gregarious, herbivorous (except for placentophagy), nonburrowing, crepuscular animals. In the sixteenth century they were taken as curiosities to Europe, where they were bred selectively by fanciers, resulting in several coat colors and hair lengths.

The most common pet and laboratory variety is the English, American, or short-haired guinea pig, which has a uniformly short-haired coat. The Duncan-Hartley and Hartley strains are representative lines of the English variety. Inbred strains 2 and 13 are popular research animals. Other varieties or

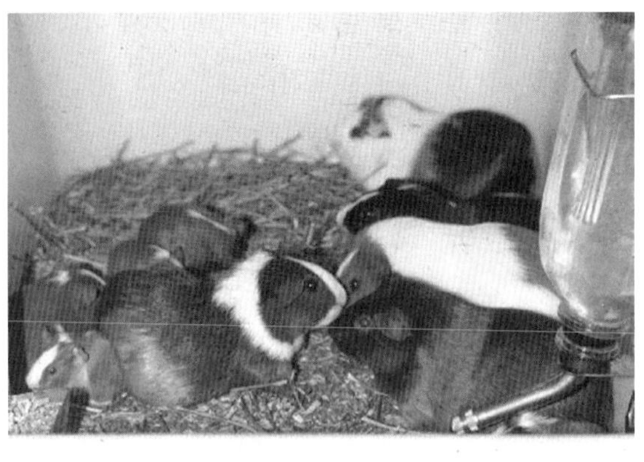

A

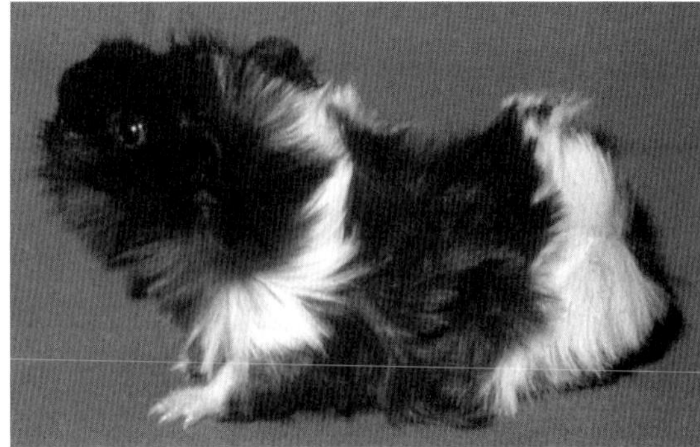

B

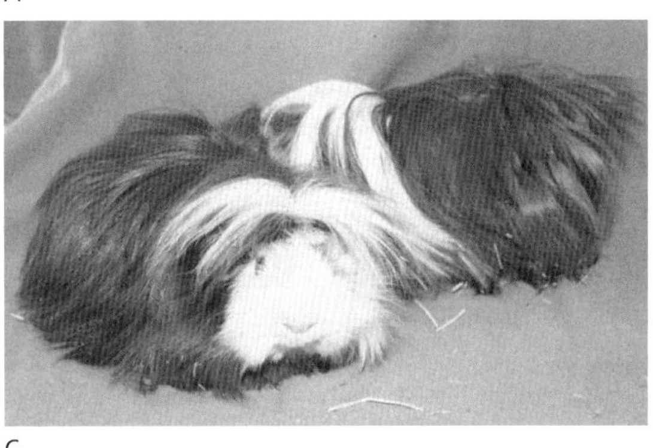

C

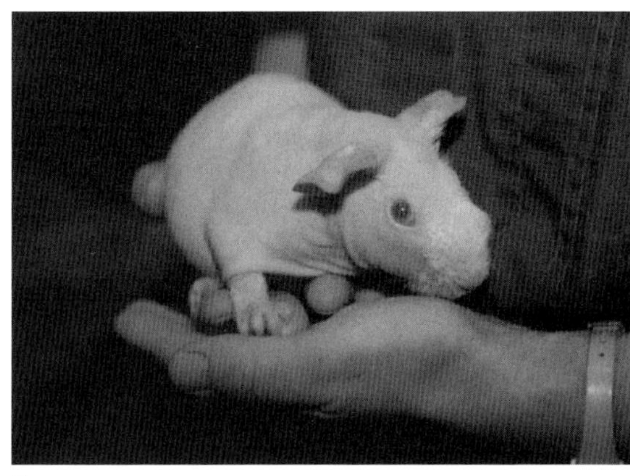

D

FIGURE 2.21. Typical appearance of several guinea pig breeds. A: English short hair*, B: Abyssinian, C: Peruvian*, and D: Skinny pig*. *Courtesy of Ernest D. Olfert.

breeds are the Abyssinian, with short, rough hair arranged in whorls or rosettes, the Silky, which has medium-length, soft hair, and the Peruvian long hair or "rag mop" variety (Figure 2.21). Guinea pigs may be monocolored, bicolored, or tricolored. The varieties interbreed, and a profusion of colors and hair coats is possible, but accurate predictions of coat color inheritance are not. The American Cavy Breeders Association currently recognizes at least 13 different breeds of guinea pig. In addition, two hairless varieties, the Skinny and the Baldwin, which are born with hair but lose it at weaning, have also been developed (see Figure 2.21).

Anatomic and Physiologic Characteristics

Guinea pigs have compact stocky bodies, short legs, round hairless pinnae, and no tails. They have four digits on the front feet and three digits on the hind feet. Their dental formula is 2(I1/1 C0/0 P1/1 M3/3) with a diastema or gap between the incisors and premolar teeth. All teeth are open rooted and grow continuously (hypsodontic). The oral cavity is relatively long and narrow with a small gape, large tongue, and fleshy cheeks that invaginate, making examination and intubation difficult (Figures 2.22–2.24). The soft palate is continuous with the base of the tongue and has a hole in it, the palatal ostium, which connects the oropharynx with the rest of the pharynx.

Guinea pigs are monogastric hindgut fermenters, with a long colon and a very large cecum, which can hold up to 65% of the total gut contents. The stomach is undivided and lined entirely with glandular endothelium. The small intestine lies primarily on the right side of the abdomen, whereas the cecum occupies most of the central and left side of the abdominal cavity. Total gastrointestinal transit time is approxi-

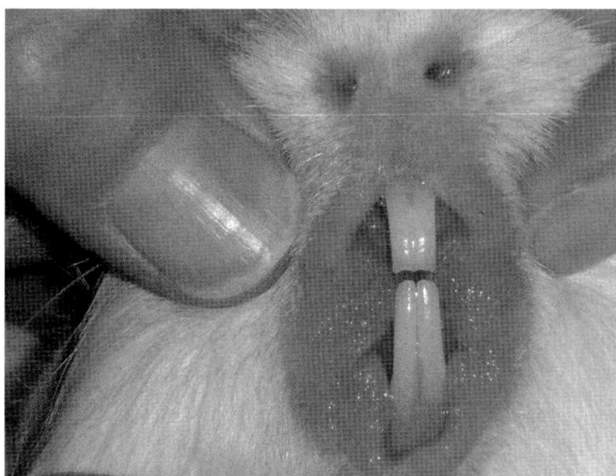

FIGURE 2.22. Normal guinea pig incisors. Note the relative lengths of the maxillary and mandibular incisors and the fleshy cheeks.

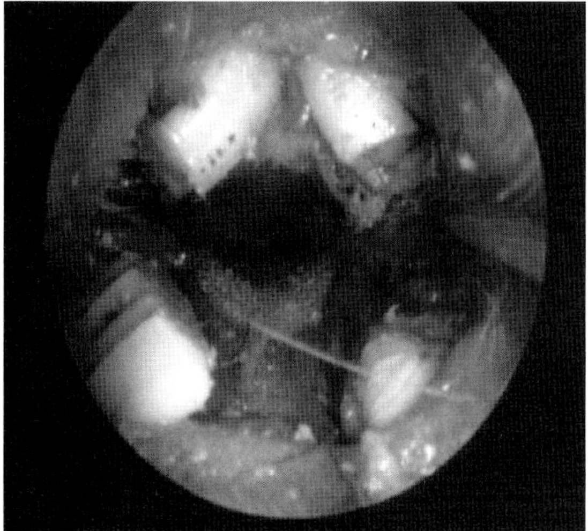

FIGURE 2.23. Normal guinea pig cheek teeth anatomy as visualized with an otoscope. Courtesy of Michael Taylor.

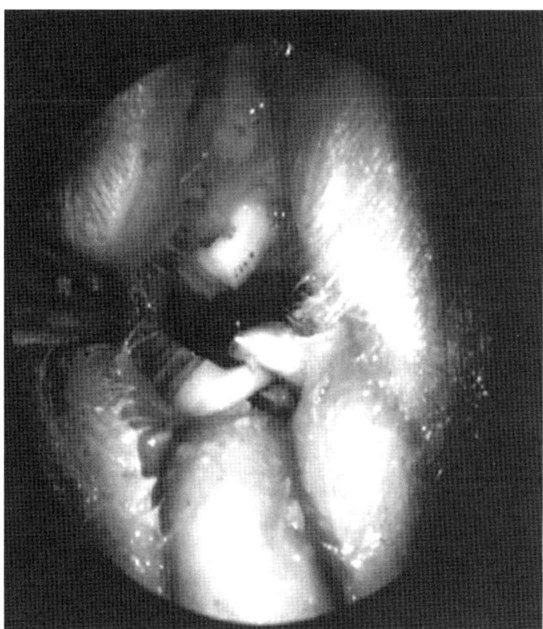

FIGURE 2.24. The lingual side of the lower molars are overgrown in this animal, with entrapment of the tongue. Courtesy of Michael Taylor.

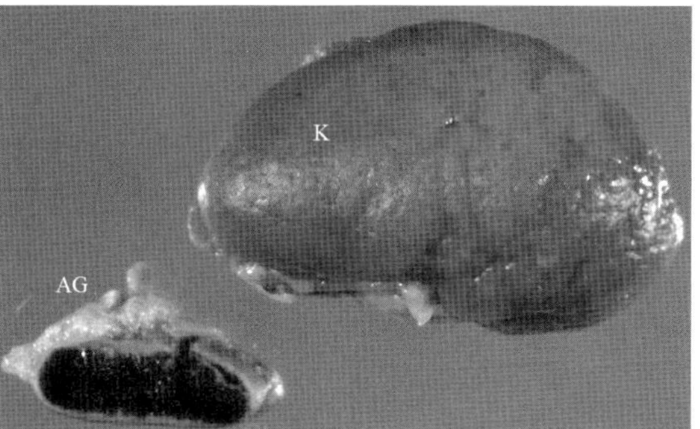

FIGURE 2.25. Adrenal gland (AG) (cut section) and kidney (K) from a guinea pig. The normal guinea pig adrenal gland may be up to one-third the size of the kidneys. Courtesy of Dean H. Percy.

mately 20 hours. Guinea pigs are vigorously coprophagic, with somewhere between 150 and 200 incidences per day. Guinea pigs are prone to potentially lethal dysbiosis following administration of certain antibiotics (see chapter 3).

Guinea pigs have large tympanic bullae, and the cochlea and blood vessels protrude into the cavity of the middle ear, allowing for examination of the microcirculation of the inner ear. They have a well-developed intracoronary collateral network, making it difficult to produce cardiac infarct by acute coronary artery occlusion. They are also noted for their large, bilobed adrenal glands (Figure 2.25). In immature animals, the functional thymus lies subcutaneously, on either side of the trachea, and within the neck, although in some guinea pigs, a portion extends caudally into the precardial mediastinum. The thymus may be located easily and removed, if necessary.

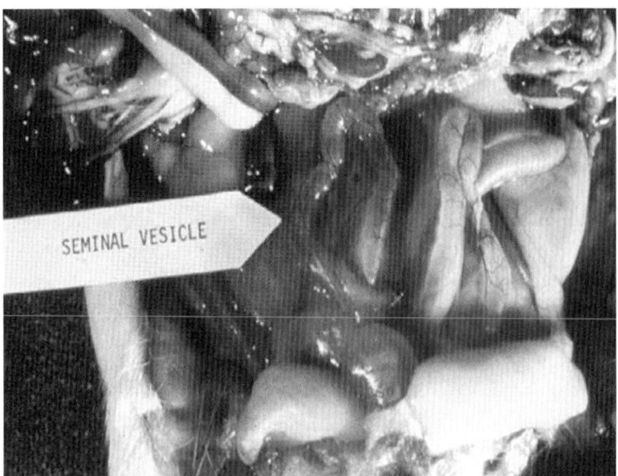

FIGURE 2.26. Seminal vesicles from a mature boar. Courtesy of Dean H. Percy.

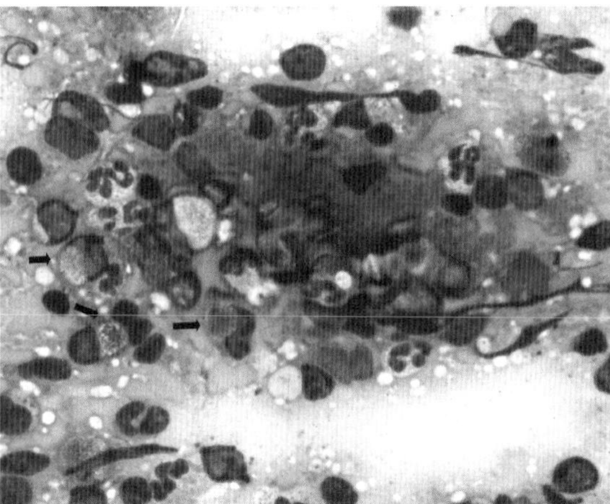

FIGURE 2.27. Kurloff cells (arrows) in a peripheral blood smear from a mature sow. Courtesy of Dean H. Percy.

Both male and female guinea pigs have two inguinal nipples, although sow nipples are longer and more prominent and mammary glands themselves are confined to the sow. Sebaceous glands are located circumanally and on the rump. Guinea pigs often walk or sit with these marking glands pressed against a surface.

The uterine artery provides the major blood supply to the ovary. The large seminal vesicles of the boar are bilateral, smooth, and transparent and extend approximately 10 cm into the abdominal cavity from their base in the accessory sex glands. To a casual observer, these elongated organs resemble a uterus (Figure 2.26).

Guinea pigs exhibit lethal bronchiolar smooth muscle contraction after histamine administration. Mature sows are an excellent source of serum complement, the protein complex involved naturally in immune and endotoxin reactions and used experimentally in serologic testing. Guinea pigs produce antibodies to specific proteins, and induction of anaphylaxis is an indicator of the presence of small amounts of antigen. Unlike the rabbit or chicken, the guinea pig injected with antibodies is protected from anaphylaxis.

Kurloff cells are large, mononuclear, granular lymphocytes, specifically NK effector cells with T-lymphocyte subset markers, and contain large intracytoplasmic inclusions of glycoproteins and acid hydrolases (Figure 2.27). These cells proliferate during estrogenic stimulation and are found in highest numbers in the placenta, where they may function to protect fetal antigens from sensitized maternal lymphocytes and immune globulins. They may also be seen in peripheral blood smears on occasion. Another postulated function is surveillance against leukemic or other neoplastic cells.

Guinea Pigs as Pets

Behavior

Guinea pigs are gentle, docile animals that are relatively easy to maintain. They rarely bite or scratch but when excited will race around their pens, scattering feed and bedding. Guinea pigs seldom climb or jump out of pens with open tops, and a 25 cm (10 inch) barrier will usually confine all but sexually mature males. They respond favorably to frequent handling and readily become conditioned to squeal when they hear the refrigerator door open, in anticipation of a treat. They have a variety of vocalizations that correlate with at least 11 social behaviors, including social interactions (chut or purr call), aversion (chutter and whine), and injury or fear (whistle, squeal, scream). Guinea pigs are excellent swimmers.

Guinea pigs have certain behavioral characteristics that have important implications for both health and husbandry. Guinea pigs, as they mature, develop rigid habits that must be accommodated if the animal

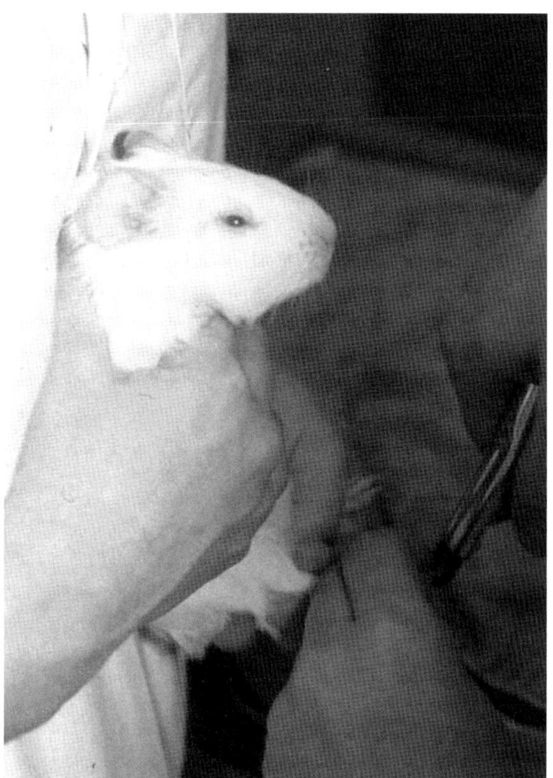

FIGURE 2.28. Guinea pig being restrained in an upright position for a nail trim. Holding the guinea pig against the handler's body increases animal comfort.

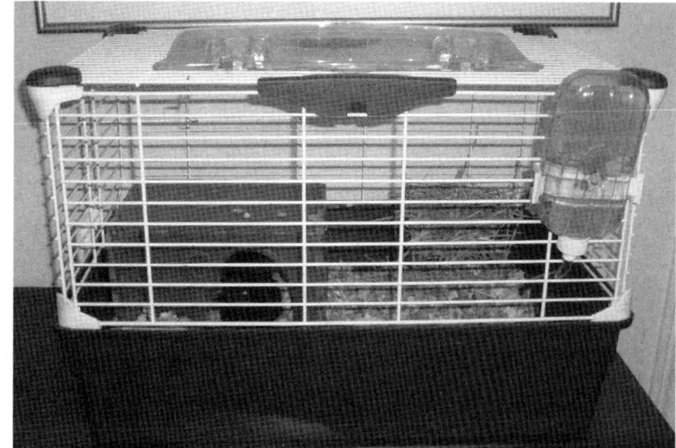

FIGURE 2.29. Typical housing for pet guinea pig. The open plastic-coated wire sides and top permit air circulation within the cage.

is to thrive. Any changes in feed (taste, odor, texture, form), water, feeder, or watering device may cause the guinea pig to stop eating or drinking. This may result in fatal consequences, especially in pregnant females. Excited guinea pigs may stampede or "circle" and either trample the young or fall from the cage. A rectangular cage or barriers within the cage reduce circling, but stampedes still occur.

Guinea pigs establish male-dominated hierarchies, and within these hierarchies subordinate animals are chewed and barbered. Although these hierarchical colony arrangements are usually stable, strange males placed together, especially in crowded conditions or in the presence of a female in estrus, will fight.

Life Span

The breeding life of guinea pigs is from 6 to 8 months to 4 years, and they can live 8 years; however, they rarely survive in a home environment more than 5 years, and their litter size is reduced to 1–2 young per litter by 27–30 months of age.

Restraint

Guinea pigs are lifted by grasping under the trunk with one hand while supporting the rear quarters with the other hand (Figure 2.28). The two-hand support technique is particularly important with adult and pregnant animals. Injured lungs or liver may result from grabbing the animal around the thorax or abdomen without providing additional support. Holding the animal close to the handler's body will increase the animal's sense of security.

Housing

Guinea pigs may be housed individually or in colony pens on the floor, in tiered bins, or in large "shoe box" cages (Figures 2.29–2.31). Young and breeder animals occasionally will climb out of bins even with cage sides of 25 cm (10 in high), and a mesh cage lid should be used to minimize accidents from falls and unplanned breedings. Solid-bottom cages are essential to prevent leg injuries. Adult animals should be provided with at least 652 cm^2 (101 in^2) and breeders with 1,100 cm^2 (180 in^2) of floor space per animal. Beddings of wood shavings, shredded paper, or other material of plant origin may be used; however, cedar dust may cause respiratory problems, and small particles may adhere to the moist genitalia and impede breeding. A hiding area, such as a piece of

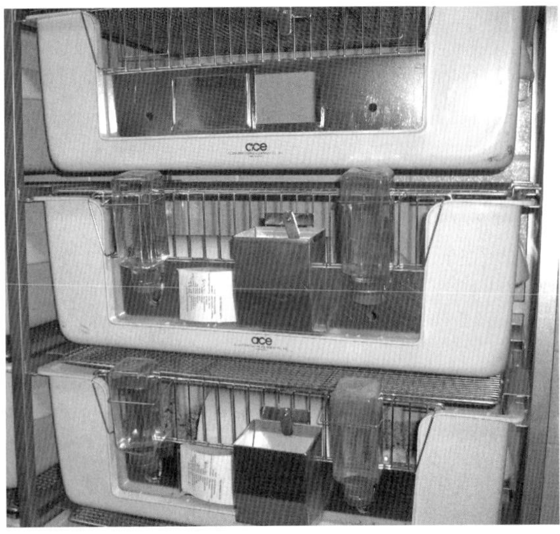
A

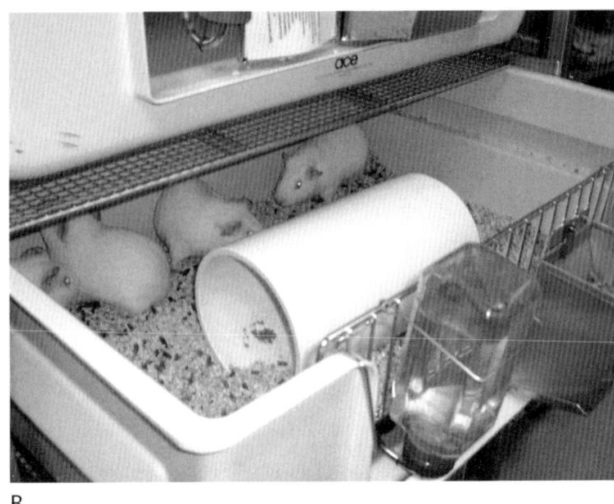
B

FIGURE 2.30. A: Rack-type group housing for laboratory guinea pigs. B: Plastic cage pulled out to demonstrate group-housed animals and tube enrichment.

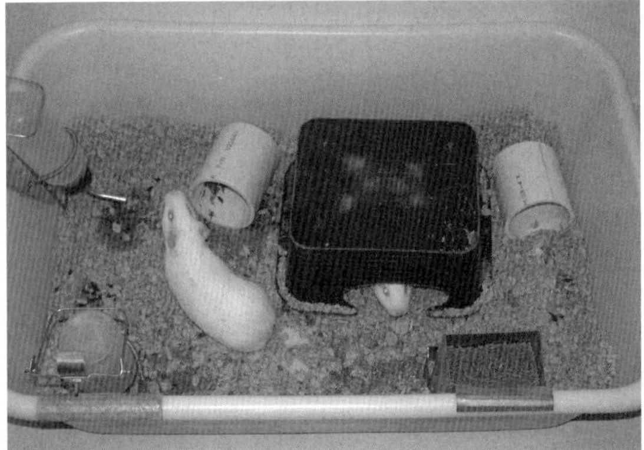

FIGURE 2.31. Typical open-topped guinea pig tub with tubes and hiding place for enrichment.

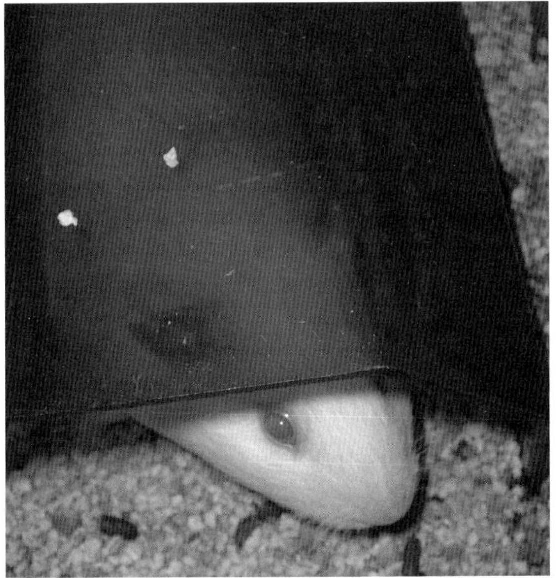

FIGURE 2.32. Male guinea pig using a commercial plastic hut as a hiding place.

large-diameter PVC tube halved longitudinally, or a commercially available house should be provided to allow a sense of security (Figure 2.32). The cage should be placed in a quiet place, out of direct sunlight, and where the ambient environment is stable.

Guinea pigs are housed at temperatures between 18° and 26°C (65–79°F), with an optimal ambient temperature at 21°C (70°F). Lower temperatures may decrease the survival rate of newborns. High ambient temperatures without adequate air flow predispose to sterility and heat stress; low temperatures and wet bedding predispose to respiratory disease. The environmental humidity should be between 40% and 70%. A 12:12 hour light:dark cycle is used commonly with 10–15 air changes per hour. Covered aquaria may not allow adequate ventilation. Guinea pigs are messy pets, scattering bedding and food; and their urine is opaque, creamy yellow, and contains crystals. Cages, pens, and feeding receptacles should be cleaned and sanitized at least once weekly. Satisfactory cleaning procedures include washing the cages with a detergent and hot water or with a disinfectant solution followed by a thorough rinse. A weakly acidic solution may be needed to remove the urine scale.

Feeding and Watering

Guinea pigs are strict herbivores and are cecal fermenters, as are horses and rabbits. Unlike rabbits, however, guinea pigs possess endogenous lactobacilli and produce propionic acid as the primary fatty acid. Food intake is controlled not by calories ingested but by bulk consumed. They require specific amounts of calcium, phosphorus, magnesium, and potassium, and regular feeding of table scraps, vitamin D–fortified cow's milk, or other animal feed is not recommended, as it may promote metastatic calcification, acidosis, ketosis, or skin disease from vitamin A or D toxicity. Deficiencies of vitamin A or tryptophan may lead to corneal lesions, and vitamin E deficiency leads to a muscular dystrophy. As described below, vitamin C deficiency is a major concern in guinea pigs, as they are unable to endogenously synthesize this nutrient.

Feeders and waterers should be suspended above the cage floor to prevent contamination with feces and bedding. Guinea pigs learn readily to drink from suspended water bottles with sipper tubes or valves, but they are notorious for chewing on and playing with these devices. They often mix dry feed with water in their mouths and pass the slurry into the sipper tube, causing it to become blocked, or to drip and empty the bottle, leaving wet bedding and no access to water. Automatic watering valves that are located outside the cage or other devices that divert spilled or leaked water to the outside of the cage are preferred. A further advantage of automatic waterers is that they ensure a continual supply of water. Automatic waterers must be checked frequently and cleaned and flushed periodically. Animals reared with water supplied in bowls or crocks may become dehydrated before finding water when it is provided by unfamiliar sipper tubes or the nipple valves of automatic watering systems.

Though herbivores, guinea pigs are fastidious eaters and may refuse to eat or drink if the feed or feeders are changed. They should receive a freshly milled, properly stored, pelleted, complete guinea pig diet, usually with hay supplementation. Such supplementation may improve production and growth and decrease obesity and dental disease, although pathogenic microorganisms may be introduced on hay or greens if they are contaminated. Adult guinea pigs will consume approximately 6 g of feed and 10–40 mL of water per 100 g body weight daily; these amounts, however, vary with ambient temperature, breeding status, food and water wastage, and relative humidity. Guinea pig chows are provided as small pellets that contain approximately 18–20% crude protein and 10–16% fiber. Large amounts of feed wastage are associated with wire-floor cages or use of feeders without inside lips. Small amounts of carrots, fresh fruits, and well-washed fresh leafy greens may be given to guinea pigs as treats but should not form more than 10% of the daily intake.

Guinea pigs, like humans and primates, lack the enzyme L-gulonolactone oxidase in the glucose-to-vitamin C pathway. Vitamin C is required for cross-linking lysine and proline in collagen fibers, necessary for forming strong bones and blood vessels. Vitamin C is water soluble and is not stored in the body, making daily supplementation essential for good health. Guinea pigs have an absolute daily requirement of ascorbic acid of 10–25 mg/kg for maintenance and up to 30 mg/kg daily for pregnancy, although 2 mg per day may prevent signs of scurvy. If ascorbic acid is not supplied in the feed, it can be added to the water (1 g/L), provided in tablet form (Oxbow, GTN-50C, 50 mg apple-flavored tablets) (Figure 2.33), or each guinea pig may be fed daily approximately one small handful or less of kale, parsley, beet greens, kiwi fruit, broccoli, orange, or cabbage. Even wood chips or shavings may contain small amounts of vitamin C. Carrots and lettuce are not good sources of vitamin C, and cabbage may contain goitrogens. The activity of vitamin C decreases as much as 50% in a 24-hour period in water in an open crock and even faster if metal or organic material is present or if the room temperature

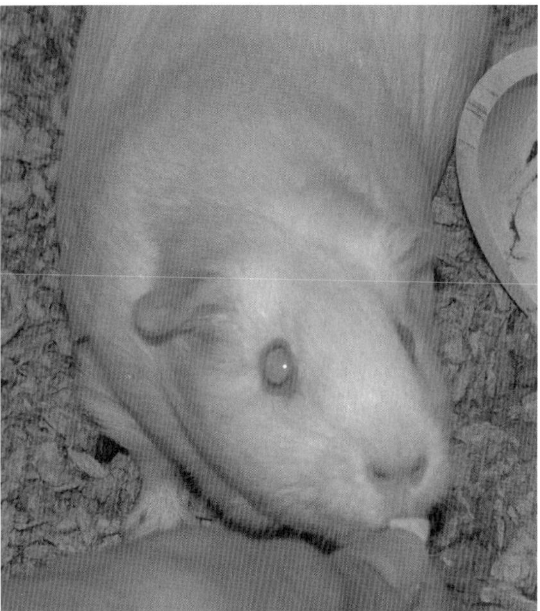

FIGURE 2.33. Guinea pig taking an orange-flavored vitamin C tablet. Once accustomed to the taste, guinea pigs consider these tablets a treat.

is elevated. Feed containing ascorbic acid should be stored properly (cool and dry) and used within 90–180 days of milling, depending on the manufacturer's instructions.

Guinea pigs should not be fed diets indicated for other species. Most pet store feeds for other rodents also have label indications for guinea pigs, which in most cases is misleading and inappropriate in that they have not been formulated taking into account the special nutritional requirements of guinea pigs. Rabbit food, for example, contains no ascorbic acid, and for guinea pigs, excess levels of vitamin D. Also, guinea pigs have higher requirements for folic acid than do rabbits or other rodents.

Reproduction

Sexing and Anatomy

Male guinea pigs (boars) are distinguished from females (sows) by their larger body size, smaller nipples, and a penis that can easily be extruded from the circular prepuce, revealing two prongs at its tip (Figure 2.34). The inguinal canals remain open throughout life, and the large 5–6 g testicles can either be withdrawn into the abdomen, or be present in scrotal swellings lateral to the anogenital line. The penis has a baculum (os penis), and accessory sex glands include long, smooth seminal vesicles (which may be mistaken by the inexperienced for a uterus), prostate, coagulating and bulbourethal glands, and vestiges of preputial glands. Mounting begins around 1 month of age, and ejaculations occur around 2 months. Boars can reach puberty at 8 weeks, but 9–10 weeks is a more realistic average.

The sow has a Y-shaped anogenital opening, with the branches of the Y representing the urogenital opening, which is usually sealed with a vaginal

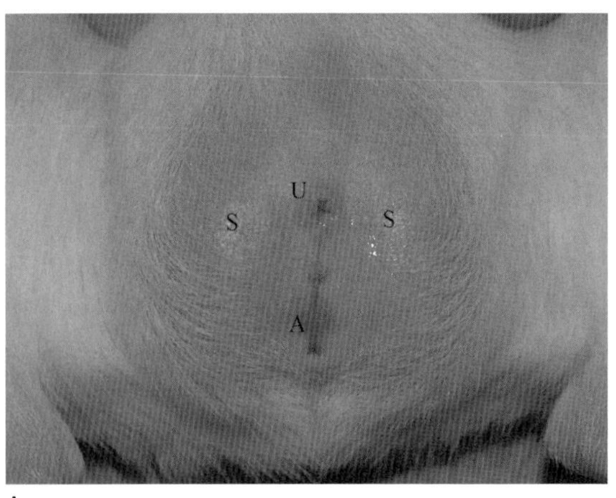

A

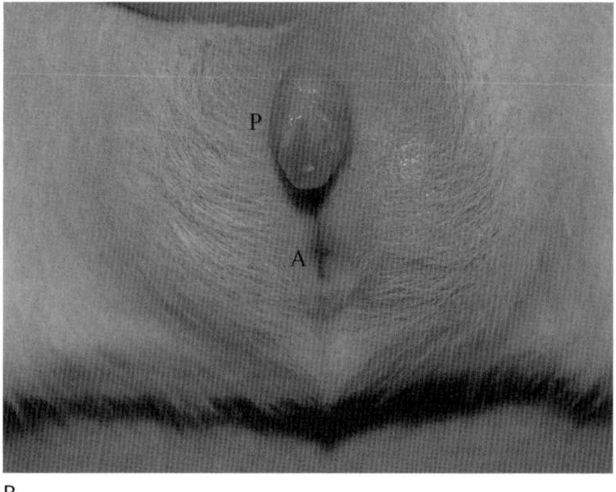

B

FIGURE 2.34. A: Male genitalia of guinea pig with penis in prepuce (U: urethral opening, A: anus, S: scrotal sac). B: External genitalia of male guinea pig with penis extruded by digital pressure (P: penis, A: anus).

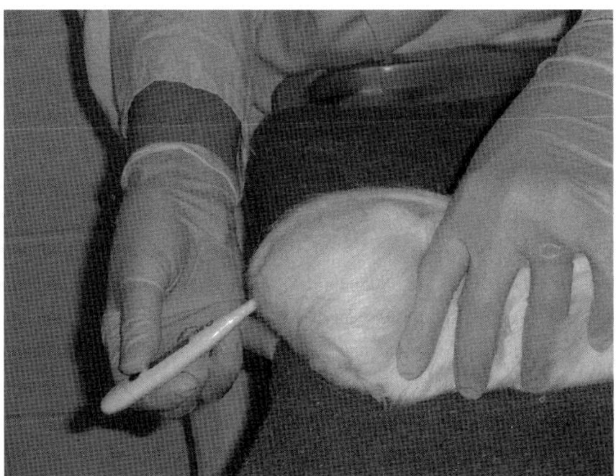

FIGURE 2.35. The anus of the guinea pig is difficult to visualize in a conscious animal. A rectal temperature may be obtained by positioning the hind end of the animal at the edge of the exam table and inserting the thermometer at an angle.

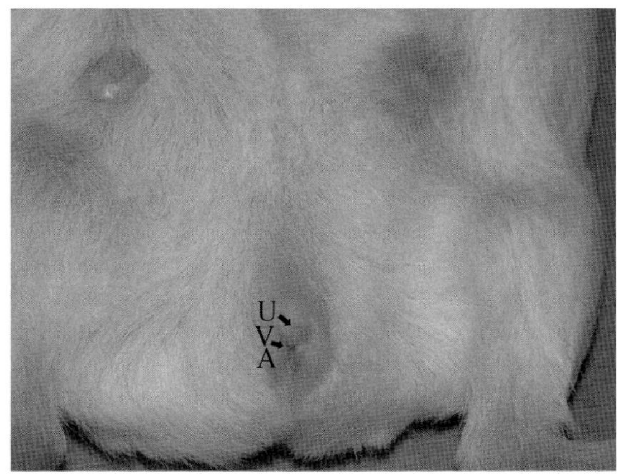

FIGURE 2.36. Female genitalia of a mature sow during estrous phase (V: vaginal opening, U: urethral opening, A: anus). The urethra opens directly to the outside via a small papilla ventral to the vaginal orifice rather than into the vestibule of the vagina, as in many other mammals. The two inguinal nipples are readily apparent.

closure membrane (Figures 2.35–2.37). The uterus is bicornate, with a single cervix.

Estrous Cycle

Sows reach puberty as early as 5–6 weeks of age. The estrous cycle lasts 15–17 days. During estrus the sow exhibits lordosis and mounts other sows. The estrous period itself lasts approximately 24–48 hours

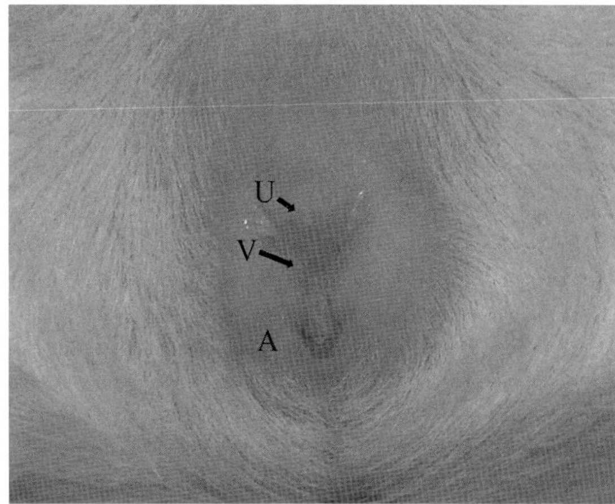

FIGURE 2.37. External genitalia of female guinea pig (V: vaginal opening, U: urethral opening, A: anus). In this animal, the genital opening is sealed with a vaginal closure membrane.

during which the intact vaginal closure membrane perforates. The female accepts the male for 6–11 hours. If timed pregnancies are desired, mating can be detected by observation of the perforated vaginal membrane, presence of a vaginal plug, which remains in the vaginal opening for several hours, or sperm in a vaginal smear. Most sows have an estrus 2–15 hours postpartum, at which time 60–80% will become pregnant if mated.

Breeding Programs

Females should weigh approximately 400 g (2–3 months of age) and the male 650 g (3–4 months of age) before breeding. One boar is housed in an adequate-sized solid-bottom pen (1,100 cm^2 per animal) with 1–10 sows. Size requirements of the pen will limit the number of females housed with a boar. In intensive harem-style breeding systems, which use the postpartum estrus, the sows and boar remain together for their entire breeding life (approximately 18 months), and the young are removed at weaning. In this "continuous" system, a sow may produce up to 5 litters (12 young) per year. In a nonintensive system, the sows are removed for delivery and are rebred after weaning (3.5 litters or 9 young per year). In the discontinuous system, remating occurs only after weaning. Another variation is to return the sow alone to the harem for 6–12 hours to permit postpartum breeding. The sow is then returned to her young. Litter intervals in guinea pig colonies range from 80 to 96 days, and 0.7–1.4 young are born per sow per month. In commercial colonies, breeders are retained for approximately 18 months, and pets may reproduce for up to 3 years.

A receptive sow prowls and runs about the cage, mounts other sows, and assumes lordosis, which can also be elicited if the rump is stroked. After one or two intromissions, mating ceases and the copulatory plug remains in the vaginal opening for several hours. Two-thirds or more of matings are fertile, and implantation occurs in 1 week. Progesterone from the corpora lutea continues for 3 weeks, then placental hormones maintain pregnancy. Artificial insemination is not a practical technique for guinea pig breeding. The placenta is hemomonochorionic, and trophoblasts are in contact with maternal blood. During the 59- to 72-day pregnancy (average 68), the normal 2 g uterus increases to 300 g, and up to one-third total maternal weight is due to fetuses (Figure 2.38). Fetal masses are palpable at 15 days to term. Animals to be palpated are food restricted for 8 hours, and the handler places a thumb on the iliac crest and the first two fingers on the ventral midline. The abdominal cavity is then palpated on one side and then the other as the hand moves anteriorly. Fetal skeletons can be seen radiographically at 6 weeks of age (Figure 2.39).

The fibrocartilaginous pubic symphysis, under the influence of the hormone relaxin, begins to separate during the latter half of gestation and continues parting until, at 48 hours prepartum, a palpable gap of around 15 mm is present. At parturition, this opening may reach 2.5 cm or more (approximately 1–1.5 in). If the first breeding is delayed past 8–10 months, the symphysis separates less easily, and fat pads occlude the pelvic canal. Such impediments may lead to dystocia, especially when small litters of large young are involved. Caesarean section, digital manipulation, or oxytocin carefully delivered at 1–3 units/kg may be needed to ensure delivery or death may result.

A normal delivery period occurs over a half-hour period, with several minutes between births. First litters are smaller. Guinea pig young are born fully furred with eyes open and teeth erupted, and within a few hours they are walking unsteadily and eating and drinking from pans (Figure 2.40). Food preferences are established and imprinted within a few days of birth. Pregnant sows may be separated or remain together, although in harems one sow's milk may be stripped by the larger young of other sows. Sows do not build nests.

Caesarean derivation is relatively easy to accomplish with late-term guinea pigs. Neonates are precocious, nearly self-sufficient, and require little hand

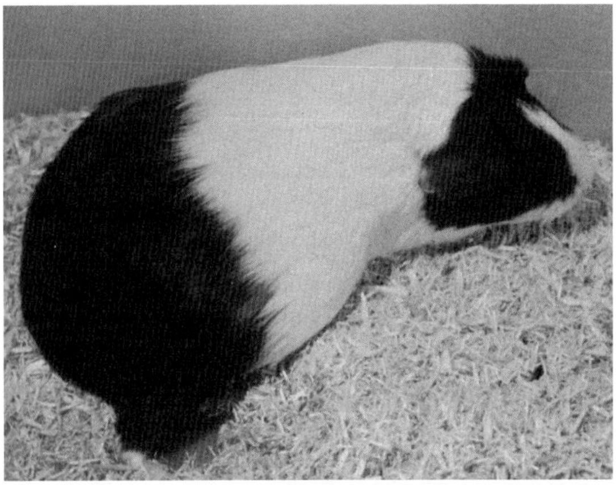

FIGURE 2.38. Pregnant sow shortly before parturition. The sow's abdomen is markedly distended with pups. Courtesy of Dale Smith.

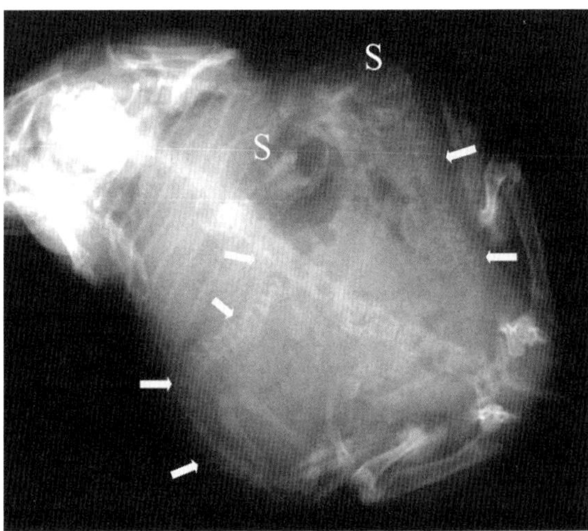

FIGURE 2.39. Radiograph of a pregnant sow with two pups. The skulls (S) and vertebral columns of the pups are clearly visible (arrows).

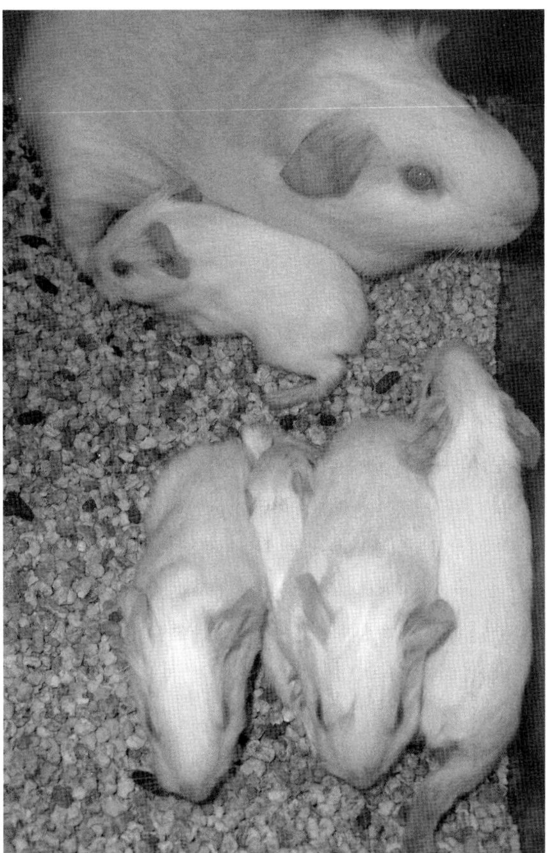

FIGURE 2.40. Five neonatal guinea pig pups within hours of birth. Pups are precocious at birth and are fully furred with open ears and eyes.

rearing if removed from the dam at birth. Although the young can eat or lap food from small bowls, bottle feeding for several days may be advantageous. The pup receives all its maternal antibody from the placenta.

Hand rearing requires regular stimulation of defecation and urination and the provision of a heat source for approximately a week. Additionally, females allow young other than their own to nurse; thus, foster nursing can be used to establish specific pathogen free colonies.

Endocrine control of gestation in the guinea pig is similar to that in the horse, monkey, and human in that the gestation period may be divided into trimesters of approximately 3 weeks. In many instances, pregnancy is maintained after ovariectomy at 25 or more days. The guinea pig has been used to study the effects of hormones and endocrine glands on pregnancy. Despite having only two nipples, guinea pigs can raise litters of 3, 4, and more young.

Neonatal Life

Young are cleaned, and the placenta is eaten, but dead (or live) fetuses rarely are attacked. The pubic symphysis closes within 24 hours. Two or three young weighing 70–100 g each are born (range: 1–6), and young weighing 60 g or less seldom survive. The young may be trampled if the adults are crowded or become excited. If the sow abandons the young before they are a week old, or if the young are weaned early, mortality may be high. Problems with ear chewing and trampling are reduced if the young and sow are removed to a nursery before or soon after birth.

Because the young will begin eating solid food during the first few days postpartum, hand rearing is not as difficult as with the altricial species, for example, rats, mice, and rabbits. One should not attempt to force-feed newborn orphaned guinea pigs during the first few hours of life, because the neonates will not be hungry until 12–24 hours of age. Young guinea pigs can attach to nipples on day 1, and during the first week more time is spent nursing in the light. The sow remains immobile during the first few minutes of nursing. Auditory signals and other cues may elicit licking by the sow. During the first few days, neonates may be fed guinea pig chow softened with water or cow's milk. Young that do not receive sow's milk during the first 3–4 days of life often do not survive. If given the opportunity, the young will nurse mothers other than their own, often to the detriment of their smaller cage mates. Milk supply does not increase with demand. Neonates imprint with specific feeds within a few days, and this impression of what is food and what is not food persists stubbornly into adulthood.

Guinea pig milk contains approximately 4% fat, 8% protein, and 3% lactose. Milk production peaks to 65 mL/kg BW/day between days 5 and 8, then ceases at approximately 18–30 days, and the young are weaned at 14–28 days or between 150 and 200 g. Males make better breeders as adults if they remain to at least 30 days of age with siblings and sow.

Disease Prevention

The general husbandry and disease prevention admonitions listed in chapter 1 should be followed for guinea pigs. Guinea pigs scatter their bedding into feeders and crocks, are susceptible to *Bordetella bronchiseptica* pneumonia, have an absolute requirement for dietary ascorbic acid, and are fastidious eaters. If the food is changed, guinea pigs may refuse to eat. Because of *Bordetella* spp susceptibility, guinea pigs should not be housed with rabbits, cats, dogs, and other species that carry this organism.

Public Health Concerns

Diseases of public health significance in guinea pigs are rare. Guinea pigs may carry bacteria (*Bordetella* spp, *Salmonella* spp, *Yersinia pseudotuberculosis, Streptococcus* spp) that are potential human pathogens, but transfer of these infections to humans would be most unusual. Allergies to guinea pig dander and proteins are common, and commercial shampoo preparations intended to remove antigens from animal fur may reduce human allergic exposures. The guinea pig sarcoptic mite can cause dermatitis in people, but this is uncommon.

Uses in Research

Approximately 207,000 guinea pigs are used annually in research in the United States and approximately 29,000 are used annually in Canada. Guinea pigs are used in studies that involve anaphylaxis, delayed hypersensitivity, genetics, ketoacidosis, several aspects of nutrition, optic neuropathies, amoebiasis, scurvy, leukemia, allergic encephalomyelitis, ulcerative colitis, immunology, auditory function, and infectious diseases including tuberculosis. Complement commonly obtained from guinea pig serum is used in complement fixation tests to diagnose infectious diseases. Various biochemical and pharmacologic tests are also conducted commonly in guinea pigs.

Table 2.3 Biodata: guinea pigs.

Adult body weight: male	900–1200 g
Adult body weight: female	700–900 g
Birth weight	70–100 g
Body surface area (cm^2)	
700–830 g	9.2 × (weight in grams)$^{2/3}$
200–680 g	10.1 × (weight in grams)$^{2/3}$
Body temperature	37.2–39.5 °C (99–103.1 °F)
Diploid number	64
Life span	5–7 yr
Food consumption	6 g/100 g/day
Water consumption	10–40 mL/100 g/day
GI transit time	13–30 hr
Breeding onset: male	600–700 g (3–4 mo)
Breeding onset: female	350–450 g (2–3 mo)
Cycle length	15–17 days
Gestation period	59–72 days
Postpartum estrus	fertile, 60–80% pregnancy
Litter size	1–6
Weaning age (lactation duration)	150–200 g 14–21 days
Breeding duration	18 mo (4–5 litters) to 4 years
Young production (index/female)	0.7–1.4/mo
Milk composition	3.9% fat, 8.1 % protein, 3.0% lactose

Biodata

The values listed in Table 2.3 are approximations only and may not represent the normal range in a given guinea pig population. Sources consulted are included among the comprehensive texts listed in chapter 1 and in the publications listed under "Sources of Information."

References

Comprehensive works on the guinea pig include Wagner JE, Manning PJ (eds.). The Biology of the Guinea Pig. New York: Academic Press, 1976; Poole TB (ed.). The UFAW Handbook on the Care and Management of Laboratory Animals, 7th ed., vol. 1. Ames, IA: Blackwell, 1999; Rowsell HC, et al. (eds.). The Guide to the Care and Use of Experimental Animals, vol. 2. Ottawa, ON: Canadian Council on Animal Care, 1984; and Richardson VC. Diseases of Domestic Guinea Pigs. Cambridge, MA: Blackwell Sciences, 1992.

Other References on Guinea Pigs

Beck W, Pantchev N. Trixacarus caviae as a cause of mange in the guinea pig and pseudoscabies in a human being—a case report. Kleintierpraxis. 2008, 53(7):424–430.

Berryman JC. Guinea-pig vocalizations: their structure, causation and function. Zeitschrift fur Tierpsychologie. 1976, 41:80–106.

Bleier R. The Hypothalamus of the Guinea Pig: A Cytoarchitectronic Atlas. Madison: University of Wisconsin Press, 1984.

Bradley Bays T. Guinea Pig Behavior. In: Exotic Pet Behavior. Bradley Bays T, Lightfoot T, Mayer J (eds.). St. Louis: Saunders Elsevier, 2006.

Cooper G, Schiller AL. Anatomy of the Guinea Pig. Cambridge, MA: Harvard University Press, 1975.

Debout C, et al. In vitro cytotoxic effect of guinea pig natural killer cells (Kurloff cells) on homologous leukemic cells (L2C). Leuk. 1993, 7:733–735.

Dunham WB, Young M, Tsao CS. Interference by bedding materials in animal test systems involving ascorbic acid depletion. Lab Anim Sci. 1994, 44(3):283–285.

Ebino KY. Studies on coprophagy in experimental animals. Exp Anim. 1992, 42(1):1–9.

Eveleigh JR. The breeding performance of the Pinbright Dunkin-Hartley guinea pig after discontinuing the feeding of green food as a supplement, with particular reference to productivity. Lab Anim. 1980, 14:55–57.

Force E, et al. Experimental study of meropenem in the therapy of cephalosporin-susceptible and -resistant pneumococcal meningitis. Eur J of Clin Microbiol Infect Dis. 2008, 27(8):685–690.

Gurney P. The Proper Care of Guinea Pigs. Neptune, NJ: T.F.H. Publications, 1999.

Harkness JE, Murray KA, Wagner JE. Biology and Diseases of Guinea Pigs. In: Laboratory Animal Medicine, 2nd ed. Fox JG, Anderson LC, Loew FM, Quimby FW (eds.). San Diego: Academic Press, 2002.

Hennessey MB, Jenkins R. A descriptive analysis of nursing behavior in the guinea pig (Cavia porcellus). J Comp Psychol. 1994, 108(1):23–28.

Hrapkiewicz K, Medina L. Clinical Laboratory Animal Medicine: An Introduction, 3rd ed. Ames, IA: Blackwell, 2007.

Huerkamp MJ, et al. Guinea Pigs. In: Handbook of Rodent and Rabbit Medicine. Laber-Laird K, Swindle M, Flecknell P (eds.). Oxford: Elsevier Science, 1996.

Jilge B. The gastrointestinal transit time in the guinea-pig. Zeitschrift fur Versuchstierkunde. 1980, 22(4):204–210.

Lin CT. Body surface areas and K values in strain 13 guinea pigs with different body weights and ages. Proc Soc Exper Biol Med. 1988, 189:285–290.

Matthews PJ, Jackson J. Pregnancy diagnosis in the guinea pig. Lab Anim Sci. 1977, 27:248–250.

Quesenberry K, Donnelly TM, Hillyer EV. Biology, Husbandry, and Clinical Techniques of Guinea Pigs and Chinchillas. In: Ferrets, Rabbits, and Rodents: Clinical Medicine and Surgery, 2nd ed. Quesenberry K, Carpenter JW (eds.). St. Louis: Saunders, 2004.

Quijandria B, de Zaldivar LC, Robison OW. Selection in guinea pigs: I. Estimation of phenotypic and genetic parameters for litter size and body weight. J Anim Sci. 1983, 56(4):814–819.

Saunte D, et al. Experimental guinea pig model of dermatophytosis: a simple and useful tool for the evaluation of new diagnostics and antifungals. Med Mycol. 2008, 46(4):303–313.

Vanderlip S. The Guinea Pig Handbook. Hauppauge, NY: Barron's, 2003.

Wolf B, et al. Taxonomical classification of the guinea pig based on its Cu/Zn superoxide dismutase sequence. Biol Chem Hoppe-Seyler. 1993, 374(8):641–649.

Websites for Guinea Pigs

http://www.oxbowanimalhealth.com/pet_care—Oxbow.

www.acbaonline.com—American Cavy Breeders Association.

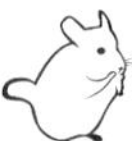

THE CHINCHILLA

Chinchillas are noted for their soft, luxurious fur, long gestation period, precocious young, and long life span. They are raised in captivity for the fur trade, as pets, and for research. Their relatively large tympanic bullae make them a useful animal model for auditory research. Chinchillas require a daily dust bath to maintain the integrity of their coat, which has approximately 60 hairs per follicle.

Origin and Description

Chinchillas are classified as caviomorph (New World hystricognath) rodents and are related to guinea pigs and degus. There are two recognized species of chinchilla: *Chinchilla brevicaudata* (short-tailed chinchilla) and *Chinchilla lanigera* (long-tailed chinchilla). *Chinchilla brevicaudata* is listed as critically endangered by the International Union for Conservation of Nature, having been hunted almost to extinction for its fur. *Chinchilla lanigera,* the species kept in captivity, is listed as vulnerable. These gregarious, nocturnal rodents are native to the dry, cool Andes Mountains of South America, and live in large colonies inhabiting burrows or rocky crevices at elevations of 3,000–5,000 m. Their natural diet is high in fiber and low in energy, consisting of grasses, cactus fruit, leaves, bark, and the occasional insect.

Anatomic and Physiologic Characteristics

Domesticated *C. lanigera* are larger than their wild counterparts, with skulls 16% longer and 6% wider, on average. Selective breeding has resulted in a variety of coat colors, including shades of black, white, beige, and blue, in addition to the wild-type gray. Some coat colors, such as white, are lethal in the homozygous state. *Chinchilla lanigera* has a large bushy tail, large head, short forelimbs, and long muscular hindlimbs. Their eyes have large corneas and a dark iris with a vertical pupillary slit. They use their long whiskers to navigate in the dark. Their large, round ears are thin-walled, and the tympanic bullae are remarkably large. Not surprisingly, chinchillas are sensitive to noise and startle easily. The dental formula is 2(I1/1 C0/0 P1/1 M3/3) and all teeth are open rooted and grow continuously, the incisors growing 4–6 cm per year (Figure 2.41). The oral cavity is narrow and the soft palate is continuous with the base of the tongue and has a hole in it leading to the rostral passage, the palatal ostium. They have four toes on the front and hind feet, each with a small claw. The gastrointestinal tract is long, with a large cecum, highly sacculated proximal colon, and smooth terminal colon. Transit time is 12–15 hours. Chinchillas have three pairs of mammary glands—one inguinal and two lateral thoracic. The thymus is located entirely within the thorax. A right coronary artery is absent.

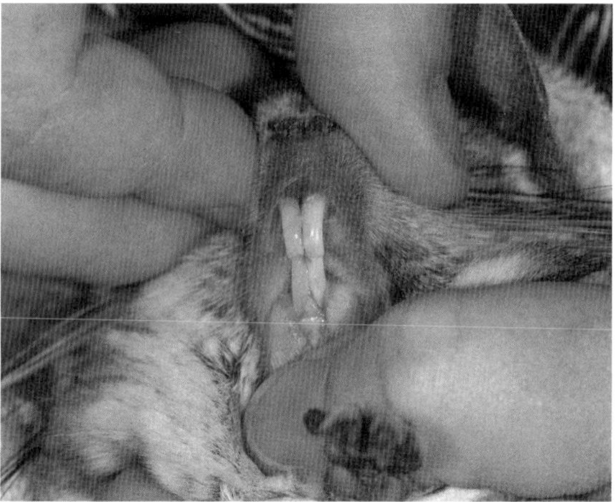

FIGURE 2.41. Normal chinchilla incisors. Note the relative lengths of the maxillary and mandibular incisors and the fleshy cheeks. Courtesy of Glen and Rebecca Grambo.

Chinchillas as Pets

Behavior

In 2000, an estimated 80,000 chinchillas were kept as household pets in the United States. Chinchillas are primarily nocturnal in the wild, but are often active during the day in captivity. They have a friendly, appealing, inquisitive nature and are not naturally aggressive toward humans. Chinchillas are odorless, quiet, and easy to maintain, provided they are fed and housed correctly. They enjoy being petted and cuddled if they are acclimated to gentle handling. Chinchillas may become stressed by loud noises and activity and should be kept in a quiet, cool area of the house. As social animals, they should be housed in same-sex pairs or groups, or if housed individually, given ample human interaction. Chinchillas are less vocal than guinea pigs and their normal communication is a soft, high-pitched grunting sound. They can also bark when angry or defensive and occasionally make a honking noise for attention. If they sense danger they will stand on their hind legs and make a warning whistle sound. Chinchillas often exercise outside their cage and are good climbers and jumpers, often banking off walls and furniture. They require safe items to chew as they are curious and will chew furnishings and cords. Chinchillas can be territorial and may aggressively defend their cage by standing and spraying urine in an upward stream toward the perceived intruder.

Life Span

The breeding life of a chinchilla lasts approximately 3 years, and their average life span is 10 years, although they can live to be 18 years of age or older and are used as a research model for longevity.

Restraint

Chinchillas can be removed from their cage by firmly grasping the base of the tail and lifting while supporting the body with the other hand. They should never be picked up by the tail alone. Alternatively, very tame animals can be gently grasped around the thorax, while supporting the hind end with the other hand (Figure 2.42). Excessive chasing around the cage, improper restraint, or even bumping into the cage may cause a phenomenon known as fur slip, where a clump of fur is released, leaving behind a patch of smooth, clean skin. Fur slip is a protective mechanism used to evade predators in the wild caused by simultaneous release of hair shafts from the follicles as a result of the "fight or flight" response. Hair regrowth following fur slip or clipping can take several months and the hair will often grow back a slightly different color.

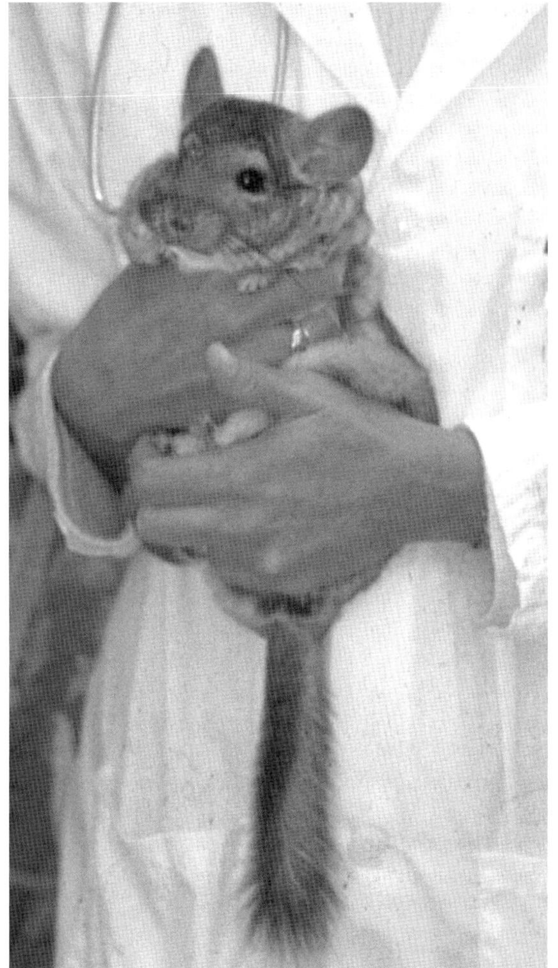

FIGURE 2.42. Two-handed restraint for a chinchilla.

Housing

Chinchillas are housed in metal or plastic solid-bottom cages. Mesh should be avoided to reduce the incidence of limb injuries, especially in young. Recycled paper products or softwood shavings may be used as bedding; however, resinous softwood or treated wood products have been associated with toxicities and should be avoided. Multilevel cages provide environmental enrichment, as the animals will move actively between the various levels (see Figures 2.43 through 2.46). Chinchillas require a dry, draft-free environment, with a temperature range between 16° and 21°C (61–70°F). They are very prone to heat stress and can die if temperatures exceed 32°C, but they can withstand temperatures of 0°C if allowed to become cold adapted. Cold temperatures stimulate production of the thick hair coat desirable for the fur trade.

A dust bath composed of nine parts silver sand and one part fuller's earth should be offered in a shallow pan at a depth of 4–6 cm for about 10 minutes

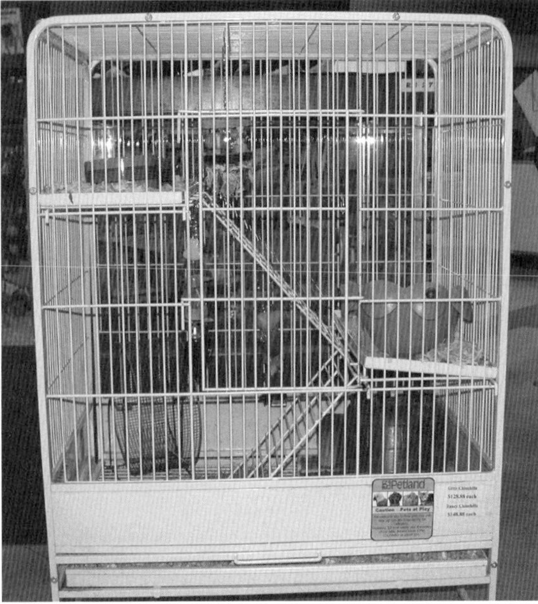

FIGURE 2.43. Typical plastic-coated wire multilevel cage for pet chinchilla.

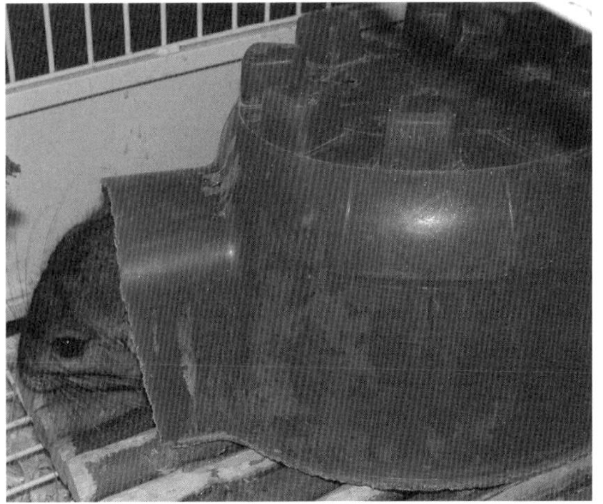

FIGURE 2.44. Igloo shelter enrichment for chinchilla.

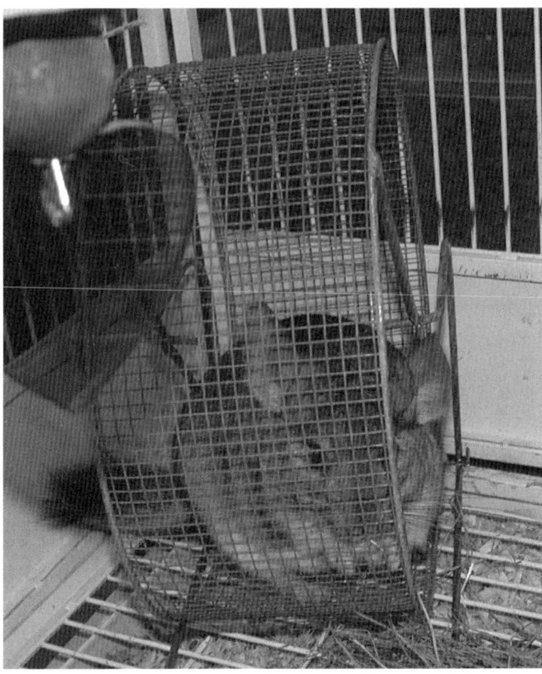

FIGURE 2.45. Running wheel for chinchilla.

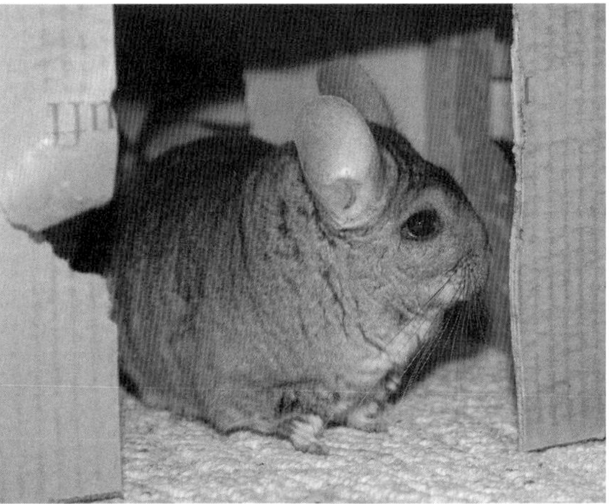

FIGURE 2.46. Cardboard box enrichment for chinchilla. Courtesy of Glen and Rebecca Grambo.

each day to prevent the fur becoming matted with oily secretions (Figure 2.47). Unlimited access to dust baths can result in dry skin and conjunctivitis. Dust baths should be withheld from near-term females and mothers with litters, as the dust may contribute to mastitis and uterine infection or get in the mouth and eyes of the young.

Chinchillas tend to choose one corner of the cage for urination, but will defecate anywhere. The fecal pellets have very little odor, and are normally well formed, dry, and easy to clean up. A light cycle of 12:12 hour light:dark with 10–15 air changes per hour is appropriate. Humidity should be kept between 30% and 60%. Cages and feeding receptacles should

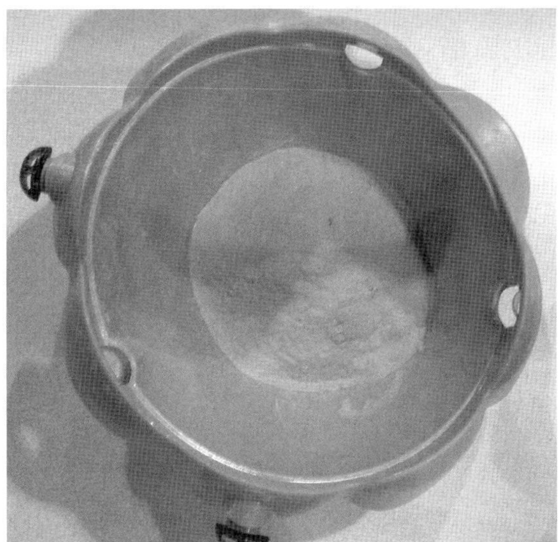

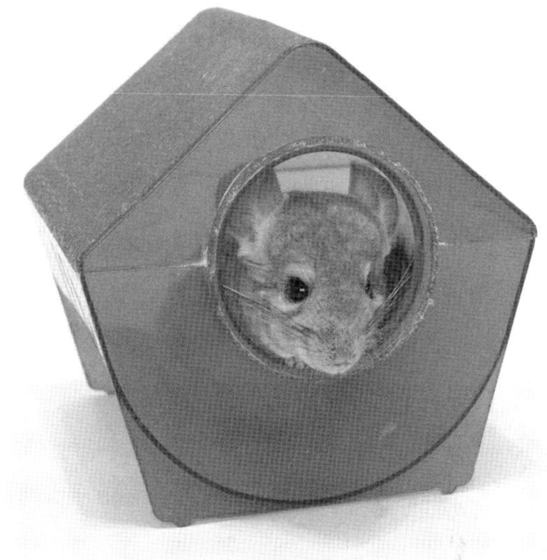

FIGURE 2.47. Examples of a chinchilla dust bath, open (left) and closed* (right). *Courtesy of Glen and Rebecca Grambo. Dust for bathing is available commercially for chinchillas.

be cleaned and sanitized at least once weekly by washing with a detergent and hot water, followed by a thorough rinse.

Feeding and Watering

Chinchillas are monogastric hindgut-fermenting herbivores. Their exact nutritional requirements have not been determined, but they thrive best with a high-fiber, low-energy diet with 16–20% protein, 25–55% fat, and 18% fiber. Chinchillas normally sit upright on their haunches to eat, holding the food with their forepaws. Commercial chinchilla pellets are larger than guinea pig pellets to facilitate holding. Commercial diets can be supplemented with free-choice grass hay. Grains and high starch or sugary treats should be avoided to prevent upsetting dietary balance. Small amounts of well-washed dark green leafy vegetables can be fed instead as treats. Suspended hoppers or heavy crocks prevent overturning and waste. Hay in elevated feeders permits individual pieces to be pulled through, and is a form of environmental enrichment. Dietary changes should be made gradually to avoid gastrointestinal upset. Salt licks with trace minerals can also be offered. Nuts should be avoided due to their high fat content. An adult chinchilla should consume approximately 30 g (1 oz) of chinchilla pellets, 5 g (1 tsp) of raw, washed vegetables, and free-choice hay each day. Unlike guinea pigs, chinchillas do not require addition of ascorbic acid to their diet. Similar to most other rodents, chinchillas are coprophagic.

Wild chinchillas rarely drink water, as they are able to maintain their hydration by licking dew drops and eating plants. Chinchillas in captivity adapt to drinking from water bottles with either valves or sipper tubes. Watering systems should be cleaned regularly to avoid contamination with *Pseudomonas aeruginosa.*

Reproduction

Sexing and Anatomy

Anogenital distance is the most reliable method for sexing chinchillas, with the distance of 1 cm in the mature male being approximately twice that of the female. Females have a large urinary papilla, ventral to the vagina, which is often mistaken for a penis (Figure 2.48). In addition, the vaginal opening is not always present due to a closure membrane that opens only during estrus and parturition. Females have a bicornate uterus with a single cervix. Females have two pairs of lateral and one pair of inguinal mammary

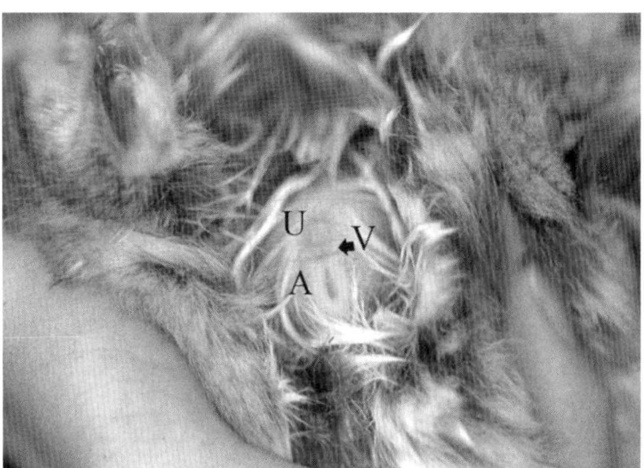

FIGURE 2.48. External genitalia of a mature female chinchilla (U: urethra, V: vaginal opening, A: anus). The urinary papilla of female chinchillas is larger than in female guinea pigs and may be mistaken for a penis.

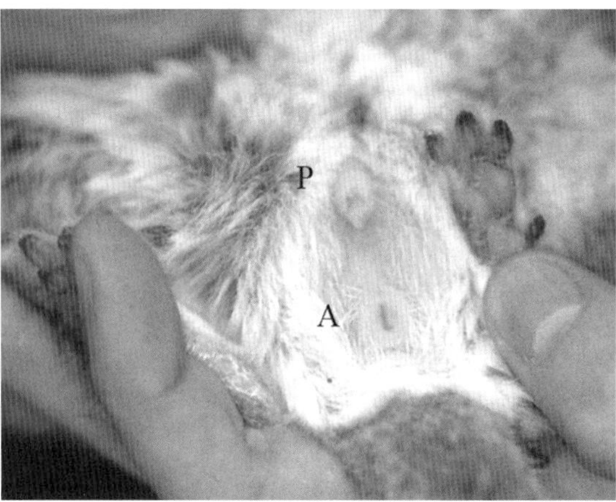

FIGURE 2.49. External genitalia of a mature male chinchilla (P: penis, A: anus).

glands. In general, the body size of females is larger than males. Males do not have a true scrotum, as the testicles can be withdrawn into the abdomen through the open inguinal canals. The penis is supported by an os penis (baculum) (Figure 2.49).

Estrous Cycle

Chinchillas are seasonally polyestrous in the northern hemisphere from November to May. The vaginal closure membrane opens during estrus, and the vaginal opening between the urethral papilla and anus appears reddened and slightly moist. Gentle pressure on the urinary papilla will usually open the vagina. If the chinchilla is not in estrus, the opening will not be present. The estrous cycle in chinchillas lasts 30–50 days, with an average of 38 days. The estrous period lasts 24–48 hours. Postpartum estrus occurs 2–48 hours after parturition, and a postlactation estrus occurs 35–84 days after parturition. A wax-like estrous plug 2.5–3 cm (1–1.2 in) diameter is normally ejected from the female at the onset of estrus, the function of which is unknown. Reddened nipples and restless behavior occasionally accompany estrus. Vaginal cytology can be used to determine stage of estrus with 70% accuracy. Generally females will have 2 litters per year.

Breeding Programs

Sexual maturity is reached at about 4–5 months of age in females and 7–9 months of age in males. Mating systems can be either monogamous or polygamous, although female chinchillas are monogamous in the wild. A polygamous breeding system is usually used. Each female resides in her own individual cage, which is connected to other cages by a tunnel. Females are restricted to their own cages by a flat metal disc attached to a collar they wear around their neck, which is slightly larger than the tunnel opening, preventing passage. Males are not fitted with collars and can move freely from cage to cage. This provides males with easy, unrestricted access to females, and an area where they can rest and escape.

If pair mating is used, new introductions should be attempted only after caging animals near each other for at least 1 week. Allowing intended mates to use the same dust bath may increase acceptance. Female chinchillas are the dominant sex, and the female should be placed into the male's cage so that she is in an unfamiliar territory. Several escape and hiding places should be available, in which only one chinchilla can fit and turn around to face the attacker. Threats are expressed by growling, chattering teeth, and spraying urine.

A quiet environment is needed for successful breeding. Mating usually occurs several times during the night. Loss of some fur from the female is normal during mating, but excessive fur slip may indicate the need to separate the pair. An ejaculatory plug is found in the vagina after mating. These plugs are approximately 3.75 cm (1.5 in) long and remain in place for several hours before falling out. Mating normally occurs at night and the best time to check for plugs is early morning.

Assisted breeding techniques, using electroejaculation and cryopreservation of spermatozoa, have also been extensively studied in the past 10 years by researchers at the University of Cordoba in Argentina to facilitate captive breeding programs for this endangered species.

The gestation period is 105–115 days, with an average of 110. Pregnancy can be detected by gentle abdominal palpation at 90 days gestation, although experienced personnel can detect pregnancy at 60 days. At about 60 days the mammary tissue and teats begin to swell and the nipples become reddened. Pregnancy can also be detected by regular weighing; weight change is minimal during the first 6 weeks, but then increases rapidly. Improper handling of a pregnant chinchilla may result in abortion or absorption of fetuses. Poor housing and severe stress can also cause loss of a litter.

The pregnant dam should be supplemented with vitamins during the last month of pregnancy. The gravid uterus occasionally puts pressure on the intestinal tract, causing constipation. Lush greens should be avoided due to the gaseous intestinal distension cause by fermentation.

Neonatal Life

The male can usually remain with the female during gestation and parturition and will participate in the care of the young. A group of chinchillas may communally raise their young. Chinchillas near parturition become inactive and anorectic and may become aggressive to a previously compatible mate. Parturition generally occurs at night or in the early morning. The strenuous phase of labor usually lasts 1–2 hours or less. During that time, the female writhes and stretches, and may vocalize. The interval between pups ranges from a few minutes to several hours and generally all pups are born within a 4-hour period. The female will continually lick her vent as each fetus emerges, and will use her teeth to pull the kits from the birth canal. The fetal membranes are normally eaten. The vagina remains open for 3–4 days before the closure membrane reforms. If the female becomes intolerant of the male during this time, he should be removed until the pups are weaned.

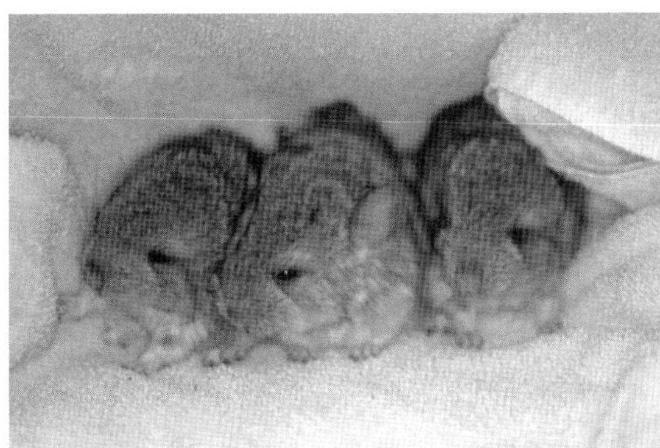

FIGURE 2.50. Two-week-old chinchilla pups. Pups are born precocious.

Dystocia is uncommon; however, Caesarean section should be considered if more than 4 hours of unproductive labor has elapsed. After labor the female should be palpated to ensure no fetuses remain, as mummified fetuses are relatively common.

Litter sizes average 2–3, although up to 6 have been reported. Dams don't normally build a nest; however, nest boxes may decrease neonatal mortality caused by cold stress. Newborns are fully furred with a complete set of teeth, and their eyes open within 24 hours. They are very vocal and normally make a continuous whimpering sound (Figure 2.50). Chinchillas sit on top of their young to nurse them and keep them warm. Weaning can occur as early as 6 weeks, although lactation can last up to 8 weeks. In the pet trade, chinchillas are separated from their mothers at 7–8 weeks of age and are usually sold at 3–6 months of age.

Orphaned kits can be fostered onto other chinchillas or even onto guinea pigs. If fostering is not possible, kits should be fed for 2–3 weeks until able to feed themselves. Feeding should occur every two to three hours and decrease as the animals get older and begin to take in food on their own. Newborn kits will begin to eat small amounts of solid food within the first week of life.

Disease Prevention

Chinchillas must be kept in a dry, cool environment to prevent respiratory problems, and should be provided with a daily dust bath for maintenance of a healthy coat.

Table 2.4. Biodata: chinchilla.

Adult body weight: male	400–500 g
Adult body weight: female	400–600 g
Birth weight	40–60 g
Body temperature	37–38 °C (98.6–100.4 °F)
Pulse	200–350 bpm
Respirations	45–80/min
Diploid number	64
Life span	9–18 yr
Food consumption	30–40 g/day; 5.5 g/100 g/day
Water consumption	10–20 ml/day; 8–9 ml/100 g/day
GI transit time	12–15 hr
Breeding onset: male	7–9 mo
Breeding onset: female	4–5 mo
Cycle length	30–50 days
Gestation period	105–120 days; average 112
Postpartum estrus	fertile
Litter size	2–6
Weaning age (lactation duration)	3–8 weeks
Breeding duration	3 yr
Milk composition	7.2% protein, 12.3%fat, 1.7 % lactose

Public Health Concerns

Diseases of public health significance include infections with *Yersinia enterocolitica, Salmonella typhimurium, Listeria monocytogenes, Rodentolepis nana, Echinococcus multilocularis,* dermatophytosis, lymphocytic choriomeningitis virus, tuberculosis, pasteurellosis, toxoplasmosis, and cryptosporidiosis. In addition, several nondermatophytic fungi and opportunistic bacteria have been isolated from chinchillas, such as *Aspergillus niger*, *Cladosporium* spp, *Rhizopus* spp, *Klebsiella pneumoniae,* and *Pseudomonas aeruginosa,* which might pose a health risk in immunocompromised people.

Uses in Research

Chinchillas are used commonly for auditory studies. Their cochlea is similar in shape to that of humans, and their range of hearing is similar. In addition, their large tympanic bullae are surrounded by thin bone that allows easy surgical access to the middle ear, cochlea, and surrounding structures. Chinchillas are also used to study the pathogenesis of Chagas disease, atherosclerosis, endocrinology of digestion, thermoregulation, cerebral blood flow, behavior, reproduction, respiratory syncytial virus, and hypothyroidism.

Biodata

(see Table 2.4)

References

Aho R. Saprophytic fungi isolated from the hair of domestic and laboratory animals with suspected dermatophytosis. Mycopathol. 1983, 83(2):65–73.

Bartoszcze M, et al. Klebsiella pneumoniae infection in chinchillas. Vet Rec. 1990, 127(5):119.

Blakeley K. Forget Fido. Forbes. 2000, 165:152.

Boussarie D. Carte d'identité chinchilla. Proceedings 27 World Small Animal Veterinary Association Congress, October 3–6, 2002, Granada (http://www.vin.com/proceedings/Proceedings.plx?CID=WSAVA2002&PID=2570).

Busso JM, et al. Electroejaculation in the chinchilla (Chinchilla lanigera): effects of anesthesia on seminal characteristics. Res Vet Sci. 2004, 78(1):93–97.

———. Year-round testicular volume and semen quality evaluations in captive Chinchilla lanigera. Anim Reprod Sci. 2005, 90(102):127–134.

Cartee R. Anatomic location and age related changes in the chinchilla thymus. Amer J Vet Res. 1979, 40(4):537–540.

Crossley DA, del Mar Miguélez M. Skull size and cheek-tooth length in wild-caught and captive-bred chinchillas. Arch Oral Biol. 2001, 46(10):919–928.

Doerning BJ, et al. Pseudomonas aeruginosa infection in a Chinchilla lanigera. Lab Anim. 1993, 27(2):131–133.

Donnelly TM, Quimby FW. Biology and Diseases of Other Rodents. In: Laboratory Animal Medicine, 2nd ed. Fox JG, Anderson LC, Loew FM, Quimby FW (eds.). San Diego: Academic Press, 2002.

Gitiban N, et al. Chinchilla and murine models of upper respiratory tract infections with respiratory syncytial virus. J Virol. 2005, 79(10):6035–6042.

Hrapkiewicz K, Medina L. Clinical Laboratory Animal Medicine: An Introduction, 3rd ed. Ames, IA: Blackwell, 2007.

IUCN Red List of Threatened Species. 2007. http://www.iucnredlist.org.

Jenkins JR. Husbandry and common diseases of the chinchilla (Chinchilla lanigera). J Small Exot Anim Med. 1992, 2:15–17.

Johnson DH. Miscellaneous Small Mammal Behavior. In: Exotic Pet Behavior. Bradley Bays T, Lightfoot T, Mayer J (eds.). St. Louis: Saunders Elsevier, 2006.

Martin LB, et al. Thyroparathyroidectomy procedures and thyroxine levels in the chinchilla. Contemp Top Lab Anim Sci. 2005, 44(6):31–36.

Nowak RM (ed.). Walker's Mammals of the World, 6th ed., vols. 1 and 2. Baltimore: Johns Hopkins, 1999.

Özdemir V, Çevik-Demirkan A, Türkmenoglu I. Right coronary artery is absent in the chinchilla (Chinchilla lanigera). Anatom, Histol Embryol. 2008, 37(2):114–117.

Ponce A, et al. Functional activity of epidiymal Chinchilla laniger spermatozoa cryopreserved in different extenders. Res Vet Sci. 1998, 64(3):239–243.

Quesenberry K, Donnelly TM, Hillyer EV. Biology, Husbandry, and Clinical Techniques of Guinea Pigs and Chinchillas. In: Ferrets, Rabbits, and Rodents: Clinical Medicine and Surgery, 2nd ed. Quesenberry K, Carpenter JW (eds.). St. Louis: Saunders, 2004.

Rosen T, Jablon J. Infectious threats from exotic pets. Dermatol Clin. 2003, 21(2):229–236.

Staebler S, et al. First description of natural Echinococcus multilocularis infections in chinchilla (Chinchilla laniger) and Prevost's squirrel (Callosciurus prevostii borneoensis). Parasitol Res. 2007, 101(6):1725–1727.

Strake JG, Davis LA, et al. Chinchillas. In: Handbook of Rodent and Rabbit Medicine. Laber-Laird K, Swindle M, Flecknell P (eds.). Oxford: Elsevier Science, 1996.

Veloso C, Keanagy GJ. Temporal dynamics of milk composition of the precocial caviomorph Octodon degus (Rodentia: Octodentidae). Revist Chilen Histor Natural. 2005, 78:247–252.

Volcani R, et al. The composition of chinchilla milk. B J Nutrit. 1973, 29(29):121–125.

Wideman WL. Pseudomonas aeruginosa otitis media and interna in a chinchilla ranch. Can Vet J. 2006, 47(8):799–800.

Wilkerson MJ, Melendy A, Stauber E. An outbreak of listeriosis in a breeding colony of chinchillas. J Vet Diagn Invest. 1997, 9(3):320–323.

Wolf P, Schröder A, Wenger A, et al. The nutrition of the chinchilla as a companion animal—basic data, influences and dependences. J Anim Physiol Anim Nutr. 2003, 87(3–4):129–133.

Websites for Chinchillas

http://exoticpets.about.com/cs/chinchillas/p/Chinchillas.htm—basic information about chinchillas and their care.

http://www.chincare.com/—care of the chinchilla.

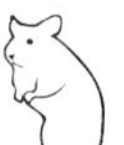

THE HAMSTER

The golden or Syrian hamster is popular both as a pet and as a research animal. These short-tailed, stocky animals weigh approximately 120 g and are known for their short gestation period, capacious cheek pouches, ability to escape confinement, and periodic pugnacious demeanor, despite their general docility. Unlike rabbits and guinea pigs, hamsters were only recently domesticated and imported as pets to North America. The Siberian or Djungarian hamster is also sold as a pet, and several other hamster species are used as animal models in studies that take advantage of unique species characteristics.

Origin and Description

The golden hamster, *Mesocricetus auratus*, is a rodent of the family Muridae and constitutes most of the hamsters used in research or kept as pets. Wild golden hamsters occur within a limited range in the Middle East, where destruction of the territory and predation by owls are threatening the species' existence. Hamsters in the Middle East, where they are called the Arabic equivalent of "originator of saddle bags" because of their often distended cheek pouches,

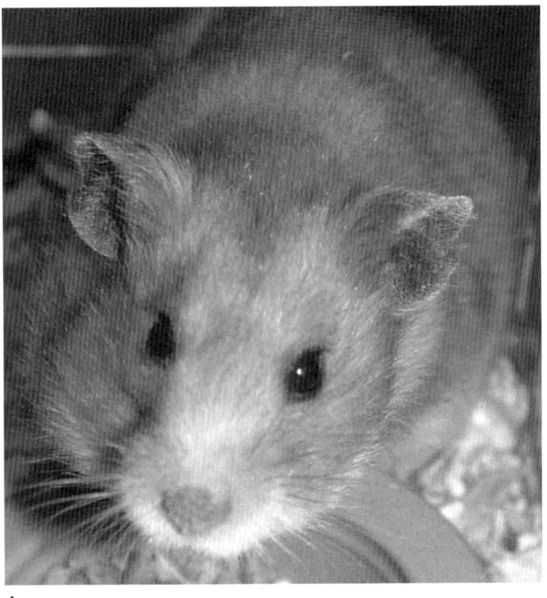
A

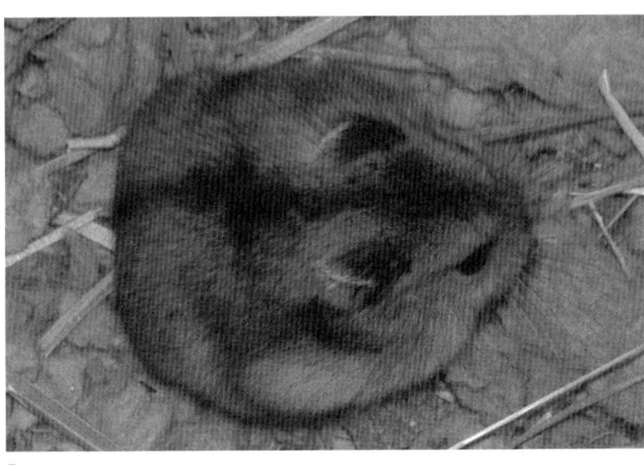
B

FIGURE 2.51. Typical appearance of hamster species. A: Syrian, and B: Chinese.

live independent lives in deep burrows, where they may store up to several pounds of grain. Hamsters are nocturnal with short periods of diurnal activity. Most hamsters used in research and sold as pets are descended from one male and two or three female littermates that survived capture and domestication in 1930.

Color varieties of domestic hamsters include the wild-type or reddish-golden brown with a gray ventrum, cinnamon, cream, white, piebald, albino, and the long-haired "teddy bear" variety. Over the past 6 decades, the number of coat color and pattern mutant genes (e.g., white spotting) encountered in hamster colonies has increased (Figure 2.51).

Other Hamster Species

Over two dozen species of hamster have been described but only a small handful of these have been domesticated. Species that are likely to be encountered other than the Syrian hamster (Siberian, Chinese, European, and Armenian) are described briefly below. All other information contained in this section and throughout the remainder of this text refers to the Syrian hamster.

The Siberian or Djungarian hamster (*Phodopsus sungorus*), known also as the hairy-footed hamster, is a small (30–50 g), colonial, nocturnal, sometimes aggressive species sold and traded by pet stores and hobbyists. This hamster has a short tail and is gray with a black dorsal stripe (except for a lighter winter coat); a satin variant also exists. Siberian hamsters have cheek pouches, lateral and ventral scent glands, and, unlike the golden hamster, can be housed in family groups. Whereas conspecific conflict occurs less often than in golden hamsters, interactions with humans may be antagonistic. Animals are highly active and move very quickly, making them skilled at escaping. Male Siberian hamsters are larger than females. Gestation is 18 days long, litter size averages 4 (range 1–9), eyes are open at 10 days, and weaning occurs at 16–18 days. Females mature at 90–130 days, whereas males mature at 150 days. The life span of the Siberian hamster is 9–24 months. These hamsters tolerate cold well, but become heat stressed at ambient temperatures of 34 °C (93 °F). They exhibit daily periods of torpor.

Diseases reported in Siberian hamsters include dermatophytosis, fight-wound abscesses, and neoplasia, especially of the oral cavity, skin, and mammary glands. Weight loss is a common nonspecific sign that accompanies pneumonia, malocclusion, or prolapsed or impacted cheek pouches.

The dark brown Chinese or striped hamster (*Cricetulus griseus*), larger common, black-bellied, or European hamster (*Cricetus cricetus*), and the grey Armenian hamster (*Cricetulus migratorius*) are sold as pets infrequently but have occasionally been used for biomedical research. For example, research on high-altitude physiology, hibernation, and tobacco-related diseases has been performed in these species. Chinese hamster ovaries are used to produce CHO cells, which have been used for in vitro cytotoxicology and karyotyping studies. *C. griseus* has also been used as a naturally occurring model for type 1 juvenile-onset diabetes.

The Chinese hamster (*Cricetulus griseus*) is gray-brown with a dark stripe down the back (Figure 2.51). Adult males weigh 30–35 g and females slightly less. The females are especially aggressive and must be housed individually. They have cheek pouches and flank glands, and are sexually mature at approximately 90 days of age and continue breeding until 12–15 months of age; life span is approximately 1.5–2 years of age. Litters average 4 offspring, and young are weaned at approximately 21 days of age. Dry nests are necessary for breeding success. Animals are easily stressed, and human interference or other factors can result in reluctance to breed. Chinese hamsters are also prone to dystocia. Tyzzer's disease has been reported as a cause of morbidity.

Anatomic and Physiologic Characteristics

This brief summary is intended only as an introduction to the several physical and functional aspects of hamsters.

Although hamsters are not true hibernators, with shortened day length, ambient temperatures less than 8 °C (48 °F), short light cycles, and isolation, pseudohibernation behavior may be observed. Hamsters remain sensitive to touch during this period, though they do exhibit a characteristic "hibernation posture" and have greatly slowed metabolism when in this state. In addition to this characteristic, hamsters can enter a period of deep sleep from which they are not easily aroused. Thus, when presented with an inactive hamster, particularly one that has been housed under cold conditions (i.e., less than 50 °F), the animal should be warmed to determine if arousal is possible—even if the animal appears to be dead!

Several inbred hamster strains have been developed using the procedures outlined for mice (see chapter 1 and Table 2.5 below). Interestingly, outbred hamsters exhibit high levels of genetic similarity in the histocompatibility complex, possibly due to the recent introduction of a small population of genetically related animals as progenitors for all domesticated hamsters. Because of this, Syrian hamsters in pet or laboratory colonies exhibit a high degree of immunologic tolerance to both homografts and heterografts of both normal and neoplastic tissue. This tolerance is even more pronounced in the tissue of the cheek pouch. Hamsters lack suppressor T cells and have atypical cytotoxic T cells.

Buccal or cheek pouches are oral-cavity evaginations reaching alongside the head and neck to the scapula. The pouches, measuring approximately 35–40 mm × 4–8 mm × 20 mm long, are muscular sacs lined with stratified squamous epithelium. They are thin walled, highly distensible, well vascularized, and devoid of lymphatic tissue other than minor vasculature. The dense subepithelial tissues underlying the oral pouches further isolate these structures from the systemic lymphatic system. These evertable pouches are functionally used to transport food and bedding and likely assist with food hoarding (Figure 2.52). Cheek pouches have been used experimentally to provide an immunologically privileged site for tumor induction and transplantation, though this once-important experimental model has recently largely been replaced by immunodeficient and genetically modified mice.

Table 2.5. Examples of inbred strains of hamsters and their characteristics.

Inbred Strain Designation	Characteristics
Bio 14.6	acromelanic white, cardiomyopathy
Bio TO-2	cardiomyopathy
UM-X7.1	cardiomyopathy
MHA	white, prone to dental caries
Bio F91 B	hypercholesterolemia, atherosclerosis
APA	glomerulosclerosis

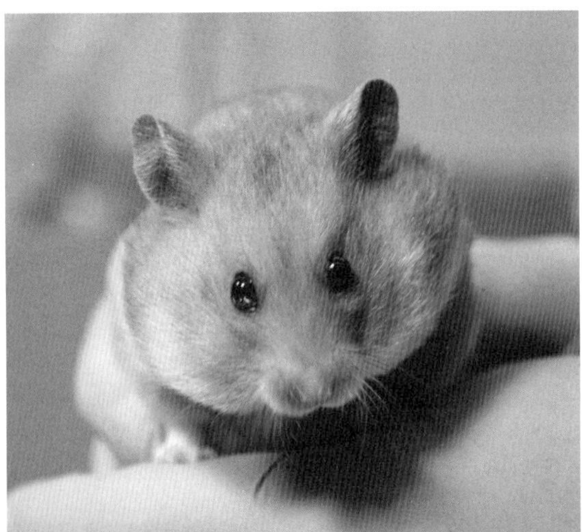

FIGURE 2.52. Syrian hamster with cheek pouches distended with food. Courtesy of A.J. Wang.

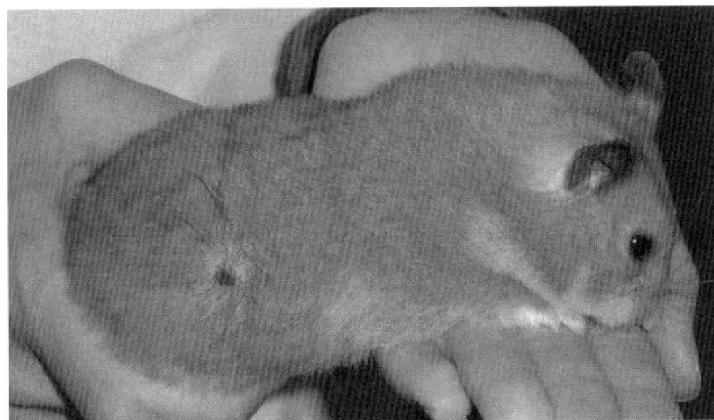

FIGURE 2.53. Flank gland on a Syrian hamster.

Other characteristics of the hamster oral cavity include a movable mandibular symphysis and molar teeth that retain food particles, promoting dental caries if *Streptococcus mutans* is present. This phenomenon has been exploited in dental research. Newborn hamsters have fully erupted incisor teeth that function during suckling to strip milk from the teats of the dam. Hamsters have 3/3 molars with fixed roots and 1/1 open-rooted incisors. There are no canine or premolar teeth.

On either flank, usually buried in hair and more prominent in intact males, are dark brown flank glands (Figure 2.53). These sebaceous glands are used to mark territory and contribute to pheromone stimuli determining mating behaviors. These glands reach a maximum size by 21 days in females and 70 days in males, and testosterone is converted to dihydrotestosterone in these glands.

The hamster stomach is separated into squamous and glandular divisions at the junction of the greater and lesser curvatures. The forestomach, anatomically linked to the esophagus, has content with neutral pH and is the site of pregastric fermentation. Their stomach and forestomach normally contain small numbers of yeast and bacteria such as staphylococci and *Enterobacteria* spp. It is likely this microflora population contributes to antibiotic toxicity in the hamster.

Hamsters produce up to 7 mL of urine per day, and the urine is high in protein levels and has a high pH (>7.5) as a result of the hamster's primarily herbivorous diet. Hamster urine is typically cloudy in appearance because of the normal crystalline precipitates. Adrenal glands in the male hamster are larger than those in the female. Group housing hamsters increases adrenal weights, but this effect may not be ACTH mediated.

Hamsters as Pets

Behavior

Hamsters have a reputation for aggressiveness toward handlers, a characteristic usually exhibited after rough handling or a sudden disturbance. This is thought to be related to the highly nocturnal nature of hamsters, as they sleep deeply during daylight hours and are difficult to arouse compared to other domesticated rodents, for example, rats, mice, and gerbils. Hamsters, even those recently captured in the wild, are tamed readily through gentle and repeated handling. They are aggressive and territorial toward other hamsters, especially when a female hamster is pregnant or lactating, although progesterone and its metabolites have been shown to inhibit aggression in female hamsters. Most aggression is ultrasound-mediated and more pronounced between females, and to the human observer, may appear with no warning. Studies on group-housed hamsters indicate that even though hamsters may prefer social contacts, such interaction can be stressful, leading to agonistic behavior and obesity.

Hamsters are remarkably adept at chewing through and escaping from their cages. Unlike rats and mice, escaped hamsters will usually not return to their cages. The use of live traps baited with peanut butter or a ramp leading into a container placed against a room wall may be necessary to catch an escaped hamster, although they may live for months hiding in a house. Pet hamsters are typically provided with running wheels for enrichment. While this provides animals with the opportunity to satisfy roaming behaviors within an enclosed environment, it can be problematic because most running activity occurs at night and may disturb human occupants of the household. This can be significant considering that some hamsters, notably pregnant females, have been reported to run up to 8 km daily.

Hamsters may be grouped by sex (males and females separated) for short periods in holding cages. They fight less often if housed together at the time of weaning or before sexual maturity, are awakened simultaneously from anesthesia in a neutral arena, or are provided with hiding places.

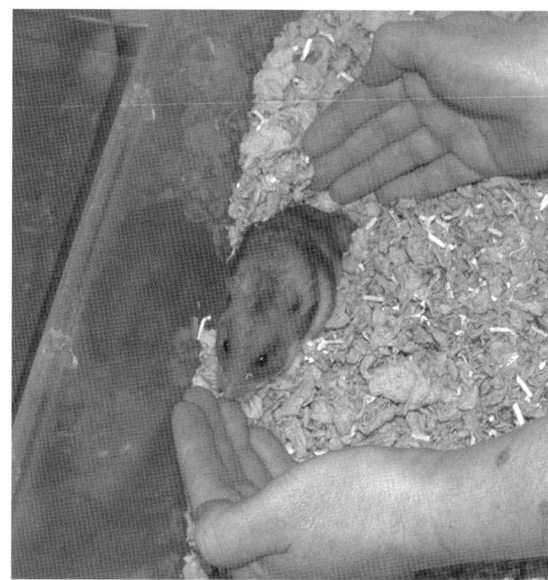

FIGURE 2.54. A method for scooping a hamster out of its cage.

Life Span

Hamsters have a life span of 18–24 months, but older individuals are reported frequently. In commercial situations, female hamsters produce 5–6 large litters during their first 6 months of life, and then produce smaller litters until the dams are 12–15 months old, and may be retired depending upon breeding capacity and objectives. Males are used for commercial breeding until 12 months of age.

Restraint

Hamsters frequently exhibit agonistic postures and may bite if roughly handled, startled, injured, or abruptly awakened. Hamsters may be picked up in a small container, by grasping the large amounts of loose skin of the neck that constitute cheek pouch capacity, or by cupping the hands and gripping over the back (Figure 2.54 and 2.55). A protective glove may be used if the animals are unaccustomed to handling or if the handler is allergic to hamsters. Gentle deliberate movements, with care taken to arouse a slumbering animal before handling, and the skill and comfort level of the handler are all factors that contribute to successful restraint.

Housing

Hamsters used in biomedical research are generally housed in plastic, solid-bottom cages with deeply piled wood shavings for bedding. For animals weighing greater than 100 g, cages should be 123 cm^2 × 15–18 cm high (ILAR and CCAC guides). More space is needed for breeding females with litters. Ambient temperatures of 18–26 °C and relative humidity between 40% and 70% are well tolerated by hamsters. Hamsters are prodigious tunnel-makers, and prefer bedded, solid-bottom cages to wire-floored cages (Figures 2.56 and 2.57). Given a deep enough cage with abundant substrate, hamsters will create an impressive system of tunnels through the bedding within their cages. Because hamsters have blunt noses, they may have difficulty eating from slotted sheet metal hoppers or wire mesh feeders if units with small spaces between bars are used. Slots should be more than 1.1 cm wide to allow the hamster to comfortably pull food into the cage.

Hamsters chew plastic, wood, and soft metals and will escape easily from poorly secured or constructed cages. Transport boxes are usually lined with mesh or light metal screening for this reason.

Hamsters produce relatively little odor and less urine than other rodents because of their desert origins. Research colony hamster cages are changed once or twice weekly, except when neonates are present. Cages are sanitized with hot (82 °C or

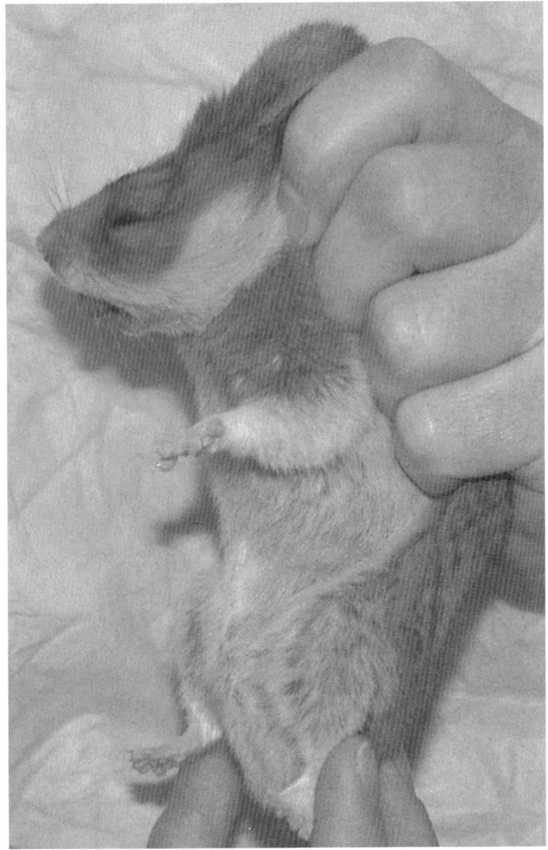

FIGURE 2.55. The hamster is being firmly restrained by grasping the loose skin around the shoulders and back (scruff grip).

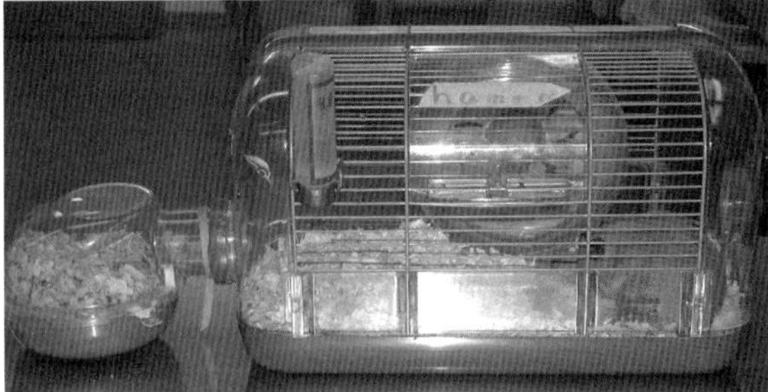

FIGURE 2.56. Typical plastic cage used for housing pet hamsters. A running wheel is provided for enrichment in the large cage and a small nest cage is attached by means of a tunnel to add complexity.

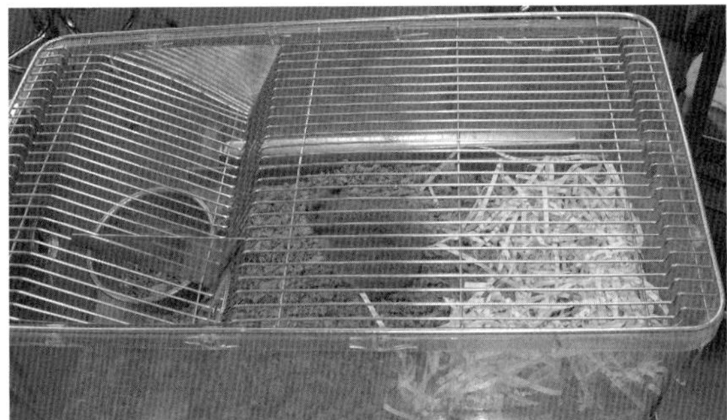

FIGURE 2.57. Shoebox-type cage used for housing laboratory hamsters. Shredded paper is supplied for tunneling and nesting enrichment.

180 °F) water with or without a detergent or with a nontoxic disinfectant followed by a thorough rinse. Bottles and hoppers are cleaned at the same time as the cages.

Whereas a number of commercial materials are available for bedding, hardwood chips are usually preferred, as they allow ample opportunities for burrowing. Soft woods, such as pine and cedar, should be avoided, as these have been associated with dermatologic conditions and respiratory irritation in hamsters, and may induce hepatic enzymes, interfering with research protocols and anesthesia. Recycled paper bedding and corncob pellets can also be used. Shredded newspaper is discouraged as a sole source of bedding, as it is minimally absorptive and contains undesirable pigments and chemicals.

Feeding and Watering

Hamsters are both granivores and insectivores. Although the nutritional requirements have not been determined specifically, a pelleted rodent diet that contains approximately 16% protein and 4–5% fat is typically provided and appears to provide a nutritionally adequate diet. Hamsters eat 8–12 g of feed and drink 8–10 mL of water per 100 g of body weight daily. They eat several small meals approximately 2 hours apart. Protein deficiency may cause alopecia, whereas dietary fat levels exceeding 7–9% may be associated with increased mortality. Vitamin E deficiency in pregnant hamsters may result in fetal death, but shouldn't occur if a balanced rodent pelleted diet is fed. Laboratory rodent feeds are often repackaged in small, unlabeled bags and sold in pet stores. The low-protein but attractively wrapped "treats" may not be adequate diets for growth and reproduction.

Seed-based diets are not appropriate, as hamsters will preferentially consume high-fat seeds, creating an unbalanced diet.

Dams with litters should receive their feed directly on the floor, as preoccupation with hopper-bound pellets may result in neglect of the young. Young hamsters begin gnawing solid food and drinking water at 7–10 days of age; therefore, the sipper tube should extend low in the cage but not into the bedding.

Hamsters are coprophagous and consume feces directly from the anus. This behavior occurs approximately 20 times each day.

Reproduction

Sexing and Anatomy

Viewed from above, the rear margin of the male hamster is rounded because of the scrotal sacs, and the female posterior is pointed toward the tail (Figures 2.58 and 2.59). Gentle pressure applied to the lower abdomen will cause the testes to protrude into the scrotal sacs. Males have a greater anogenital distance than do females and a pointed genital papilla with a round opening. Male hamsters have prominent, dark marking glands in the skin of both flanks, visible as indentations in the hair coat. These glands may be difficult to see without shaving the animal. Females have 12–17 mammary glands; nipples are readily visible on the adult female but are not seen on males.

Breeding Activity

Just as hamsters in the wild have a winter (hibernal) sexual quiescence, laboratory and pet hamsters also have a normal seasonal breeding quiescence in the winter months. During this time, fecundity decreases and litter mortality increases. Provision of a constant temperature (22–24 °C; 73 °F) and 12–14 hours of light reduces some of this effect.

Golden hamsters become sexually mature at 32–42 days, but managed breeding usually is delayed until the female is 6–10 weeks and the male is 10–14

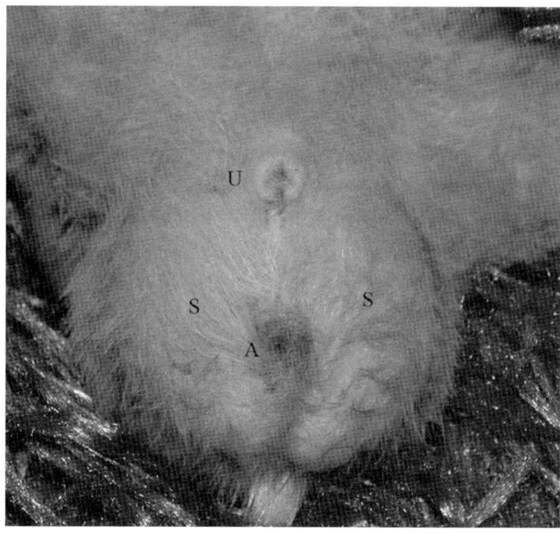

FIGURE 2.58. External genitalia of mature male hamster (U: urethral opening, S: scrotum, A: anus). Courtesy of Lorilee Sereda.

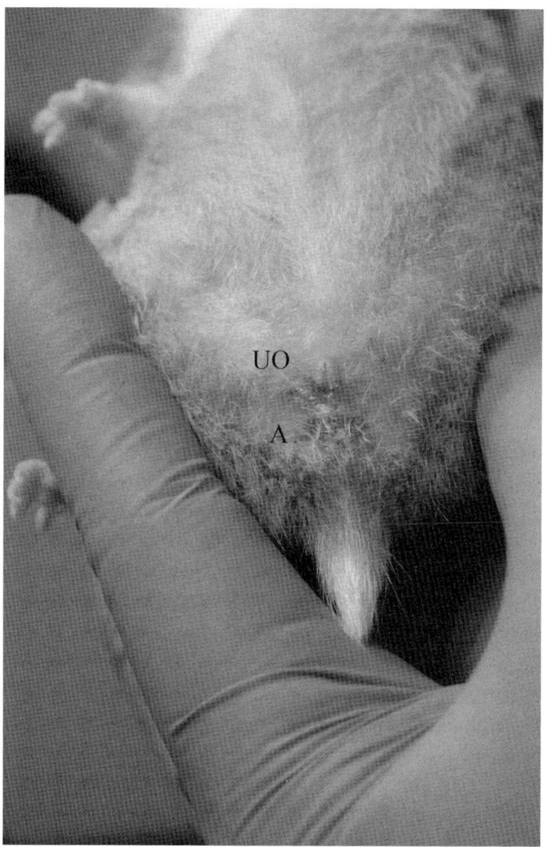

FIGURE 2.59. External genitalia of mature female hamster (UO: urogenital opening, A: anus). Courtesy of A.J. Wang.

weeks (85–130 g). Hamsters have an estrous cycle lasting approximately 4 days. Postpartum estrus is usually anovulatory but a fertile estrus follows weaning by 2–18 days. Vaginal pheromones and chemical production (dimethyl disulfide) stimulate aggression and attract males. On the morning after estrus, an opaque, tenacious and stringy vaginal discharge is produced and is referred to as the postovulatory discharge. Presence of this secretion should not be confused with a disease process and can be used to stage the estrous cycle for future breeding.

Except for the few hours of estrus occurring once during the 4-day cycle, a sexually unreceptive female will usually attack a recently introduced male. Females will demonstrate lordosis behavior approximately 8 hours prior to ovulation.

Several breeding schemes can be used. *Hand mating:* When small numbers of animals are being bred, the male can be introduced either directly to the female's cage or on top of a wire lid to gauge female acceptance about 1 hour before the start of the dark cycle. If the female does not attack and displays lordosis, the male is introduced to the cage and then removed from the breeding cage after copulation. *Monogamous pair mating:* A prepubertal male and female are introduced and housed together permanently, assuming they continue to be compatible. Although more males are required with this system than the hand mating scheme, it is labor efficient. During *sequential monogamous mating*, seven females are rotated through a male's cage in a series at weekly intervals, resulting in litter intervals of 35–40 days. After weaning of the litter, the female is returned to the male's cage for 1 week every seventh week. This method is labor efficient but places greater demands on studs if smaller numbers of males are used. *Group or harem mating*: One to five males are placed with a larger number of females. Seven to 12 days after pairing, the pregnant females are removed and housed individually until after pups have been weaned. Fighting may occur when females are returned to the cage, and additional space provisions, monitoring, and hiding areas are required for this system to be successful.

Pregnancy and Rearing

The absence of postovulatory discharge at 5 and 9 days postmating and the observation of a distended abdomen and rapid weight gain at 10 days are signs of pregnancy. The hamster's gestation period lasts 15–16 days and embryo implantation occurs on day 6.

Before delivery, the female becomes active and restless and develops a vaginal discharge. Litters contain 5–9 offspring. Infertile matings or crowding of females may produce an occasional pseudopregnancy of 7–13 days in duration. Active nest building may enhance hormonal functions associated with parturition and lactation and is more prodigious when temperatures are cooler. Nest material, such as paper tissues, should be provided to pregnant hamsters several days before parturition. Transfer of the nest that contains neonates reduces disturbances that may occur when changing cages. As neonatal hamsters are very immature and require a warm environment, the nest is essential.

Litter abandonment and cannibalism, common during the first pregnancy and the first week postpartum, may occur if the nest is scant, disturbed, or too visible; if the young are born on wire, handled, or bite the mother while nursing; or if the diet is inadequate and the dam does not produce milk. Large or small litter sizes in a noisy environment may also result in abandonment. The female hamster may conceal her newborn litter in her cheek pouches if a threat is perceived, which can result in injury to or suffocation of the offspring. To avoid disturbing the neonates, the female should be supplied with a week's supply of food and bedding 13 days after mating. This allows the mother to nest undisturbed, especially if some feed is placed on the floor of the cage and the water bottle tube can be reached by the young. Hair growth begins at 9 days and weaning occurs at 20–25 days postpartum.

Fostering is rarely successful with hamsters, as both adopted and natural litters may be cannibalized. Cross-fostering onto dams of other rodent species has not been successful because of the extreme immaturity of hamster young and their sharp incisors. Hand rearing is not successful.

Disease Prevention

The general husbandry and disease prevention measures mentioned in chapter 1 should be observed. Common husbandry problems resulting in disease in both laboratory and pet hamsters are fighting, cannibalism of young, escape from cages, susceptibility to climatic changes, and inadvertent food and water deprivation.

Public Health Concerns

Lymphocytic choriomeningitis virus (LCMV) infection has received attention because of several outbreaks in humans, most recently in 2006. Severe disease and death were recorded in individuals receiving organ donations from a donor with an active LCMV infection associated with a pet hamster. Most pet rodents are purchased from small breeders and redistributed in large centralized centers, allowing infectious agents to spread readily between animals and species. In response to this, the Centers for Disease Control and Prevention (CDC) has increased efforts to eliminate this pathogen from breeding operations selling to wholesale or retail pet suppliers in the U.S. Owners should always be reminded to wash hands carefully after holding and playing with their pets. Salmonellosis, hymenolepid tapeworm, and *Acinetobacter* spp infections are hamster diseases of potential public health significance, particularly in association with pet hamsters. *Acinetobacter* spp infection in humans can lead to osteomyelitis and tenosynovitis, conditions that are difficult to cure. The possibility of rabies occurring in pet or research rodents is extremely unlikely because they are not likely to be exposed to infected animals in the rabies virus cycle.

Uses in Research

Approximately 175,000–200,000 hamsters are used annually in research in the United States, while 5,800 are used in Canada. Most hamsters are outbred, but useful inbred strains exist as animal models for epilepsy, muscular dystrophy, and heart failure. Hamsters are used in investigations of congenital anomalies, dental caries, microcirculation, protozoal infections, gerontology, behavior, histocompatibility, infectious diseases, respiratory neoplasia, viral oncogenesis, muscular dystrophy, left-sided atrial thrombosis and ventricular hypertrophy, gallstones, amyloidosis, pancreatic neoplasia, cestodiasis, toxicology, reproductive physiology, circadian rhythms, lipid metabolism, and, in the Chinese hamster, dia-

Table 2.6. Biodata: Syrian hamsters.

Adult body weight: male	85–130 g
Adult body weight: female	95–150 g
Birth weight	2 g
Body surface area (cm^2)	11.8 × (weight in grams)$^{2/3}$
Body temperature	37–38 °C (98.6–100.4 °F)
Diploid number	44
Life span	18–24 mo
Food consumption	8–12 g/100 g/day
Water consumption	8–10 mL/100 g/day
Breeding onset: male	10–14 wk
Breeding onset: female	6–10 wk
Cycle length	4 days
Gestation period	15–16 days
Postpartum estrus	infertile; nonovulatory (golden hamster) fertile (Siberian hamster)
Litter size	5–9
Weaning age (lactation duration)	20–25 days
Breeding duration	10–12 mo
Commercial	5–7 litters
Young production (index/female)	3/mo
Milk composition	12.0% fat, 9.0% protein, 3.4% lactose

betes mellitus. Hamsters are used in various infectious disease studies, as they are relatively susceptible to infection with a wide range of bacterial, viral, and prion diseases.

Biodata

The values listed in Table 2.6 are approximations only and may not represent the normal range in a given population.

References

More comprehensive works on hamsters include Van Hoosier GL, Jr., McPherson CW (eds.). The Hamster in Biomedical Research. Orlando: Academic Press, 1987; Poole TB (ed.). The UFAW Handbook on the Care and Management of Laboratory Animals, 7th ed., vol. 1. Ames, IA: Blackwell, 1999; Rowsell HC, et al. (eds.). The Guide to the Care and Use of Experimental Animals, vol. 2. Ottawa, ON: Canadian Council on Animal Care, 1984; Bays T, Lightfoot T, Mayer J. Exotic Pet Behavior: Birds, Reptiles and Small Mammals. St. Louis: Saunders Elsevier, 2006; and Hoffman R, et al. (eds.). The Golden Hamster: Its Biology and Use in Medical Research. Ames: Iowa State University Press, 1968.

Other References on Hamsters

Aoki S, et al. On the flank gland in Syrian hamsters. Exp Anim. 1993, 42:93–97.

Arnold C, Gillaspy S. Assessing laboratory life for golden hamsters: Social preference, caging selection, and human interaction. Lab Anim. 1994, 23(2):34–37.

Barlett P. The Hamster Handbook. Hauppauge, NY: Barron's, 2003.

Brain PF. Understanding the behaviors of feral species may facilitate design of optimal living conditions for common laboratory rodents. Anim Technol. 1992, 43:99–105.

Bucsis G, Somerville B. Training Your Pet Hamster. Hauppauge, NY, Barron's, 2005.

Ebino KY. Studies on coprophagy in experimental animals. Exp Anim. 1993, 42:1–9.

Field KL, Sibold AL. The Laboratory Hamster and Gerbil. Boca Raton, FL: CRC Press, 1998.

Ghosal NG, Bal HS. Histomorphology of the hamster cheek pouch. Lab Anim Sci. 1990, 24:228–233.

Kress DW, et al. Mating suppresses splenic natural killer cell activity in male golden hamsters. Brain Behav Immunol. 1989, 3:274–280.

Martin RW, Martin DL, Levy CS. Acinetobacter osteomyelitis from a hamster bite. Pediatr Infect Dis J. 1988, 7:364–365.

Nowak RM. Walker's Mammals of the World, 6th ed. Baltimore: Johns Hopkins, 1999.

Ohwada K. Body surface area of the golden Syrian hamster. Exp Anim. 1992, 41:221–224.

Quesenberry K, Donnelly TM, Hillyer EV. Small Rodents. In: Ferrets, Rabbits, and Rodents: Clinical Medicine and Surgery, 2nd ed. Quesenberry K, Carpenter JW (eds.). St. Louis: Saunders, 2004.

Reznik G, et al. Clinical Anatomy of the European Hamster Cricetus. New York: State Mutual Book and Periodical Service, 1978.

Robinson R. Synergistic action of white spotting genes in the Syrian hamster (Rodentia, Cricetidae). Genetica. 1990, 82:135–137.

Streilein JW, et al. (eds.). Hamster Immune Responses in Infectious and Oncologic Diseases. New York: Plenum, 1981.

Vanderlip S. Dwarf Hamsters (Complete Pet Owner's Manual). Hauppauge, NY: Barron, 2009.

Werner RG, Ehie FR. Nutritional idiosyncrasies of the golden hamster (Mesocricetus auratus). Lab Anim Sci. 1976, 26:670–673.

Websites for Hamsters

http://exoticpets.about.com/od/hamsters/tp/hamsterguide.htm—choosing and caring for pet hamsters.

http://www.ask-the-vet.com/hamster-care.htm—health information for hamsters.

http://www.hsus.org/pets/pet_care/rabbit_horse_and_other_pet_care/how_to_care_for_hamsters.html—site for hamster care.

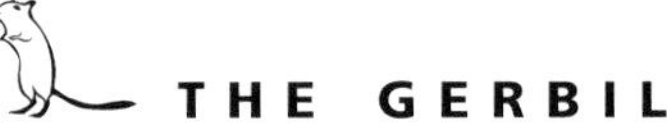

THE GERBIL

The Mongolian gerbil or jird is an active, generally easy to handle, and nonaggressive rodent distinguished by its monogamous mating behavior, water and temperature conservation mechanisms, spontaneous epileptiform seizures, and relative freedom from other spontaneous diseases.

Origin and Description

The Mongolian gerbil, *Meriones unguiculatus*, is a rodent of the family Muridae. There are 14 genera and 110 species of gerbil-like rodents within the subfamily Gerbillinae, and all are characterized by movement via jumping or hopping actions. Although species other than the Mongolian gerbil are rarely used as research subjects in North America, in other countries *M. libycus*, *M. shawii*, and *M. tristami* continue to be used as research models.

The Mongolian gerbil is native to desert regions of Mongolia and northeastern China, and is an active, curious, burrowing, social animal with cycles of activity, feeding, and rest during day and night, although in captivity peak activity may occur in the middle of the dark cycle. They consume equal amounts of food day and night. In the wild, gerbils are diurnal with crepuscular tendencies and may hibernate. Their burrows are elaborate tunnels with multiple entrances, nesting rooms, and food chambers for storing seeds over the winter. Social groups of gerbils may include 10–20 entrances, and in the wild, gerbils remain near an entrance. Gerbils retain a "mental map" of their burrows and when threatened by a predator bolt to the most accessible hole.

All Mongolian gerbils used for research in North America came from 20 breeding pairs that were originally trapped in Mongolia and taken to Japan. Of these, four breeding pairs were sent to the United States in 1954 to the laboratory of Dr. Viktor Schwentker, who established the first commercial breeding colony. Most laboratory gerbils today are highly related, making gene mapping studies with this species difficult because of the low allelic polymorphisms that are typically used to map genes.

The agouti or banded brown-haired Mongolian gerbil is the color variety sold commonly as pets or research animals, but gerbils with over 20 different hair coat colors are available (Figure 2.60). The agouti coloration is the dominant color pattern. Black gerbils frequently have a white stripe or patch that extends from the chin to the chest and white spots on the feet. White, dove, piebald, and cinnamon color mutations exist as well as a hairless mutation.

Anatomic and Physiologic Characteristics

Gerbils of both sexes have a distinct midventral abdominal pad, which is larger in males, composed of large sebaceous glands under control of sex hormones. Secretions from this gland are used in territorial marking and pup identification. Both sexes mark by sliding on the belly or rubbing the abdomen against surfaces, but males mark more frequently, especially if raised in a naturalistic environment or with reproductively active females. The female gerbil has four pairs of teats, two thoracic and two inguinal. Spontaneous, convulsive (epileptiform) seizures occur in approximately 30% of pet or laboratory gerbils. These seizures, which begin at approximately 2 months of age, may be hereditary. The seizures range from mild to severe and can be induced by various stressors such as unfamiliar surroundings or loud noises.

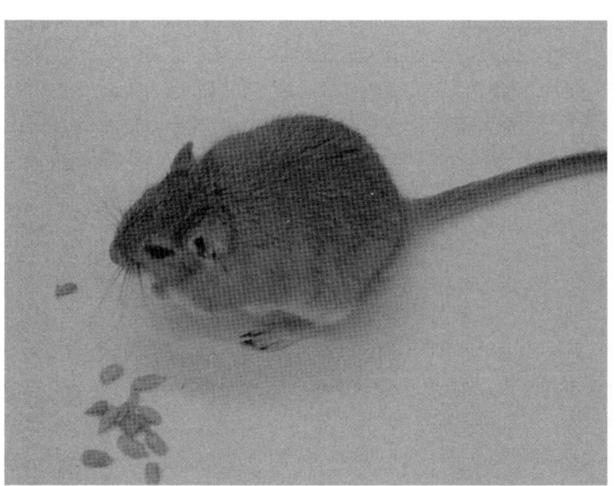

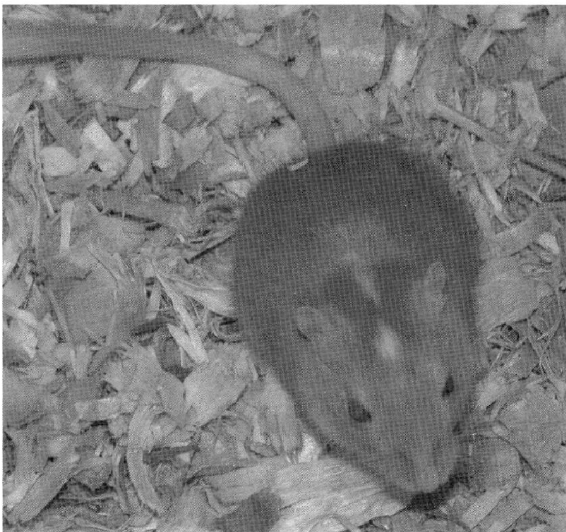

FIGURE 2.60. Agouti gerbils (left) are most common, but solid coat colors are also seen (right). Left photo Courtesy of Phyllis Paterson.

Grooming using normal red-tinged protoporphyrin and lipid secretions from the Harderian gland and saliva may provide means of chemocommunication and pelage insulation. In addition, Harderian gland secretions provide lubrication to the eye and are thought to be photoprotective. Accumulation of porphyrin secretions may be an indication of stress or poor health.

Gerbils exhibit lipemia more frequently than other rodent species. The lipemia is probably of dietary origin and is accentuated by feeding high-fat chows or sunflower seeds. Gerbils appear to develop lipemia even on diets with standard fat levels (4–6%). High serum cholesterol levels, for example, 1,590 mg/dL, have resulted from feeding gerbils standard rodent diets plus 1% cholesterol. Hypercholesterolemia is associated primarily with low-density lipoproteins. Hepatic lipidosis and gallstones, but not atherosclerosis, develop in gerbils on the high-fat diet.

Similar to other rodent species, there is some sexual dimorphism in gerbil erythrocyte parameters. Compared with female gerbils, males have higher packed red cell volumes, hemoglobin levels, total leukocyte counts, and circulating lymphocyte counts. Some erythrocytes of both sexes have prominent polychromasia and basophilic stippling. As for guinea pigs, hamsters, and rabbits, in gerbils the neutrophils are termed heterophils because they are seen to contain eosinophilic cytoplasmic granules with Romanowsky (Wright's) stains.

Compared with other rodents, gerbils have a higher adrenal gland weight–to–body weight ratio, which may contribute to their unique water-conserving capability. They have developed adaptive mechanisms for temperature extremes, such as spreading saliva on their pelage to promote evaporative heat loss. The thymus is within the thorax and persists in adults, as in rats and mice. The body weight of gerbils varies from animal to animal and among colonies, ranging from 50 to 80 g for females and 80 to 130 g for males. Although such variability may be a genetic phenomenon, diet is a likely major contributing factor, that is, higher fat content and diets of better nutritional quality lead to heavier body weights. The hind legs of gerbils are adapted for jumping.

Gerbils as Pets

Behavior

Gerbils are clean, friendly, curious, and quiet, produce little waste and odor, rarely bite or fight, and adapt to gentle handling easily. Gerbils are more exploratory and less thigmotaxic than other small rodents. An escaped gerbil prefers an open space or its cage to hiding, although escaped gerbils may be difficult to capture. Gerbils rarely vocalize but often sit upright, or when threatened or excited, drum their rear legs on the floor.

Although gerbils are social animals that live in either mixed or same-sex groups, they can be aggressive toward intruders. Gerbils may fight if crowded or mixed as adults, but the usual social interactions are grooming, wrestling, and communal sleeping. Incessant digging with the forepaws in the corners of the cage is a characteristic of gerbils and may be an indication of a stereotypic behavior due to lack of appropriate stimulation. Old gerbils or gerbils that are experiencing pain are more inclined to bite than are young or breeding adults.

Pain may be difficult to detect in gerbils because they are prey species. Close observation for subtle behavioral changes is necessary to detect distress or states of disease. Piloerection, hunched posture, reduced locomotion, reduced food consumption and feces production, and lack of interaction with cagemates may all be indicators of poor health or pain.

Gerbils paired after reaching puberty (10 weeks) or reunited after prolonged separation may fight. Fighting is reduced if the gerbils reach maturity in the same cage or if the animals are allowed to recover simultaneously from anesthesia in a neutral cage. It may not be possible to mix adults from different established pairs without serious fighting. Agouti female gerbils prefer agouti mates, whereas sandy and black females prefer non-agouti mates.

Other behavioral characteristics of gerbils are their stable monogamous matings, rapid learning of avoidance responses but poor maze performances (perhaps because they are too curious), and epileptiform seizures in some gerbils older than 2 months after excitement, sudden noise, handling, or introduction to a strange environment.

Life Span

The reproductive life of a female gerbil ranges from 15 to 20 months, during which time 4–10 litters may be produced. The average life span is 3 years, but 4-year-old gerbils are common.

Restraint

The gerbil is grasped firmly at the base of the tail and the neck at the nape; the animal is then lifted and cradled in the hand. The tail is long and relatively inflexible. Extreme care must be taken not to pull on the tail because the skin on the caudal tail comes off readily (degloving injury or "tailslip"). The gerbil may be restrained more securely with an over-the-back grip (Figures 2.61–2.63). Gerbils resist being placed on their backs and, while struggling, may be dropped accidentally, especially by small children or those unaccustomed to handling rodents. The immobility response is elicited readily by grasping the nape of the neck.

Housing

Plastic or metal rodent cages with a solid floor and deep bedding are the usual housing arrangement and are preferred to wire cages without bedding (Figure 2.64). Bedding should be of sufficient depth (2 cm) to facilitate nest building and should be clean, dry, absorbent, and nonabrasive. Provision of an opaque cage, material for nest building, or a hiding place within the cage may improve reproductive and maternal performance (Figure 2.65). Gerbils are active gnawers and burrowers, and cages should be designed to prevent escape. Pet or laboratory gerbils exposed to a naturalistic environment (stones, sand, water dish) find food more readily, rear up, mark,

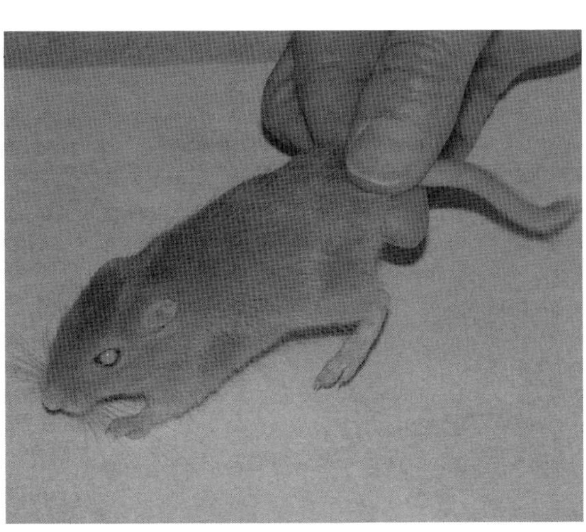

FIGURE 2.61. A safe method of restraining the gerbil by the base of the tail.

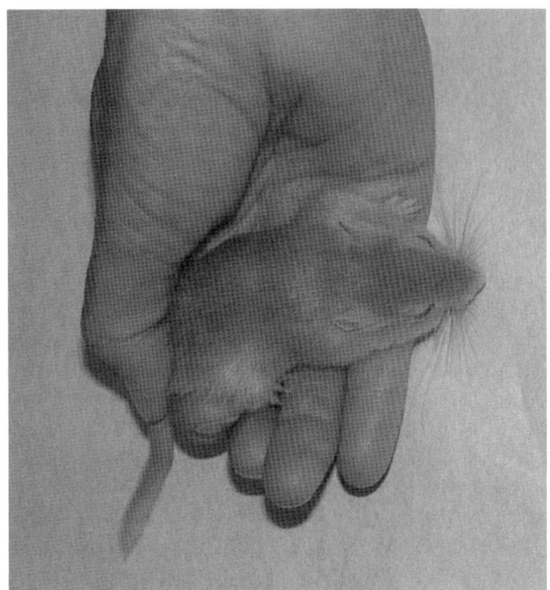

FIGURE 2.62. While carrying a gerbil in the hand, a firm grasp should be maintained on the base of the tail.

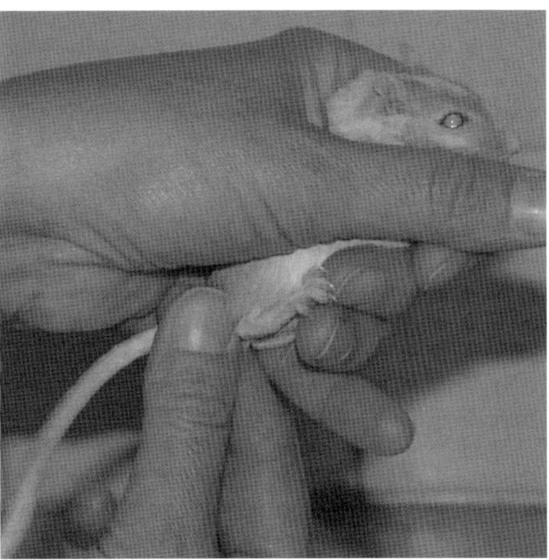

FIGURE 2.63. An "over-the-back" grip for a gerbil.

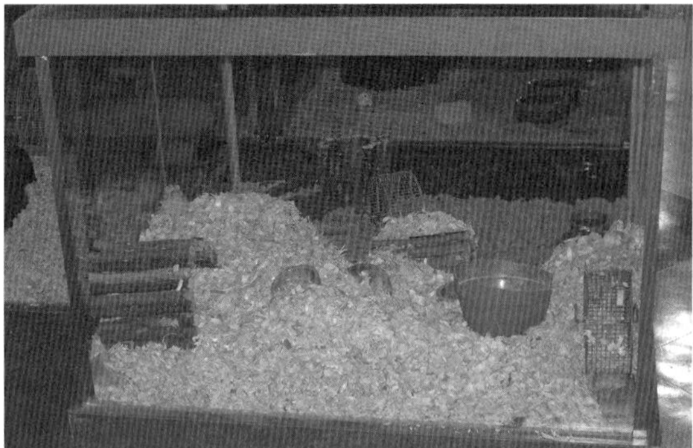

FIGURE 2.64. A large glass aquarium with a perforated lid used for housing gerbils. Animals may perform a range of behaviors and should have access to running wheels as well as hiding places.

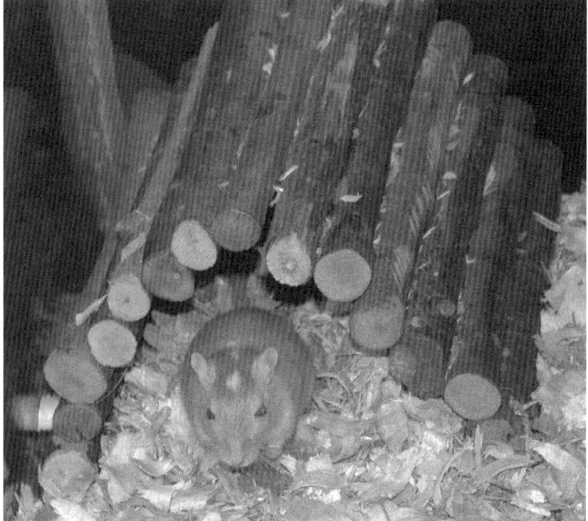

FIGURE 2.65. A naturalistic shelter used to provide a hiding place for gerbils within the cage.

and move more often than do controls. Access to a dust bath assists with grooming (Figure 2.66).

Current U.S. guide requirements suggest that mature gerbils older than 12 weeks require a floor area of 230 cm^2 (36 in^2) per animal. A breeding pair requires a cage area of 1300 cm^2 (180 in^2). Cage sides should be at least 15 cm (6 in) high. Cages suitable for rats and hamsters may be satisfactory for gerbils, although they may not provide enough room for gerbils to perform normal hopping or jumping actions.

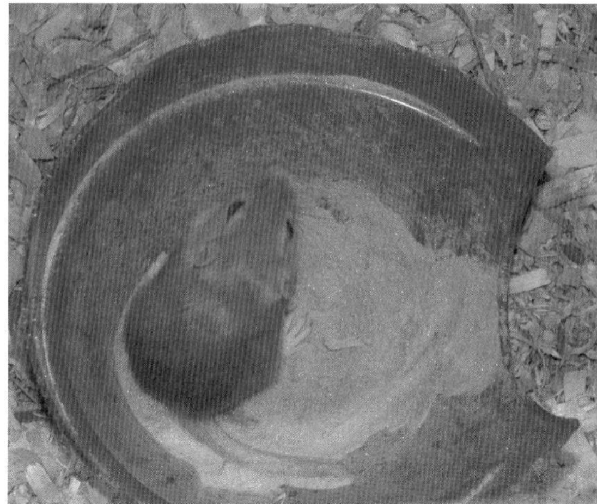

FIGURE 2.66. A sand bath will assist with grooming and maintaining the pelage in good condition. Sand or dust for bathing is available commercially for gerbils.

Gerbils tolerate a range of temperatures, but they become uncomfortable at temperatures above 35 °C. They possess greater capacity for heat regulation than do other pets and laboratory rodents because of their desert origin. Their tolerance of heat decreases as humidity increases. In the wild, their habitat of deep burrows provides a cool respite against the higher humidity and temperatures experienced in the summer. Gerbils are usually housed at temperatures between 18° and 29 °C (65–85 °F) with a temperature at 22 °C (72 °F) accepted as a compromise. The environmental humidity should be above 30%, but at approximately 50% R.H. or higher, the gerbil's hair coat becomes roughened and damp. A 12:12 hour light:dark cycle is the usual light cycle for laboratory housing.

Gerbils have efficient urine concentrating abilities and fecal pellets are small, dry, and hard. In gerbil colonies, the bedding is usually changed when dirty or every 1–2 weeks. Nests of lactating females should be disturbed as little as possible to minimize cannibalism. Nests may be transferred intact to new clean cages. Cages should be washed with hot water and detergent, disinfected, and rinsed.

Feeding and Watering

Gerbils are granivorous or herbivorous and may be fed ad libitum using a food hopper. Gerbils should be fed a complete, freshly milled, pelleted rodent chow containing approximately 16–22% protein. Young begin eating at approximately 15 days of age. Mortality ensues when food in hoppers or water is inaccessible; therefore, supplementary food provided on the cage floor may be necessary for younger animals. Quality hamster and gerbil pelleted feeds (not seeds only) are usually available in pet stores. Adult gerbils consume 5–8 g of feed daily. Females display more food hoarding behavior than do males.

Gerbils may prefer sunflower seeds to pelleted chows, but such seeds, with low-calcium and high-fat content, are not a complete diet. Gerbils 2–5 weeks old may have difficulty opening the sunflower seeds or gnawing the hard pellets, so the pellets should be softened by presoaking in water. Although gerbils in the wild feed on seeds and succulents and require little water, gerbils that are water deprived stabilize at approximately 86% of hydrated weight.

Caged gerbils should be supplied continuously with clean water. Inadequate water consumption may result in infertility, reduced body weight, and death secondary to dehydration. Although gerbils maintain weight when receiving as little as 2 mL of water daily, adult gerbils will consume approximately 4–10 mL daily. Older males drink more water than do females or younger males. Sipper tubes should reach to and be operable by the smallest cage inhabitant. Increased drinking behavior in gerbils may be an indication of disease, for example, chronic renal failure.

Reproduction

Sexing

Weanling and older males have a dark scrotum, and the anogenital distance is substantially greater in males (10 mm) than in females (5 mm), which makes sexing relatively straightforward (Figures 2.67 and 2.68). Both sexes have a genital papilla. The midventral marking (sebaceous) or scent gland is androgen-sensitive and approximately twice as large in the male.

Estrous Cycle

Gerbils are nonseasonally polyestrous and generally breed throughout the year. They are mated at 10–12 weeks of age when they weigh approximately 55–70 g; however, the testes may descend and the vagina may open as early as 28 and 40 days, respectively. Because gerbils are often permanently paired, the detection of estrus is rarely a factor in breeding.

The gerbil's estrous cycle lasts 4–6 days, and a fertile, postpartum estrus occurs within 18 hours of parturition in approximately 60% of gerbils. As a rule, the gestation period of lactating gerbils is increased by up to 2 days for each young nursed. Estrus lasts approximately 24 hours, and gerbils in estrus are restless and may have a congested vulva. Estrus may be induced by vaginal stimulation or by pairing adult males and females.

Breeding Programs

Gerbils breed readily in the home or laboratory environment. Breeding pairs established before sexual maturity, at approximately 7–8 weeks of age, are usually stable, monogamous, lifelong arrangements in which one partner's removal or death may render the other sexually and socially incompatible in subsequent pairings or may induce pregnancy failure. The affiliative behavior within pairs may be due to discrimination of a mate's urine odor, although initial pair formation may be determined by pheromones in parotid gland saliva.

The male participates in the care of young and is left in the cage at all times. Separation of breeding pairs should follow fighting, rejection, or aggression toward the young. Some breeders remove the male gerbil for 2 weeks postpartum to eliminate postpartum mating and reduce disturbance of the female and young. The 2-week period should not be lengthened because of the increased potential for fighting when they are reunited. Polygamous (trio) harem groups have been used successfully, but fighting may result.

Pregnancy and Rearing

During pregnancy a mature gerbil will gain between 10 and 30 g. The gestation period of nonlactating gerbils lasts 24–26 days, although both shorter (19–21 days) and longer periods have been reported. Use of the postpartum estrus will lead to concomitant pregnancy and lactation, a situation that leads to delayed implantation and therefore prolonged gestation. In this case, gestation may be as long as 48 days.

Nest-building behavior occurs in both pregnant and nonpregnant gerbils. This activity is accentuated

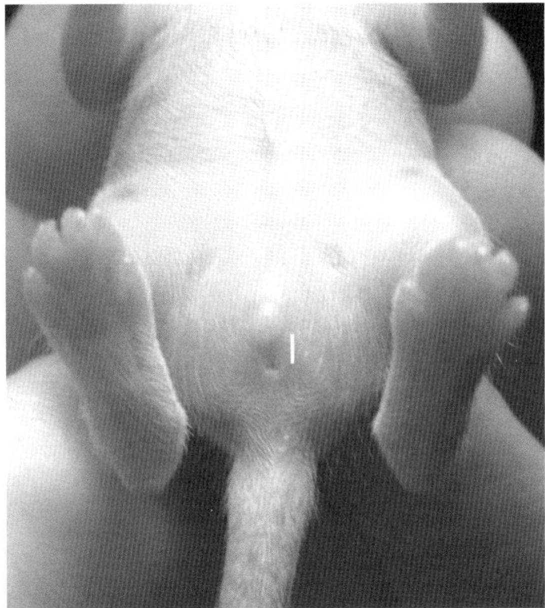

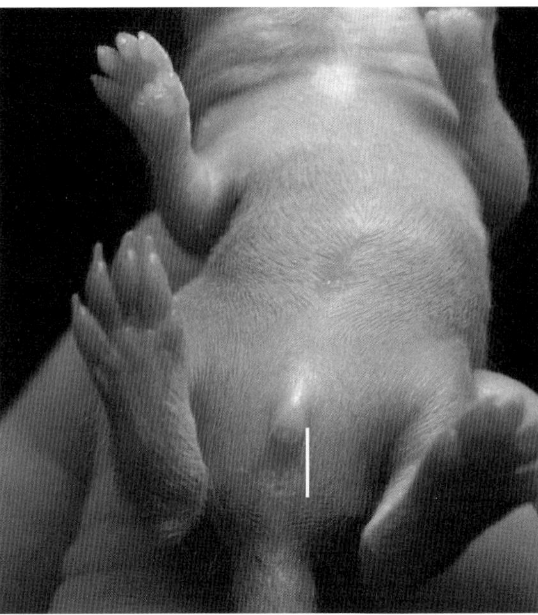

FIGURE 2.67. External genitalia of an 11-day-old female (left) and male (right) pup. The distance between the urogenital papilla and the anus (white bar) is longer in the male even at this age. Nipples are clearly visible on the ventral abdomen of the female pup but not on the male pup. As for many rodent species, pups are born hairless and begin to develop a hair coat between 10 and 14 days. Courtesy of Leah Frei.

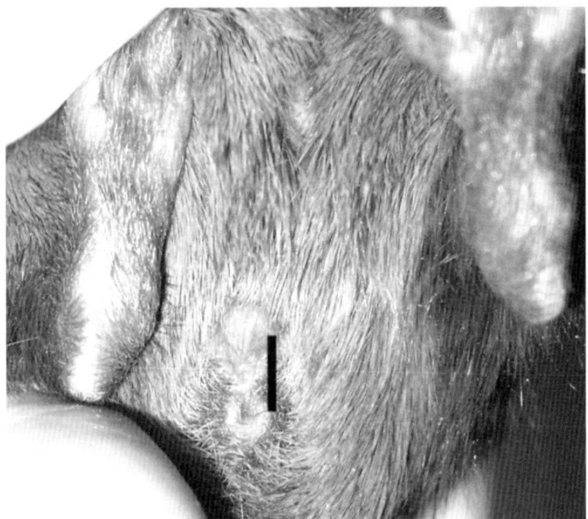

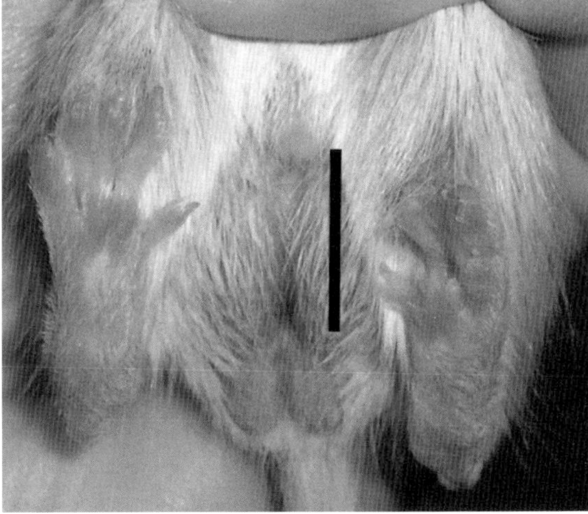

FIGURE 2.68. External genitalia of an adult female (left) and adult male (right) gerbil. The anogenital distance (black bar) is much longer for the male, compared with the female. Scrotal sacs are also present in the male. Courtesy of Leah Frei.

in cooler temperatures. Nests may be constructed from a variety of materials such as paper, cardboard, wooden wool, or commercial nesting materials, which gerbils are adept at shredding. Maternal nests are often covered. A hardwood box, ceramic container, or plastic tube or igloo placed in the cage facilitates nest building.

Usually 3–7 (1–12) gerbils are born per litter, and delivery is almost always at night. Neonates weigh approximately 2.5–3 g at birth and are altricial (naked with sealed eyes and ears). Neonates from small litters tend to weigh more than those from large litters. Ears open in approximately 5 days, hair appears in 6 days, incisors erupt in 12–14 days, and eyes open in 16–17 days. If the litter is destroyed and lactation ceases, the female will resume cycling. There may be a selective advantage in the wild for destroying smaller litters and rebreeding.

Young rarely are abandoned or cannibalized. Factors that contribute to abandonment include small litters (3 or fewer young), excessive handling of the young, lack of nesting material, and cages without provision for hiding. Fostering is possible if the orphaned and host litters are born within a few days of each other. Hand feeding of neonatal rodents is difficult, usually because animals cannot be fed frequently enough. This results in overfeeding and subsequent regurgitation and aspiration of stomach content.

Disease Prevention

General husbandry practices to minimize and prevent disease are listed in chapter 1. Gerbils' fondness for sunflower seeds can produce the false impression of good dietary habits; however, sunflower seeds are high in fat, low in calcium, and are not a complete diet for rodents.

Public Health Concerns

Gerbils in captivity have few spontaneous diseases and even fewer diseases of public health significance. *Salmonella* spp and *Rodentolepis/Hymenolepis* spp infections are potential health problems for humans. Both conditions are rare in gerbil colonies. Gerbils could become feral in North America and cause extensive damage to crops, and it is illegal to breed, own, or sell gerbils as pets in California.

Uses in Research

It is difficult to gauge how many gerbils are used in research annually in the United States, as gerbils are lumped together as "other species" in annual audit reports. In Canada, approximately a thousand gerbils are used annually. Studies in which gerbils are used include cerebral infarction and stroke, auditory phenomena, parasite infections, epilepsy, infectious diseases, histocompatibility, dental disease, behavior, radiobiology, endocrinology, water conservation, and lipid metabolism. Gerbils are more resistant to radiation exposure than are other laboratory rodents. Cerebral ischemia and infarction can be produced in gerbils through unilateral carotid ligation, and this technique is frequently used for surgical modeling of

Table 2.7. Biodata: gerbils.

Adult body weight: male	80–130 g
Adult body weight: female	55–85 g
Birth weight (depends on litter size)	2.5–3.0 g
Blood volume	7.7 mL/100 g
Body surface area (cm^2)	10.5 × (weight in grams)$^{2/3}$
Body temperature	37.0–38.5 °C (98.6–101.3 °F)
Diploid number	44
Life span	3–4 yr
Food consumption	5–8 g/100 g/day
Water consumption	4–7 mL/100 g/day
Vaginal opening	41 days or 28 g
Breeding onset: male	70–85 days
Breeding onset: female	65–85 days
Estrous cycle length	4–6 days
Gestation period (nonlactating)	24–26 days
Gestation period (concurrent lactation)	27–48 days
Postpartum estrus	fertile
Litter size	3–7; 5 average
Weaning age	20–26 days
Breeding duration	12–17 mo
Commercial	4–10 litters
Litters per year	7 avg
Young production	>l/wk per breeding pair

stroke. In such animals, the posterior communicating artery is ligated, and because the right and left cerebral vascular supplies are poorly connected, an ipsilateral stroke syndrome may be produced.

Biodata

The values listed in Table 2.7 are approximations only and may not represent the normal range in a given population.

References

More comprehensive works on gerbils include Poole TB (ed.). The UFAW Handbook on the Care and Management of Laboratory Animals, 7th ed., vol. 1. Ames, IA: Blackwell, 1999; Rowsell HC, et al. (eds.). The Guide to the Care and Use of Experimental Animals, vol. 2. Ottawa, ON: Canadian Council on Animal Care, 1984; and Bays T, Lightfoot T, Mayer J. Exotic Pet Behavior: Birds, Reptiles and Small Mammals. St Louis: Saunders Elsevier, 2006.

Other References on Gerbils

Agren G. Pair formation in the Mongolian gerbil. Anim Behav. 1984, 32:528–535.

Anastasi D. Gerbils: The Complete Guide to Gerbil Care. Irvine, CA: Bowtie Press, 2005.

Arrington LR, Ammerman CB, Franke DE. Protein requirement of growing gerbils. Lab Anim Sci. 1973, 23:851–854.

Brown RE, et al. Mate recognition by urine odors in the Mongolian gerbil (Meriones unguiculatus). Behav Neurol Biol. 1988, 49:174–183.

Cheal M. The gerbil: a unique model for research in aging. Exp Aging Res. 1986, 12:3–21.

———. Lifespan environmental influences on species typical behavior of Meriones unguiculatus. Basic Life Sci. 1987, 42:145–159.

———. Lifespan ontogeny of breeding and reproductive success in Mongolian gerbils. Lab Anim. 1983, 17:240–245.

Clark MM, Crews D, Galef BG, Jr. Androgen mediated effects of male fetuses on the behavior of dams late in pregnancy. Dev Psychobiol. 1993, 26:25–35.

Clark MM, Spencer CA, Galef BG, Jr. Improving the productivity of breeding colonies of Mongolian gerbils (Meriones unguiculatus). Lab Anim. 1986, 20:313–315.

De la Cruz F, Junquera J. The immobility response elicited by clamping, bandaging, and grasping in the Mongolian gerbil (Meriones unguiculatus). Behav Brain Res. 1993, 54:165–169.

Ellard CG. Organization of escape movements from overhead threats in the Mongolian gerbil (Meriones unguiculatus). J Comp Psychol. 1993, 107:242–249.

Field KL, Sibold AL. The Laboratory Hamster and Gerbil. Boca Raton, FL: CRC Press, 1998.

Grant M, Thiessen D. The possible interaction of harderian material and saliva for thermoregulation in the Mongolian gerbil, Meriones unguiculatus. Percep Motor Skills. 1989, 68:3–10.

Kotter E. Gerbils. Hauppauge, NY: Barron's, 1999.

Matsuzaki T, Yasuda Y, Nonaka S. The genetics of coat colors in the Mongolian gerbil (Meriones unguiculatus). Exp Anim. 1989, 38:337–341.

Noms ML. Disruption of pair bonding induces pregnancy failure in newly mated Mongolian gerbils (Meriones unguiculatus). J Reprod Fertil. 1985, 75:43–47.

Nowak RN. Walker's Mammals of the World, vol. II. Baltimore: Johns Hopkins, 1999.

Ordken CC, Scott SE. Feeding characteristics of Mongolian gerbils (Meriones unguiculatus). Lab Anim Sci. 1984, 34:181–184.

Pendergrass M, Thiessen D, Friend P. Ventral marking in the male Mongolian gerbil reflects present and future reproductive investments. Percep Motor Skills. 1989, 69:355–367.

Petrij F, et al. A second acromelanistic allelomorph at the albino locus of the Mongolian gerbil (Meriones unguiculatus). J Hered. 2001, 92:74–78.

Quesenberry K, Donnelly TM, Hillyer EV. Small Rodents. In: Ferrets, Rabbits, and Rodents: Clinical Medicine and Surgery, 2nd ed. Quesenberry K, Carpenter JW (eds.). St. Louis: Saunders, 2004.

Sabry I, Al-Azemi M, Al-Ghaith L. The Harderian gland of the Cheesman's gerbil (Gerbillus cheesmani) of the Kuwaiti desert. Eur J Morphol. 2000, 38(2):97–108.

Smith BA, Block ML. Male saliva cues and female social choice in Mongolian gerbils. Physiol Behav. 1991, 50:379–384.

Thiessen DD. Body temperature and grooming in the Mongolian gerbil. Ann NY Acad Sci. 1988, 525:27–39.

Van der Linden W, Bergman F. Change in bile composition during gallstone formation in gerbils. Z Ernahrungswiss. 1977, 16(2):115–119.

Williams WM. The Anatomy of the Mongolian Gerbil (Meriones unguiculatus). West Brookfield, MA: Tumblebrook Farm, 1974.

Wong R, et al. Social preference of female gerbils (Meriones unguiculatus) as influenced by coat color of males. Behav Neural Biol. 1990, 54:184–190.

Websites for Gerbils

http://www.agsgerbils.org/Learn/Gerbil_Care_Handbook/index.php—The American Gerbil Society.

http://www.aspca.org/pet-care/small-pet-care/gerbil-care.html—basics of gerbil care.

THE MOUSE

Commensal and wild mice have spread around the world, and the laboratory or house mouse is kept occasionally as a pet. Because mice are small prolific breeders that are easily and economically maintained in large populations, possess great genetic diversity, can be readily manipulated genetically, and are well characterized anatomically and physiologically, they are the most widely used mammal in biomedical research and testing. Because of intensive study by scientists and common use in research colonies, more is known about mouse biology and disease than any other nonhuman species. Mice are also reared as pets by fanciers, and for production of food sources for reptile and raptor colonies.

Origin and Description

The mouse, *Mus musculus*, is a rodent (order Rodentia) of the family Muridae. In recent times ancestors of these mice spread worldwide from a presumed origin in temperate Asia stretching from modern-day Turkey to China, probably interbreeding with closely related species along the way. Mice can live permanently caged and managed by humans for generations, commensally in human habitations, or entirely in the wild. "Wild" mice undergo periodic population expansions, and at all times they may cause extensive damage to human food supplies and directly or indirectly transmit infectious diseases to people.

The domestication and breeding of mice by fanciers led to the genetic diversity of mouse populations that are seen today and to increasing research interest of scientists in the nineteenth century. The long-established Swiss albino or CD-1 mouse became the source of many outbred, white laboratory stocks, although there are several other origins for both white and pigmented mice. Several genera of wild mice other than *Mus* are encountered in research colonies, including field mice, *Microtus* spp; grasshopper mice, *Onychomys* spp; cane mice, *Zygodontomys* spp; and white-footed mice, *Peromyscus* spp.

Pygmy Mice

Pygmy mice, *Mus minutoides*, are the smallest members of the *Mus* family, originate in sub-Saharan Africa, and in recent years have become a trendy small mammal pet. They weigh approximately 1 g at birth and up to 12 g as adults. Their color is blackish brown to red with bellies of white, buff, or gray. They are nocturnal, breed year round, and have litters of 1–5 after a 20-day gestation. Both parents raise the young and sexual maturity occurs at 10 weeks. These mice do well in captivity, even in groups.

Research mice, as well as other research animals, may be conveniently classified into two broad categories based on host microbiology and genetic characteristics. The microbiological classification includes (1) germ-free (axenic) mice, which are free from detectable microorganisms; (2) defined flora (gnotobiotic) mice, which possess a specified flora and fauna; (3) specific pathogen free mice, which are free of specified viral, bacterial, and parasitic microorganisms; and (4) conventional mice, which include almost all other mice housed under a variety of conditions.

Genetic classification includes (1) outbred mice, derived from mating unrelated mice, referred to as stocks; (2) inbred mice, genetically homogeneous descendents of at least 20 consecutive brother-sister matings, referred to as strains; (3) Fl hybrids, produced by mating mice of two different inbred strains; and (4) genetically engineered or modified mice. It is not the intent of this book to discuss the myriad ways in which genetically modified mice may be produced; however, a number of recent references have been published on this subject.

The development of successful genetic engineering techniques for mice over 30 years ago, combined with the high fertility, fecundity, and ease of housing, have together led to the contemporary dominance of this species in biomedical research. The ability to compare genetic similarity between humans and another mammalian species has been an extremely useful tool to study gene function, interactions, disease, and evolution. A complete sequence of the mouse genome was produced in 2002, with more recent work focusing on genetic polymorphisms between inbred strains and specific gene function (http://www.informatics.jax.org/).

Several inbreeding schemes exist, and brother-sister mating schemes in each successive generation tend to maximize the speed at which genetic differences (heterozygosity) are eliminated in a new strain. In general, at least 20 brother-sister matings are required to produce a new inbred strain. Genetic mapping of microsatellite markers can be used to select the animals with the genetic traits of interest, which can sometimes reduce the number of matings required for producing inbred strains. Because random mutations will occur spontaneously with time, strains maintained away from the original breeding colony will diverge genetically from the original colony over time and become sublines. This is particularly true if mice are separated before 60 generations of backcrossing.

Selective breeding and inbreeding have produced the diversity of mice encountered today as pets and research animals, with over 450 recognized inbred strains of mice. Because of this enormous variety, in addition to the thousands of genetically engineered strains, it is critical that new strains of mice be named according to conventional nomenclature rules to allow veterinarians and scientists to communicate effectively about mouse strains at a global level.

Inbreeding of mice has resulted in a variety of attractive, strain-specific coat colors. These different inbred variants can possess less desirable genetic predispositions, including tendencies toward immunodegenerative diseases and increased tumor incidence. Regardless of their use, such mice often develop complex abnormalities characteristic of the parent strains. This diversity in disease profiles among strains presents the investigator, animal facility manager, and small animal practitioner with multiple differential diagnostic challenges.

Anatomic and Physiologic Characteristics

The conventional, outbred white mouse is distinguished by its small size and the physiologic accommodations necessary for that size. The rapid heart rate (500–600 bpm), high oxygen consumption (1.7 mL O_2/g/hr), and extraordinary fecundity (potentially one million descendants after 425 days) are notable mouse characteristics.

More than a hundred years of inbreeding and strain development have produced a considerable reservoir of strain variations (Figure 2.69) and

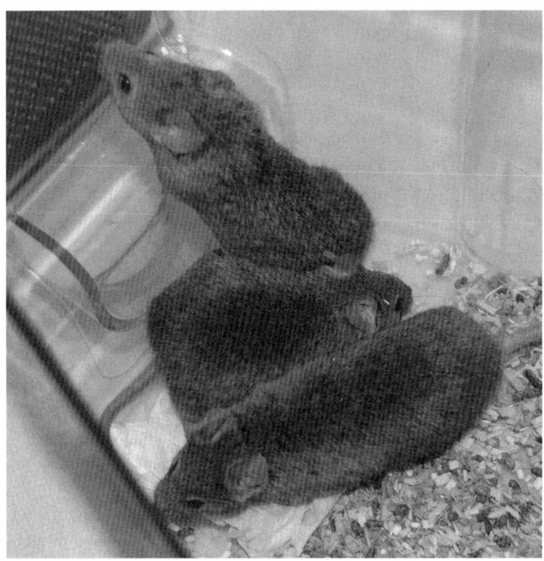

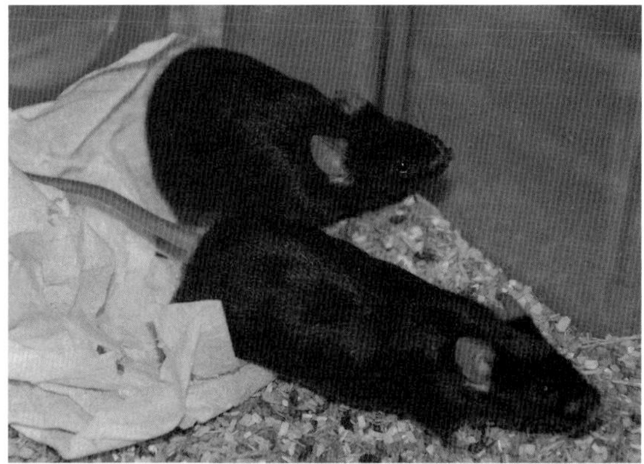

FIGURE 2.69. Numerous mouse strain variations exist with a variety of coat color patterns. Depicted are agouti mice (left) and C57BL/6 mice (right).

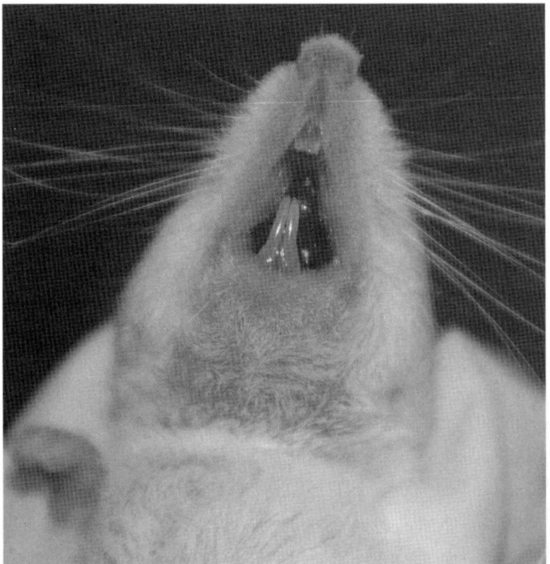

FIGURE 2.70. Normal mouse incisors. Note the relative lengths of the maxillary and mandibular incisors.

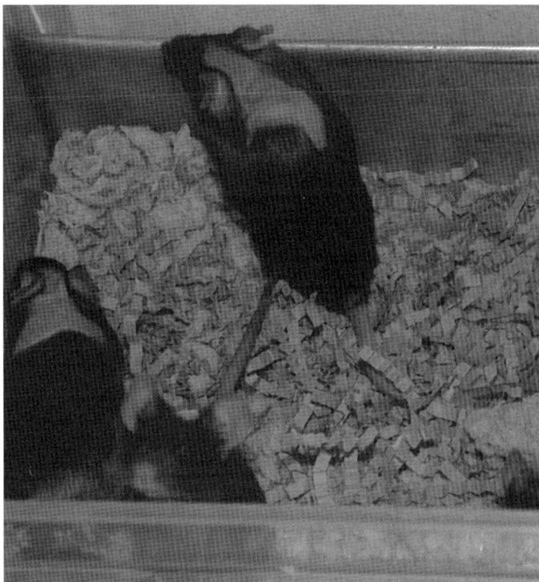

FIGURE 2.71. Barbering seen in a cage of black (C57BL/6) mice. Although barbering doesn't generally harm the affected animals, it may be indicative of a problem within the social group.

mutants, which are used by the millions in the investigation of a vast array of normal and abnormal phenomena. The following characteristics provide a small sample of available mutants: anemic, athymic, bent tail, diabetic, frizzy, fuzzy, grizzled, jolting, naked, nervous, radiation sensitive, and tottering. A wide variety of spontaneous neoplasms occur in inbred strains, listings of which can be obtained from the Mouse Tumor Biology Database (http://tumor.informatics.jax.org/mtbwi/index.do).

Some anatomic characteristics of mice include sexual dimorphism in splenic size (50% larger in males than in females); inability to vomit; a lack of deciduous dentition and open-rooted incisors (Figure 2.70); three pairs of thoracic mammary glands and two pairs of inguinal, all reaching from the ventral midline over the flank, thorax, and portions of the neck; a stomach divided into squamous nonglandular and glandular portions; and inguinal canals that remain open for the life of the male.

Mice as Pets

Behavior

Because of their small size and rapid movements, mice are not good pets for small children, but if gently handled, they can become good, albeit small pets for the older child or adult. Mice are timid, social, omnivorous, territorial, and escape-prone rodents that may be housed in small cage spaces and require relatively small quantities of food and water. Although wild mice are distinctly nocturnal, laboratory mice and pet mice are active and resting alternately throughout the day and night. In the wild, mice live in compatible, single male–dominated groups, called demes. The size and complexity of these social structures and the degree to which neighboring demes overlap are highly dependent on the availability of food supplies.

Adult mice, especially males or those previously housed alone, newly mixed in the same cage, usually barber one another or fight, as do those existing in unstable hierarchies (Figure 2.71). The hierarchical status in a cage can often be determined from the number and severity of bite wounds over the rump and back (Figure 2.72). Adult male mice, particularly those from different litters, often need to be housed separately to prevent fighting and the resulting abscesses, dermatitis, septicemia, and death. This male aggression is influenced by both testosterone and training, and both innate and

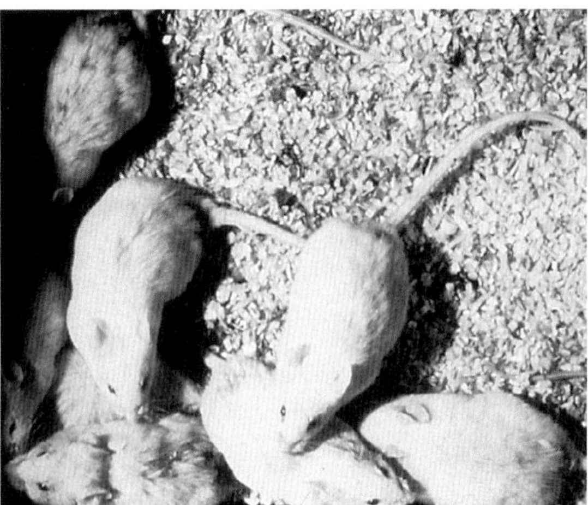

FIGURE 2.72. Fighting injuries seen in a cage of CD-1 mice.

learned components are necessary for the full demonstration of aggression. Intermale aggression can be avoided by early castration or by destroying the sense of smell, as territories are defined by urine marking. Mouse urine odor is determined by both genetics and environment and is strain-specific. Female mice seldom fight, but may do so to defend their nests. Mice housed alone tend to be more aggressive than their group-housed counterparts. If roughly handled or startled, mice will bite or pinch with their teeth. Barbering or hair chewing is a learned behavior that when seen generally indicates inappropriate housing or social groupings. The mouse doing the barbering in a cage is not necessarily the most dominant mouse, and barbering patterns may be strain-specific.

Life Span

Mice may live 2–3 years, but there are major differences in longevity among strains, owing mainly to differential tumor and disease susceptibilities. For example, AKR (white) and OH (agouti) mice live shorter lives than do A (white) and C57BL (black) strains. Pet mice are typically not inbred and thus life span and disease susceptibility are more difficult to predict. The breeding life of female mice is approximately 8 months and they can produce 6–10 litters during this period, although few inbred strains will produce more than 5 litters in a lifetime.

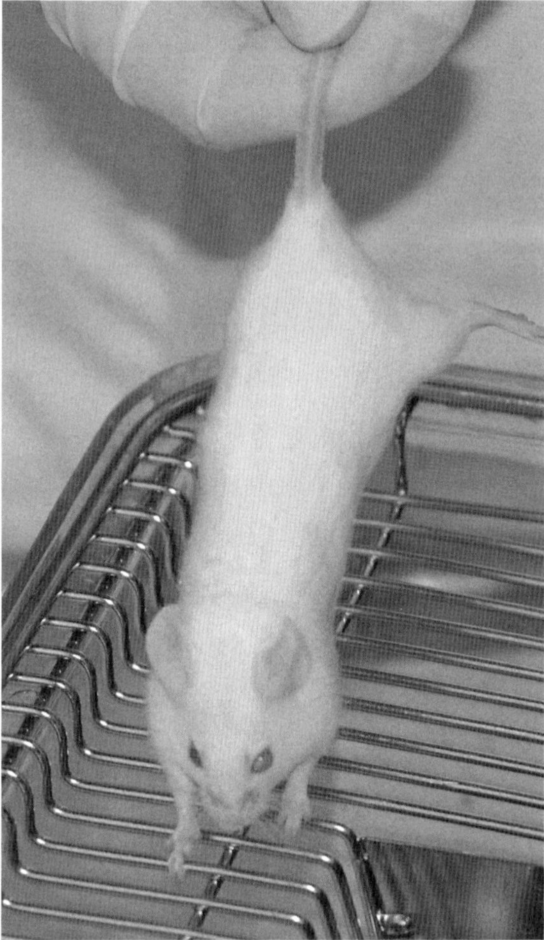

FIGURE 2.73. The cage top may be used to stabilize the mouse for scruff restraint.

Restraint

Mice may be picked up by grasping the base of the tail with fingers (Figure 2.73). If inspection or manipulation is intended, the mouse is lifted by the tail, placed on a rough, toe-gripping surface, grasped on the scruff of the neck by thumb and forefinger and inverted, and then the tail is held between the palm and little finger (Figure 2.74). Grasping and pulling the tip of the tail may strip the skin from the tail. Mice can also be scooped up using a small plastic container, and tared plastic containers are convenient for weighing (Figure 2.75).

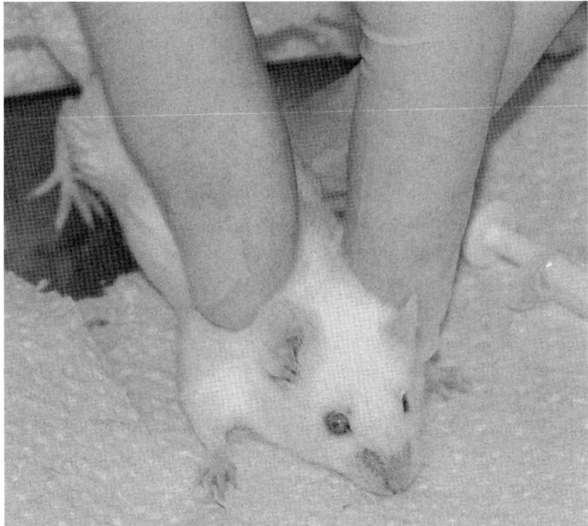
A

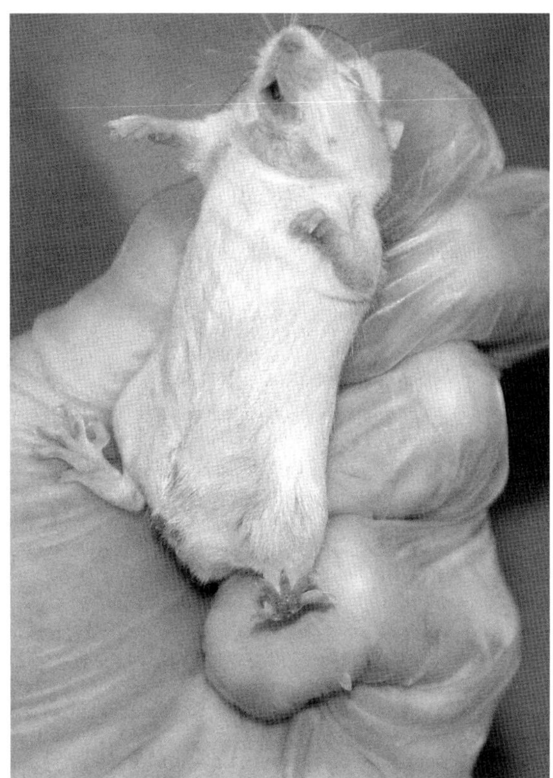
B

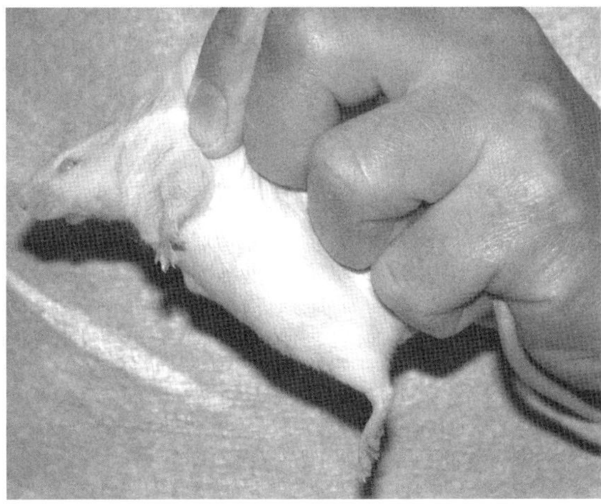
C

FIGURE 2.74. To scruff a mouse, the base of the tail is held firmly and the loose skin around the neck and shoulders is firmly scruffed (A). A well-restrained mouse is unable to turn around and bite or scratch the handler (B and C).

Housing

Mice used in research or as pets are usually housed in either metal or plastic cages with wire mesh or slotted bar tops (Figure 2.76). A homemade shoebox cage with a hardware cloth top is satisfactory for pet mice, as are the several wire and plastic cages available in pet stores. Large mice may have difficulty eating through 0.65 cm (1/4 in) mesh, and weanling mice may escape through larger meshes. Care should be taken to choose housing that will prevent escape, loss of young, and fractured limbs.

According to the ILAR guide, mouse cages should provide at least 97 cm^2 (15 in^2) floor space per adult (>25 g) mouse and be at least 13 cm (5 in) high. The CCAC recommends 100 cm^2 (25 in^2) by 15 cm high per adult mouse and 160 cm^2 for dams with litters.

Bedding, which may be paperchip, sawdust, corncob, or hardwood chip or shavings, should be hypoallergenic, dust-free, inedible, absorbent (but not cause dehydration of newborn mice), nontoxic, and free of pathogenic organisms. Softwoods, such as pine and cedar wood shavings, are used for pet rodent bedding because of their pleasant aroma and low cost. Because volatile hydrocarbons from these shavings may stimulate hepatic microsomal enzymes and may induce dermatitis and nasal irritation and sneezing, they should be avoided as a bedding material for research animals or kiln dried at high temperatures prior to use, which evaporates the volatile oils. Wood wool, paper towels, and commercial cotton nesting materials make excellent rodent nesting material. Complexity can be added to cages through the use of hardwood blocks or tunnels, plastic or paper tunnels or igloos, small nylon chew toys, and running wheels (Figures 2.77 and 2.78). Owners should use caution when adding running wheels, as mice may catch their limbs between the wheel spokes if they are set too far apart and may fracture their legs.

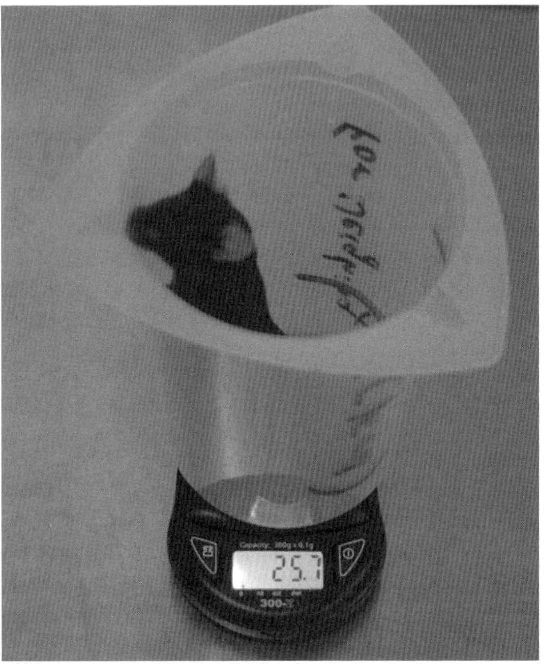

FIGURE 2.75. Small plastic containers may be used to accurately weigh mice. Courtesy of Amanda Martyn.

Temperatures in mouse rooms should be maintained between 18 °C and 26 °C (64–79 °F), with an approximate average of 22 °C (72 °F). The relative humidity in mouse rooms usually should be between 40% and 70%. Cage filter lids or covers of any type that retard diffusion of air may increase ambient cage temperature and humidity, making temperature and odor control more difficult. In research settings, these filter lids are placed on cages to minimize cross-contamination of pathogens among cages. Ventilated cage racks overcome the problem of increased temperature and humidity within covered cages by increasing the number of air changes per hour. The increased air flow may sometimes result in chilling of young or hairless animals.

Mouse caging, as for all animal caging and bedding, should be cleaned or changed as often as necessary to prevent accumulation of odor and waste and to keep the animals dry and clean. Timing of

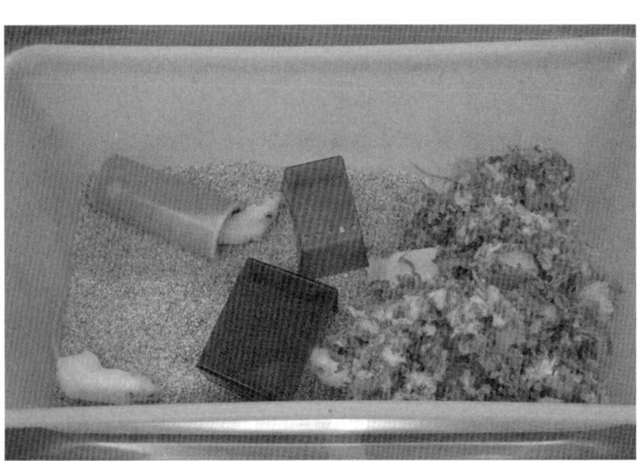

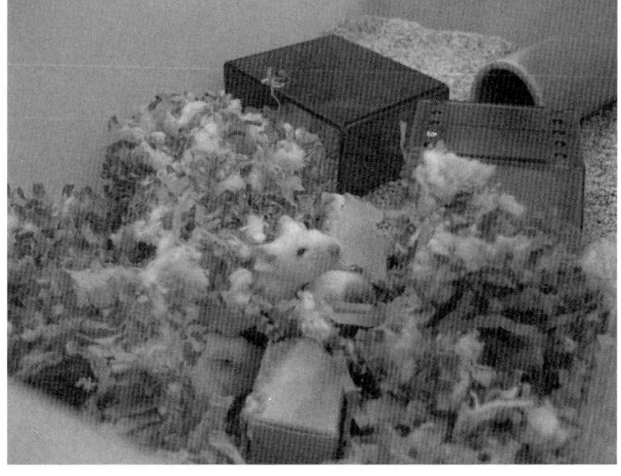

FIGURE 2.76. Large shoebox mouse cage for housing five mice. Complexity is provided through the use of shelters, tunnels, and nesting material (left). Close-up of the nest created from a paper towel and cotton nesting material; three mice are visible (right).

changes will depend on the cage population and type of cage system being used. Static cages may require cleaning twice weekly, whereas individually ventilated cages may only require changing once every 2 weeks.

Mice reared in colonies used for "pinkie" production for reptile or raptor feeding are often housed in large multifamily units with as many as a hundred or more animals per enclosure. These groupings can lead to significant amplification of endemic diseases, especially if new mice are added, and if husbandry provisions are suboptimal.

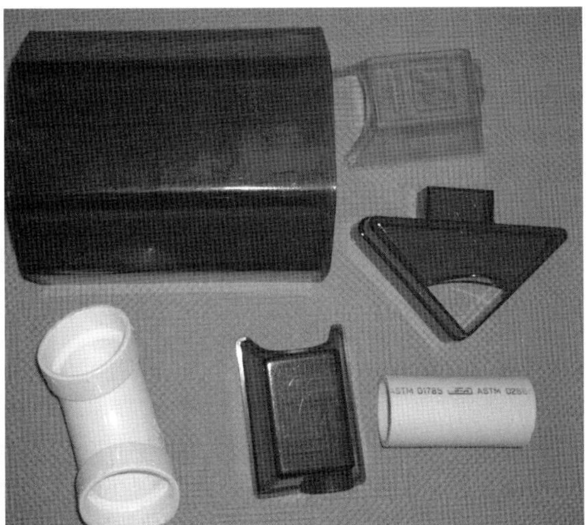

FIGURE 2.77. A variety of commercial enrichment devices are available for mice and may be used to create cage complexity.

Feeding and Watering

Mice should be fed a clean, wholesome, and nutritious pelleted rodent diet ad libitum and watered with an automatic watering system, water bottles with sipper tubes, disposable water bottles or pouches, or water-based gel packs. An appropriate source of fresh water is critical, and young animals may die within 24 hours if water is not available.

Several types of special-purpose rodent diets are available, including a wide variety of pet "treats" and feeds. While mice enjoy treats, as for other pet species, to minimize the development of obesity and other health-related disorders, treats should not make up more than 5–10% of the daily diet. The most balanced diet for rodents, including rats and mice, is commercially available pelleted rodent laboratory or pet diets. Regardless of the source, to ensure high nutrient content, the food should be purchased in small quantities, stored in a dark, dry, and cool place, and used within 6 months of milling. Special diets that have been irradiated or are suitable for autoclaving can be used for immunodeficient or barrier-reared mice in laboratory settings. While most commercial rodent pellets are produced by open-formula process, closed-formula diets and those certified free of contaminants are also available for use in research colonies.

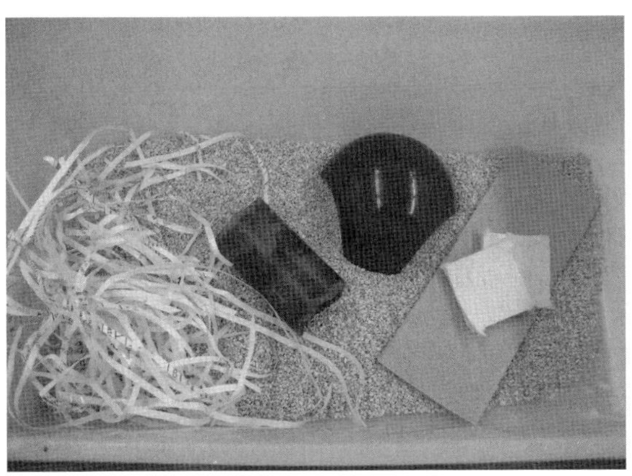

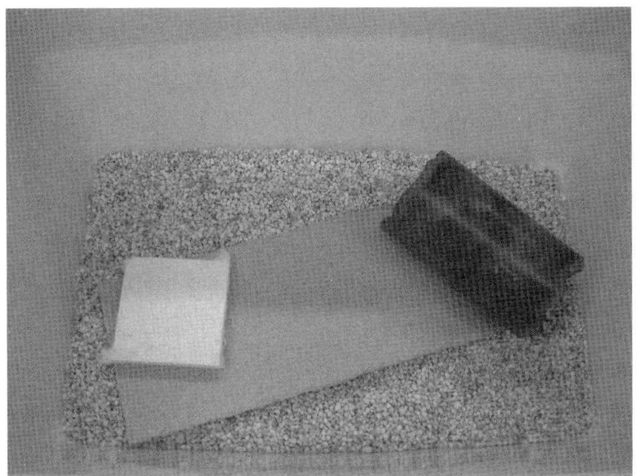

FIGURE 2.78. Enrichment may be tailored to cage size, as shown for a large breeding cage (left) and a smaller cage (right). Both cages contain inexpensive nesting material and at least one shelter for the mice.

Diets for maintenance usually contain 4–5% fat and approximately 14% protein. Diets for growth and reproduction contain 7–11% fat and 17–19% protein. Because these feeds vary in price, freshness, protein content, and quality, careful shopping is necessary. Fresh water and a high-quality pelleted feed provide a complete diet; sweets, low-protein treats, supplemental vitamins, salt blocks, and vegetables are usually not necessary and may even lead to illness.

An adult mouse will consume approximately 15 g of feed and 15 mL of water per 100 g body weight per day. Water and feed consumption vary with the ambient temperature, humidity, water availability, dryness of the feed, breeding status, feed quality, and state of health.

Reproduction

Sexing

Neonatal males may be distinguished from females by a greater anogenital distance in males (1.5–2 times), the pale testes visible through the abdominal wall, and the larger genital papilla. In females, the conspicuous row of teats at 9–13 days of age is a distinguishing feature, because, as for male rats, gerbils, and rabbits, there is no teat development in male mice (Figures 2.79–2.81).

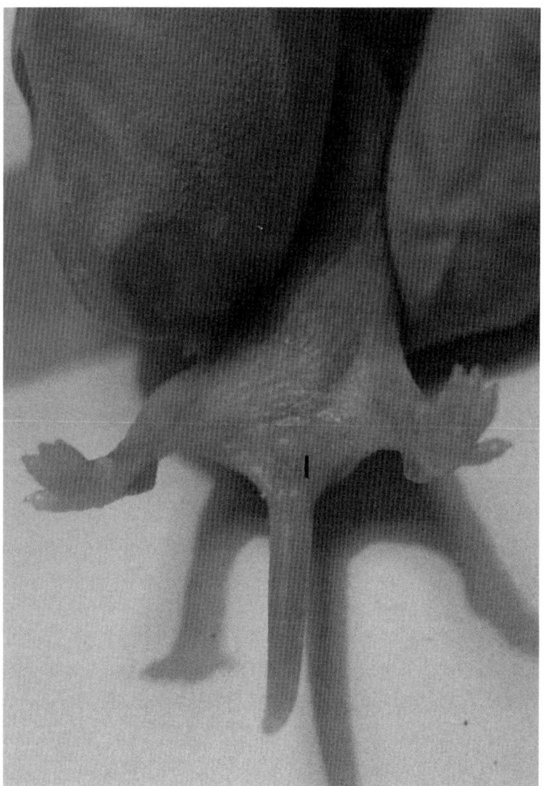

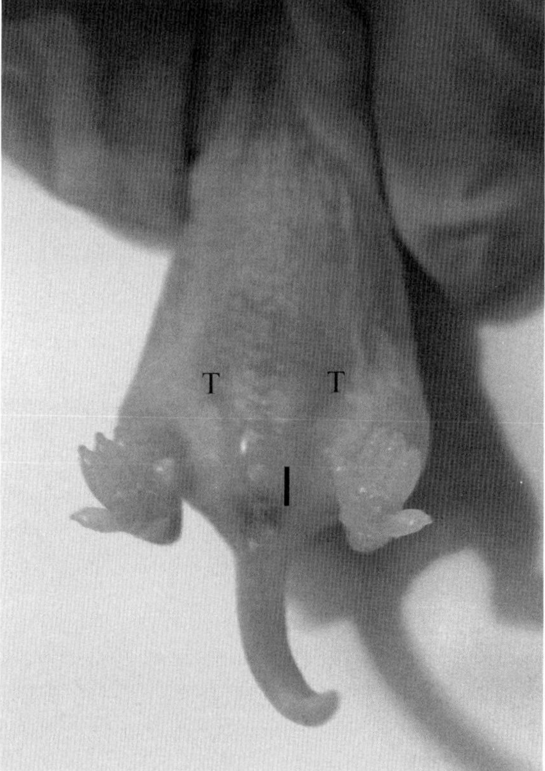

FIGURE 2.79. External genitalia of 5-day-old female (left) and male (right) mouse pups. The distance between the urogenital papilla and the anus (black bar) is longer in the male at this age. The testes can be seen through the abdominal skin of the male (T). Courtesy of Amanda Martyn.

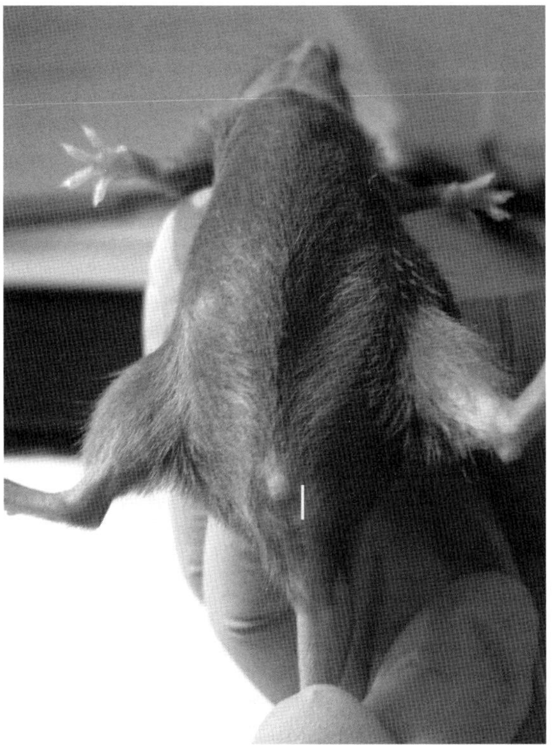

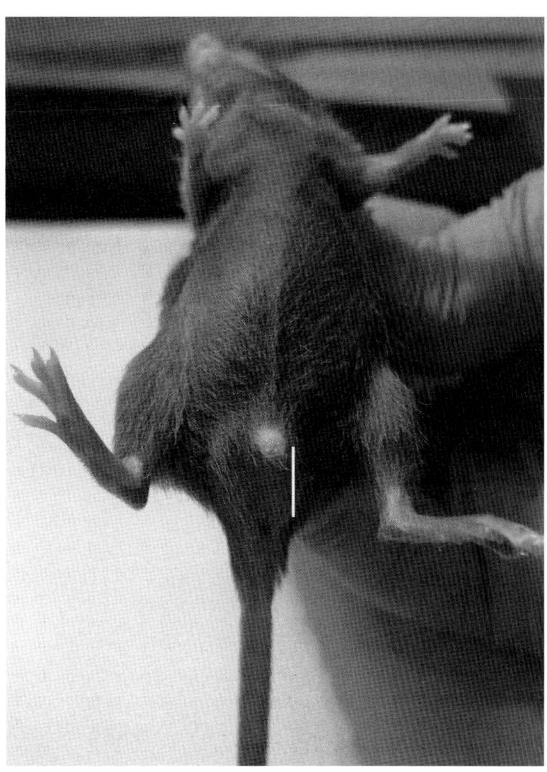

FIGURE 2.80. External genitalia of 5-week-old female (left) and male (right) mouse pups. The distance between the urogenital papilla and the anus (white bar) is longer in the male. Courtesy of Amanda Martyn.

Estrous Cycle

Although mice may have a first estrus at 28–40 days, they are generally first bred when age 50 or more days (20–30 g). Mice bred too young or after 10 weeks have reduced fertility. The onset of sexual maturity varies with strain, season, growth rate, litter size, and level of nutrition. The estrous cycle lasts 4–5 days, with an average evening estrus period of 12 hours. Except for postpartum estrus, estrus does not occur during lactation. Group-caged female mice may enter a period of continuous anestrus, which is terminated by the odor or presence of a male. Most females will then come into sexual receptivity in approximately 72 hours, a synchronization of estrous cycles known as the Whitten effect. Pseudopregnancy may prolong the interval between estrous periods.

During proestrus the vaginal smear contains epithelial cells with some cornified cells and leukocytes; in estrus, cornified cells predominate. In late metestrus and diestrus, cornification decreases and lymphocytes increase.

Breeding Programs

Considerations in mouse breeding programs include space availability, strain fecundity, inbreeding schemes, concerns about maintenance of a specific pathogen free colony, and production requirements. Mice are continuously polyestrous with minor seasonal variations. Mice have a fertile, postpartum estrus occurring 14–28 hours after parturition, and many breeding schemes use this estrus for increased production. Representative breeding systems for mice include colony, monogamous, and polygamous mating schemes. In colony mating, one male and two to six females are housed together continuously, and the young are removed at weaning. This system is the most efficient of all for use of space and labor, but record keeping is difficult.

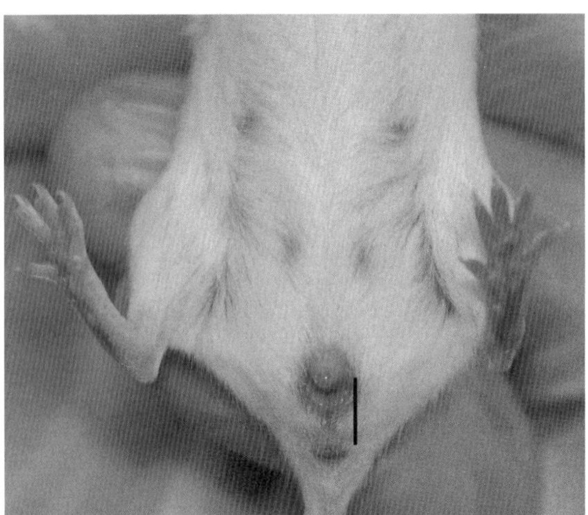

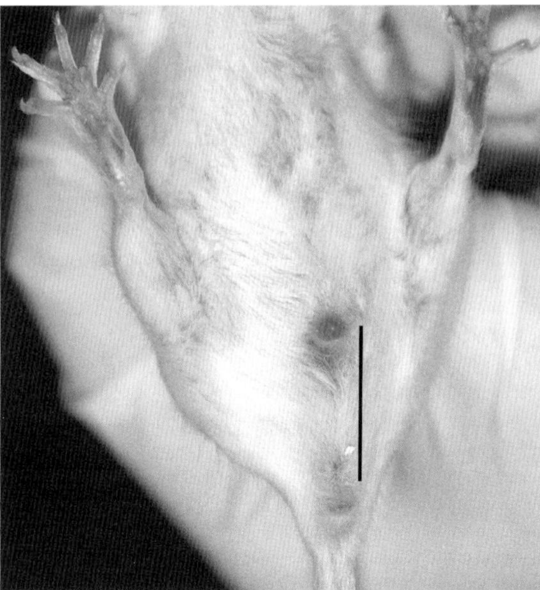

FIGURE 2.81. External genitalia of 10-week-old (mature) female (left) and male (right) mice. The distance between the urogenital papilla and the anus (black bar) is almost twice as long in the male, nipples are clearly seen on the ventral abdomen of the female, and scrotal sacs are present in the male. As in other female rodents, the mouse has three external openings: the urethral opening, the vaginal opening, and the anus.

The monogamous system involves the constant pairing of one male and one female. The young are removed before the next parturition. This system, which also uses the postpartum estrus, produces the maximum number of litters per female in the shortest time and provides for ease of record keeping and evaluation of individual production. Disadvantages of monogamous breeding include the need to maintain a larger population of males and the increased need for labor, space, and equipment to service the increased populations.

A polygamous or harem scheme combines one male and two to six females. Females are removed to separate cages before parturition and the postpartum estrus is not used. In this system, each female provides more milk, larger young, and more young weaned per litter. Dams and sires are also readily identified for breeding records. Disadvantages include lower total litter numbers and increased labor time per cage.

Pregnancy and Rearing

Detection of sperm by vaginal examination or the presence of a coagulation or postcopulatory plug (a small waxy coagulum) in the vagina is evidence of mating within the past 24 hours. Note that it is not uncommon for the plug to fall out before it can be detected, and it can be difficult to see in the bedding. Checking for plugs early in the morning will increase the chance of observing them in situ. As gestation proceeds, the mammary structures develop, and the fetuses can be palpated. Daily weighing will reveal an increased rate of weight gain approximately 13 days into gestation. Mammary development is pronounced at 14 days.

In dams without current litters, the gestation period ranges from 19 to 21 days. Simultaneous lactation and pregnancy delays uterine implantation of conceptuses and prolongs the gestation period 3–10 days, depending on the size of the nursing litter. The gestation period in hybrid mice tends to be shorter than the period in inbred mice. If a mouse bred within the previous 24 hours is exposed to a strange male, the implantation may be blocked. This phenomenon is called the Bruce effect.

Pseudopregnancy in mice is noticed rarely but may follow male overuse and sterile matings. Pseudopregnancy may last 1–3 weeks. Mice routinely prepare small sleeping nests in the bedding. The hollowed brood nest, which may contain one or more families, depending on the housing and breeding scheme, is prepared in late gestation. The female spends much time with the young and usually will retrieve scattered young to the nest. In harem breeding arrangements young may suckle several lactating dams. In large-scale group housing used by noncommercial hobbyists, the young from several litters may be piled together in a nursery and managed by one of several dams sequentially.

Litter size varies considerably with strain and age. The first litter is usually smaller, with optimal production (10–12 pups) occurring between the second and eighth litters. Inbred strains usually produce smaller litters than do hybrid, outbred, or randombred animals. Predictably, disease and nutrition status also influence productivity.

Young mice are weaned at approximately 21–28 days (10–12 g). Small mice of slower-growing inbred strains may be weaned as late as 28 days of age. In the wild, litters of mice disperse from their nest at 4–6 weeks of age. If the postpartum estrus is not used, the female resumes cycling 2–5 days postweaning. Mutilation and cannibalism of the young are uncommon among mice, but whelping or recently whelped female mice should remain undisturbed for at least 2 days postpartum. These aggressive behaviors may be strain related. Mice have a highly developed sense of smell and acute hearing. High-pitched sounds (ultrasonic) may cause audiogenic seizures in some strains (e.g., DBA/2) and interfere with communication between dams and pups, leading to associated destruction of litters.

Disease Prevention

In addition to the routine husbandry precautions listed in chapter 1, systematic diagnostic evaluation of colony animals should be conducted at regular intervals to screen for subclinical infections. Filter cage covers on static or individually ventilated cages prevent or reduce airborne transmission of microorganisms within a densely populated laboratory mouse room, although such covers may increase intracage ammonia level, humidity, and cage temperature. In laboratory settings, chlorination (10–12 ppm) or acidification (pH 2.5) of the drinking water will reduce the level of *Pseudomonas* spp contamination, which commonly occurs in biofilms and standing water, as will regular cleaning of water bottles and flushing of rack and room water lines used for automatic watering. A 10 ppm Cl_2 solution is prepared by mixing 2 mL of 5.25% sodium hypochlorite solution in 10 L of water. A solution with a pH of 2.5 is prepared by mixing 10 L of water with approximately 2.6 mL of concentrated hydrochloric acid (37.5% HCl by weight). Because of variations in the pH and hardness of local water supplies, the pH of the final mixture should be monitored and titrated to a pH of 2.5. Dental caries and reduced water consumption may occur following acidification or chlorination, and colonies should be monitored closely after instituting this type of change to ensure that animals have acclimated appropriately.

Wild mice carry several diseases of clinical significance and should be excluded from areas housing pet or laboratory stock.

Stress involved in shipment of mice (packing, unpacking, loading, and unloading) may cause immune function depression. A posttransport stabilization period of a minimum of 48 hours prior to initiation of research studies using animals allows the immune system to return toward normal. Studies using reversed light cycles may require longer periods for animal acclimation.

Public Health Concerns

Salmonellosis and lymphocytic choriomeningitis are zoonotic diseases of rare occurrence in laboratory mouse colonies. The pathogens of these diseases are more common in noncommercial settings or in pet store stock. Over 35 diseases may be transmitted by pet and wild rodents and good hygiene practices, including appropriate hand washing, should always occur after handling these species. Rabies vaccinations usually are not indicated for persons bitten by pet or laboratory rodents because these animals have reduced opportunity for exposure to commonly infected animals, such as skunks, raccoons, or bats. The exception to this is wild rodents that may occasionally be adopted as pets. There is no currently approved rabies vaccine for pet rodents.

Cutaneous and respiratory allergies to rodent dander or urinary proteins commonly develop in people who own or work with mice for extended periods of time. Such allergies are not always accompanied by a positive skin reaction to injected dander, and a physician's advice should be sought if itching, reddening, runny nose, sneezing, or difficult breathing follows exposure to rodents. Allergies can become life threatening and appropriate personal protective equipment—such as dedicated lab clothing, lab coats, gloves, and face or respirator masks—is advisable to minimize exposure and personnel risk.

Table 2.8. Biodata: mice.

Adult body weight: male	20–40 g
Adult body weight: female	25–40 g
Birth weight	0.75–2.0 g
Body surface area (cm^2)	10.5 × (weight in grams)$^{2/3}$
Rectal temperature	36.5–38.0 °C (97.7–100.4 °F)
Diploid number	40
Life span	1.5–3 yr
Food consumption	12–18 g/100 g/day
Water consumption	15 mL/100 g/day
GI transit time	8–14 hr
Breeding onset: male	50 days
Breeding onset: female	50–60 days
Cycle length	4–5 days
Gestation period	19–21 days
Postpartum estrus	fertile
Litter size	10–12
Weaning age	21–28 days
Breeding duration	7–9 mo
Commercial	6–10 litters
Young production	8/mo
Milk composition	12.1% fat, 9.0% protein, 3.2% lactose

Uses in Research

It is difficult to accurately estimate the numbers of mice used annually in research in the United States because these numbers aren't formally tracked. Estimates range from 10 to 30 million per year. Approximately 1 million mice are used annually in Canada for research, education, and testing. Uses include safety testing of new therapeutics, genetics, aging, infectious disease, histocompatibility, hemolytic anemia, congenital defects, neoplasia, radiobiology, amyloidosis, autoimmune disease, congenital athymia, obesity, dwarfism, monoclonal antibody production, diabetes mellitus, renal disease, and behavior.

Biodata

The values listed in Table 2.8 are approximations only and may not represent the normal range in a given population.

References

Comprehensive works on the mouse include Fox, JG, Barthold, S, Davisson M, Newcomer, CE (eds.). The Mouse in Biomedical Research (4 vols.). Orlando: Academic Press, 2006; Poole TB (ed.). The UFAW Handbook on the Care and Management of Laboratory Animals, 7th ed., vol. 1. Ames, IA: Blackwell, 1999; Rowsell HC, et al. (eds.). The Guide to the Care and Use of Experimental Animals, vol. 2. Ottawa, ON: Canadian Council on Animal Care, 1984; and JAX Newsletter, the Jackson Laboratory, Bar Harbor, ME.

Other References on Mice

American Association for Laboratory Animal Science. The Laboratory Mouse. Memphis, TN: AALAS, 2006.

Blake JA, et al. Mouse Genome Database Group. The Mouse Genome Database genotypes:phenotypes. Nucleic Acids Res. 2009, 37 (Database issue):D712–D719.

Cook M. The Anatomy of the Laboratory Mouse. Orlando: Academic Press, 1976.

Frith CH, Ward JM. Color Atlas of Neoplastic and Non-Neoplastic Lesions in Aging Mice. New York: Elsevier, 1988.

Green MC, Witham BA (eds.). Handbook on Genetically Standardized JAX Mice, 4th ed. Bar Harbor, ME: Jackson Laboratory, 1991.

Gude WD, et al. Histological Atlas of the Laboratory Mouse. New York: Plenum, 1982.

Hedrich H, ed. The Laboratory Mouse. San Diego: Academic Press, 2004.

Hogan B, et al. Manipulating the Mouse Embryo: A Laboratory Manual. F. Constantini and E. Lacy, eds. Cold Spring Harbor, NY: Cold Spring Harbor, 1986.

Kaufman MH. An Atlas of Mouse Development. Orlando: Academic Press, 1992.

Maltais LJ, et al. Rules and guidelines for mouse gene nomenclature: a condensed version. International Committee on Standardized Genetic Nomenclature for Mice. Genom. 1997, 45(2):471–476.

Morozov A. Conditional gene expression and targeting in neuroscience research. Curr Protoc Neurosci. 2008, Chapter 4: Unit 4.31.

Mouse Genome Sequencing Consortium. Initial sequencing and characterization of the mouse genome. Nature. 2002, 420:520–562.

Nowak RM. Mammals of the World, 6th ed. Baltimore: Johns Hopkins, 1999.

Percy DH, Barthold SA. Pathology of Laboratory Rabbits and Rodents, 3rd ed. Ames, IA: Blackwell, 2007.

Prosser H, Rastan S. Manipulation of the mouse genome: a multiple impact resource for drug discovery and development. Trends Biotechnol. 2003, 21(5): 224–232.

Quesenberry K, Donnelly TM, Hillyer EV. Small Rodents. In: Ferrets, Rabbits, and Rodents: Clinical Medicine and Surgery, 2nd ed. Quesenberry K, Carpenter JW (eds.). St. Louis: Saunders, 2004.

Röck F, et al. Quantitative analysis of mouse urine volatiles: in search of MHC-dependent differences. PLoS ONE. 2007, 2(5):e429.

Sidman RL, Angevine JB, Jr, Pierce ET. Atlas of the Mouse Brain and Spinal Cord. Cambridge, MA: Harvard University Press, 1971.

Suckow M, Danneman P, Brayton C. The Laboratory Mouse. Boca Raton, FL: CRC Press, 2000.

Theiler K. The House Mouse: Development and Normal Stages from Fertilization to Four Weeks of Age. New York: Springer-Verlag, 1972.

Van den Broek, Omtzight CM, Beynen AC. Whisker trimming behaviour in A2G mice is not prevented by offering means of withdrawal from it. Lab Anim. 1993, 27:270–272.

Vanderlip S. Mice: Complete Pet Owner's Manual. Hauppauge, NY: Barron's, 2001.

Wirtschafter ZT. The Genesis of the Mouse Skeleton: A Laboratory Atlas. Springfield, IL: Charles C. Thomas, 1960.

Websites for Mice

http://www.aspca.org/pet-care/small-pet-care/mouse-care.html—care of pet mice.

http://www.cdc.gov/rodents/diseases/index.htm—a listing of zoonotic diseases of rodents.

http://www.expertvillage.com/video-series/885_pet-mice.htm—videos on care and selection of pet mice.

http://www.mbl.org/mbl_main/atlas.html—mouse brain atlas.

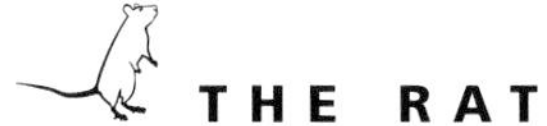

THE RAT

The domesticated variety of the brown or Norway rat, usually represented by the albino or piebald animal in pet stores or research colonies, is an Old World import that occupies a long-standing and important place in biomedical and behavioral research. Rats are easily maintained and handled, inexpensive, relatively disease resistant, and suited for a range of research endeavors. They make excellent pets, being able to learn their names, come when they are called, and readily distinguish between two human caregivers.

Origin and Description

The laboratory rat, *Rattus norvegicus*, is a rodent of the family Muridae. Wild rats originated, in recent times at least, in the temperate regions of central Asia, from southern Russia through northern China, and are burrowing colonial animals. Through migration along trade and military routes, the cosmopolitan rat has spread around the world. The rat has no special connection with Norway, likely acquiring this connotation when seen centuries ago on seafaring Norwegian ships.

Domesticated rats were raised by fanciers in the seventeenth century and for combat with terriers (rat-baiting) in subsequent centuries. By the mid-nineteenth century, rats were being used in scientific experimentation. Rats, similar to mice, are available in various microbiologic (germ-free, gnotobiotic, specific pathogen free, and conventional) and genetic varieties; however, most research rats are barrier-raised in specific pathogen free colonies. Commonly available stocks (outbred animals) include Sprague-Dawley and Wistar, and common strains include

Long-Evans and Fischer 344 rats, although numerous other types are available. There are six breeds of fancy rats recognized by the American Fancy Rat and Mouse Association and these, as well as crosses of common laboratory strains, are kept as pets.

The Sprague-Dawley rat, an albino, has a narrow head and tail longer than the body, whereas the Wistar rat has a wide head and shorter tail. The Long-Evans and other hooded varieties are smaller than the albino strains and have darker hair (tan to black) over portions of the head and anterior body. Proportions of darker to white hair vary (Figure 2.82). Strain-related aggressiveness and disease susceptibilities exist among the several varieties of domestic rats, but the variation is so great that dogmatic statements would have innumerable exceptions.

Examples of outbred and mutant stocks and inbred strains of rats of biomedical interest include N:OM (Osborne-Mendel), highly susceptible to murine mycoplasmosis; SDN:SD (Sprague-Dawley), high incidence of spontaneous mammary tumors; BUF/N (Buffalo rats), thyroiditis and resistance to nephrosis; Rochester/Wistar, interstitial cell tumors; Long-Evans cinnamon, Wilson's disease; SHR/N, spontaneously hypertensive rat; Brattleboro rat, diabetes inspidus; and the Gunn rat, hepatic jaundice.

The black or roof rat, *Rattus rattus*, is seen occasionally in research colonies. This rat is smaller than *R. norvegicus* and is better adapted to tropical climates. Rats native to North America include the cotton rat, *Sigmondon* spp; and the kangaroo rat, *Dipodomys* spp.

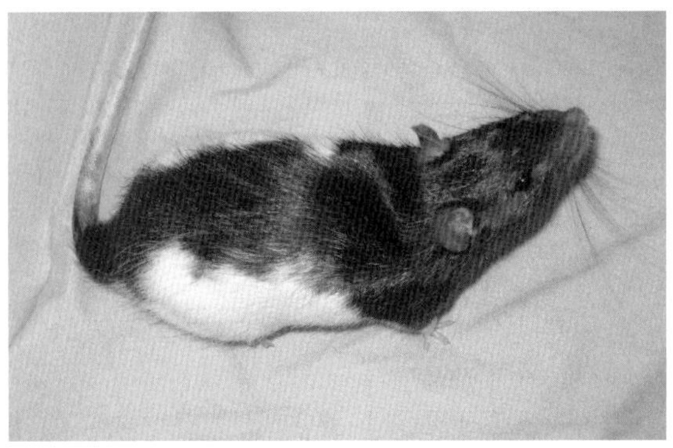

FIGURE 2.82. A Long-Evans rat.

Anatomic and Physiologic Characteristics

Rats, similar to other laboratory murine rodents, have a baculum or os penis, a (unilateral) dental formula of 1/1 incisors and 3/3 molars with continuously erupting incisors, cheeks that close into the diastema separating incisors from the oral cavity, an open inguinal canal, a divided stomach and large cecum, an articulated mandibular symphysis, both pectoral and inguinal mammary glands extending dorsally, and a diffuse pancreas. Rats have no gallbladder. They have a tapered head with pinnae relatively smaller than those of the mouse, a long often hairless tail, and an anus usually pressed against the ground.

The gnawing apparatus, shared with other rodents, is remarkable. The continuously erupting (hypsodontic), chisel-like incisors and powerful jaw muscles all contribute to the rat's omnivorous habits and gnawing ability (Figure 2.83). The 12 molars are

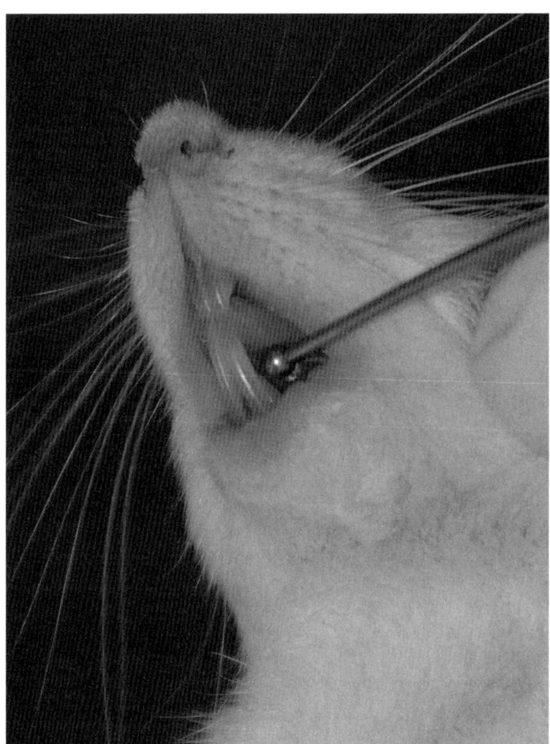

FIGURE 2.83. Normal rat incisors. Note the relative lengths of the maxillary and mandibular incisors.

rooted permanently (brachiodontic), located far back in the mouth, and are used for grinding.

Rats and other rodents have masses of brown fat in various cervical locations and between the scapulae, particularly in young animals. This fat serves neonatal and cold-stressed rodents as thermogenic material for metabolic regulation. The quantity and significance of brown fat diminish into puberty and adulthood.

Albino rats have poor eyesight and depend on facial vibrissae, hearing, and acute olfaction for sensory input. Blinded rats may appear essentially normal, although these animals may have diminished capacity to learn behaviors associated with visual cues. Behind the rat's eyeball lies a pigmented lacrimal gland called the Harderian gland, after the seventeenth-century anatomist Jakob Harder. This red-brown gland, larger than the eyeball itself, produces lipid and red porphyrin-rich secretions that lubricate the eye and lids and may play a role in determining neonatal pineal rhythms. In some stressful situations, for example, restraint or lack of access to food, or in acute illnesses, these red tears may not be groomed over the pelage but instead may accumulate and stain the face, nose, and forepaws, termed chromodacryorrhea. The dried red porphyrin crust fluoresces bright red under ultraviolet light and contains no blood.

Male rats exhibit a prolonged period of growth, and ossification of the long bones is not complete until into the second year. Murine rodents, however, mature in the first several months of life. The rat genome has been recently sequenced, and this information, in addition to that of the mouse, has been very useful in relating genetic structure to phenotype and function (http://rgd.mcw.edu/).

Rats as Pets

Behavior

Despite a well-known association with plagues, garbage, and sorcery, domestic rats, if handled gently, make excellent quiet, clean, easily trained pets that rarely bite. Rats are highly sociable and several males and females may be combined in a single, large cage. Young are raised communally with shared nursing responsibilities. Fighting occurs rarely among sexually mature adults that have been raised in close association, although sires may bother the young, and postparturient dams may fight among themselves. Rats are burrowers, omnivorous, usually nocturnal, and are year-round breeders in captivity. Escaped rats often will return to their cages.

Life Span

Rats generally live at least 24 months, although some may live longer than 3 years. They have a productive breeding life of approximately 9–12 or more months, during which time they may bear 7–10 litters with 6–14 offspring per litter. Life span is extended by caloric restriction and by feeding soy protein rather than casein. After 12 months, litter size decreases, and litter interval increases until sexual senescence at 450–500 days.

Restraint

Rats gently handled become tame and will bite rarely unless startled or hurt (Figure 2.84). Because the tail skin may deglove, the tail should be grasped only at the base and for short periods (Figure 2.85). Rats in wire-bottom cages, in particular, should not be pulled by the tail because the animal can grasp the wire and injure its feet or tear the tail skin. Rats are picked up by placing the hand firmly over the back and rib cage and restraining the head with thumb and forefinger immediately behind the mandibles (Figure 2.86). Rats held upside down are more involved with right-

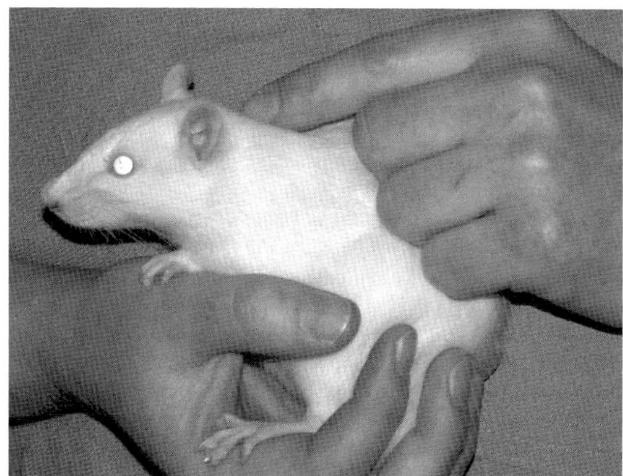

FIGURE 2.84. Gentling a rat. Holding newly acquired rats for 30–60 seconds several times in 1 day or over the course of a week will allow the animals to rapidly habituate to handling.

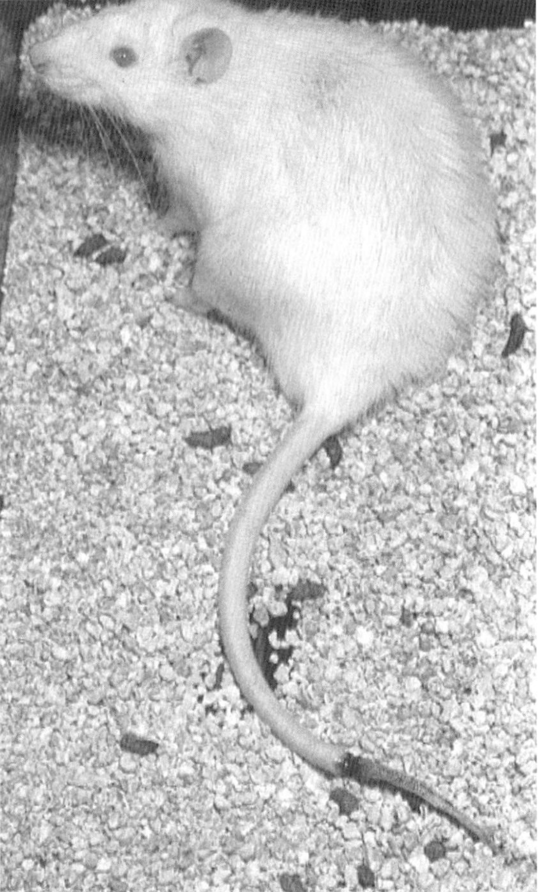

FIGURE 2.85. Tail degloving injury in an animal incorrectly restrained by the tip of the tail. Treatment included tail tip amputation under anesthesia.

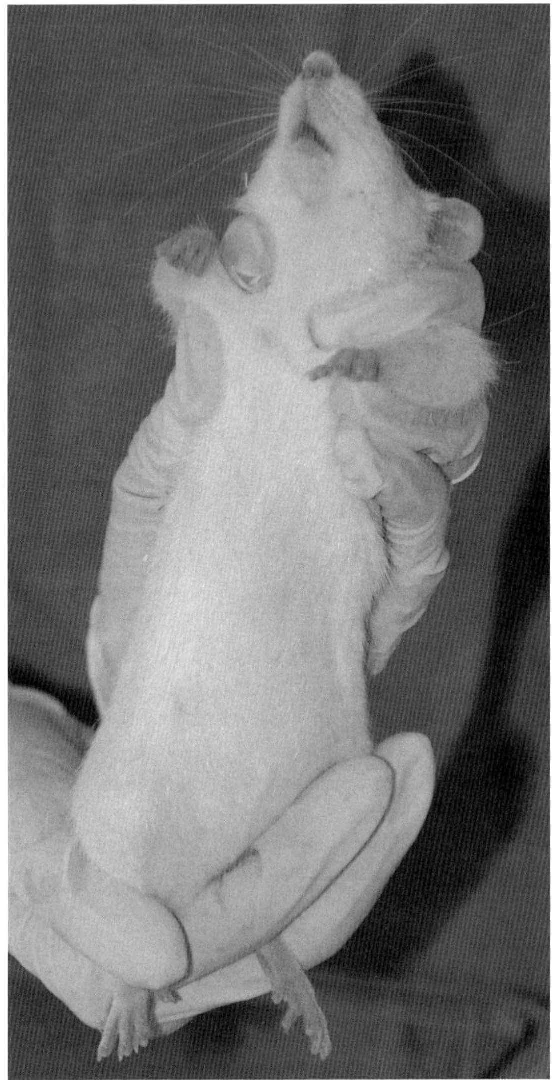

FIGURE 2.86. Over-the-back restraint of a rat. For larger animals, the hind end should be supported by the second hand.

ing themselves than with biting. A variety of commercial restraint devices are also available for use with various rat procedures (Figure 2.87). Small plastic containers or tubing may be used to remove fractious animals from their cage. Plastic containers are also useful for obtaining accurate body weights for drug dosages (Figure 2.88).

Housing

Rats are housed preferentially in plastic or wire-sided cages with solid floors (Figure 2.89). Rat cages with mesh floors, whether used for research or pet animal caging, should have grids of 1.6 cm^2 or 2 wires per inch to minimize damage to the feet, and are not generally recommended. Rats housed on wire floors longer than 6 months may develop ulcerative foot lesions that are difficult to resolve. A homemade, shoebox-shaped cage with a hardware cloth top is satisfactory for pet rats, as are the several open plasticized wire-type rodent cages available in pet stores. Terraria are used commonly to house pet rodents, but care must be taken to ensure accessibility to water and feed, and high ammonia levels may occur if the cages are not cleaned regularly. Care should be taken to

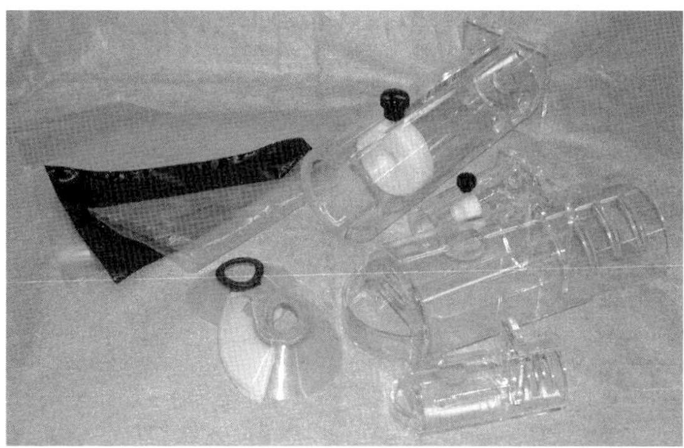

FIGURE 2.87. Various commercial restraint devices available for rats include (clockwise from top left) Decapicones®, plastic restrainers of varying sizes, and Elizabethan collars.

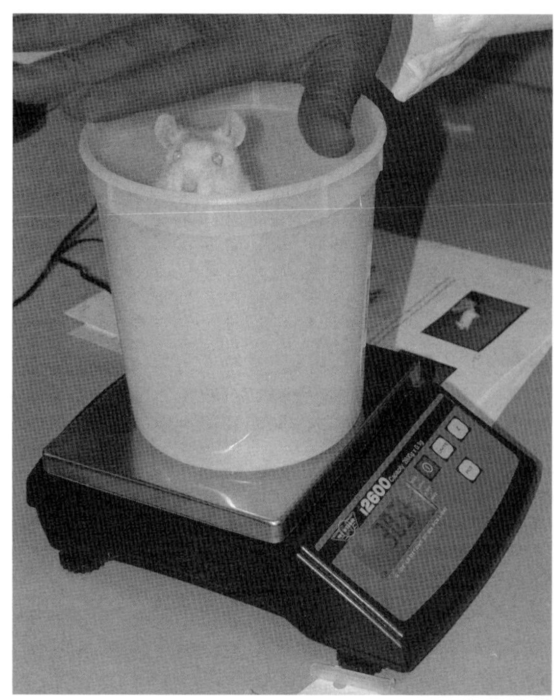

FIGURE 2.88. A small plastic container may be useful for obtaining accurate body weights of rats. Courtesy of Amanda Martyn.

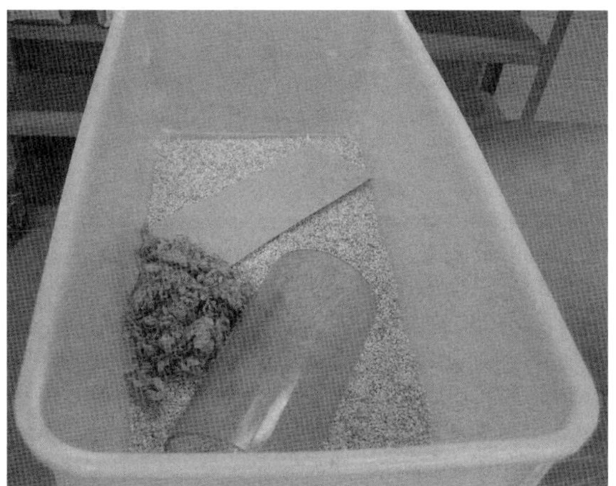

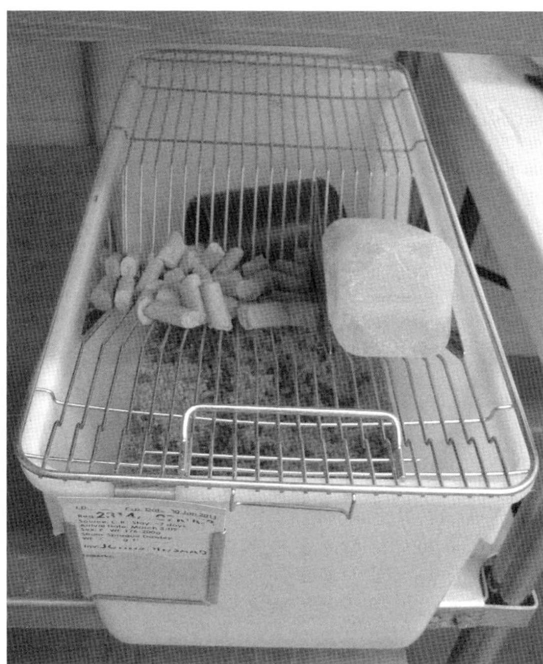

FIGURE 2.89. Typical shoebox cage used for laboratory rat housing. To increase cage complexity, a plastic tube, paper towel, and shredded paper have been added (left). Shoebox cages are typically kept on cage racks within an animal room (right).

prevent escape, loss of neonates through wire floors, and fractured limbs from floor grids that are too small. Young rats housed on wire and deprived of the nest may become dehydrated, especially during months when ambient humidity is low. Low humidity and ambient temperatures can contribute to a condition of dehydration and vascular shunting in neonates and weanlings known as "ringtail" (Figure 2.90).

According to the ILAR guide, rat cages should provide at least 259 cm^2 (40 in^2) of floor space per adult (300 g) rat. A female with litter requires 1,000 cm^2 (155 in^2) of floor space. Rat cages should be at least 18 cm (7 in) high. The CCAC recommends a minimum of 250 cm^2 (39 in^2) by 18 cm for rats over 150 g and at least 800 cm^2 (129 in^2) for dams with litter.

Bedding for rats, which may be paper, hardwood chip or shavings, ground corncob, or sawdust, should be hypoallergenic, dust-free, absorptive, nontoxic, and clean. Soft shavings, shredded paper, and wood wool are formed more easily into nests.

Temperatures in rat rooms should be maintained between 18 °C and 27 °C (65–79 °F), with the optimal ambient temperature at 22 °C (72 °F), and the relative humidity should be between 40% and 70%. The use of cage filter covers (or aquarium covers) raises the ambient temperature, ammonia, and humidity levels in the cage above those of the room. Light intensity is reduced within translucent or covered cages. A 12 : 12 hour dark:light cycle is used in rat colonies; continuous light will depress cycling. Rodents, especially nocturnal rodents like rats, do very well in dimly lighted rooms and should not be housed in direct sunlight. To effect energy conservation and to promote both good animal health and sanitation, lights in animal rooms can be controlled by a rheostat and timer, and reduced following room sanitation and animal observation. Bright lighting may promote retinal degeneration and should be avoided.

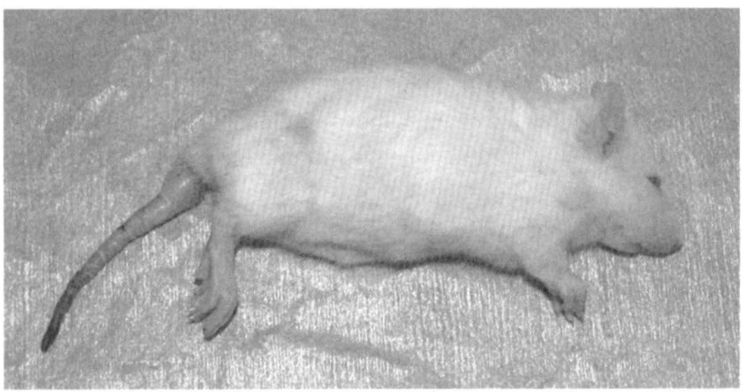

FIGURE 2.90. Ringtail, as depicted, may occur in suckling and weanling rats and mice when the ambient temperature or relative humidity is too low. The tail tip develops dry gangrene and will slough.

Litter or bedding should be changed as often as necessary to keep odor minimal and the rats dry and clean; one to three bedding changes per week are usually sufficient. Cages, feeders, and water bottles should be washed once or twice weekly. Rats can be litter trained, and some pet animals are allowed free access to areas of the house that have been structured to eliminate hazards and escape areas.

Cage complexity can be enhanced with wooden or plastic tubes, nylon or hardwood chew toys (Figure 2.91), structures to climb on, and the addition of multiple levels within the cage (Figure 2.92).

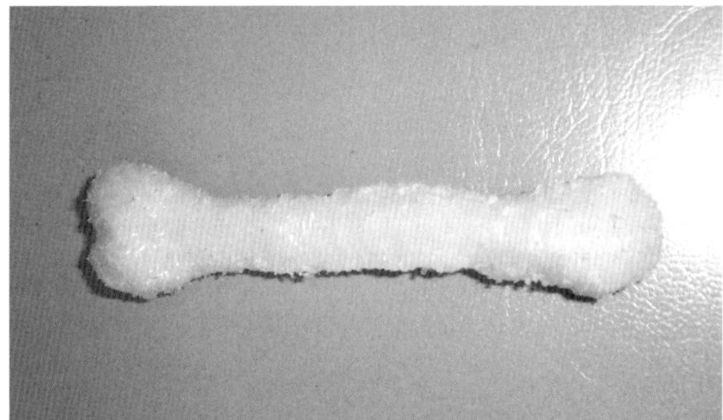

FIGURE 2.91 Nylon or wooden chew toys, such as this well-used Nylabone®, can be added to the cage for complexity. Rats may vary in their preferences for chew toys.

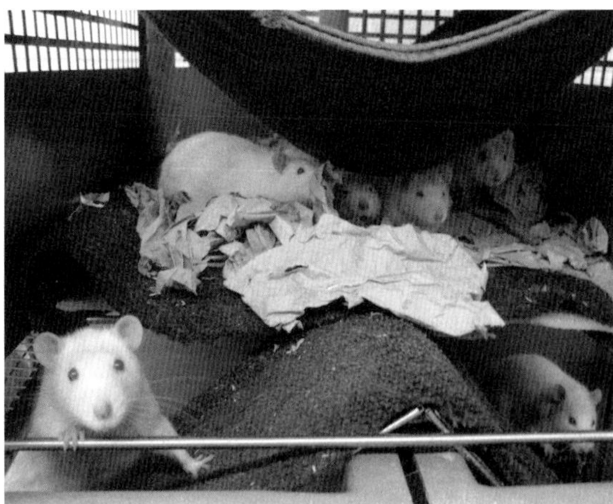

FIGURE 2.92. Multilevel rat cage with hammocks, nesting materials, and small pieces of carpet added for complexity.

Feeding and Watering

Rats should be provided with a clean, wholesome, fresh, and nutritious pelleted rodent free-choice diet. These commercially available pelleted diets for both pet and research rodents are complete and don't require supplementation. High-sugar and -fat treats should be avoided and dietary supplements should not consist of greater than 5–10% of the daily food intake. Special formulations discussed for mice can also be used for rats. Food should be kept in a cool, dark, dry place and used within 6 months of milling to ensure appropriate nutrient content. Rats should be watered from water bottles with sipper tubes or through an automatic watering system. Rats can be cautious feeders (neophobic) if not introduced to a range of foods as young animals and may avoid strange foods or consume very small quantities initially to ensure that they are safe. This is a protective mechanism for wild rats, allowing them to escape poisoning induced by gorging on potentially toxic substances. Some of the small rodent feed found in pet stores, despite attractive packaging, is inadequate in protein and energy and it can be difficult to distinguish actual manufacturing dates. It is always recommended to buy small quantities of food at more frequent intervals than to stockpile large amounts of feed. An adult rat (300 g) will consume approximately 5 g of feed and 10 mL of water per 100 g body weight per day. Consumption varies with the ambient temperature, humidity, health status, breeding stage, diet, and time of day. Rats will display distinct dietary preferences and are attracted to odors of black pepper, milk, and coffee over those of cheese. Rats are nocturnal and feed primarily at night, consuming most of their food ration within the first few hours of the dark phase.

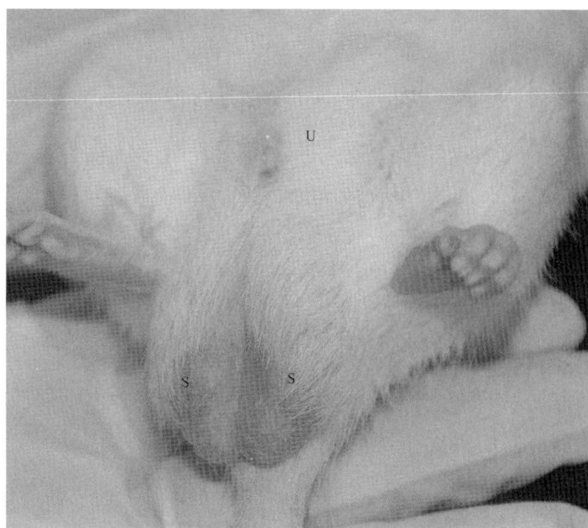

FIGURE 2.93. External genitalia of an adult male rat. The paired scrotal sacs (S) are clearly visible as well as the urethral opening (U). The anus is hidden under the scrotal sacs.

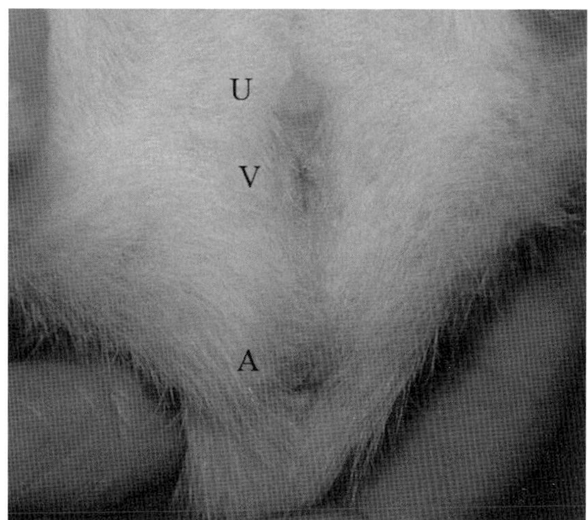

FIGURE 2.94. External genitalia of a female rat. As in the other rodent species, the anogenital distance is much shorter than in males and there are three external openings: the urethral opening (U), the vaginal opening (V), and the anus (A).

Reproduction

Sexing

The testicles are evident at an early age, especially if the male rat is held head up, as the testes will drop from the inguinal canal into the scrotum. Males have a larger genital papilla and greater anogenital distance than do females (5 mm in males and 2.5 mm in females at 7 days) (Figure 2.93). Female nipples are visible when the young are between 8 and 15 days old. A rapid way to sex immature murine rodents is to lift tails and compare genitalia among littermates (Figure 2.94).

Estrous Cycle

Rats reach puberty at 50–60 days, with the vagina opening at 35–90 days, and the testes descending at

20–50 days. Copulation may occur early in puberty. Strong, healthy, vigorous offspring are produced if the rats are mated first at 65–110 days of age, when the females weigh approximately 250 g and the males 300 g. The age at first mating depends on the strain and growth rate of the rat.

The rat's estrous cycle lasts 4–5 days, with an estrous period of approximately 12 hours, which, as in mice, occurs in the evening. The Whitten effect, an induction and synchronization of estrus in some females after exposure to male odor, is less pronounced in rats than in mice. Occasional induced ovulations may occur in rats.

The short estrous cycle and the relative docility of rats allowing group housing reduce the necessity for cycle monitoring. During proestrus, the vaginal smear contains epithelial cells with some cornified cells and leukocytes. In estrus, cornified cells become prominent. In late metestrus and during diestrus, cornification decreases and lymphocytes increase.

Breeding Programs

Considerations in rat breeding programs include space availability, strain fecundity, inbreeding systems, epidemiologic concerns, and production requirements. Rats are continuously polyestrous, with minor seasonal variations, and they have a fertile, postpartum estrus occurring within 48 hours of parturition. Although approximately half the females bred postpartum have live births, most rat breeders do not use the postpartum estrus because the sire may bother the neonates. The male is removed from the cage before parturition and returned after weaning. Simultaneous lactation and pregnancy may delay implantation 3–7 days and lengthen gestation.

Representative breeding systems for rats include monogamous and polygamous systems. The monogamous system involves permanently pairing one male and one female, with the young removed at weaning or before the next delivery. This system requires a large male population and increased labor and equipment. The postpartum estrus, however, would be fertile in approximately half the rats, and, if used, would maximize the number of litters per female per unit time.

The polygamous or harem system combines one male and two to six females. Females are removed to separate cages before parturition (usually at about 16 days of gestation), and the postpartum estrus is not used. In this system, the undisturbed females provide more milk and have larger young and litters. The female is returned to the harem after the young have been weaned. If a colony system involves leaving the males and females together after delivery, removal of the young for 12 hours on the first postpartum day may facilitate postpartum mating and increase the survivability of the young.

Some commercial rat producers move the male from cage to cage; each cage contains a single female. The male remains 1 week in each cage and is reintroduced just after weaning. One male can be used for every seven females. If the male is not removed before parturition, cannibalism, litter desertion, and agalactia may result. A similar system is used for hamsters, but the females are moved through the male's cage.

Pregnancy and Rearing

After rats mate, a white, waxy copulatory plug is present in the vagina for 12–24 hours postcoitum. A discharged plug may be found in the cage or litter pan. The copulatory plugs of rats tend to be dislodged more quickly than do those of mice. If mating occurs, sperm will also be present in a vaginal smear. Rats can be palpated, observed, or weighed to detect pregnancy. Mammary development is evident at 14 days.

Rats have a gestation period between 21 and 23 days, unless there is concomitant lactation, in which case gestation may be prolonged by several days. Exposure to a strange male within 24 hours of a fertile mating will not prevent implantation and luteotropic activity (Bruce effect), as may occur in mice. Pseudopregnancy is uncommon in rats, but when it occurs, it lasts approximately 13 days.

Rats build scant, shallow nests from bedding. Cotton, tissue paper, wood shavings, and shredded paper make good nesting materials. Pups born on ground corncob bedding are often exposed to the cage floor, which may cool the young and cause the dam to abandon the litter.

A few hours before delivery, the dam licks her perineum and a clear vaginal mucus appears. An average rat litter contains 6–12 young. Eyes open and hair is evident about 1 week postpartum. For the first few days after delivery, such disturbances as excessive handling, loud noises, vibration, and lack of nesting material may cause the female rat to cannibalize her young. If the cage must be cleaned or changed, some of the nest and dirty bedding should be transferred to the new cage.

Young rats are weaned at 21 days (40–50 g). If the postpartum estrus is not used, the female rat resumes cycling 2–4 days postweaning.

Germ-free rats have been produced by hand raising under sterile conditions, and presumably rats younger than 16 days could be fed a warmed formula from a pipette. Young rats are chilled easily, and the food may be aspirated. Simulated maternal stimulation to induce defecation and micturition must also be provided by swabbing the perineum with a moistened cotton swab after feeding. Precautions must be taken to ensure that rodent diseases are not introduced in utero or via personnel, water, feed, cages, air, and equipment.

Disease Prevention

In addition to the usual husbandry precautions listed in chapter 1, a systematic diagnostic evaluation of colony animals should be conducted routinely to screen for subclinical infections (i.e., a quality assurance program for monitoring animal health; see chapter 3). Filter cage covers prevent or reduce airborne transmission of microorganisms within a densely populated rat room, although such covers also alter the cage environment. Insects and wild rodents should be excluded from rodent colonies.

Public Health Concerns

Allergies to animal dander and urinary proteins occur commonly in humans, and cutaneous and upper and lower respiratory allergies to rats are very common. The urine of all rats contains a number of allergenic urine proteins (predominantly alpha2mu-globulin, also known as prealbumen), which may induce severe pulmonary and cutaneous allergies in people. Appropriate personal protective equipment such as masks, lab coats, and gloves should be considered when working with rats to minimize exposures to allergens. Large, crowded rat populations, poor air circulation, and infrequent cage changing and cleaning that lead to accumulation of ammonia gas compound the allergy problem in humans.

Zoonotic diseases carried or transmitted by rats include leptospirosis, streptococcal infections, salmonellosis, cestodiasis, hemorrhagic fever with renal syndrome, and rat bite or Haverhill fevers. Sylvatic plague (*Yersinia pestis*) is carried by rat fleas. The rat mite *Liponyssus sylviarum* can transmit St. Louis encephalitis virus, and *L. bacoti* attacks humans directly. Rat bite fever is caused by *Streptobacillus moniliformis*, which can be carried in the nasopharynx of asymptomatic rats. People who are experiencing rat bite fever may develop recurrent fever with petechial hemorrhages, endocarditis, and polyarthritis. Although these diseases and infections may occur in wild rats brought into a laboratory, they are rare in domestic rats, as is rabies. Excellent hygiene, including hand washing and not eating or drinking around the animals, should always

Table 2.9. Biodata: rats.

Adult body weight: male	450–520 g
Adult body weight: female	250–300 g
Birth weight	5–6 g
Body surface area (cm^2)	10.5 × (weight in grams)$^{2/3}$
Rectal temperature	35.9–37.5 °C (96.6–99.5 °F)
Diploid number	42
Life span	2.5–3.5 yr
Food consumption	5–6 g/100 g/day
Water consumption	10–12 mL/100 g/day or more
GI transit time	12–24 hr
Breeding onset: male	65–110 days
Breeding onset: female	65–110 days
Cycle length	4–5 days
Gestation period	21–23 days
Postpartum estrus	fertile
Litter size	6–12
Weaning age	21 days
Breeding duration	350–440 days
Commercial	7–10 litters
Young production	4–5/mo
Milk composition	13.0% fat, 9.7% protein, 3.2% lactose

be encouraged amongst clients, staff, and other personnel handling rats, to minimize exposure risks.

Uses in Research

Formal tracking of rat numbers used in research does not occur in the United States; however, estimates of research rat use approach four to five million annually. In Canada, the CCAC reports annual research rat use at approximately 310,000 per year. Uses of laboratory rats include studies of aging, neoplasia, drug effects and toxicity, gnotobiology, dental caries, lipid metabolism, nutrition, behavior, alcoholism and cirrhosis, arthritis, metabolism, jaundice, hypertension, embryology, teratology, diabetes insipidus, genetics, and infectious disease.

Biodata

The values listed in Table 2.9 are approximations only and may not represent the normal range in a given population.

References

Comprehensive works on the rat include Suckow MA, Weisbroth SH, Franklin CL (eds.). The Laboratory Rat. Orlando: Academic Press, 2005; Poole TB (ed.). The UFAW Handbook on the Care and Management of Laboratory Animals, 7th ed., vol. 1. Ames, IA: Blackwell, 1999; and Rowsell HC, et al. (eds.). The Guide to the Care and Use of Experimental Animals, vol. 2. Ottawa, ON: Canadian Council on Animal Care, 1984.

Other References on Rats

Barnett SA. The Rat: A Study in Behavior, 3rd ed. Chicago: University of Chicago Press, 1976.

Bays T, Lightfoot T, Mayer J. Exotic Pet Behavior. St. Louis: Saunders Elsevier, 2006.

Bazin H (ed.). Rat Hybridimas and Rat Monoclonal Antibodies. Boca Raton, FL: CRC Press, 1989.

Bohensky F. Photo Manual and Dissection Guide of the Rat: With Sheep Eye. Garden City Park, NY: Avery, 1986.

Boorman GA, et al. (eds.). Pathology of the Fischer Rat: Reference and Atlas. Orlando: Academic Press, 1990.

Brain PF. Understanding the behaviours of feral species may facilitate design of optimal living conditions for common laboratory rodents. Anim Technol. 1992, 43:99–105.

Burek JD (ed.). Pathology of Aging Rats. Boca Raton, FL: CRC Press, 1978.

Chiasson RB. Laboratory Anatomy of the White Rat, 4th ed. New York: William C. Brown, 1980.

Ducommun D. The Complete Guide to Rat Training. Neptune, NJ: TFH Publications, 2008.

Emmers R. Somesthetic System of the Rat. New York: Raven, 1988.

Everett JW. Neurobiology of Reproduction in the Female Rat. New York: Springer-Verlag, 1989.

Gordon S, Tee RD, Taylor AJN. Analysis of rat urine proteins and allergies by sodium dodecyl sulfate-polyacrylamide gel electrophoresis and immunoblotting. J Allergy Clin Immunol. 1993, 92:290–305.

Greene EG. Anatomy of the Rat. New York: Hafner Press, 1935 (reprinted 1971).

Hebel R, Stromberg MW. Anatomy and Embryology of the Laboratory Rat. Worthsee, Germany: BioMed Verlag, Birgit, Hebel, 1986.

Himsel C. Rats. Hauppange, NY: Barron's, 2005.

Koib B, Tees RC (eds.). The Cerebral Cortex of the Rat. Cambridge, MA: MIT Press, 1990.

Konig J, Klippell RA. The Rat Brain: A Stereotaxic Atlas of the Forebrain and the Lower Parts of the Brain Stem. Melbourne, FL: Robert E. Krieger, 1974.

Krinke GJ, Bullock GR, Bunton T. The Laboratory Rat. Orlando: Academic Press, 2000.

Paxinos G. The Rat Nervous System: Forebrain and Midbrain, vols. 1 and 2. Orlando: Academic Press, 1986.

Paxinos G, Watson C. The Rat Brain, 2nd ed. Orlando: Academic Press, 1986.

Peace TA, et al. Effects of caging type and animal source on the development of foot lesions in Sprague Dawley rats (Rattus norvegicus). Contemp Top Lab Anim Sci. 2001, 40(5):17–21.

Pellegnno LJ, et al. A Stereotaxic Atlas of the Rat Brain, 2nd ed. New York: Plenum, 1979.

Quesenberry K, Donnelly TM, Hillyer EV. Small Rodents. In: Ferrets, Rabbits, and Rodents: Clinical Medicine and Surgery, 2nd ed. Quesenberry K, Carpenter JW (eds.). St. Louis: Saunders, 2004.

Robinson R. Genetics of the Norway Rat. Ellens Park, PA: Franklin, 1965.

Sharp PE, LaRegina MC. The Laboratory Rat. Boca Raton, FL: CRC Press, 1998.

Stinson SF, et al. (eds.). Atlas of Tumor Pathology of the Fischer Rat. Boca Raton, FL: CRC Press, 1989.

Tabuchi E, et al. Rat preference for food-related odors. Brain Res Bull. 1991, 27:387–391.

Wayneforth HB, Flecknell PA. Experimental and Surgical Techniques in the Rat, 2nd ed. Orlando: Academic Press, 1992.

Yu BP. How diet influences the aging process. Proc Soc Exp Biol Med. 1994, 205:97–105.

Websites for Rats

http://www.aspca.org/pet-care/small-pet-care/rat-care.html—care of pet rats.

http://ratguide.com/care/—articles about rat behavior and care.

http://www.biologycorner.com/bio3/anatomy/rat_guide.html—online rat dissection guide.

http://www.loni.ucla.edu/Atlases/Atlas_Detail.jsp?atlas_id=1/Rat.html—online rat brain atlas.

http://www.ratcare.org/—care of pet rats.

Chapter 3

Clinical Procedures

Clinical procedures used to diagnose and treat diseases in rabbits and rodents include sample collection and clinical pathology, medical imaging, ophthalmology, administration of drugs, anesthesia, analgesia, surgery, serologic techniques, other special techniques, and euthanasia. Specific treatments are discussed for the diseases described in chapter 5. Treatments for rabbits and rodents are often based on extrapolation from other species, on clinical experience and trials, and on hearsay. In some cases, treatments with drugs and regimens efficacious in larger animals may be ineffective or even harmful in small mammals; nevertheless, for the benefit of the pet, the owner, and the researcher with the valuable subject, a treatment should at least be considered and attempted, when reasonable.

SAMPLE COLLECTION

Sample collection is a cornerstone of both research and clinical practice. Many diagnostic tests available for other animals are also applicable to pet rabbits and rodents. Limitations exist in the amount of sample that may be collected and the size of the collection devices; however, many of these limitations have been overcome with development of microanalysis techniques.

Rabbits and rodents are prey species and become stressed by activities such as transport, separation from cagemates, predator odors (e.g., dog, cat, ferret), handling, and restraint. Many prey species, such as the rabbit, will exhibit a "fight or flight" response, which is a display of anxiety, fear, or panic when an unfamiliar person (veterinarian or technician) or animal approaches, causing them to freeze or bolt unexpectedly. It is important to be aware of these tendencies, to avoid injury to the animal and the handler during sample collection. Sedation or anesthesia should be used if necessary and when appropriate.

Blood Collection

Collection of blood is the most common procedure performed both in laboratory animals and in small mammal pets. Samples can be challenging to obtain, especially in small rodents. Clinically useful information can be gleaned from a microhematocrit tube of blood and a well-prepared blood smear, including hematocrit, total protein, blood urea nitrogen (BUN), glucose, white blood cell (WBC) count, and a differential analysis. Some diagnostic laboratories can run a complete blood count (CBC), hematocrit, and several plasma chemistries with as little as 150 uL of whole blood, making this level of diagnostic medicine available to patients as small as 15 g. Proper selection of needle size, minimizing force when transferring blood from a syringe into a sample tube, and immediately separating blood cells from plasma or serum will reduce artifact caused by hemolysis.

Refinement of blood collection procedures used for laboratory rodents and greater expectations for delivery of medicine to all species from pet owners have motivated practitioners to become more proficient at safely collecting samples from small mammal pets. The choice of procedure depends on the species, volume of blood required, intended frequency of bleeding, whether or not anesthesia can be used, and whether the animal is a pet or a laboratory subject.

The blood volume of rabbits and rodents is 6–8% of body weight, and approximately 10% of that can be removed at one time. Up to 25% of total blood volume can be collected in a 2-week period. Blood volume is restored in 24 hours, but red blood cells (RBCs) and reticulocytes take up to 2 weeks to return to normal levels. Replacement of blood with fluids (sterile 0.9% saline) should be considered, especially if >10% of blood volume is taken. With 20–25% blood loss, the arterial blood pressure, cardiac output, and oxygen delivery to vital organs decreases, leading to hypovolemia and shock. Table

Table 3.1. Approximate adult blood volumes (BV) and suggested sample sizes for rabbits and rodents.

Species	Adult Total Blood Volume (mL)	Single Sample Volume (10% BV) (mL)	Exsanguination Volume (mL)
Rabbit	160–480	20–40	60–160
Guinea pig	40–80	4–8	15–30
Chinchilla	27–48	3–5	10–18
Hamster	6.8–12	0.5–1.2	3–5
Gerbil	4.4–8.0	0.5–1.0	2–4
Mouse	1.6–3.2	0.2–0.3	1–1.5
Rat	20–40	2–3	8–12

Table 3.2. Common sites and suggested equipment for use in blood collection in rabbits.

	Recommended Equipment		
Site	Needle	Syringe	Comments
Marginal ear vein	28 g–25 g	0.5–1 mL	Use of topical anesthetic facilitates collection For <1 mL of blood Dilate with warmth Pinna sloughing reported
Central ear artery	25 g–20 g	3–5 mL	Use of topical anesthetic facilitates collection For large amounts of blood Oil of wintergreen dilates vessel
Cephalic vein	27 g–25 g	1 mL	For <1 mL of blood
Jugular vein	25 g–22 g	3 mL	For large amounts of blood Avoid overextending neck Approach either cranial to caudal or caudal to cranial
Lateral saphenous vein	25 g–22 g	3 mL	For larger amounts of blood Collapses easily
Toenail clip	N/A	N/A	Not recommended
Cardiac puncture	22 g–20 g; 2.5–3 cm (1–1.5″)	5–35 mL	Anesthesia required Terminal procedure

3.1 gives approximate blood volumes and lists suggested blood sample sizes for rabbits and rodents.

Rabbits

Common sites for blood collection in rabbits, along with recommended equipment, are listed in Table 3.2. Many rabbits can be manually restrained for blood collection, especially if it is done in a quiet, stress-free environment by competent handlers. Wrapping the rabbit in a towel facilitates restraint. Several variations of the "towel-wrap" have been described, but the goals of each is to prevent the rabbit from backing out of the towel and to minimize the rabbit's ability to kick. A cat bag may be useful for larger rabbits. Commercially available restraint jackets, such as the Bunny Snuggle® (Lomir Biomedical, Inc.), are also available. Sedation may be necessary for fractious or stressed rabbits.

With gentle aspiration, the marginal ear vein can be used to collect small amounts of blood. Gently rubbing or warming the ear will improve the blood flow. The vessel can be occluded by pinching or applying an elastic band or paper clip to the base of the ear. It is imperative to remember to remove any tourniquet device when bleeding has been completed. Thrombosis of the ear vein and subsequent sloughing of ear tissue has been reported after blood collection or catheter placement, especially in breeds with small ears. Larger amounts of blood can be collected from the central ear artery either with a syringe and needle or by allowing blood to flow freely into a collection tube directly from a needle. If necessary, a small amount of oil of wintergreen can be applied to the skin over the artery to facilitate dilation. A topical anesthetic such as EMLA® or Maxilene® cream applied over the vessel at least 10 minutes prior to arterial puncture will minimize pain and avoidance behavior, such as head movement. If necessary, midazolam at 0.5–2 mg/kg, acepromazine at 1–2 mg/kg IM, or Hypnorm® at 0.15–0.5 mL/kg IM will facilitate restraint, vasodilatation (acepromazine), and relaxation.

The jugular vein is a common site for collection of blood volumes greater than 1 mL. Sternal restraint, with the head extended and front legs pulled downward over the edge of the table, similar to restraint for jugular bleeds from cats, and a lateral or dorsal restraint position, with front legs pulled caudally, have all been described. Care must be taken not to overextend the neck, or acute respiratory distress may occur. The vein is occluded at the thoracic inlet and entered from either a cranial to caudal or caudal to cranial direction, depending on the ease of access. In does, the dewlap may need to be pushed laterally or ventrally prior to venipuncture.

The "football" hold (see Figure 2.7) is useful for accessing the lateral saphenous vein. The rabbit's head can be tucked under one elbow to reduce visual stimulation while the leg is extended and presented to the bleeder. The vein runs diagonally across the mid-tibia and is occluded by encircling the stifle. More than 1 mL of blood can be collected with gentle aspiration. Pressure must be applied after needle withdrawal to prevent hematoma formation. The cephalic vein can yield a small amount of blood, and restraint is similar to that for dogs and cats. The vessel can be occluded by encircling the elbow with a thumb and finger, or by using a tourniquet. Covering the rabbit's eyes with a towel may help reduce stress.

Cardiac puncture requires anesthesia and is used for terminal blood collection in research animals (see below). It is not an appropriate method of blood collection for pets.

Alcohol used sparingly to wet the fur over the vein, plucking the hair from the venipuncture site, or careful clipping may be necessary to increase visibility and facilitate collection. Rabbit blood clots quickly and it should be mixed with anticoagulant immediately. To help prevent clotting, sterile heparin or sodium EDTA can be aspirated through the needle, into the syringe, and then expelled, leaving a residual amount in the needle hub. Several air-dried blood smears made with fresh blood at the time of venipuncture will prevent cell morphology changes caused by the anticoagulant in the tube during transport to a laboratory. In addition, minimizing force when transferring blood into a collection tube, removing the rubber stopper from vacuum-sealed collection tubes before expelling blood into them, and immediately separating blood cells from plasma or serum will help minimize artifact caused by hemolysis. Firm clot formation takes 30–45 minutes in rabbits. Automated flow cytometry is reliable for analyzing most hematological parameters in rabbits.

Rodents

Common sites for blood collection in rodents, along with recommended equipment, are listed in Table 3.3. A variety of commercially available and homemade restraint devices are utilized for blood collection in laboratory rodents, including acrylic tubes, plastic bags and jackets, cloth "envelopes," and Rodent Snuggles® (Lomir Biomedical, Inc.), which can be adapted to clinical practice. Isoflurane anesthesia is generally safe, and may be required, especially in highly stressed individuals. Tuberculin syringes (0.5 or 1.0 mL) are useful to prevent collapse of small veins. Microcollection tubes such as

Table 3.3. Common sites and suggested equipment for blood collection in rodents.

Site/Species	Recommended Equipment: Needle	Recommended Equipment: Syringe	Comments
Lateral saphenous vein: Guinea pig	28 g attached	0.5 mL insulin	Direct aspiration possible in larger guinea pigs and chinchillas
Chinchilla, Hamster, Gerbil, Rat, Mouse	25 g–20 g	No syringe	Clip fur and apply thin coat of petroleum jelly; use MHC tube or allow blood to drip into container
Femoral vein: Guinea pig, Chinchilla, Hamster, Gerbil, Rat, Mouse	27 g–22 g	1–3 mL	Located medially Anesthesia usually required Can place needle and collect from hub with MHC tubes in small rodents
Cephalic vein: Guinea pig	25 g	No syringe	Collect blood from needle hub as above
Jugular vein: Guinea pig, Chinchilla, Hamster, Gerbil, Rat	25 g–22 g	1–3 mL	Can attempt in the awake guinea pig or chinchilla Anesthesia required for smaller rodents
Cranial vena cava: Guinea pig, Chinchilla, Rat	25 g–22 g; 1.6–2.5 cm	3–5 mL	Anesthesia required Risk of death from bleeding into thoracic cavity
Tail vein/artery: Chinchilla, Gerbil, Rat, Mouse	25 g–27 g	1 mL	Warm tail to vasodilate vessels Can place needle and collect from hub with MHC tubes in small rodents
Lateral tarsal vein: Hamster	25 g–27 g	No syringe	Collect blood from needle hub as above
Facial vein: Mouse	22 g–18 g	N/A	Allow blood to drip into container
Toenail clip: Guinea pig	N/A	N/A	Not recommended
Cardiac puncture: All	Varies	Varies	Anesthesia required Terminal procedure

Microtainer® (Becton Dickinson) or Microvette® (Sarstedt) are available. For tests that can be run on either serum or plasma, the yield of plasma is higher than serum for a given sample (i.e., 0.4 mL blood yields 0.2 mL plasma and 0.15 mL serum). Collection tubes with gel separators improve the plasma or serum volume recovery.

Guinea Pigs

Guinea pigs become distressed when restrained in lateral or dorsal recumbency, and they prefer to be held upright and close to the restrainer's body, or cupped reassuringly on an exam table. Small amounts of blood can be collected from the lateral saphenous vein by cradling the animal and presenting the leg to the bleeder while occluding the vein by encircling the limb (Figure 3.1). After clipping the fur and applying petroleum jelly to the site, a 20-gauge needle is used to quickly puncture the vessel. The blood is collected into microhematocrit (MHC) tubes or into a container as it beads off the petroleum jelly. In very large guinea pigs and some chinchillas, direct aspiration may be successful with a 0.5 or 1.0 mL insulin syringe, using gentle suction.

The caudal branch of the medial saphenous vein can provide up to 3.0 mL of blood via puncture with a 25-gauge, 1.6 cm (5/8 in) needle on a 3.0 mL syringe.

Jugular venipuncture can be attempted in unanesthetized animals using sternal restraint with the head and neck extended upward and forward to avoid respiratory distress. The vein is usually not visible or palpable, and the skin is relatively thick in this area. If anesthesia is used, the guinea pig is positioned in dorsal recumbency, and a length of gauze looped around the upper incisors used to extend the neck. The vein is then accessed in a cranial to caudal direction.

The cranial vena cava may be used to collect large amounts of blood; however, this technique carries with it the risk of death from bleeding into the thoracic cavity (Figure 3.2). The anesthetized guinea pig is restrained in dorsal recumbency, with the front legs pulled caudally and apart. The notch between the junction of the first rib and the manubrium is palpated, and the needle inserted at a 30–40° angle to the body, aimed toward the opposite hip. Slight suction is applied as the needle is advanced. Alternatively, for terminal bleeding, blood may be collected by cardiac puncture (Figure 3.3)

Collection of blood from the cephalic vein can be difficult due to the guinea pig's short forearm. It may be possible to use a microhematocrit tube to collect blood directly from the hub of a needle placed in the vein. Because clipping the toenail is painful and the sample quality is poor, this method should be used

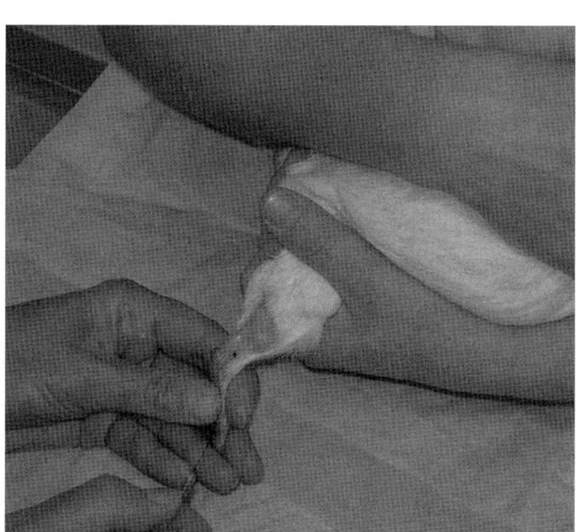

FIGURE 3.1. Collection of blood from the lateral saphenous vein of an awake guinea pig.

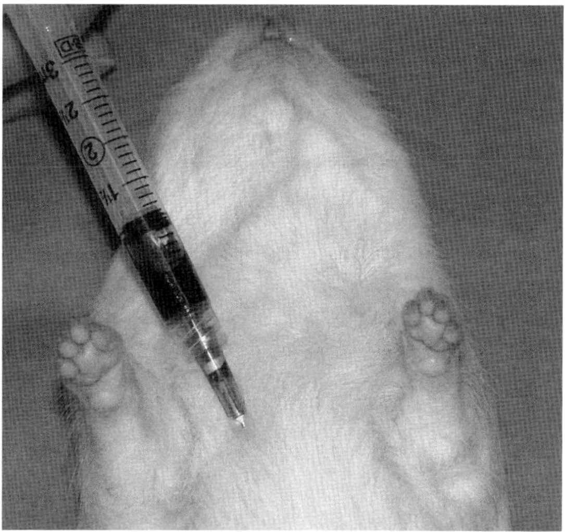

FIGURE 3.2. Cranial vena cava approach for blood collection from an anesthetized guinea pig.

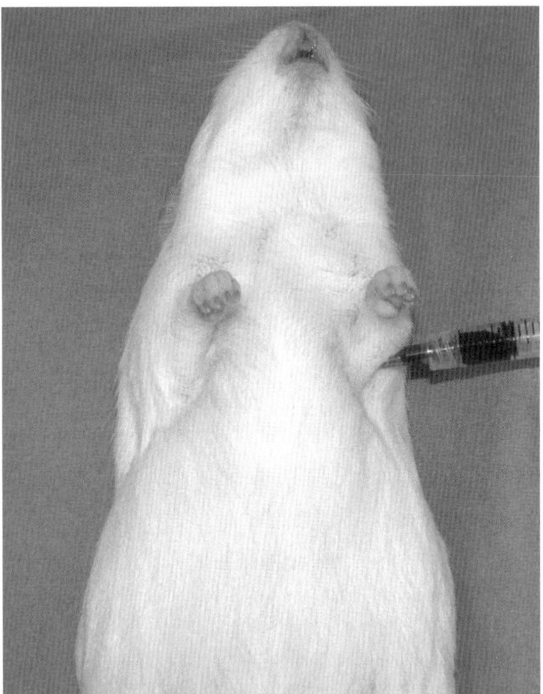

FIGURE 3.3. Cardiac puncture may be used for terminal blood collection in anesthetized rodents.

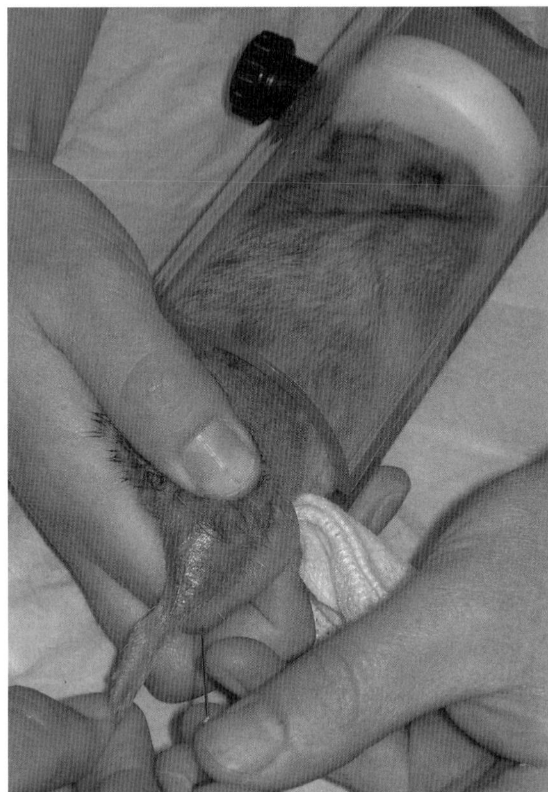

FIGURE 3.4. Hamster within a plastic restrainer for lateral saphenous venipuncture.

only as a last resort. In laboratory animals, implantable catheters for multiple blood sampling can be placed in the carotid, jugular, and femoral veins.

Chinchillas

Blood can be collected from the lateral saphenous vein, jugular vein, and cranial vena cava of chinchillas in a manner similar to the guinea pig. The jugular vein is very superficial and the skin is thinner than in guinea pigs. Blood can also be collected from the ventral tail artery. The chinchilla is restrained in an upright position against the restrainer's body, with the ventrum toward the bleeder. The bleeder holds the tail in one hand, and advances the needle at a 30–40° angle, directly on the ventral midline one-third to halfway between the base and tail tip, applying gentle suction.

Hamsters and Gerbils

Anesthesia is almost always required for blood collection in hamsters and gerbils. With practice, blood can be collected from the jugular vein by positioning the rodent in dorsal recumbency, looping a length of suture around the upper incisors to assist in straightening the neck, and entering the vein from a cranial to caudal direction. Blood can be collected directly from the hub of the needle with a microhematocrit tube. In awake animals, blood can be collected from the lateral saphenous vein (Figure 3.4), as described for the guinea pig, or, in hamsters, a needle can be placed in the lateral tarsal vein on the lateral aspect of the hind foot, and blood collected directly from the hub. The ventral tail artery and lateral tail vein of gerbils may also yield small amounts of blood. Use of the cranial vena cava presents more risk than with larger rodents but is also used (Figure 3.5).

Rats and Mice

Lateral tail veins are easily accessed in rats and mice (Figure 3.6). When collecting blood by this route, always attempt venipuncture more distally on the tail

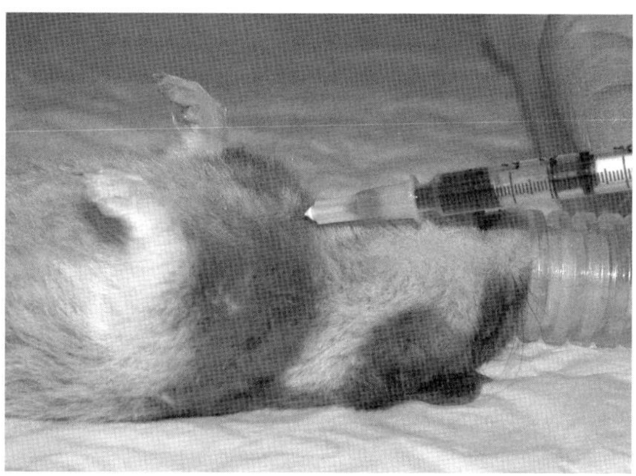

FIGURE 3.5. Cranial vena cava puncture in an anesthetized hamster.

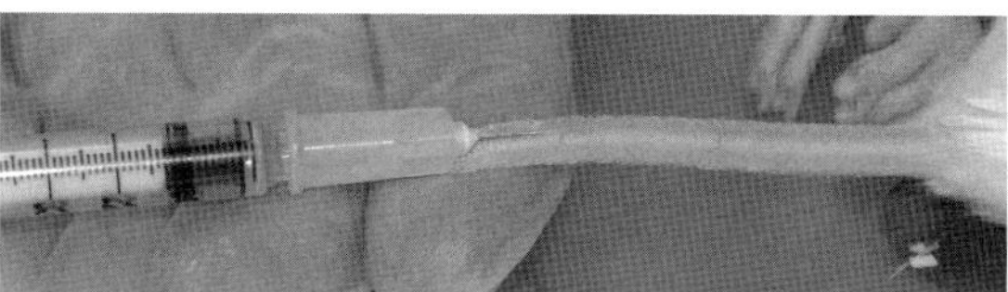

FIGURE 3.6. The lateral tail vein of the mouse can be used to collect small amounts of blood from a conscious animal or can be used for injection.

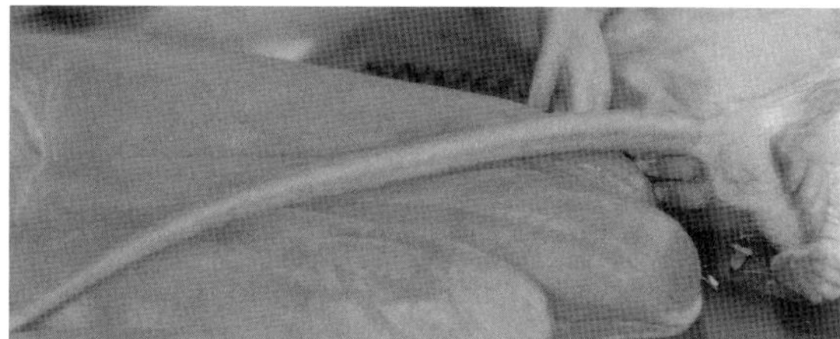

FIGURE 3.7. Both the mouse (depicted) and rat have ventral tail arteries that can be used for collection of small amounts of blood in a conscious animal. Pressure must be applied for several minutes after bleeding to ensure adequate hemostasis.

and move proximally if the first attempt is unsuccessful. Doing the reverse may result in hematoma formation and vessel collapse, making future attempts more difficult. Warming the animal with a heating pad or a heatlamp or immersing the tail in warm water will help vasodilate the vessels (Figure 3.8). Use of a tourniquet and an appropriately sized butterfly catheter with most of the tubing cut off allows the blood to drip directly into the collection

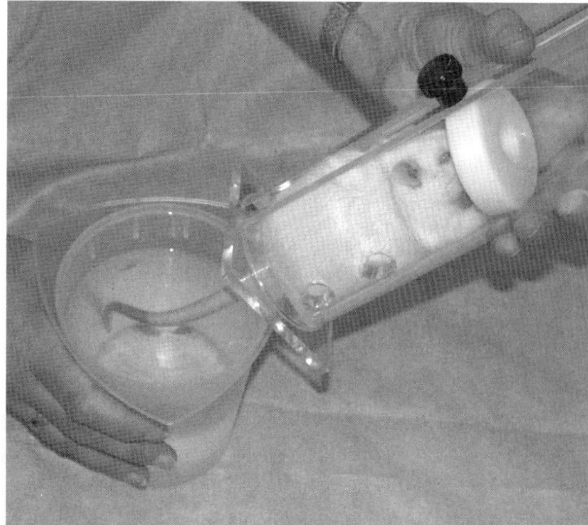

FIGURE 3.8. Vasodilatation of the tail vein can be accomplished by immersing the tail in warm water prior to bleeding. Care must be taken to ensure the water is not too hot, which may induce tissue damage.

tube. Puncture of the ventral tail artery in its distal half can also be performed in rats using a 27-gauge needle at a 30° angle, collecting blood directly from the hub with microhematocrit tubes (Figure 3.7). An alternative is to nick the vessel with a #15 scalpel blade, taking care not to cut too deeply. Use of a topical anesthetic, such as EMLA® or Maxilene® cream, may reduce the discomfort of these procedures.

The lateral saphenous vein can be used for blood collection, as described for the guinea pig, using the appropriate rat or mouse restraint device. Jugular and cranial vena cava venipuncture can be used in anesthetized rats, with the latter being more risky for bleeding into the thoracic cavity and death.

In mice, blood collection from the facial vein is rapid, does not require anesthesia, and is relatively easy to master. The restraint necessary to accomplish this procedure may lead to respiratory distress, especially when learning the procedure as it may take longer to perform (Figure 3.9). The mouse is very firmly grasped by the nape of the neck and the skin pulled taut so that the forelimbs are pulled back behind the head. A point at the junction of the mandible and a line extending from the lateral canthus of the eye (often marked by a sensory vibrissa or dimple on the side of the face) is punctured with an

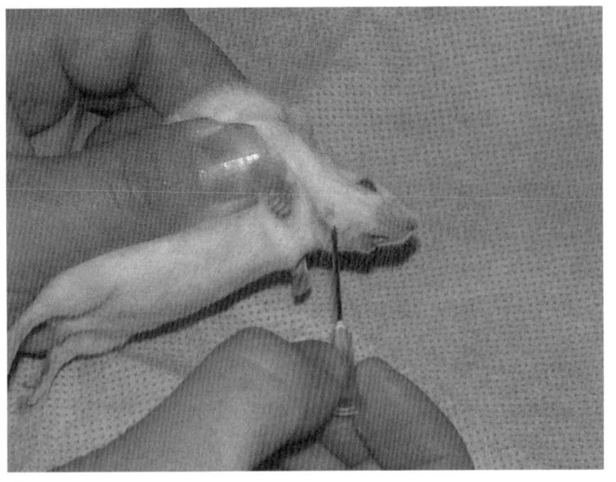

A

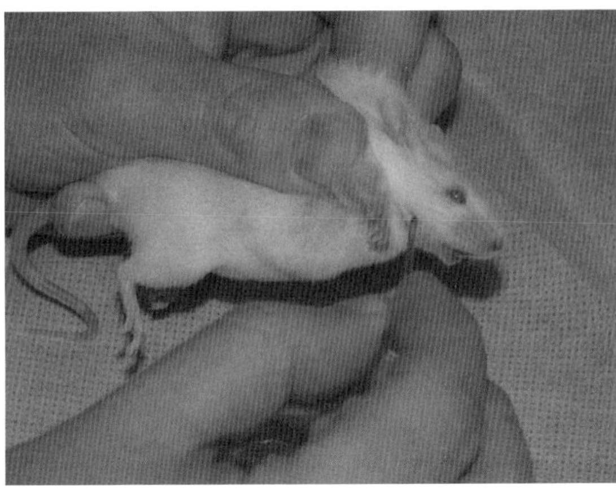

B

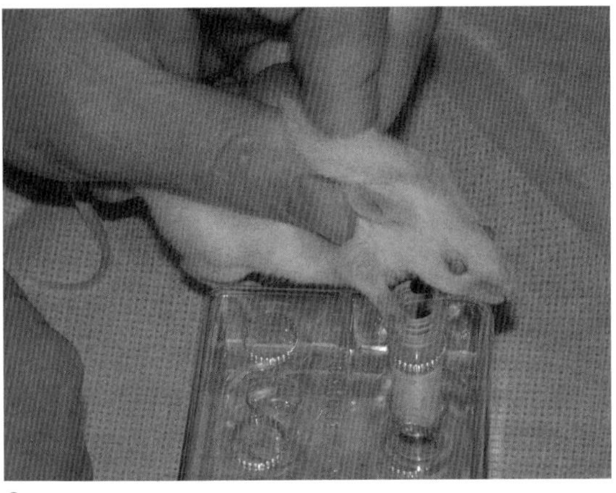

C

FIGURE 3.9. Facial vein bleeding in a conscious mouse. The mouse is firmly restrained (A). A needle or lancet is directed into the facial vein as demonstrated (B). After venipuncture, the mouse is held over a collection tube and the blood is allowed to drip into the tube (C).

18-gauge needle or lancet, using a determined stabbing motion. The mouse is held over the collection tube, allowing the blood to drip freely until the desired amount has been collected. Release of the mouse from the restraint is usually enough to stop the bleeding. Caution must be exercised when bleeding via this technique, however, as overbleeding and shock may occur if greater than 10–12 drops of blood are collected from any given animal. This is diagnosed by generalized pallor in an albino mouse and unsteadiness. These animals should be placed in a warmed environment and treated with 1–2 mL of warmed lactated Ringer's solution given subcutaneously (SC) or intraperitoneally (IP).

Retroorbital Sinus Bleeding

Historically, retroorbital sinus bleeding was the method of choice for small laboratory rodents. Alternative sites, such as the lateral saphenous vein, tail artery and vein, and facial vein have largely replaced this method of blood collection. Retroorbital sinus bleeding is not permitted by many animal care programs without strong scientific justification and general anesthesia. To perform this technique, the anesthetized rodent is held on a flat surface in lateral recumbency or restrained in the hand. A microhematocrit tube or small-bore Pasteur pipette is rotated and directed caudally and medially at the angle of the medial canthus of the eye into the infraorbital venous vessels, which vary considerably in location and size. Blood from the ruptured sinus will flow into the tube. When the blood ceases to flow or the required amount is obtained, the tube is withdrawn. Local anesthesia can be used to provide postprocedural pain relief. Eye trauma, Harderian gland lesions, and nasal hemorrhage may occur with this technique; however, the extent of trauma is often inversely proportional to the skill of the bleeder. Some institutions allow this technique to be performed in the awake animal by trained and experienced personnel with use of a topical anesthesia, but this technique has fallen out of favor because of several viable alternative methods that have fewer complications. Orbital sinus bleeding is not appropriate for the pet rodent.

Terminal Blood Collection

Cardiac Puncture

Large volumes of blood may be collected rapidly by cardiac puncture in anesthetized rabbits and rodents. This procedure is usually performed terminally in anesthetized animals, although it may be performed as a survival procedure under certain circumstances and with general anesthesia. Cardiac puncture is useful in smaller species without otherwise accessible sites for collecting large volumes of blood. The needle is inserted into the notch formed by the last rib and the xiphoid process, and directed toward the heart at a 10–30° angle above the ventral body wall. Alternatively, the needle can be inserted into the lateral thoracic region toward the area of maximal heartbeat. In rats, for example, a 24-gauge 2.5-cm (1-in) needle inserted between the fifth and sixth ribs is directed at the left ventricle (see Figure 3.3). A direct cardiac puncture may also be performed in deeply anesthetized rodents after opening the chest cavity. Large volumes of blood can also be collected by severing the brachial vessels or by collection from the posterior vena cava.

Saline Perfusion in Rabbits

Saline perfusion allows for collection of a much greater percentage of the blood volume of a rabbit compared to cardiac puncture. A 22-gauge catheter is placed in the marginal ear vein of the anesthetized rabbit and a 0.9% NaCl drip started at maintenance rate. The carotid artery is isolated lateral to the trachea, and a 3–4 French (Fr) × 70 cm open-ended urethral catheter is introduced 8 cm into the artery and secured. The saline line is opened fully and an IV pressure bag is inflated to 150 mm Hg, while at the same time blood is removed from the arterial catheter with a 60 mL syringe and placed in the appropriate containers.

Urine Collection

Rabbits

Rabbit urine samples can be collected during voluntary micturition, by housing in a metabolic cage, using direct bladder expression in the awake or anesthetized animal, via catheterization under sedation or general anesthesia, or by cystocentesis. The bladder is located just cranial to the pelvic rim and can be flaccid and difficult to palpate. Manual expression should be performed carefully as the bladder wall is thin and ruptures easily. Catheterization of both males and females is more successful if sedation (e.g., 1 mg/kg midazolam IM) is used. Passage of a 3.5–9 Fr catheter can be accomplished in the male rabbit by positioning the animal in a sitting position to extrude the penis. The urethral opening of the female is located on the floor of the vagina and is best accessed with the rabbit in sternal recumbency. Cystocentesis by ventral midline approach is performed using a 22-gauge, 2.5-cm (1-in) needle, with the rabbit held upright against the restrainer's body.

Rodents

Rats and mice often urinate upon restraint and this response can be used to opportunistically collect a small sample into a collection tube or from a plastic surface prepared for this purpose. Rodents placed on a cold, clean surface will also often urinate. Manual expression in the unanesthetized animal should be performed cautiously to prevent bladder rupture. Manual expression or free-catch samples may be contaminated with vaginal, preputial, or environmental contaminants. Cystocentesis by ventral midline approach is the preferred method of urine collection if urine culture is intended. Sedation and use of a 25- to 27-gauge needle is recommended. If sedation is not used, restraint of the animal in an upright position against the handler's body is preferable to restraint in dorsal or lateral recumbency on an examination table. Urethral catheterization is possible in female rats and mice. Animals must be fully anesthetized, placed in ventral recumbency, and held up by their tails to access the urethral papilla. A 24-gauge IV catheter (with stylet removed) is used for mice, and a 3.5 Fr tomcat catheter for rats. Metabolic cages are often used in experimental animals for repeated urine collection.

Bone Marrow Collection

Bone marrow collection can be performed in rabbits in a similar manner to dogs and cats. The proximal femur is surgically prepared, and a small incision made over the intertrochanteric fossa. A spinal needle is inserted into the fossa through the cortical bone into the intermedullary space, by rotating back and forth. Once in place, the stylet is removed and a syringe is attached. Gentle negative pressure is applied until marrow appears in the hub.

Cerebrospinal Fluid Collection

In rabbits, small amounts of fluid can be collected from the cisterna magna, similar to methods for dogs. Care must be taken not to obstruct the airway during flexion of the neck; general anesthesia and intubation are recommended. A 22-gauge, 3.8-cm (1.5-in) spinal needle is used. Fluid is allowed to drip into the collection tube. A lumbosacral approach can also be used similar to the canine. There is little information available regarding interpretation of cellular constituents of cerebrospinal fluid in rabbits.

References

Benson KG, Paul-Murphy J. Clinical pathology of the domestic rabbit. Vet Clin Exot Anim. 1999, 2:539–551.

Carraway JH, Gray LD. Blood collection and intravenous injection in the guinea pig via the medial saphenous vein. Lab Anim Sci. 1989, 39:523–624.

Chew JL, Chua KY. Collection of mouse urine for bioassays. Lab Anim. 2003, 32:7.

Diehl K-H, et al. A good practice guide to the administration of substances and removal of blood, including routes and volumes. J Appl Toxicol. 2001, 21:15–23.

Dyer SM, Cervasio EL. An overview of restraint and blood collection techniques in exotic pet practice. Vet Clin Exot Anim. 2008, 11:423–443.

Field KJ, Sibold AL. The Laboratory Hamster and Gerbil. Boca Raton, FL: CRC Press, 1999; 110–111.

Fisher PG. Exotic mammal renal disease: diagnosis and treatment. Vet Clin Exot Anim. 2006, 9:69–96.

Golde WT, Gollobin P, Rodriguez LL. A rapid, simple, and humane method for submandibular bleeding of mice using a lancet. Lab Anim. 2005, 34:39–43.

Graham J. Common procedures in rabbits. Vet Clin Exot Anim. 2006, 9:367–388.

Hem A, Smith AK, Solberg P. Saphenous vein puncture for blood sampling of the mouse, rat, hamster, gerbil, guinea pig, ferret and mink. Lab Anim. 1998, 32:364–368.

Jenkins JR. Rabbit diagnostic testing. J Exot Pet Med. 2008, 17:4–15.

———. Rodent diagnostic testing. J Exot Pet Med. 2008, 17:16–25.

Marshall K. Rabbit hematology. Vet Clin Exot Anim. 2008, 11:551–567.

McClure DE. Clinical pathology and sample collection in the laboratory rodent. Vet Clin Exot Anim. 1999, 2:565–590.

Murray MJ. Rabbit and Ferret Sampling and Artifact Considerations. In: Laboratory Medicine: Avian and Exotic Pets. Fudge AM (ed.). Philadelphia: Saunders, 2000; 265–268.

Ness RD. Clinical pathology and sample collection of exotic small mammals. Vet Clin Exot Anim. 1999, 2:591–620.

Pliny A. Clinical hematology of rodent species. Vet Clin Exot Anim. 2008, 11:523–533.

St. Clair MB, Sowers AL, Davis JA, et al. Urinary bladder catheterization of female mice and rats. Contemp Top Lab Anim Sci. 1999, 38:78–79.

Timm KI. Orbital venous anatomy of the Mongolian gerbil with comparison to the mouse, hamster and rat. Lab Anim Sci. 1989, 39:262–264.

———. Orbital venous anatomy of the rat. Lab Anim Sci. 1979, 29:636–638.

Van Herck H, et al. Histological changes in the orbital region of rats after orbital puncture. Lab Anim. 1992, 26:53–58.

HEMATOLOGY, CLINICAL CHEMISTRY, AND URINALYSIS

Analysis of laboratory animal blood and urine for research purposes is commonly done, and encompasses all known aspects and analytical techniques. Historically, in companion rabbit and rodent medicine, analysis of blood and urine was performed infrequently, and most diagnoses were based on history, clinical signs, and necropsy findings. Today, blood and urine analysis is quite common as an adjunct to diagnosis, surgery, and treatment in rabbits and some rodents.

Hematology, clinical chemistry, and urinary values may vary significantly with strain or breed of animal, nutritional status, sex, sampling site or frequency, time of day, stressors, age, disease status, environment, and drug exposure. As a consequence of these influences and others, normal value ranges can be both broad and misleading when applied to a specific population of animals or to an individual animal.

Rabbits: Clinical Pathology

Most reference ranges in the literature have been developed from research studies using homogenous groups of rabbits belonging to the same breed, age, and environmental conditions. This differs from companion pets, in which a diverse group of breeds are encountered, some of which are suffering from underlying chronic problems, such as malnutrition, improper husbandry, or subclinical disease. Increased expectations from pet owners and a recent emphasis on wellness examinations have enabled reference laboratories to include larger numbers of rabbits in development of normal reference ranges, which may more accurately reflect the companion pet population. Table 3.4 lists normal physiologic values in rabbits.

Hematology

Specific pathogen free (SPF) New Zealand white rabbits undergo significant age-related changes during the first 4 weeks of life, with a gradual increase in RBCs, WBCs, and total eosinophil and basophil counts, and a reversal of the heterophil:lymphocyte ratio to favor lymphocytes. After 6 weeks of age, these parameters become comparable to those of adult rabbits. Hemoglobin concentration peaks at 4–7 months of age, and females have significantly lower hemoglobin concentrations and lower hematocrit values than do males (mean 140 vs. 127 g/L and mean 43% vs. 39% for males and females, respectively). Males have higher WBC (mostly lymphocyte) populations than do female rabbits. In addition, total WBC and lymphocyte counts are lowest in the late afternoon and evening, when the heterophil and eosinophil counts rise. These variations should be kept in mind when interpreting results. There are no recognized blood groups in rabbits. Transfusions are well tolerated; however, cross-matching should be done beforehand.

Erythrocytes

Rabbit RBCs normally exhibit anisocytosis, varying in diameter from 5.0 to 7.8 um. In addition, normal blood has 2–4% reticulocytes (polychromatic erythrocytes), due to the short RBC life span (average 57 days) and subsequent high turnover. Rouleau formation and platelet clumping are commonly seen on smears. Male and older animals tend to have higher cell counts than female and younger animals. A marked increase in nucleated RBCs may indicate endothelial damage or a regenerative response. Regenerative anemia may be associated with trauma, fleas, or hemorrhage secondary to conditions such as uterine adenocarcinoma. Clinically healthy rabbits mount a rapid reticulocytic response after hemorrhage. Lead toxicosis results in regenerative anemia, often with nucleated erythrocytes, hypochromasia, poikilocytosis, and cytoplasmic basophilic stippling. Nonregenerative anemia can be seen with chronic conditions, such as infection, renal disease, or neoplasia. Dehydration is the primary reason for an RBC increase as polycythemia vera is not reported in rabbits. Cold stress in rabbits causes increases in platelet and RBC counts, packed cell volume, and total plasma protein, and a decrease in serum albumin.

Leukocytes

The rabbit heterophil functions like the neutrophil of other species but is histochemically distinct. The heterophil measures 9–15 um in diameter and the cytoplasm contains large, orange, nonrefractile granules against a scattering of smaller red-staining cytoplasmic granules.

Rabbit eosinophils stain dull pink-orange with Wright's (Romanovsky) stains and are 12–16 um in diameter. The eosinophilic granules often completely fill the cytoplasm. Eosinophils are primarily involved in the inactivation of histamine or histamine-like toxic substances and are capable of phagocytosis. They also play a role in tissue healing. Low-grade eosinophilia has been associated with chronic parasitism. Basophils are present in higher numbers (2–10%, and up to 30% of WBCs) than are encountered

Table 3.4. Reference physiologic values for rabbits (SI units are in parentheses, where appropriate).

Body weight	2–6 kg
Respiratory rate	30–60/min
Tidal volume	4–6 mL/kg
Oxygen use	0.47–0.85 mL/g/hr
Heart rate	130–325/min
Blood volume	57–78 mL/kg
Blood pressure	90–30/60–90 mm Hg
Erythrocytes	4–7.2 × 10^6/mm^3 (4–7.2 × 10^{12}/L)
Hematocrit	36–48% (0.36–0.48 L/L)
Hemoglobin	10.0–15.5 g/dl (100–155 g/L)
Leukocytes	7.5–13.5 × 10^3/mm^3 (7.5–13.5 × 10^9/L)
Neutrophils	20–35%
Lymphocytes	55–80%
Eosinophils	0–4%
Monocytes	1–4%
Basophils	2–10%
Platelets	200–1000 × 10^3/mm^3 (200–1000 × 10^9/L)
Serum protein	2.8–10.0 g/dl (28–100 g/L)
Albumin	2.7–4.6 g/dl (27–46 g/L)
Globulin	1.5–2.8 g/dl (15–28 g/L)
Fibrinogen	0.2–0.4 g/dl (2–4 g/L)
Sodium	131–155 mEq/L (131–155 mmol/L)
Potassium	3.6–6.9 mEq/L (3.6–6.9 mmol/L)
Chloride	92–112 mEq/L (92–112 mmol/L)
Serum calcium	12.5–16.0 mg/dl (3.12–4.0 mmol/L)
Serum phosphate	2.7–7.3 mg/dl (0.87–2.36 mmol/L)
Serum glucose	75–150 mg/dl (4.2–8.3 mmol/L)
Blood urea nitrogen	15.0–23.5 mg/dl (5.4–8.4 mmol/L)
Creatinine	0.8–1.8 mg/dl (71–159 umol/L)
Total bilirubin	0.25–0.74 mg/dl (4–13 umol/L)
Serum lipids	280–350 mg/dl (2.8–3.5 g/L)
Phospholipids	75–113 mg/dl (0.8–1.1 g/L)
Triglycerides	124–156 mg/dl (1.2–1.6 g/L)
Cholesterol	18–35 mg/dl (0.46–0.91 mmol/L)
AST	6.5–31.0 U/L
Alkaline phosphatase	112–350 U/L

in other species, and rabbits are the only laboratory species in which peripheral basophils are seen normally in circulation. They are similar in size to heterophils, measuring 8–12 um, and contain purple or black metachromatic granules. Their function is not fully understood; basophilia with concurrent eosinophilia has been described in rabbits with chronic skin problems.

Lymphocytes are the predominant WBC in peripheral rabbit circulation. Rabbit lymphocytes are similar to those of other mammals. Most circulating lymphocytes are small, measuring 7–10 um. The less common large lymphocytes measure 10–15 um and may show azurophilic cytoplasmic granules.

Rabbit monocytes are the largest of the leukocytes. Large, dark red granules in monocyte cytoplasm have been associated with toxicity. Monocytosis is linked with chronic inflammation (abscesses, mastitis, tympanic bulla empyema); however, the absence of a monocytosis does not rule out inflammation.

White blood cell differential percentages rather than changes in total WBC number are the best indication of inflammation or infectious disease in rabbits, as a leukocytosis does not typically develop. An increase in the absolute heterophil concentration and decrease in the absolute lymphocyte concentration alter the normal ratio of approximately 1:1 lymphocytes:heterophils. Rabbits with an acute infection may present with 60% or greater heterophils and 30% or less lymphocytes. Occasionally rabbits with an acute infectious process will have a normal differential and a decrease in total WBC numbers. Bands are uncommon in clinical infection, and the absence of a left shift does not rule out an infectious problem.

Adrenocortical stress or exogenous steroids can also affect the differential, and even restraint for clinical examination can alter the heterophil to lymphocyte ratio. An acute stress response is characterized by increased plasma cortisol concentrations and leukocytosis with heterophilia, lymphopenia, and eosinopenia. Total WBC can be used to further characterize acute stress from chronic stress, as both leukopenia and lymphopenia are more common with chronic stress.

Experimentally induced viral infections cause normal to increased lymphocyte counts. Rabbit coagulation has short prothrombin times, long thrombin times, and very high levels of factor V.

Clinical Chemistry

Aspartate Aminotransferase

In rabbits, aspartate aminotransferase (AST, also known as SGOT: serum glutamic oxaloacetic transaminase) is widely distributed in many tissues, including cardiac muscle and liver. The half-life is only 5 hours. Hemolysis or struggling during sample collection will elevate AST levels. Creatine phosphokinase levels also increase after restraint and are purely muscular in origin. Elevated AST levels may also be seen with liver damage. Diarrhea is associated with increases in AST, cholesterol, phosphorus, and BUN, and decreases in serum calcium, alkaline phosphatase (ALP), total protein, glucose, and albumin. Hepatic function also may be reduced in diarrheic rabbits.

Alanine Aminotransferase

In rabbits, alanine aminotransferase (ALT, also known as SGPT: serum glutamic pyruvic transaminase) is not as useful an indicator of liver disease as with other species because, as in other herbivores, it is not liver-specific. ALT is not affected by restraint. Mildly increased levels are common in apparently healthy rabbits. Mild increases have been attributed to exposure to low concentrations of toxic substances, such as resins in wood-based litter or aflatoxins in food. The half-life is approximately 5 hours.

Both ALT and AST levels increase from 8 to 36 days after experimental infection with *Eimeria stiedae*; bilirubinemia and lipemia increase from day 22, and glycemia and total proteins decrease from days 22 to 29.

Lactate Dehydrogenase

Lactate dehydrogenase (LDH) is nonspecific and not valuable for diagnostic use in rabbits.

Akaline phosphatase

Akaline phosphatase (ALP) is found in high concentration in liver and bone and is also found in bowel epithelium, kidney tubules, and placenta. Rabbits produce two ALP isoenzymes in the liver and also have an intestinal isoenzyme, for a total of three ALP isoenzymes. Young growing animals exhibit physiologic increases in ALP activity due to osteoblastic activity. ALP is not altered by restraint and can be used to differentiate real tissue damage. Bile stasis caused by conditions such as hepatic coccidiosis, liver abscesses, neoplasia, or lipidosis will elevate ALP. ALT, bilirubin, and GGT are also usually elevated with these conditions.

Creatine Kinase (Creatine Phosphokinase)

Creatine kinase (CK) is a rapid and sensitive indicator of muscle degeneration, which precedes histologic changes in the muscle by up to 3 days. It increases more rapidly and to a greater extent than AST and lactate dehydrogenase in rabbits undergoing surgery. This enzyme may also increase with myopathies.

Gamma Glutamyltransferase

Gamma glutamyltransferase (GGT) activity is low in rabbit serum. Activity of this enzyme is high in the kidney but doesn't reach the circulation because it is eliminated with the urine. Elevated GGT in rabbits is often linked to obstructive lesions of the bile ducts but with a lower sensitivity than that of other species.

Bile Pigments

Rabbits produce a large quantity of bile for their weight, and the main component is biliverdin. Biliverdin can not be directly assayed and approximately 30% of biliverdin is converted to bilirubin, which can be measured in the blood. The main cause of elevated levels of biliverdin is bile flow obstruction, seen with hepatic coccidiosis, especially in young rabbits, or biliary neoplasia. Aflatoxicosis from eating moldy food may cause hepatic fibrosis with increased bilirubin and ALT levels. Viral hemorrhagic disease causes marked acute hepatic necrosis and increased bilirubin, concurrent with high levels of all hepatocellular enzymes.

Bile Acids

Cecotrophy makes it difficult to obtain a fasted blood sample in rabbits, and because of this bile acid measurement is not a routine procedure in clinical practice.

Cholesterol and Triglycerides

Cholesterol is either synthesized in the liver or obtained from the diet and is a precursor of steroids. It is metabolized by the liver and excreted in the bile. Fasting is needed for accurate measurement, which limits its diagnostic value in rabbits because of cecotrophy. Abnormal levels of cholesterol and triglycerides (TG) can be related to a diet rich in fats, obesity, or hepatic disease. In anorexic rabbits, elevated cholesterol carries a poor prognosis, because it indicates end-stage hepatic lipidosis. Elevated cholesterol has also been linked to pancreatitis, diabetes mellitus, nephrotic syndrome, and chronic renal failure.

Amylase and Lipase

Amylase is derived almost exclusively from the pancreas in rabbits, and elevated levels indicate damage from pancreatitis, pancreatic duct obstruction, peritonitis, or abdominal trauma. Renal failure results in elevated levels because the enzyme is cleared by renal filtration. The half-life of amylase in rabbits is 97 minutes. Corticosteroids can increase serum amylase concentration while hemolysis decreases levels. The function and diagnostic value of lipase in rabbits are unknown; like amylase, it is elevated by corticosteroid administration.

Urea and Creatinine

Urea levels in rabbits are dependent on a number of factors, including circadian rhythm, amount and type of protein in the diet, nutritional status, liver function, intestinal absorption, urease activity of cecal flora, and hydration status. Small changes in urea levels are often hard to interpret, and mild elevations in BUN are a common finding. BUN levels below the reference range indicate hepatic insufficiency or muscle mass loss.

Creatinine level may be a more reliable indication of renal function than BUN in the rabbit, as it is not influenced by nonrenal factors. Rabbits have a limited ability to concentrate urine, and only a few hours without drinking or diarrhea may cause an increase in urea and creatinine levels suggestive of renal failure. Levels rapidly return to normal once dehydration is corrected. Prerenal azotemia can occur with stress, fright, water deprivation, dehydration, heat stroke, toxic insults, and gastrointestinal hemorrhage due to increased protein digestion. In most cases of prerenal azotemia, elevations of BUN are less than 100 mg/dL and are accompanied by urine specific gravity values greater than 1.03.

Renal azotemia, in association with hyper- or hypokalemia, hypercalcemia, hyperphosphatemia, nonregenerative anemia, and isosthenuric urine, can be seen with clinical *Encephalitozoon cuniculi* infection, chronic interstitial nephritis, glomerulonephritis, pyelonephritis, neprolithiasis, renal cysts, and lymphosarcoma. Variable increases in BUN and creatinine levels occur with isosthenuric urine. Levels of serum urea and creatinine do not increase until approximately 75% of renal function has been lost, making early diagnosis of renal disease difficult.

Postrenal azotemia can occur with obstruction of urine flow due to bladder sludge or urolithiasis, and urine specific gravity will vary with these conditions.

Glucose

Glucose metabolism in rabbits is different than in dogs or cats. Because rabbits ingest cecal pellets, a fasting blood sample is difficult to obtain. Diabetes mellitus is rare in rabbits, but hyperglycemia induced by stress is common and may be associated with glucosuria. Other causes of hyperglycemia include acute intestinal obstruction, early mucoid enteropathy, hepatic lipidosis, hypovolemic shock, hyperthermia, stress, exogenous glucocorticoids, and other drugs such as halothane and xylazine.

Hypoglycemia in anorexic rabbits indicates a risk of hepatic lipidosis. It may also occur in acute sepsis or terminal mucoid enteropathy, liver failure, or other chronic disease.

Electrolytes

Sodium levels have low diagnostic value in rabbits. Hypernatremia may be due to dehydration or loss of fluids. Hyponatremia can be associated with polyuric renal failure. Lipemia or hyperproteinemia can artifactually decrease sodium levels.

Hypoadrenocorticism has not been reported in rabbits. Elevated potassium levels are more often due to acute renal failure or urine flow obstruction. Severe tissue damage may also cause hyperkalemia while hemolysis can artifactually elevate levels.

Hypokalemia in rabbits can be caused by dietary insufficiency and loss of fluids from the gastrointestinal system or kidneys. Stress-induced increases in catecholamines can also cause hypokalemia. Hyperproteinemia and lipemia may artifactually decrease blood potassium levels and affected animals may present with muscle weakness.

Calcium metabolism in rabbits is different than in other species. Blood calcium levels are influenced more by the calcium content of the diet than in dogs or cats. Rabbits absorb calcium in proportion to the concentration of the ion in the gut and the kidney eliminates the excess. Vitamin D is not important in calcium absorption if dietary levels are high, yet it does play a role if levels are low and is important in calcium distribution throughout the body. Parathyroid hormone regulates blood calcium levels, but the level at which calcium is moved from blood to bone is high in the rabbit, and blood calcium levels are higher and the range is broader than in other species. The urinary excretion rate of calcium is approximately 45–60%, whereas most mammals excrete no more than 2% of their calcium through renal filtration. This predisposes the rabbit to accumulation of calcium precipitates in the bladder ("urinary sludge") as well as renal and urinary calculi. Renal failure compromises calcium excretion but not absorption, resulting in hypercalcemia in conjunction with clear urine. Excessive mineralization of bones and kidneys and calcification of the aorta are often seen in rabbits with chronic renal failure. Measurement of blood calcium is essential to diagnose renal disease in rabbits, which carries a poor prognosis. The most common cause of hypercalcemia in pet rabbits is excessive dietary calcium. Thymoma may also produce hypercalcemia. Hypocalcemia is rarely reported in rabbits and can be caused by hypoalbuminemia due to poor nutrition. Hypocalcemic seizures have been reported in late pregnant and lactating does.

Phosphorus is intracellular, and blood phosphorus levels are easily increased by hemolysis. Blood phosphate levels should always be evaluated with calcium to determine the mineral balance in patients diagnosed with urinary calculi, dental disease, or nutritional secondary hyperparathyroidism. The kidney is the main organ involved in phosphorus balance by regulation of glomerular filtration and tubular reabsorption, so blood phosphate levels can be an indirect measurement of kidney function and general azotemia. Serum phosphorus levels can be elevated as a result of prerenal, renal, or postrenal effects. Hyperphosphatemia usually indicates chronic kidney failure with a loss of >75% of nephrons and may also be an indicator of soft tissue trauma. The clinical significance of hypophosphatemia is not known.

Protein Disorders

The main cause of hyperproteinemia in rabbits is dehydration, but it can also be seen with chronic infectious or metabolic processes. Hypoproteinemia is usually attributable to chronic malnutrition or protein loss. If both albumin and globulin are low, hemorrhage or protein loss through exudative skin lesions, such as burns or primary or secondary myiasis, should be considered. The liver is the only site of albumin synthesis, so hypoalbuminemia may indicate an advanced hepatic disease, such as may result from hepatic coccidiosis or scarring and necrosis secondary to migrations of *Cysticercus (Taenia) pisiformis* larvae. A common cause of hypoalbuminemia in rabbits is chronic malnutrion either from poor diet or advanced dental disease. Reduced cecotrophy due to obesity, trauma, or dental disease will also cause hypoproteinemia.

Serum electrophoresis, which divides the globulins into distinct fractions, may show elevated alpha-globulins, indicative of acute disease such as bacterial infection or abscess. Elevated gamma globulins indicate a subacute to chronic inflammation. Coronavirus infections lead to a significant increase in rabbit globulins similar to that seen in cats.

Urinalysis

Rabbits urinate infrequently but in large volumes, averaging 130 mL/kg/day (range 20–350). Normal rabbit urine is turbid and rich in minerals, and it requires centrifugation or filtration for biochemical analysis or examinations. Suckling rabbits have clear urine. Color may range from light yellow to reddish-brown, because of dietary pigments. Pigments should be distinquished from hematuria, which is common with cystitis, cystic calculi, and uterine adenocarcinoma. Urine preserved by refrigeration is suitable for examination for up to 2–3 hours.

Urine test dipsticks work well to evaluate blood, glucose, ketone, and pH levels in rabbit urine but are not accurate for other parameters. Stress hyperglycemia may cause glucosuria. The presence of ketones in urine is always abnormal and indicates anorexia, hepatic lipidosis, pregnancy toxemia, or, rarely, diabetes mellitus. Urine pH tends to be high (7.5–9) in rabbits fed a proper diet. Acidic urine indicates acidosis due to anorexia, fever, pregnancy toxemia, or hepatic lipidosis.

The specific gravity (SG) of normal rabbit urine is often quite low, with an average of 1.015 (range 1.003–1.036). Prerenal azotemia is associated with an elevated SG (>1.030), whereas true azotemia due to renal failure is associated with dilute urine (SG < 1.013).

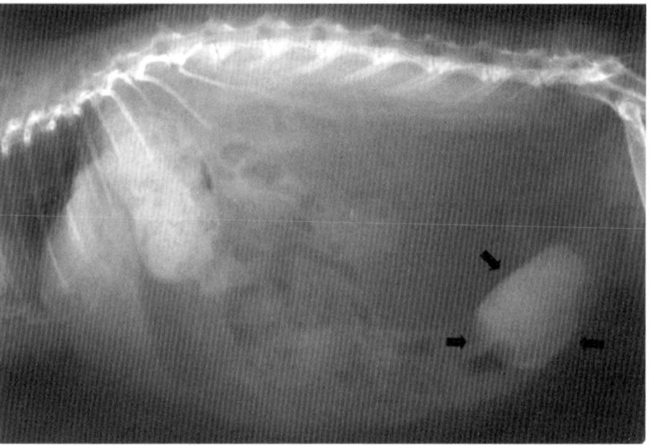

FIGURE 3.10. Rabbit urine frequently contains calcium crystals and the urinary bladder may normally appear radioopaque with survey radiographs (arrows).

Trace protein in the urine of clinically normal rabbits is not significant, but dilute urine (<1.020) with protein is highly significant. Proteinuria appears earlier than other biochemical changes in renal disease, making this test useful in clinical practice.

Sediment examination can differentiate normal urine that is rich in crystals from sludge (Figure 3.10). Rabbit urine typically contains a large amount of crystals. Calcium oxalate crystals are numerous and calcium carbonate and ammonium magnesium phosphate (struvite) crystal crystals are common. After centrifugation, normal crystals should resuspend when shaken, while urine sludge remains a solid mass.

Cytology is similar to that for other mammals, and a small number of leukocytes is considered normal. Gram or trichrome stains can reveal *E. cuniculi* spores.

Rodents: Clinical Pathology

The extensive use of rodents in biomedical research has allowed clinically useful information to become available to the companion pet community. As standards of veterinary care are constantly rising for companion pets, rodent owners are also expecting higher levels of medicine and surgery than ever before. Tables 3.5–3.10 give normal physiologic values for rodents.

Hematology

Erythrocytes

Similar to rabbits, the RBCs of most rodents have a short half-life compared with larger domestic

Table 3.5. Reference physiologic values for guinea pigs (SI units are in parentheses, where appropriate).

Body weight	700–1200 g
Respiratory rate	40–130/min
Tidal volume	2.3–5.3 mL/kg
Heart rate	230–380/min
Blood volume	65–85 mL/kg
Blood pressure	80–94/55–58 mm Hg
Erythrocytes	4.5–7.0 × 10^6/mm^3 (4.5–7.0 × 10^{12}/L)
Hematocrit	37–48% (0.37–0.48 L/L)
Hemoglobin	11–15 g/dl (110–150 g/L)
Leukocytes	7–18 × 10^3/mm^3 (7–18 × 10^9/L)
Neutrophils	28–44%
Lymphocytes	39–72%
Eosinophils	1–5%
Monocytes	3–12%
Basophils	0–3%
Platelets	250–850 × 10^3/mm^3 (250–850 × 10^9/L)
Serum protein	4.6–6.2 g/dl (46–62 g/L)
Albumin	2.1–3.9 g/dl (21–39 g/L)
Globulin	1.7–2.6 g/dl (17–26 g/L)
Sodium	132–156 mEq/L (132–156 mmol/L)
Potassium	4.5–8.9 mEq/L (4.5–8.9 mmol/L)
Chloride	98–115 mEq/L (98–115 mmol/L)
Serum calcium	5.3–12 mg/dl (1.32–3.00 mmol/L)
Serum phosphate	3.0–12 mg/dl (0.97–3.87 mmol/L)
Serum glucose	60–125 mg/dl (3.3–6.9 mmol/L)
Blood urea nitrogen	9.0–31.5 mg/dl (3.2–11.2 mmol/L)
Creatinine	0.6–2.2 mg/dl (53–194 umol/L)
Total bilirubin	0.3–0.9 mg/dl (5–15 umol/L)
Serum lipids	95–240 mg/dl (1.0–2.4 g/L)
Phospholipids	25–75 mg/dl (0.3–0.8 g/L)
Triglycerides	0–145 mg/dl (0–1.4 g/L)
Cholesterol	20–43 mg/dl (0.52–1.11 mmol/L)
ALT	10–25 IU/L
Alkaline phosphatase	18–28 IU/L

mammals, ranging from 45 to 68 days. Polychromasia is commonly observed. Guinea pigs and chinchillas have larger RBCs compared with other rodents. Rouleau formation and polychromasia are more common in very young animals. Polychromasia and macrocytosis are characteristic of regenerative anemias. There is no significant difference between male and female guinea pigs' RBCs and hemoglobin. Blood samples from chinchillas anesthetized with ketamine and xylazine have an increased packed cell volume (PCV), hemoglobin, mean corpuscular hemoglobin concentration (MCHC), and WBC, and a decreased monocyte, basophil, and eosinophil count than in unanesthetized animals.

Newborn hamsters may have up to 10–30% nucleated erythrocytes while adults have 2% or fewer. Red blood cell levels decrease after castration. Erythrocytic measures increase during esti-

Table 3.6. Reference physiologic values for chinchillas (SI units are in parentheses, where appropriate).

Body weight	450–800 g
Respiratory rate	40–80/min
Heart rate	40–100/min
Erythrocytes	5.2–10.7 × 10^6/mm^3 (5.2–10.7 × 10^{12}/L)
Hematocrit	27–54% (0.27–0.54 L/L)
Hemoglobin	8–15.4 g/dl (80–154 g/L)
Leukocytes	4–11.5 × 10^3/mm^3 (4–11.5 × 10^9/L)
Neutrophils	9–45%
Lymphocytes	19–98%
Eosinophils	0–9%
Monocytes	0–6%
Basophils	0–1%
Platelets	254–740 × 10^3/mm^3 (254–740 × 10^9/L)
Serum protein	5.0–6.0 g/dl (50–60 g/L)
Albumin	2.4–4.2 g/dl (24–42 g/L)
Sodium	130–155 mEq/L (130–155 mmol/L)
Potassium	5–6.5 mEq/L (5–6.5 mmol/L)
Chloride	105–115 mEq/L (105–115 mmol/L)
Serum calcium	5.6–12.1 mg/dl (1.40–3.02 mmol/L)
Serum phosphate	4–8 mg/dl (1.29–2.58 mmol/L)
Serum glucose	60–120 mg/dl (3.3–6.7 mmol/L)
Blood urea nitrogen	10–25 mg/dl (3.6–8.9 mmol/L)
Total bilirubin	0.4 mg/dl (7 umol/L)
Cholesterol	40–100 mg/dl (1.03–2.59 mmol/L)
AST	96 IU/L
ALT	10–35 IU/L
Alkaline phosphatase	3–47 IU/L

CLINICAL PROCEDURES

vation, perhaps due in part to an extended RBC life span.

Red cell life span in the gerbil is approximately 9–10 days, which is short compared with that of other domestic rodents and may result in up to 40% of circulating RBCs with stippling as well as the presence of reticulocytes in healthy young gerbils, and lower levels of both in adults.

In rats and mice, Howell Jolly bodies are common in small numbers of RBCs, and rouleau formation is rarely seen. The mouse red blood cell has a life span of approximately 40–47 days.

In rats, hematologic values vary depending on site of blood withdrawal. For example, PCV, hemoglobin (Hb), and WBCs are increased in tail vein blood compared with blood obtained by cardiac puncture, likely due to decreased flow rates and sludging of blood through smaller vessels in the tail. RBCs are smaller in rats compared with rabbits and guinea pigs, and reticulocytes are relatively high in young rats and then decrease, although polychromasia remains a constant feature. Other hematologic changes that occur as rats age include increases of Hb, RBC, and PCV levels from 2 to 8 weeks, and decreases to a stable level at 8 weeks of mean corpuscular volume (MCV), mean corpuscular hemoglobin (MCH), and reticulocytes. Reticulocyte numbers increase and MCHC decreases between 66 and 121 weeks, and neutrophils and lymphocytes increase between 66 and 121 weeks. The hematocrit

Table 3.7. Reference physiologic values for hamsters (SI units are in parentheses, where appropriate).

Body weight	85–150 g
Respiratory rate	35–135/min
Tidal volume	0.6–1.4 mL
Oxygen use	0.6–1.4 mL/g/hr
Heart rate	250–500/min
Blood volume	65–80 mL/kg
Blood pressure	150/100 mm Hg
Erythrocytes	6–10 × 10^6/mm^3 (6–10 × 10^{12}/L)
Hematocrit	36–55% (0.36–0.55 L/L)
Hemoglobin	10–16 g/dl (100–160 g/L)
Leukocytes	3–11 × 10^3/mm^3 (3–11 × 10^9/L)
Neutrophils	10–42%
Lymphocytes	50–94%
Eosinophils	0–4.5%
Monocytes	0–3%
Basophils	0–1%
Platelets	200–500 × 10^3/mm^3 (200–500 × 10^9/L)
Serum protein	4.5–7.5 g/dl (45–75 g/L)
Albumin	2.6–4.1 g/dl (26–41 g/L)
Globulin	2.7–4.2 g/dl (27–42 g/L)
Sodium	128–144 mEq/L (128–144 mmol/L)
Potassium	3.9–5.5 mEq/L (3.9–5.5 mmol/L)
Serum calcium	5–12 mg/dl (1.25–3.00 mmol/L)
Serum phosphate	3.4–8.2 mg/dl (1.10–2.65 mmol/L)
Serum glucose	60–150 mg/dl (3.3–8.3 mmol/L)
Blood urea nitrogen	12–25 mg/dl (4.3–8.9 mmol/L)
Creatinine	0.91–0.99 mg/dl (80–88 umol/L)
Total bilirubin	0.25–0.60 mg/dl (4–10 umol/L)
Cholesterol	25–135 mg/dl (0.66–3.49 mmol/L)
AST	28–122 IU/L
ALT	22–128 IU/L
Alkaline phosphatase	45–187 IU/L

is not an accurate indicator of blood loss because fluid dilution of the cell component is not complete for up to 72 hours postbleeding. Red blood cell life span in rats is approximately 45–68 days.

Leukocytes

The function of rodent neutrophils is similar to that of other mammals, although they may differ in cytochemistry and ultrastructure. For example, hamster neutrophils have no lysozyme activity and mouse neutrophils have decreased alkaline phosphatase activity, compared with other mammalian neutrophils. Neutrophils of most rodents except rats and mice are referred to as heterophils because their granules are eosinophilic in color with Romanowsky stains. As in other mammals, the nucleus may be segmented or band-shaped (immature).

Guinea pig heterophils contain round granules, and the nucleus may normally be segmented or band-shaped. In sows, sex chromatin lobes ("drumsticks" or Barr bodies) may be seen occasionally in the heterophil nucleus. Chinchilla heterophils usually

Table 3.8. Reference physiologic values for gerbils (SI units are in parentheses, where appropriate).

Body weight	55–100 g
Respiratory rate	90/min
Oxygen use	1.4 mL/g/hr
Heart rate	360/min
Blood volume	65–80 mL/kg
Erythrocytes	$8–9 \times 10^6/mm^3$ ($8–9 \times 10^{12}/L$)
Reticulocytes	21–54/1000 RBC
Stippled RBC	2–16/1000 RBC
Polychromatophilic RBC	5–30/1000 RBC
Hematocrit	43–49% (0.43–0.49 L/L)
Hemoglobin	12.6–16.2 g/dl (126–162 g/L)
Leukocytes	$7–15 \times 10^3/mm^3$ ($7–15 \times 10^9/L$)
Neutrophils	5–34%
Lymphocytes	60–95%
Eosinophils	0–4%
Monocytes	0–3%
Basophils	0–1%
Platelets	$400–600 \times 10^3/mm^3$ ($400–600 \times 10^9/L$)
Serum protein	4.3–12.5 g/dl (43–125 g/L)
Albumin	1.8–5.5 g/dl (18–55 g/L)
Globulin	1.2–6.0 g/dl (12–60 g/L)
Sodium	144–158 mEq/L (144–158 mmol/L)
Potassium	3.8–5.2 mEq/L (3.8–5.2 mmol/L)
Serum calcium	3.7–6.2 mg/dl (0.92–1.55 mmol/L)
Serum phosphate	3.7–7.0 mg/dl (1.19–2.26 mmol/L
Serum glucose	50–135 mg/dl (2.8–7.5 mmol/L)
Blood urea nitrogen	17–27 mg/dl (6.1–9.6 mmol/L)
Creatinine	0.6–1.4 mg/dl (53–124 umol/L)
Total bilirubin	0.2–0.6 mg/dl (3–10 umol/L)
Cholesterol	90–150 mg/dl (2.38–3.88 mmol/L)

exhibit a hypersegmented nucleus. The nuclei of mature gerbil, rat, and mouse granulocytes may lack distinct lobes and be horseshoe-, sausage-, or donut-shaped. Rats and mice have neutrophils with colorless cytoplasm, although some fine red granules may be present such that the cytoplasm is diffusely eosinophilic with Romanowsky stains.

Eosinophils make up 1–9% of total leukocytes in rodent blood and contain large cytoplamic granules that become increasingly eosinophilic as the cell matures. Eosinophils increase in number when there is a chronic antigenic stimulus such as occurs with parasite larva and allergic reactions associated with mast cells and basophilic degranulation. In rats, *Trichosomoides crassicauda*, a urinary bladder nematode, may induce a peripheral eosinophilia. Eosinophils may be distinguished from heterophils and neutrophils by their larger size, round to rod-shaped granules, pale basophilic cytoplasm, and ring- or U-shaped nucleus. In chinchillas, eosinophils are the only granulocyte with eosinophilic cytoplasmic granules.

Rodent basophils make up 0–4% of total leukocytes and have characteristic reddish-purple to black staining granules on Romanovsky-stained films. Morphologically, granules of rodent basophils are

Table 3.9. Reference physiologic values for mice (SI units are in parentheses, where appropriate).

Body weight	20–40 g
Respiratory rate	60–220/min
Tidal volume	0.09–0.23 mL
Oxygen use	1.63–2.17 mL/g/hr
Heart rate	325–780/min
Blood volume	70–80 mL/kg
Erythrocytes	7.0–12.5 × 10^6/mm^3 (7.0–12.5 × 10^{12}/L)
Hematocrit	39–49% (0.39–0.49 L/L)
Hemoglobin	10.2–16.6 g/dl (102–166 g/L)
Leukocytes	6–15 × 10^3/mm^3 (6–15 × 10^9/L)
Neutrophils	10–40%
Lymphocytes	55–95%
Eosinophils	0–4%
Monocytes	0.1–3.5%
Basophils	0–0.3%
Platelets	800–1100 × 10^3/mm^3 (800–1100 × 10^9/L)
Serum protein	3.5–7.2 g/dl (35–72 g/L)
Albumin	2.5–4.8 g/dl (25–48 g/L)
Globulin	0.6 g/dl (6 g/L)
Sodium	112–193 mEq/L (112–193 mmol/L)
Potassium	5.1–10.4 mEq/L (5.1–10.4 mmol/L)
Chloride	82–114 mEq/L (82–114 mmol/L)
Serum calcium	3.2–8.5 mg/dl (0.80–2.12 mmol/L)
Serum phosphate	2.3–9.2 mg/dl (0.74–2.97 mmol/L)
Serum glucose	62–175 mg/dl (33.4–9.7 mmol/L)
Blood urea nitrogen	12–28 mg/dl (4.3–1.0 mmol/L)
Creatinine	0.3–1.0 mg/dl (27–88 umol/L)
Total bilirubin	0.1–0.9 mg/dl (2.0–15 umol/L)
Cholesterol	26–82 mg/dl (0.67–2.12 mmol/L)
AST	54–269 IU/L
ALT	26–77 IU/L
Alkaline phosphatase	45–222 IU/L

homogeneous. The basophils of rodents must be differentiated from mast cells, which are more common in the sample when blood is taken by cardiac puncture.

Monocytes are the largest leukocyte in peripheral blood films and are similar in all rodents. The nuclei vary from round to oval to lobed. The cytoplasm is moderately abundant, pale blue-gray, and may contain azurophilic granules.

Lymphocyte morphology is variable in rodents with respect to size, cytoplasmic color (pale to dark basophilia), and degree of nuclear chromatin condensation. The size falls between that of an RBC and a neutrophil. Smaller cells are thought to be inactive. Reactive lymphocytes have more abundant cytoplasm with deeper basophilic staining and nuclei with clefts. These cells are thought to be B cells involved in immunoglobulin production.

Both large and small lymphocytes are present normally in guinea pigs. The distinctive Foa-Kurloff or Kurloff cell is a large lymphocyte containing a single large intracytoplasmic inclusion 1–8 um in diameter

Table 3.10. Reference physiologic values for rats (SI units are in parentheses, where appropriate).

Body weight	250–520 g
Respiratory rate	70–115/min
Tidal volume	0.6–2.0 mL
Oxygen use	0.68–1.10 mL/g/hr
Heart rate	250–450/min
Blood volume	50–70 mL/kg
Blood pressure	84–134/60 mm Hg
Erythrocytes	7–10 × 10^6/mm^3 (7–10 × 10^{12}/L)
Hematocrit	36–48% (0.36–0.48 L/L)
Hemoglobin	11–18 g/dl (110–180 g/L)
Leukocytes	6–17 × 10^3/mm^3 (6–17 × 10^9/L)
Neutrophils	9–34%
Lymphocytes	65–85%
Eosinophils	0–6%
Monocytes	0–5%
Basophils	0–1.5%
Platelets	500–1300 × 10^3/mm^3 (500–1300 × 10^9/L)
Serum protein	5.6–7.6 g/dl (56–76 g/L)
Albumin	3.8–4.8 g/dl (38–48 g/L)
Globulin	1.8–3.0 g/dl (18–30 g/L)
Sodium	135–155 mEq/L (135–155 mmol/L)
Potassium	4–8 mEq/L (4–8 mmol/L)
Serum calcium	5.3–13.0 mg/dl (1.32–3.24 mmol/L)
Serum phosphate	5.3–8.3 mg/dl (1.71–2.68 mmol/L)
Serum glucose	50–135 mg/dl (2.8–7.5 mmol/L)
Blood urea nitrogen	15–21 mg/dl (5.4–7.5 mmol/L)
Creatinine	0.2–0.8 mg/dl (18–71 umol/L)
Total bilirubin	0.20–0.55 mg/dl (3–9 umol/L)
Serum lipids	70–415 mg/dl (0.7–4.2 g/L)
Phospholipids	36–130 mg/dl (0.4–1.3 g/L)
Triglycerides	26–145 mg/dl (0.3–1.4 g/L)
Cholesterol	34–130 mg/dl (0.88–3.36 mmol/L)
ALT	16–89 IU/L
Alkaline phosphatase	16–125 IU/L

referred to as a Kurloff body (see Figure 2.27). They are more common in sexually immature male and pregnant guinea pigs, suggesting that their presence is influenced by sex hormones. These cells are thought to function as natural killer (NK) cells, a type of lymphocyte. Kurloff cells may be found in the peripheral circulation as well as in fixed tissue sections, for example, spleen, and should not be misinterpreted as neoplastic cells. In female rats, removal of the ovaries and to a lesser extent the uterus increases circulating T and B lymphocyte numbers in peripheral blood.

In general, the differential WBC count of rodents tends to be predominantly lymphocytic. The WBC response to disease tends to result in an increase in immature leukocytes, toxic neutrophils, and Dohle bodies (aggregates of endoplasmic reticulum that appear as gray-blue cytoplasmic inclusions) rather than increases in the total and differential leukocyte counts. Leukocytosis in rodents may be associated with chronic, closed-cavity inflammation, such as abscesses. Epinephrine induces neutrophils to leave the marginating pool in response to the increased heart rate and blood flow, resulting in a neutrophilia. Exogenously administered corticosteroids as well as increased circulating endogenous corticosteroids associated with physiological stress will result in lymphopenia, and occasionally, a mature neutrophilia. In hamsters, the WBC counts decrease during estivation.

WBC count can be estimated from a well-prepared smear of fresh blood. The numbers of WBCs per high-power (×40) objective from at least five fields are counted. The average number is multiplied by 1,000 to give an estimated total WBC.

Clinical Chemistry

Rodent clinical chemistry interpretation does not differ greatly from that of rabbits. In guinea pigs and rats, ALT has little organ specificity, but it may still be useful for assessing liver damage. In mice, ALT has the highest activity in the liver, and increased levels of ALT are attributable to hepatic injury. AST is nonspecific in mice. Fasted rats may exhibit a marked increase (five- to seven-fold) in hepatic-origin ALT, which may also increase in response to handling or liver disease. ALP in healthy hamsters is composed mostly of the isoenzyme from bone and intestine. Elevated levels may be seen in hamsters with liver disease, but dramatic increases are usually associated with bile duct obstructions. High levels of ALP are also associated with leukemia and prostatic tumors. The guinea pig liver contains higher levels of GGT compared with other rodents.

Unlike in the rabbit, bilirubin is the end-product of hemaglobin metabolism in rodents. Total bilirubin levels are a sensitive indicator of liver damage or hemolysis in rodents.

High serum cholesterol levels develop in gerbils even when they are fed diets that contain normal levels of fat. Gerbils have higher serum lipid values than other rodents and lipemia is common.

BUN levels are highly variable in rodents and may be affected by diet. Creatinine levels may be influenced by the assay method. Picric acid–based tests, which are commonly used in automated assays, may overestimate creatinine levels in rodents, necessitating the use of alternate methods for accurate determinations (i.e., high-performance liquid chromatography). In hamsters, high-protein diets (20% or more) may be accompanied by elevated BUN levels. In mice, significant increases in BUN occur when the host has lost approximately 70% of renal function.

Glucose levels are affected by the nutritional, hormonal, and affective state of the animal. Hyperglycemia has been reported in hamsters during estivation. Administration of thiobarbiturates may also lead to hyperglycemia.

Amyloidosis, a malady common to hamsters, mice, gerbils, and guinea pigs, is associated with decreased plasma albumin and increased globulin levels. In mice and rats, hyperproteinemia occurs with dehydration, whereas hypoproteinemia (hypoalbuminemia) occurs with renal disease.

Urinalysis

Normal rodent urine is variable in color, ranging from colorless to yellowish to light brown. Diet or antibiotics may cause porphyrin excretion, resulting in a reddish tinge. Rodent urine specific gravity values range from 1.003 to 1.060. Rats may concentrate urine to twice that measured in humans, and specific gravities of 1.020–1.050 are normal. The volume of urine produced is approximately 3.3–4.2 mL/100 g/day. Rodent urine may be acidic or alkaline (pH 5–8.4). There is marked circadian fluctuation in rodent urine pH and the diet and protein source greatly influence the pH. Urine should always be collected at the same time of day for comparisons.

Urine protein levels may be significant in some rodents. Mice produce approximately 0.5–2.5 mL of urine every 24 hours, and males are normally mildly proteinuric, with higher levels seen in sexually mature mice. Proteinuria is normal in rats due to tubular production of alpha-globulins, and urine protein levels can be as high as 30 mg/dL. Hamsters excrete an average of 9.7 mg protein in the urine weekly, approximately 10× the urinary protein excretion rate of normal humans. Both normal hamsters and those with advanced renal disease may have proteinuria. Hamsters produce approximately 5–8 mL of urine per day, with calcium phosphate and carbonate crystals contributing to turbidity. Gerbils produce scant concentrated urine that may contain trace protein. Glomerulonephritis and amyloidosis are the most common causes of renal disease–associated proteinuria for rodent species.

Glucose is not normally present in rodent urine. Guinea pigs with diabetes mellitus may have urine glucose levels of 3–6 g/L. Guinea pigs with diabetes mellitus often present in a state of ketosis. Ketones are always interpreted to be abnormal when present in rodent urine and may be seen after prolonged anorexia or starvation or during pregnancy. Guinea pigs and chinchillas with dental disease and those with severely impacted ceca are common examples of patients with conditions inducing ketonuria.

Positive urine bilirubin is associated with destruction of heme from blood cells or muscle or disease of the biliary tree. Normal rodent urine has very few RBCs (0–3 cells/hpf). An increase may be seen with inflammation or damage to the urinary or reproductive system, such as occurs with infection, calculi, or neoplasia. Guinea pigs are particularly susceptible to urinary tract infections.

Urine from normal guinea pigs and chinchillas usually contains large amounts of light-colored sediment. Cloudy urine is usually caused by calciuria, which is normal to some extent in rodents. Amorphous calcium carbonate, struvite, and triple phosphate crystals are most common. Rodents being treated with sulfonamide drugs may have sulfur crystals. RBCs, WBCs, casts, and bacteria may be found in rodent urine and have the same interpretation and importance as in other mammals, that is, the presence of WBCs suggests infection, while casts suggest renal tubular disease.

References

Anderson NL. Pet Rodents. In: Saunders Manual of Small Animal Practice, 3rd ed. Birchard SJ, Sherding RG (eds.). St. Louis: Saunders Elsevier, 2006; 1881–1909.

Barriga OO, Arnoni JV. Eimeria stiedae: weight, oocyst output, and hepatic function of rabbits with graded infections. Exp Parasitol. 1979, 48:407–414.

Benson KG, Paul-Murphy J. Clinical pathology of the domestic rabbit. Vet Clin Exot Anim. 1999, 2:539–551.

Bortolotti A, Castelli D, Bonati M. Hematology and serum chemistry values of adult, pregnant and newborn New Zealand rabbits (Oryctolagus cuniculus). Lab Anim Sci. 1989, 39:437–439.

Breitweiser B. Practical approach to hamster urinary analysis. J Small Exotic Anim Med. 1992, 1:104–105.

Campbell TW, Ellis CK. Avian and Exotic Hematology and Cytology, 3rd ed. Ames, IA: Blackwell, 2007.

Chen SI, Quesenberry KE. Rabbits. In: Saunders Manual of Small Animal Practice, 3rd ed. Birchard SJ, Sherding RG (eds.). St. Louis: Saunders Elsevier, 2006; 1858–1880.

Fisher PG. Exotic mammal renal disease: diagnosis and treatment. Vet Clin Exot Anim. 2006, 9:69–96.

Fox RR, Laird CW. Biochemical parameters of clinical significance in rabbits: II. Diurnal variations. J Hered. 1970, 61:265–268.

Fudge AM. Rabbit Hematology. In: Laboratory Medicine: Avian and Exotic Pets. Fudge AM (ed.). Philadelphia: Saunders, 2000; 273–275.

Harcourt-Brown F. Textbook of Rabbit Medicine. Oxford: Butterworth Heinemann, 2002.

Harkness JE. Rabbit husbandry and medicine. Vet Clin Small Anim. 1987, 17:1019–1044.

Hewitt CD, et al. Normal biochemical and hematological values in New Zealand white rabbits. Clin Chem. 1989, 35:1777–1779.

Hillyer EV. Pet rabbits. Vet Clin Small Anim. 1995, 24:25–66.

Hinton M, Jones DRE, Festing MFW. Haematological findings in healthy and diseased rabbits, a multivariate analysis. Lab Anim. 1982; 16:123–129.

Hoefer H. Rabbit and Ferret Renal Disease Diagnosis. In: Laboratory Medicine: Avian and Exotic Pets. Fudge AM (ed.). Philadelphia: Saunders, 2000; 311–318.

Jenkins JR. Rabbit and Ferret Liver and Gastrointestinal Testing. In: Laboratory Medicine: Avian and Exotic Pets. Fudge AM (ed.). Philadelphia: Saunders, 2000, 291–304.

———. Rabbit diagnostic testing. J Exot Pet Med. 2008, 17:4–15.

———. Rodent diagnostic testing. J Exot Pet Med. 2008, 17:16–25.

Kabata J, et al. Hematologic values of New Zealand white rabbits determined by automated flow cytometry. Lab Anim Sci. 1991, 41:613–619.

Kuhn G, Hardegg W. Quantitative studies of haematological values in long-term ovariectomized, ovariohysterectomized and hysterectomized rats. Lab Anim. 1991, 25:40–45.

Lewis JH. Rabbits. In: Comparative Hemostasis in Vertebrates. New York: Plenum Press, 1996; 182–193.

Loeb WF, Quimby FW. The Clinical Chemistry of Laboratory Animals. Oxford: Pergamon Press, 1989.
Mader DR. Basic Approach to Veterinary Care. In: Ferrets, Rabbits, and Rodents: Clinical Medicine and Surgery, 2nd ed. Quesenberry KE, Carpenter JW (eds.). St. Louis: Saunders, 2004; 147–154.
Marshall K. Rabbit hematology. Vet Clin Exot Anim. 2008, 11:551–567.
McClure DE. Clinical pathology and sample collection in the laboratory rodent. Vet Clin Exot Anim. 1999, 2:565–590.
Mclaughlin RM, Fish RE. Clinical Biochemistry and Hematology. In: The Biology of the Laboratory Rabbit, 2nd ed. Manning PF, Ringler DR, Newcomer CE (eds.). San Diego: Academic Press, 1994; 111–127.
Melillo A. Rabbit clinical pathology. J Exot Pet Med. 2007, 16:135–145.
Meyer MH, Meyer RA, Jr, Gray RW, et al. Picric acid methods greatly overestimate serum creatinine in mice: more accurate results with high-performance liquid chromatography. Anal Biochem. 1985, 144(1):285–290.
Morgan RV, Moore FM, Pearce LK, et al. Clinical and laboratory findings in small companion animals with lead poisoning: 347 cases (1977–1986). J Am Vet Med Assoc. 1991, 199:93–97.
Ness RD. Clinical pathology and sample collection of exotic small mammals. Vet Clin Exot Anim. 1999, 2:591–620.
Pliny A. Clinical hematology of rodent species. Vet Clin Exot Anim. 2008, 11:523–533.
Reavill D, Joseph V. Clinical Pathology of the Rabbit. In: Rabbit Medicine and Procedures for Practitioners Program and Abstracts. Berkeley, CA: House Rabbit Society, 1997; 157–170.
Rosenthal KL. Diagnostic and Therapeutic Techniques in Rabbits. In: Rabbit Medicine and Procedures for Practitioners Program and Abstracts. Berkeley, CA: House Rabbit Society, 1997; 157–170.
Saunders RA, Davies RR. Notes on Rabbit Internal Medicine. Oxford: Blackwell, 2005.
Schock A, Reid HW. Characterisation of the lymphoproliferation in rabbits experimentally affected with malignant catarrhal fever. Vet Microbiol. 1996, 53:111–119.
Shanklin WM, Sheppard LB, Burke GW. Staining of rabbit eosinophil and pseudoeosinophil leukocytes. Acta Anat. 1977, 97:147–150.
Silva TO, et al. Reference values for chinchilla (Chinchilla laniger) blood cells and serum biochemical parameters. Ciencia Rural, Santa Maria. 2005, 35:602–606.
Song BZ, Donoff RB, Tsuji T, et al. Identification of rabbit eosinophils and heterophils in cutaneous healing wounds. Histochem J. 1993, 25:762–771.
St. Clair MB, Sowers AL, Davis JA, et al. Urinary bladder catheterization of female mice and rats. Contemp Top Lab Anim Sci. 1999, 38:78–79.
Suckow MA, Douglas FA. The Laboratory Rabbit. Boca Raton, FL: CRC Press, 1997; 9.
Turton JA, et al. Age-related changes in the haematology of female F344 rats. Lab Anim. 1989, 23:295–301.
Vernau KM, Grahn BH, Clarke-Scott HA, et al. Thymoma in a geriatric rabbit with hypercalcemia and periodic exophthalmos. J Am Vet Med Assoc. 1995, 206:820–822.

MEDICAL IMAGING

Diagnostic imaging of rabbits and rodents may facilitate diagnosis, assessment, and treatment of skeletal injury or disease, foreign body presence, dental abnormalities, neoplasia, otitis media, pregnancy, urolithiasis, and many other conditions. Radiography and ultrasonography are the most common and least expensive imaging techniques used; however, computed tomography, magnetic resonance imaging, and, more recently, synchrotron imaging are also used, especially in research settings. It is beyond the scope of this book to delve into specifics for each of the various imaging modalities. Interested readers are referred to the resources listed in the reference section.

Radiography

For rabbits and rodents, equipment should be capable of short exposure times (1/30–1/120 of a second), 5.0–7.5 milliampere second (mAs) exposures, and a range of 40–100 kilovoltage peak (kVp), adjustable in 1–2 kVp increments. A focal film distance of 90 cm is used commonly with detailed screen/film combinations.

Immobilization of patients is essential, as is a fast exposure time because of the rapid respiratory rate of rabbits and rodents. Radiolucent foam or tape is helpful for correct animal positioning. The fur should be clean and dry, as dirt or water may produce artifacts. Soft tissues in small mammals have a low density, so methods to enhance contrast are useful. High-resolution film screens, such as high-detail rare earth intensifying screens with appropriate film, can be used to obtain diagnostic radiographs in small patients. Cassettes and screens designed for human extremities may be useful.

Radiography of Rabbits

Rabbits may be anesthetized for thoracic or abdominal radiography with 10 mg/kg propofol IV (gives approximately 5 minutes of anesthesia), isoflurane, or ketamine at 20–25 mg/kg combined with acepromazine at 2 mg/kg IM. The animal may be positioned directly on the cassette with limbs extended.

Ventrodorsal and lateral views are standard for the spine, pelvis, thorax, and abdomen (Figure 3.11). Both right and left lateral views of the thorax should be taken to optimize information gained. The thoracic cavity of adult rabbits contains a large amount of fat, which may be superimposed over the cardiac apex and may mimic pleural fluid. Contrast in the thoracic cavity can be increased by exposing the film at maximal inspiration, or using positive pressure inflation, if the animal is intubated.

For skull radiographs, the dorsoventral view provides better evaluation of the tympanic bullae. In addition to the lateral view, rostrocaudal and oblique views may facilitate examination of other areas of interest, such as the teeth, orbits, or sinuses (Figure 3.12). Dorsopalmar and dorsoplantar views are used for the front and rear legs, respectively, along with mediolateral views for the appendicular skeleton.

Variations in both normal and abnormal animals make interpretation of abdominal radiographs challenging. Large fatty livers and gastrointestinal gas accumulation are common findings, and the cecum may be large and fluid-filled. Rabbits excrete large amounts of calcium via the kidneys, and these calcium salts are often visible radiographically in the bladder as a normal finding.

Radiography of Rodents

Small rodents may be immobilized for radiography by injections of ketamine with xylazine or acepromazine, or with isoflurane in oxygen given by face mask.

A sedated animal can be placed directly on the cassette or can be restrained in any of several positions using radiolucent tape or foam. The dorsoventral (sternum down) position is preferred over ventrodorsal, and masking tape can be used to flatten the neck, limbs, and tail. Other views are taken as for rabbits. A radiolucent tube can be used to contain and restrain a rodent. With any restraint method, tape

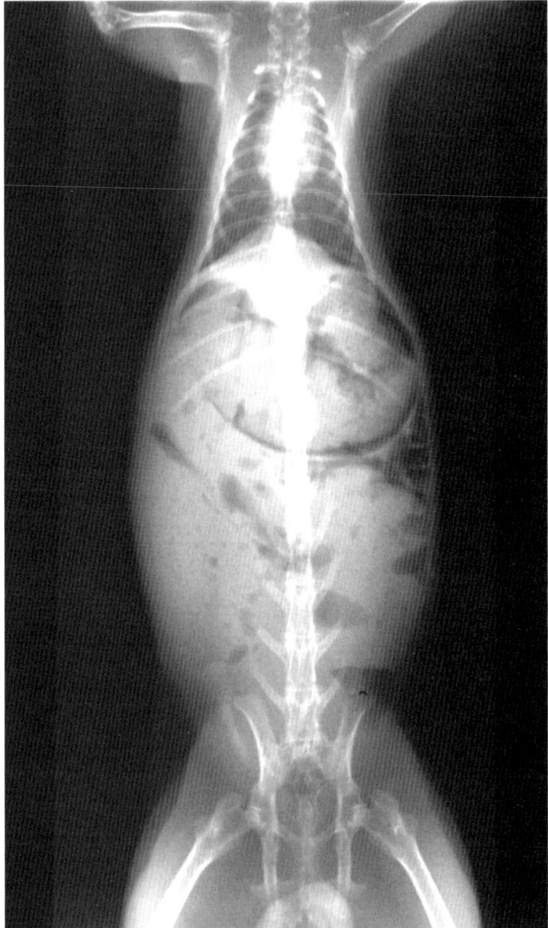

A

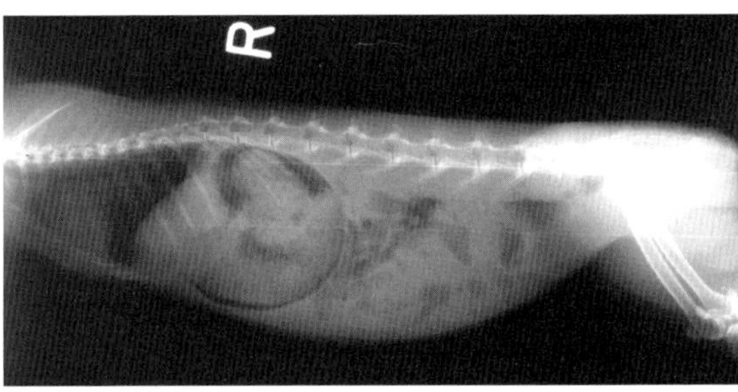

B

FIGURE 3.11. Ventrodorsal (A) and lateral (B) survey radiographs of the thorax and abdomen of a normal rabbit.

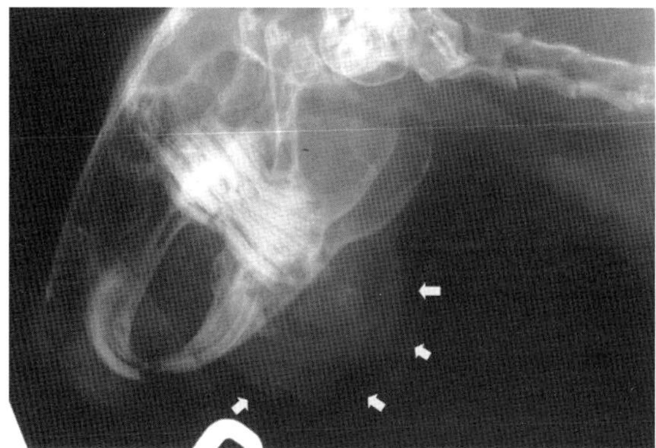

FIGURE 3.12. Lateral skull radiograph of a pet rabbit demonstrating soft tissue swelling and mineralization associated with submandibular osteomyelitis (arrows).

can be applied circumferentially to the limbs and then to the cassette or table for extension.

The abdomen is large compared with the thorax, and the large gastrointestinal tract shows little contrast but usually contains ample gas. In guinea pigs and chinchillas, the cecum takes up much of the abdomen, whereas the abdominal anatomy of hamsters, gerbils, mice, and rats is more similar to that of the dog or cat. Guinea pigs, chinchillas, and rats have an os penis, which should not be confused with a urolith.

Contrast Radiography

Contrast radiography by various methods allows visualization of the gastrointestinal tract, bladder, and other organs. In rodents, soft tissues of the upper respiratory and upper digestive tracts have low density, and on radiographs, these tissues are poorly defined. For assessment of the stomach, pneumogastrography can be used, which involves introducing 5 mL air/kg body weight into the stomach through a tube, to evaluate the position or identify extraluminal masses. Positive contrast studies can be performed with appropriate radioopaque material given at 3–20 mL/kg body weight to investigate stomach position, shape, and emptying time. Contrast studies should be performed with the stomach empty, if possible; however, rabbit stomachs are never completely empty, so ingesta present after fasting is normal. In rodents, emptying times vary between species, but in general gastric emptying begins within 30 minutes of feeding and is complete by 3 hours. In rabbits, contrast reaches the cecum in approximately 4 hours and is retained there for prolonged periods. Contrast may stay in the stomach for days. Colonic radiography involves retrograde infusion of a contrast medium into the colon with a catheter.

Both negative (installation of air or carbon dioxide) and positive (installation of radioopaque material, such as an iodine-based solution) contrast can be used for retrograde cystography, provided a urinary catheter can be placed. An intravenous pyelogram may be possible if catheterization of the cephalic, lateral saphenous, or tail vein can be accomplished for injection of contrast media. Excretory urography is useful for evaluation of size, shape, position, and internal structure of the kidneys, ureters, and urinary bladder.

Contrast radiography of the nasolacrimal duct in rabbits can be performed by cannulating the duct and flushing with radioopaque material.

Ultrasonography

Ultrasonography is a valuable adjunct to radiography and can be used to further investigate radiographic findings. Ultrasonography allows differentiation of fluid from soft tissues and also permits visualization of the organ parenchyma, so it is particularly useful for evaluating the urinary bladder, heart, uterus, liver, spleen, kidneys, and ovaries. Sound waves are obstructed by gas, and because of this ultrasonography of the abdomen of small herbivores is often unrewarding. The dynamic nature of ultrasonography allows for assessment of cardiac movement and blood flow, using Doppler mode. Ultrasound-guided biopsies can also be performed, as needed.

For small mammals, a minimum requirement is a high-definition transducer with a footprint of less than 2 cm. Anesthesia is required for most species and body hair must be clipped to exclude air between the transducer and the skin. Acoustic coupling gel should be applied liberally to both the transducer and the skin. Hypothermia is a concern due to hair loss, wetting of the skin surface, and general anesthesia, and must be guarded against, particularly in very small animals.

Artifacts and overdiagnosis are common in ultrasonography, and it is important that the operator be familiar with the normal anatomy of the species being imaged.

Computed Tomography Scanning

A computed tomography (CT) image is created by rotating an x-ray tube around an anesthetized animal while a computer generates a two-dimensional cross-section of the area being scanned and displays it on a computer screen in shades of gray. Contrast resolution is very good, allowing differentiation between fluids and soft tissues. CT scanning is particularly useful for investigation of bone, intracranial lesions, nasal cavity, teeth, sinuses, orbit, middle ear, and metastases within organs. Intravenous contrast media can be used to enhance various structures, especially those associated with abnormal vasculature.

Magnetic Resonance Imaging

Magnetic resonance imaging (MRI) uses computer-generated images that measure the hydrogen content of the tissues. Spatial resolution and soft tissue contrast are greater with this technique than with CT, and the tissues can be viewed in any plane. The animal must be completely immobilized, as any movement will blur the image. MRI is very useful for musculoskeletal, articular, and cerebral imaging, and for longitudinal studies of soft tissue, as well as for viewing inflammation and neoplasia. MRI is primarily used in experimental animals.

Synchrotron Imaging

Synchrotron imaging is a relatively new medical imaging modality used in experimental studies, and it is increasingly being used as a powerful clinical and basic research tool around the world at facilities with biomedical beamlines (Figure 3.13). The technique of diffraction-enhanced imaging (DEI) uses monochromatic x-rays from a synchrotron to produce images of both soft tissues and bone that are far superior to traditional imaging techniques. K-edge digital subtraction angiography (KEDSA) is another synchrotron-based technique that uses monochromatic radiation, permitting acquisition of high-quality angiography images after intravenous administration of as little as 0.5 mL/kg iodinated contrast material. Real-time imaging of the vascular networks of any organ system in vivo is possible with synchrotron radiation angiography, and high-resolution imaging of the microcirculation in experimental animals is providing new insights into vasomotor regulation within intact organ systems such as the brain, kidney, lung, and heart. Future applications of synchrotron techniques are expected to rapidly advance the understanding of the pathogenesis, diagnosis, and treatment of many diseases.

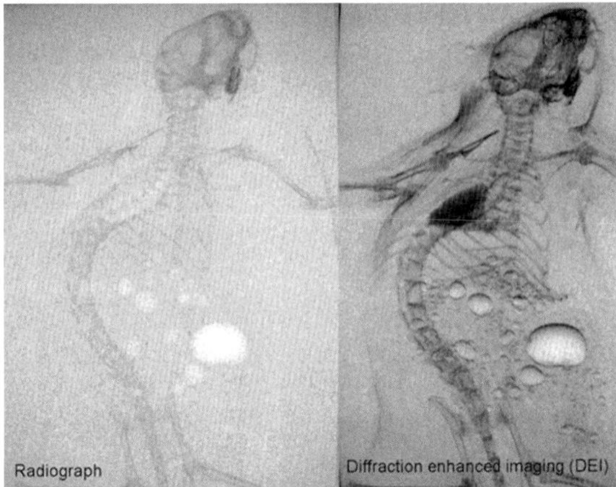

FIGURE 3.13. Images of a dead mouse taken on the bend magnet part of the Biomedical and Imaging Therapy (BMIT) synchrotron beamline at the Canadian Light Source Inc. in Saskatoon. The mouse has been immersed in water to improve the ability to "see inside" the body with either conventional radiography (left) or diffraction enhanced imaging (DEI) (right). The images were taken with an incident exposure of ~2 milliGrays at an imaging energy of 41 keV (kilo-electron volts). The DEI system used Si (3,3,3) for the monochromator and analyzer, which gives very good soft tissue definition. Note the enhanced contrast from structured tissues such as lung and bone as well as bubbles in the abdomen, which are highlighted by the DEI method. Both images are unprocessed and are presented as acquired. Courtesy of L. Dean Chapman.

References

Capello V, Lennox AM. Clinical Radiology of Exotic Companion Animals. Ames, IA: Wiley-Blackwell, 2008.

Kelly ME, et al. Diffraction-enhanced imaging of the rat spine. Can Assoc Radiol J. 2006, 57:204–210.

———. Synchrotron-based intravenous cerebral angiograpy in a small animal model. Phys Med Biol. 2007, 52:1001–1012.

Margulis AR, Carlsson E, McAlister WH. Angiography of malignant tumors in mice. Acta Radiol. 1961, 56:179–192.

Morgan JP, Silverman S. Techniques of Veterinary Radiography, 5th ed. Ames: Iowa State University Press, 1993; 266–267.

Redrobe S. Imaging techniques in small mammals. Sem Av Exot Pet Med. 2001, 10:187–197.

Reidenberg JS, Laitman JT. A new method for radiographically locating upper respiratory and upper digestive tract structures in rats. Lab Anim Sci. 1990, 40:72–76.

Rubel GA, Isenbugel E, Wolvekamp P. Atlas of Diagnostic Radiology of Exotic Pets. Philadelphia: Saunders, 1991.

Serota KS, Jeffcoat MK, Kaplan ML. Intraoral radiography of molar teeth in rats. Lab Anim Sci. 1981, 31:507–509.

Shirai M, et al. Synchrotron-based angiography for investigation of the regulation of vasomotor function in the microcirculation in vivo. Clin Exp Pharmacol Physiol. 2009, 36:107–116.

Silverman S. Diagnostic Imaging of Exotic Pets. In: Exotic Pet Medicine I. Quesenberry KE, Hillyer EV. Vet Clin North Am. 1993, 23:1287–1299.

Silverman S, Tell LA. Radiology of Rodents, Rabbits, and Ferrets. An Atlas of Normal Anatomy and Positioning. St Louis: Saunders, 2005.

Wagner JE, et al. Otitis media of guinea pigs. Lab Anim Sci. 1976, 26:902–907.

OPHTHALMOLOGY

Ocular disease of rabbits and rodents is evidenced by watery or mucoid discharge, blepharospasm, erythema or vascular injection, exophthalmos, or corneal and lens opacities. Less conspicuous changes in the uvea, vitreous, or retina are not readily observed. Orbital lesions may result from infections, nutritional deficiencies, injury, congenital malformations, husbandry practices, and as a sequela to technical procedures, such as retroorbital bleeding. The lateral placement and bulbous nature of the eyes of rabbits and rodents, which is typical of prey species, predisposes them to traumatic or iatrogenic ulcers, especially during sedation and anesthesia, when they may be placed in lateral recumbency.

Vision assessment of these animals can be difficult because many are nocturnal and depend (especially albinos) on olfactory and tactile cues. Most are housed in familiar quarters and rarely venture into novel areas. In addition, the small size of the eye in rodents and difficulty in restraint of the head can hinder examination of conscious animals.

Equipment and Methods

Equipment needed for ophthalmologic examination optimally includes a 20–40 diopter (D) condensing lens and a pocket magnifier, or head loupe. A systematic approach should be used, starting with tests of vision, examination of eyelids, surrounding skin (including nares), visible eye structures (conjunctiva, sclera, and cornea), and comparison of the two globes. Assessment of tear production is difficult due to the small size of the globe. A Schirmer tear test or phenol red thread tear test can be performed in most rabbits and guinea pigs. Topical anesthetics should be used sparingly in rabbits and rodents to prevent systemic toxicity, but they are necessary for manipulations of the eye and adnexa. The lids can be retracted to examine the conjunctival sac, and in rabbits, the single large nasolacrimal punctum, which lies ventrally at the fornix. Tonometry is possible in most rabbits; a range of 15–25 mm Hg has been reported in normal animals. Examination of the cornea, anterior chamber, lens, and vitreous should be performed, if possible, with a slit lamp. The pupils can be dilated with a mydriatic such as 1% tropicamide for examination of the fundus. Animals with pigmented irises (usually brown) may bind the mydriatic agent to uveal melanin. In these animals, a drop of 1% atropine combined with one drop of 10% phenylephrine can be given three to four times over a 15-minute period. Fundic examination is conducted using indirect ophthalmoscopy with a 30–40 diopter indirect condensing lens. Rabbits may have plasma atropinesterase, which may preclude pupillary dilatation with alkaloid mydriatics.

Other useful procedures include fluorescein dye staining, to evaluate the cornea and nasolacrimal system, bacterial culture, and conjunctival scrapings.

Rabbits

The rabbit eyeball has a large cornea, large rounded lens, and poorly developed ciliary body. Eyelids separate completely at approximately 10 days after birth. The fundus is merangiotic (partially vascularized) with intravitreal vessels at a level nasal and temporal to the optic disc. The myelinated optic disc is depressed centrally and lies above the horizontal midline, which necessitates looking "up" into the rabbit's eye to see the disc. The superior rectus muscle is normally visible through the superior bulbar conjuctiva. The orbit contains four glands: lacrimal, intraorbital, Harderian, and gland of the nictitating membrane. The nictitating membrane (third eyelid) is functional and extends from the medial canthus. Flushing of the nasolacrimal duct is not difficult and is described in the section "Other Special Techniques." Normal Schirmer tear test values for the rabbit range from 0 to 11.22 mm/min (mean of 5.30 ± 2.96 mm/min) without topical anesthetic. Low values can be obtained in healthy rabbits and the significance of this test has been questioned. The phenol red thread tear test requires less tear volume and a shorter testing time and may be more appropriate. Values of 20.88 mm/15 seconds (range 15–27 ± 2.90 mm/15 seconds) have been reported. Normal intraocular pressure ranges from 15 to 25 mm Hg.

Ocular problems in rabbits include epiphora, conjunctivitis or blepharoconjunctivitis (Figure 3.14), glaucoma, uveitis, exophthalmos due to orbital abscess or neoplasm (Figure 3.15), and conjunctival overgrowth (pseudopterygium). Prolapse of the gland of the third eyelid ("cherry eye"), congenital abnormalities, cataract, corneal opacities, and ocular colobomas have also been reported.

Epiphora is seen with either excessive tear production from ocular irritation or infection, or inadequate tear drainage due to an obstructed nasolacrimal duct. The condition manifests as crusting and matting of the hair at the medial canthus. Dystichiasis (abnormally positioned eyelashes) and trichiasis (ingrown eyelashes) have been reported in rabbits and are treated as in dogs. Nasolacrimal duct obstruction is a common sequela to chronic rhinitis or dacryocystitis caused by *Pasteurella multocida* and may also occur secondary to dental disease. Flushing of the duct may relieve the obstruction but care must be taken not to apply too much pressure, as rupture of the duct and subsequent abscess formation may occur (Figure 3.16). If the obstruction cannot be relieved by flushing, twice-daily warm compresses and massage over the rostrum for several days may help.

Conjunctivitis is most commonly caused by *P. multocida*, although other bacteria, such as *Staphylococcus aureus*, *Pseudomonas* spp, and *Chlamydophila* spp, are sometimes present. The bacteria may be present in the conjunctival sac or extend from the nasal cavity through the nasolacrimal duct. Purulent material can often be expressed into the conjunctival sac from the duct by applying digital pressure to the skin ventral to the medial canthus of the eye. *Pasteurella multocida* infections can also result in orbital cellulitis, uveitis, and conjunctivitis. Ammonia accumulation due to poor husbandry practices or inadequate ventilation may also induce conjunctivitis. Other causes of conjunctivitis, blepharitis,

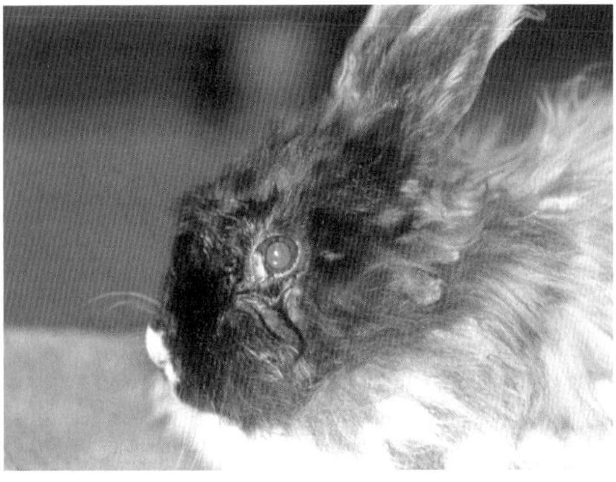

FIGURE 3.14. Conjunctivitis in a rabbit with prolapse of the nictitating membrane.

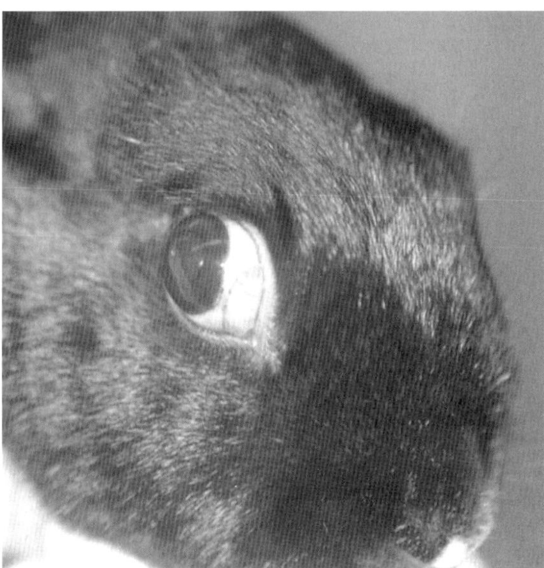

FIGURE 3.15. Exophthalmos in a pet rabbit secondary to a retrobulbar abscess.

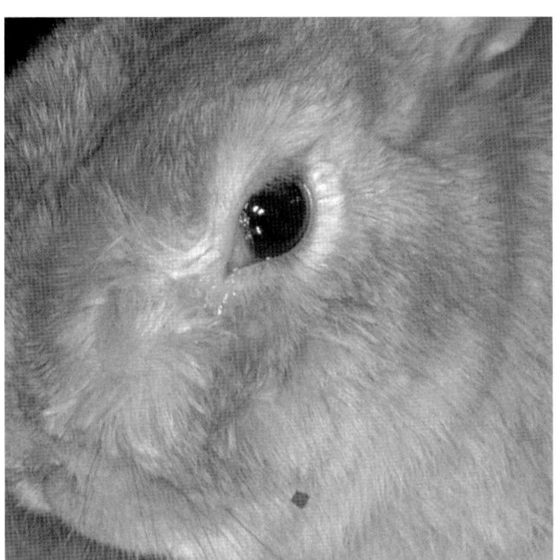

FIGURE 3.16. Epiphora and facial swelling secondary to rupture of the nasolacrimal duct in a pet rabbit.

and epiphora include trauma, eyelid malformations, dystichiasis, and trichiasis.

Blepharitis may be seen in cases of rabbit syphilis, caused by *Treponema cuniculi*. Spirochetes may be seen on scrapings of the infected area. Myxomatosis may also cause blepharitis.

Congenital buphthalmia (enlargement of the eye from excessive intraocular fluid accumulation), often with secondary glaucoma, occurs in New Zealand white (NZW), and some cross-bred rabbits. In NZW rabbits, it is an inherited autosomal recessive trait with incomplete penetrance and is characterized as uni- or bilateral buphthalmia that may progress to include corneal edema and blindness. The onset may be as early as 1 month of age, but more typically it occurs at 3–6 months. Treatment is unrewarding as the effects of topical miotic and beta-blocking drugs are usually not sufficient to preserve vision. Newer carbonic anhydrase inhibitors such as dorzolamide and brinzolamide or prostaglandin analogues such as latanoprost may be effective in reducing intraocular pressure. Surgical therapies include cyclocryotherapy and diode laser cycloablation for potentially sighted eyes, and evisceration with prosthesis implantation or enucleation for blind eyes. Intraoperative hemorrhage from the orbital venous sinus is a possible complication of enucleation but is often self-limiting before serious consequences occur.

Uveitis is associated with ocular trauma, ulcerative keratitis, systemic infection, and spontaneous lens rupture (phacoclastic uveitis) sometimes attributable to *Encephalitozoon cuniculi* infection. Treatment involves use of topical antiinflammatory and antimicrobial agents, similar to those for other species. Severe infections and phacoclastic uveitis often require enucleation.

Unilateral exophthalmos in rabbits is most often caused by orbital abscesses associated with dental disease. In advanced cases, enucleation, tooth extraction, and draining of the orbit may be successful if hemorrhage is appropriately controlled. In early cases, it may be possible to spare the globe by using a periocular approach. Marsupialization of the abscess cavity, packing with antibiotic impregnated polymethylmethacrylate beads, or packing with iodoform-impregnated gauze are some treatment options, but prognosis is always guarded. Other reported causes of unilateral exophthalmos include presence of *Taenia serialis* coenurus, orbital neoplasia, cellulitis, retrobulbar fat prolapse, and salivary mucocele. Bilateral exophthalmos has been associated with mediastinal masses such as thymoma or lymphoma, and as a consequence of chronic external jugular catheter placement.

Conjunctival overgrowth (pseudopterygium) is an uncommon, idiopathic condition, characterized by bilaterally symmetrical annular conjunctival overgrowth of the cornea. Treatment involves surgical excision of the conjunctival tissue; however, recurrence is common. A newer technique involving centrifugal incisions of the overgrowing conjunctiva to the limbus followed by eversion and transpalpebral fixation may result in fewer recurrences.

Prolapse of the gland of the third eyelid may be uni- or bilateral in rabbits. The cause is unknown, and surgical correction is usually successful in uncomplicated cases. Corneal opacities may be caused by keratitis, inherited corneal dystrophy (in Dutch rabbits), and dietary and inherited ocular lipidosis. Spontaneous juvenile cataracts have been reported to occur at an incidence of 5.7% in New Zealand white rabbits, which is consistent with an autosomal recessive mode of transmission. Secondary cataract formation can be seen after chronic uveitis.

Diabetic rabbits may develop osmotic cataracts similar to those in dogs. Cataract removal by phacoemulsification is possible.

Watanabe heritable hyperlipidemic (WHHL) rabbits exhibit ocular lesions consistent with lipid keratopathy. The condition is characterized by accumulation of lipid-laden macrophages in the cornea, iris, and ciliary body.

Congenital abnormalities of the rabbit eye are rare. Entropion and ectropion have been reported and can be surgically corrected. Cyclopia, persistent hyperplastic primary vitreous, lens coloboma, and optic nerve coloboma have been reported.

Guinea Pigs

Guinea pigs have a paurangiotic (nearly avascular) fundus, with only a few capillary loops near the central optic disc. The nictitating membrane is rudimentary and consists of a fold of conjunctiva near the medial canthus. Intraorbital glands include a large intraorbital lacrimal gland and an extensive zygomatic salivary gland. Guinea pigs are precocious and the eyelids are separated at birth. The retina is mottled red-brown. Small amounts of tears are normally produced. Schirmer tear test values without and with topical anesthetic are 0.36 mm ± 1.09 mm (wetting/min) and 0.43 mm ± 1.29 mm (wetting/min), respectively, while phenol red thread tear test values are reported to be 16 mm ± 4.7 mm (wetting/15 s). Guinea pigs have reduced corneal sensitivity compared to other species.

Ocular disorders include blepharitis, conjunctivitis, "pea eye" (an inferior conjunctival mass), scleral and corneal mineralization, cataract (Figure 3.17), and panophthalmitis. Lymphosarcoma with conjunctival involvement has been reported.

Blepharitis may be caused by dermatophytes, especially in young animals. Conjunctivitis can be seen with infectious agents, such as *Chlamydophila psittaci*, streptocci, *Micrococcus* spp, *Staphylococcus aureus*, *Pasteurella multocida, Bordetella bronchiseptica, Proteus* spp, and pneumococci, but may also be seen secondary to ascorbic acid deficiency. *Chlamydophila psittaci* infection can be enzootic and transmission is primarily venereal, with neonates infected at birth. Lesions usually resolve in approximately 1 month and treatment is considered unnecessary, unless the animal is severely affected. Conjunctival scrapings may yield typical intracytoplasmic chlamydial inclusions with Jiminez or Macchiavello's stain. Conjunctival cytology characteristic of bacterial conjunctivitis typically consists of numerous heterophils with or without intracellular bacteria. Corneal and scleral calcification occurs in guinea pigs with or without simultaneous mineralization elsewhere.

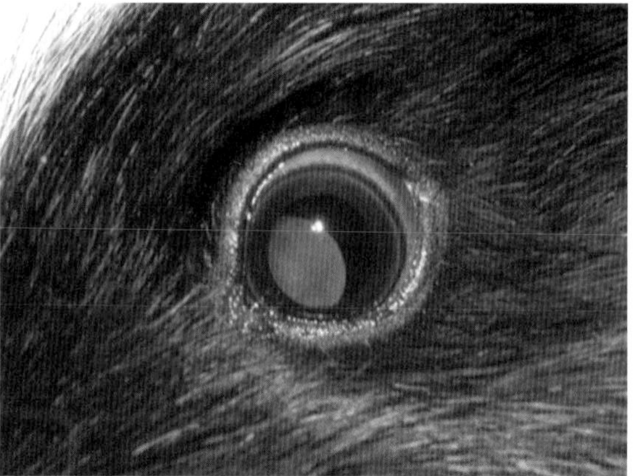

FIGURE 3.17. Aphakic crescent in a guinea pig. The crescent-shaped tapetal reflex is seen between the iris margin and a subluxated lens.

"Pea eye" describes a condition in which a ventral subconjunctival nodule protrudes from the conjunctival sac in one or both eyes. The enlargement is thought to be a portion of the lacrimal or zygomatic glands. Concurrent ventral ectropion may result, but treatment is usually unnecessary. Cortical cataracts are not uncommon and are suspected to be genetic in origin. Panopthalmitis may occur secondary to *Streptococcus zooepidemicus* abscess formation and bacteremia.

Chinchillas

Chinchillas have an anangiotic retina (without blood vessels), a rudimentary third eyelid, and a vertical pupillary slit. Like guinea pigs, they are precocial, and the eyelids are separated at birth. Asteroid hyalosis and cataracts have been reported in older animals. Exophthalmos caused by orbital *Taenia* spp coenurus has been reported in the chinchilla.

Hamsters and Gerbils

Syrian hamster eyelid separation occurs at approximately 15 days, Chinese hamster eyelid separation occurs between 10 and 14 days, and gerbil eyelid separation occurs 16–22 days after birth. Small rodents have a holangiotic retina (central blood supply) with radial vessels and a centrally located optic disc. Light entering the eye is focused on the entire retina. The shallow anterior chamber loses fluid rapidly with continuous eyelid opening, as occurs during surgery. Anterior chamber fluid loss may lead to corneal and lens opacities, which are reversible with rehydration and eyelid closure. The cornea is large and the lens round. The retina is rod dominated as expected in nocturnally active species.

Similar ocular disorders have been reported for hamsters and gerbils as for other rodent species (Figure 3.18). Keratoconjunctivitis may be caused by infections, environmental dryness, or cagemate trauma. Prolapse of the globe is not uncommon in hamsters due to the shallow orbits. Because of their nocturnal nature, the globe is usually severely damaged by the time the problem is detected, and enucleation is often necessary. Some laboratory strains of Chinese hamsters spontaneously develop diabetes mellitus and secondary cataracts. Facial dermatitis is common in gerbils and is characterized by erythema, alopecia, and crusting of the external nares, muzzle, and periocular areas. The cause is unclear but a multifactorial etiology is suspected, including reduced grooming and inappropriate cage bedding.

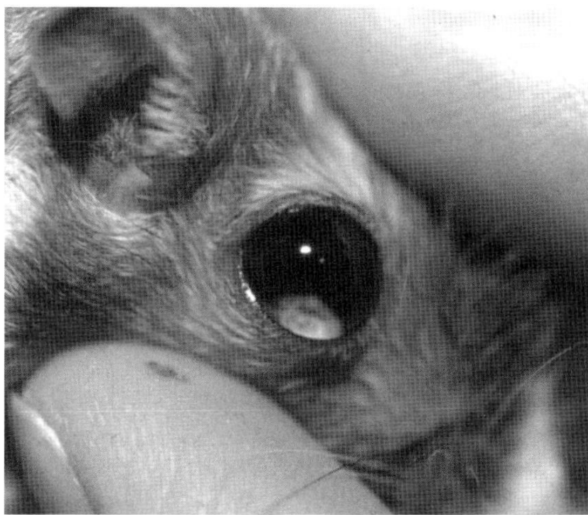

FIGURE 3.18. Cataract in a gerbil eye.

Mice and Rats

Mice and rats also have a holangiotic retina. Rats have three tear-producing glands, the intraorbital, exorbital, and Harderian, which is associated with the third eyelid. Porphyrin-pigmented tears are normally produced, predominantly by the Harderian gland, and production is controlled by parasympathetic innervation. Factors that increase parasympathetic activation increase the level of Harderian gland porphyrin production and may result in chromodacryorrhea or red tear production. Physiological stress and diseases such as mycoplasmosis and sialodacryoadenitis are important causes of chromodacryorrhea.

The most common cause of conjunctivitis in pet rats and mice is mycoplasmosis. Purulent conjunctivitis has been associated with *Pasteurella* spp in rats with an underlying mycoplasma infection. Poor ventilation and improper handling can also contribute to conjunctivitis.

In rats, sialodacryoadenitis caused by coronaviral infection leads to conjunctivitis and periorbital swelling, followed by lymphadenopathy and salivary gland swelling. The disease is highly contagious but usually self-limiting. Permanent damage to the lacrimal gland and reduced tear production may occur postinfection. In addition, keratitis and conjunctivitis may lead to chromodacryorrhea and self-mutilation. Diagnosis is made by classic pathognomonic signs, detection of coronavirus antigen, or serological testing of the animals.

Keratitis, corneal ulceration, and hypopyon have been reported in rats and mice following injectable anesthesia with ketamine/xylazine combinations, even when intraoperative eye lubricants are used (Figure 3.19). The cornea and subcorneal structures receive oxygenation from the anterior chamber. Injectable anesthetic agents may induce profound hypoxemia as well as hypotension, and it is hypothesized that this may result in corneal damage during anesthesia and prolonged postoperative recumbency. Animals undergoing injectable anesthesia should be supplemented with oxygen by face mask and reversed with specific pharmacologic agents

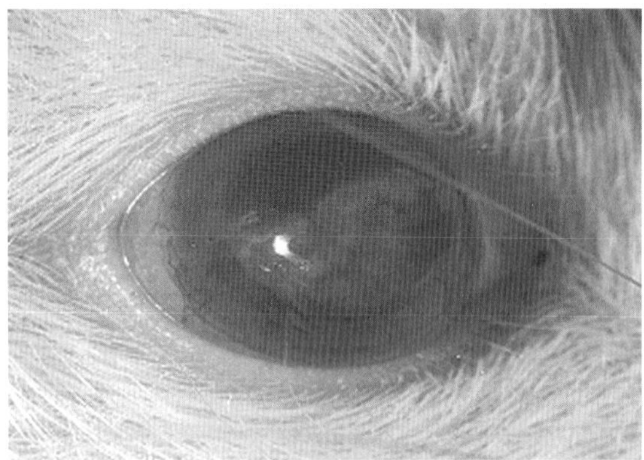

FIGURE 3.19. Corneal scarring and neovascularization in a rat as a sequela to ulceration. Reprinted with permission from AALAS.

whenever possible, to minimize the risk of corneal hypoxia and injury.

Spontaneous microphthalmia occurs incidentally in rats, notably in the F344 rat, as well as various strains of mice, such as the C57BL/6. Defective tear drainage and microbial contamination of the conjunctival sacs can result.

Retinal degeneration can be seen in rats and mice under constant illumination and has also been reported as a spontaneous defect in albino rats and a number of different mouse strains, such as black Swiss and NIH Swiss mice. Strain-specific ophthalmic characteristics may have important implications for animal performance during behavioral tests that have a visual component. It is important to ensure that animals that perform poorly on these tests are sighted.

Subepithelial mineralization of the cornea, apparent as focal corneal opacities, has been reported in both rats and mice, and persistent hyaloid vessels are commonly noted during fundic examination. Other conditions reported in rats include glaucoma, cataracts, and coloboma.

References

Abrams KL, et al. Evaluation of the Schirmer tear test in clinically normal rabbits. Amer J Vet Res. 1990, 51:1912–1913.

Allgoewer I, Ewringmann A, Pfleghaar S. Lymphosarcoma with conjunctival manifestation in a guinea pig. Vet Ophth. 1999, 2:117–119.

Allgoewer I, Malho P, Schulze H, et al. Aberrant conjunctival stricture and overgrowth in rabbits. Vet Ophth. 2008, 11:18–22.

Bagely LH, Lavach D. Ophthalmic diseases of rabbits. Calif Vet. 1995, 49:7–9.

Bauck L. Ophthalmic conditions in pet rabbits and rodents. Comp Cont Educ Pract Vet. 1989, 11:258–267.

Bellhorn RW. Laboratory Animal Ophthalmology. In: Veterinary Ophthalmology, 2nd ed. Gelatt KN (ed.). Philadelphia: Lea & Febiger, 1991, 656–679.

Biricik HS, et al. Evaluation of the Schirmer and phenol red thread tests for measuring tear secretion in rabbits. Vet Rec. 2005, 156:485–487.

Brayton C, Justice M, Montgomery CA. Evaluating mutant mice: anatomic pathology. Vet Pathol. 2001, 38:1–19.

Clapcote SJ, Lazar NL, Bechard AR, et al. NIH Swiss and black Swiss mice have retinal degeneration and performance deficits in cognitive tests. Comp Med. 2005, 55(4):310–316.

Davidson MG. Ophthalmology of exotic pets. Comp Cont Educ Pract Vet. 1985, 7:724–737.

Felchle LM, Sigler RL. Phacoemulsification for the management of Encephalitozoon cuniculi-induced phacoclastic uveitis in a rabbit. Vet Ophth. 2002, 5:211–215.

Giordano C, et al. Immunohistochemical identification of Encephalitozoon cuniculi in phacoclastic uveitis in four rabbits. Vet Ophth. 2005, 8:271–275.

Gwin RM, Gelatt KN. Bilateral ocular lipidosis in a cottontail rabbit fed an all-milk diet. J Am Vet Med Assoc. 1977, 171:887.

Holmberg BJ, Hollingsworgh SR, Osofsky A, Tell LA. Taenia coenurus in the orbit of a chincilla. Vet Ophth. 2007, 10:53–59.

Kern TJ. Rabbit and rodent ophthalmology. Sem Av Exot Pet Med. 1997, 6:138–145.

Kostolich M, Panciera RJ. Thymoma in a domestic rabbit. Cornell Vet. 2005, 82:259–263.

Kouchi M, Ueda Y, Horie H, et al. Ocular lesions in Watanabe heritable hyperlipidemic rabbits. Vet Ophth. 2006, 9:145–148.

Millichamp NJ. Management of ocular disease in exotic species. Sem Av Exot Pet Med. 1997, 6:152–159.

Munger RJ, Langevin NL, Podval J. Spontaneous cataracts in laboratory rabbits. Vet Ophth. 2002, 5:177–181.

Ninomiya H, Kuno H, Inagaki S. Vacular changes associated with chorioretinal and optic nerve colobomas in rats (Crj:CD9SD), IGS. Vet Ophth. 2005, 8:319–323.

O'Reilly A, et al. Taenia serialis causing exophthalmos in a pet rabbit. Vet Ophth. 2002, 5:227–230.

Sebesteny A, et al. Lipid keratopathy and atheromatosis in a SPF rabbit colony attributable to diet. Lab Anim. 1985, 19:180–188.

Trost K, Skalicky M, Nell B. Schirmer tear test, phenol red thread tear test, eye blink frequency and corneal sensitivity in the guinea pig. Vet Ophth. 2007, 10:143–146.

Turner PV, Albassam MA. Susceptibility of rats to corneal lesions following anesthesia. Comp Med. 2005, 55(2):182–189.

Vernau KM, Grahn BH, Clarke-Scott HA, et al. Thymoma in a geriatric rabbit with hypercalcemia and periodic exophthalmos. J Am Vet Med Assoc. 1995, 206:820–822.

Volopich S, Gruber A, Hassan J, et al. Malignant B-cell lymphoma of the Harder's gland in a rabbit. Vet Ophth. 2005, 8:259–263.

Wagner F, et al. Recurrent bilateral exopththalmos associated with metastatic thymic carcinoma in a pet rabbit. J Small Anim Pract. 2005, 46:393–397.

Wagner F, Fehr M. Common ophthalmic problems in pet rabbits. J Exot Pet Med. 2007, 16:158–167.

Williams DL. Laboratory Animal Ophthalmology. In: Veterinary Ophthalmology, 3rd ed. Gelatt KN (ed.). Baltimore: Lippincott Williams and Wilkins, 1999; 1209–1236.

———. Ocular disease in rats: A review. Vet Ophth. 2002, 5:183–191.

Wolfer J, et al. Spontaneous lens rupture in the rabbit. Vet Pathol. 1992, 29:478.

ADMINISTRATION OF DRUGS AND FORMULARY

Few drugs used in clinical practice are approved specifically in the United States by the Food and Drug Administration (FDA) for use in rabbits and rodents, a consideration that presents both legal and therapeutic complications (Tables 3.11 and 3.12). Apart from shortcomings resulting from interspecies extrapolations and limited clinical trials, several factors influence the pharmacologic effects of any given drug. Sex, strain or breed, age, diet, health status, time of day, breeding status, metabolic rate, presence of pathogenic organisms among intestinal flora, and nutritional level of the subjects, as well as composition of the bedding, experimental protocol, concomitant administration of other drugs, type of caging, and ambient temperature, all can affect a therapeutic outcome. In experimental studies, the use of antibiotics and other drugs should be carefully evaluated to ensure that any potentially confounding effects of the drug will not interfere with the experiment and ultimately render the animal useless. In addition to these concerns, some drugs that are safe and efficacious in other animals are toxic in rabbits or rodents or will change an active, clinical infection to a chronic, subclinical, carrier state.

Antibiotic therapy should include consideration of microbial sensitivity, cost of treatment, toxicity of the antibiotic to animals, toxicity of the antiobiotic to humans from ingestion of rabbit meat or handling the agent, public health significance of the pathogen involved, compatibility with other drugs or fluids, and the experimental protocol of the research study.

Fatal reactions to antibiotic administration are a major concern in the therapy of rabbit, guinea pig, chinchilla, gerbil, and hamster diseases, particularly with beta lactam antibiotics (penicillins and cephalosporins), macrolides (erythromycin and azithromycin), and lincosamides (lincomycin and clindamycin). An alteration in normal enteric flora (dysbiosis) may occur, followed by clostridial or coliform proliferation, and subsequent release of toxins into the cecum. Deaths from enterotoxemia begin within 48 hours of initiating antibiotic therapy and continue for a week or more. The morphologic effect caused by oral doses of at least 10,000 U of penicillin G is a hemorrhagic cecitis and colitis. Not all treated animals die after drug administration and rats and mice are resistant to these side effects. Many other antibiotics have been associated with fatal enterotoxemias in rabbits and rodents, and even those considered safe can sometimes cause problems.

Aminoglycosides (streptomycins, dihydrostreptomycin, gentamicin, amikacin, neomycin, kanamycin, and tobramycin) can cause an ascending flaccid paralysis with respiratory arrest, coma, and death. The effects are due to neuromuscular blockade of skeletal muscle as aminoglycosides are thought to be calcium channel blockers. This reaction occurs most commonly when the drug is given at high doses, but anesthesia may be a predisposing factor. All members of the family are also potentially nephrotoxic and ototoxic. Gentamicin-induced retinal toxic effects may occur in rabbits after intravitreal injection of the antibiotic. Streptomycin is frequently toxic in gerbils.

Table 3.11. Drug formulary for rabbits, guinea pigs, and chinchillas. (Caution: Most uses and dosages are extralabel. Units are mg/kg unless otherwise specified.)

Drug	Rabbit	Guinea Pig	Chinchilla
Antimicrobials			
Amikacin	2–5 q8–12h SC,IM	2–5 q8–12h SC,IM	2–5 q8–12h SC,IM,IV
Ampicillin	Toxic	Toxic	Toxic
Captan powder			1 tsp/2 cups dust
Cephalexin	11–22 q8–12h PO,SC	50 q24h IM	
Chloramphenicol	30 q8–12h PO,SC,IM,IV	50 q12h PO,SC,IM	50 q12h PO,SC,IM
Chlortetracycline	50 q24h PO		50 q12h PO
Ciprofloxacin	5–20 q12h PO	7–20 q12h PO	5–15 q12h PO
Doxycycline	2.5 q12h PO	2.5 q12h PO	2.5 q12h PO
Enrofloxacin	5–10 q12h PO,SC,IM or 200 mg/L dw × 14 d	0.05–0.2 mg/mL dw × 14 d or 5–10 q12h PO,SC,IM	10 q12h PO,SC,IM
Gentamycin	1.5–2.5 q8h SC,IM,IV	2–4 q8–12h SC,IM	2 q12h SC,IM,IV
Griseofulvin	25 q24h × 30–45 d PO	25–50 q12h × 14–60 d PO or 1.5% in DMSO for 5–7 d; topically	25 q24h × 30–60 d PO
Ketoconazole	10–40 q24h PO		
Lime sulfur dip	Dilute 1:40 with water, dip q7d for 4–6 wk	Dilute 1:40 with water, dip q7d for 4–6 wk	Dilute 1:40 with water, dip q7d for 4–6 wk
Metronidazole	20 q12h PO	20 q12h PO	10–20 q12h PO; use with caution
Neomycin	30 q12h PO	12–16 q12h PO	15 q24h PO
Oxytetracycline	50 q12h PO, or 1 mg/mL dw		50 q12h PO
Penicillin G, benzathine	42,000–60,000 IU/kg q48h SC,IM	Toxic	Toxic
Penicillin G, procaine	42,000–60,000 IU/kg q24h SC,IM	Toxic	Toxic
Sulfadimethoxine	10–15 q12h × 10 days PO	10–15 q12h PO	25–50 q24h × 10–14 d PO
Sulfamethazine	1 mg/mL drinking water (dw)	1 mg/mL dw	1 mg/mL dw
Sulfaquinoxaline	1 mg/mL dw	1 mg/mL dw	
Tetracycline	50 q8–12h PO or 250–1000 mg/L dw	10–20 q8–12h PO	0.3–2 mg/mL dw or 10–20 q8–12h PO
Trimethoprim/sulfa	30 q12–24h PO,SC,IM	15–30 q12h PO,SC	30 q12h PO,SC,IM
Tylosin	10 q12h PO,SC	10 q24h PO,SC; use with caution	10 q24h PO,SC
Vancomycin	50 q8h IV,IM		

(continued)

Table 3.11. ***(continued, units are mg/kg unless otherwise specified)***

Drug	Rabbit	Guinea Pig	Chinchilla
Antiparasitic Agents			
Albendazole	7.5–20 × 3–14 d PO		25 q12h × 2d PO
Amprolium (96% oral solution)	0.5 mL/500 mL dw × 10 d		
Amitraz		0.3% solution q7d topically	
Carbaryl powder 5%	Twice weekly	Topically q7d × 3 wk	In dust q7d × 3 wk
Fenbendazole	10, repeat in 2 wk, prn PO, or 50 ppm in feed × 2–6 wk	20 q24h × 5 d PO	20 q24h × 3–5 d PO
Imidacloprid	1 cat dose q30d, topical		
Ivermectin	0.4 q7–14d PO,SC	0.2–0.5 q7d × 3 wk PO,SC	0.2 q7d × 3 wk PO,SC
Lime sulfur	2–3% dip q7d × 4–6 wk	Dilute 1:40 in water, dip q7d × 6 wk	
Lufenuron	30 q30d PO		
Metronidazole	20 q12h PO	10–40 q24h PO	50–60 q12h × 5 d PO
Monensin	0.002–0.004% in feed		
Piperazine	200 mg/kg, repeat in 2–3 wk or 2–5 mg/mL dw × 7 d	2–5 mg/mL dw for 7 d, off 7 d, repeat	100 q24h × 2 d PO
Praziquantel	5–10 repeat in 10 d PO,SC,IM	6–10 PO	5–10 repeat in 10 d PO,SC,IM
Pyrantel pamoate	5–10 repeat in 2–3 wk PO		
Pyrethrin shampoo or powder	Weekly × 4–6 wk	Weekly × 3 wk	Weekly × 3 wk
Selemectin	6 topical	6 topical	
Sulfadimethoxine	50 once then 25 q24h × 10–20 d PO	25–50 q24h × 10 d PO	25–50 q24h × 10 d PO
Sulfamethazine	100 q24h PO, or 0.77 g/L dw or 0.5–1% in feed		
Sulfaquinoxaline	0.04–0.1% dw or 125–250 ppm in feed		
Thiabendazole	25–50 PO	100 q24h × 5 d PO	50–100 q24h × 5 d PO

Table 3.12. **Drug formulary for hamsters, gerbils, mice, and rats. (Caution: Most uses and dosages are extralabel. Units are mg/kg unless otherwise specified.)**

Drug	Hamster	Gerbil	Rat	Mouse
Antimicrobials				
Amikacin	2–5 q8–12h SC	2–5 q8–12h SC	10 q12h SC	10 q8–12h SC
Ampicillin	Toxic	6–30 q8h PO	20–100 q12h PO,SC	20–100 q12h PO,SC or 500 mg/L dw
Amphotericin B	1 mg/animal q12h × 5 d/wk × 3 wk SC			
Cephalexin		25 q24h SC	15 q12h SC	60 q12h PO
Cephaloridine	10–25 q24h SC	30 q12h IM	10–25 q24h SC	10–25 q24h SC
Cephalosporin				30 q12h SC
Chloramphenicol	50–200 q8h PO, or 30–50 q12h SC	50–200 q8h PO, or 30–50 q12h SC	50–200 q8h PO, or 30–50 q12h SC	0.5 mg/mL dw or 50–200 q8h PO, or 30–50 q12h SC
Chlortetracycline	20 q12h PO,SC			25 q12h PO,SC
Ciprofloxacin	7–20 q12h PO	7–20 q12h PO	7–20 q12h PO	7–20 q12h PO
Doxycycline	2.5 q12h PO	2.5 q12h PO	5 q12h PO	2.5–5 q12h PO
Enrofloxacin	0.05–0.2 mg/mL dw × 14 d or 5–10 q12h PO SC	0.05–0.2 mg/mL dw × 14 d or 5–10 q12h PO SC	0.05–0.2 mg/mL dw × 14 d or 5–10 q12h PO SC	0.05–0.2 mg/mL dw × 14 d or 5–10 q12h PO SC
Erythromycin			20 q12h PO	20 q12h PO
Gentamicin	5 q24h SC	2–4 q8h SC	5–10 divided q8–12h	2–4 q8–12h SC
Griseofulvin	25–50 q12h × 14–60 d PO, or 1.5% in DMSO for 5–7 d; topically	25–50 q12h × 14–60 d PO, or 1.5% in DMSO for 5–7 d; topically	25–50 q12h × 14–60 d PO, or 1.5% in DMSO for 5–7 d; topically	25–50 q12h × 14–60 d PO, or 1.5% in DMSO for 5–7 d; topically
Ketoconazole	10–40 q24h × 14 d PO	10–40 q24h × 14 d PO	10–40 q24h × 14 d PO	10–40 q24h × 14 d PO
Metronidazole	7.5 mg/70–90 gm animal q8h	7.5 mg/70–90 gm animal q8h	10–40 q24h PO	2.5 mg/mL dw × 5 d or 20–60 q8–12h PO
Neomycin	0.5 mg/mL dw or 100 q24h PO	2.6 mg/mL dw or 100 q24h PO	2.6 mg/mL dw or 25 q12h PO	2.6 mg/mL dw
Oxytetracycline	0.25–1 mg/mL dw or 16 q24h SC	0.8 mg/mL dw or 10 q8h PO, or 20 q24h SC	0.4 mg/mL dw or 10–20 q8h PO	0.4 mg/mL dw or 10–20 q8h PO
Sulfadimethoxine	10–15 q12h PO	10–15 q12h PO	10–15 q12h PO	10–15 q12h PO

(continued)

Table 3.12. ***(continued, units are in mg/kg unless otherwise specified)***

Drug	Hamster	Gerbil	Rat	Mouse
Antimicrobials *(continued)*				
Sulfamerazine	1 mg/mL dw	0.8 mg/mL dw	1 mg/mL dw	1 mg/mL dw or 500 mg/L dw
Sulfamethazine	1 mg/mL dw	0.8 mg/mL dw	1 mg/mL dw	1 mg/mL dw
Tetracycline	0.4 mg/mL dw or 10–20 q8–12h PO	2–5 mg/mL dw or 10–20 q8–12h PO	2–5 mg/mL dw or 10–20 q8h PO	2–5 mg/mL dw or 10–20 q8h PO
Trimethoprim/ sulfa	15–30 q12–24h PO,SC	30 q12–24h PO,SC	15–30 q12h PO,SC	30 q12h PO,SC
Tylosin	2–8 q12h SC,PO, or 0.5 mg/mL dw	0.5 mg/mL dw or 10 q24h PO,SC	0.5 mg/mL dw or 10 q24h PO,SC	0.5 mg/mL dw or 10 q24h PO,SC
Vancomycin	20 × 3+ mo PO			
Antiparastitic Agents				
Amitraz	1.4 mL/L water using cottonball application q14d for 3–6 tx	1.4 mL/L water using cottonball application q14d for 3–6 tx		
Carbamate(5%)	Twice weekly		Twice weekly	Twice weekly
Fenbendazole	20 q24h × 5 d PO	20 q24h × 5 d PO	20 q24h × 5 d PO, or 150 mg/kg feed for 7 d on, 7 d off for 3 tx	20 q24h × 5 d PO, or 150 mg/kg feed for 7 d on, 7 d off for 3 tx
Fipronil	7.5 q30–60g topically		7.5 q30–60g topically	7.5 q30–60g topically
Ivermectin	0.2–0.4 q7–10d × 3 tx PO,SC		0.2–0.4 q7–10d × 3 tx PO,SC	0.2–.5 q7d × 3 wk PO SC topically
Mebendazole			40 q7d × 21 d	40 q7d × 21 d
Metronidazole			10–40 mg/animal or 2.5 mg/mL dw × 5 d	30–40 q8–12h PO
Moxidectin				0.5 mg/kg of 0.5% pour-on applied to dorsum
Niclosamide		1 mg/10 gm PO		
Permethrin			0.25% dust in cage or cottonball soaked in 5% solution in cage for 4–5 wk	4 g of 0.25% dust once weekly in bedding for 4 wk

(continued)

CLINICAL PROCEDURES

Table 3.12. ***(continued, units are in mg/kg unless otherwise specified)***

Drug	Hamster	Gerbil	Rat	Mouse
Antiparastitic Agents *(continued)*				
Piperazine citrate	2–5 mg/mL dw × 7 d, off 7 d, then repeat	2–5 mg/mL dw × 7 d, off 7 d, then repeat or 20–60 mg/100 gm PO	2–5 mg/mL dw × 7 d, off 7 d, then repeat	2–5 mg/mL dw × 7 d, off 7 d, then repeat
Pyrantel pamoate	50 PO	50 PO		
Praziquantel	6–10 PO	30 q14d × 3 tx PO	6–10 PO	6–10 PO, or 140 ppm in feed for 5 d
Pyrethrin powder	3×/wk × 3 wk	3×/wk × 3 wk	3×/wk × 3 wk	3×/wk × 3 wk
Thiabendazole	100–200 PO	100 q24h × 5d PO	100–200 PO	100–200 PO, or 0.3% in feed for 7–10 d, use repeated tx

Although generally safe in rabbits and rodents, quinolone antibiotics (e.g., enrofloxacin) may cause arthropathies in young animals. Many bacteria infecting these species are highly sensitive to chloramphenicol. Chloramphenicol has rarely been associated with nondose-dependent irreversible aplastic anemia in humans and appropriate directions for hand washing after handling must be given when this antibiotic is dispensed.

Often there is limited information available on species-specific pharmacokinetics of certain drugs for rabbits and rodents, and dosages must be extrapolated from those used for dogs and cats. Several approaches exist to adjust drug dosages from one species to another. Linear extrapolations based on body weight alone tend to result in overdosing of larger animals and underdosing of smaller ones. If this method is selected, drug doses should be extrapolated from those used for ferrets or cats.

Methods such as allometric (metabolic) scaling take basal metabolic rate and surface area into consideration and are rooted in the concept that smaller species tend to have higher metabolic rates and organ blood flow rates. Comparisons of allometric scaling among these species give scaling ratios of 2.8 for a mouse, 1.5 for a hamster, 1.3 for a rat, 1.2 for a guinea pig, and 1.0 for a rabbit. Drugs that are best estimated by allometric scaling include antibiotics, compounds that are not highly protein bound, and compounds that rely largely on renal elimination rather than hepatic metabolism. This method does not take into account species- or strain-specific differences in specific hepatocellular metabolic pathways, which can not always be predicted based on animal size or rate of basal metabolism.

Another comparison for developing approximate drug dosages is surface area/body weight or surface area/body volume ratios, as these ratios tend to increase more gradually than changes in body weight alone. For example, surface area to body weight ratio comparisons are 5.7 for a mouse, 3.7 for a hamster, 2.5 for a rat, 1.7 for a guinea pig, and 1.0 for a rabbit. This calculation is particularly useful for estimating drug dosages for cancer chemotherapeutics.

References

Adams HR. Veterinary Pharmacology and Therapeutics, 8th ed. Ames: Iowa State University Press, 2001.

Allen DG, et al. Handbook of Veterinary Drugs, 2nd ed. Philadelphia: Lippincott Williams and Wilkins, 1998.

Bendele AM, et al. Passive role of articular chondrocytes in quinolone-induced arthropathy in guinea pigs. Toxicol Pathol. 1990, 11:304–312.

Blakeley BR, Rousseaux CG. Effect of ivermectin on the immune response in mice. Amer J Vet Res. 1991, 52:593–595.

Broome RL, et al. Pharmacokinetic properties of enrofloxacin in rabbits. Amer J Vet Res. 1991, 52:1835–1841.

Conlee JW, et al. Differential susceptibility to gentamicin ototoxicity between albino and pigmented guinea pigs. Hearing Res. 1989, 41:43–52.

Curl JL, Curl JS. Pharmacokinetics of gentamicin in laboratory rabbits. Amer J Vet Res. 1988, 49:2065–2067.

Curl JL, Curl JS, Harrison JK. Pharmacokinetics of long acting oxytetracycline in the laboratory rat. Lab Anim Sci. 1988, 38:430–434.

Diggs HE, et al. Effect of chronic ivermectin treatment on GABA receptor function in ethanol withdrawal-seizure prone and resistant mice. Lab Anim Sci. 1990, 40:68–71.

Flecknell PA. Laboratory Animal Anaesthesia, 2nd ed. London: Academic Press, 1996.

Gaertner DJ. Comparison of penicillin and gentamicin for treatment of pasteurellosis in rabbits. Lab Anim Sci. 1991, 41:78–80.

Hara-Kudo Y, et al. Incidence of diarrhea with antibiotics and the increase of clostridia in rabbits. J Vet Med Sci. 1996, 58:1181–1185.

Hunter RP, Isaza R. Concepts and issues with interspecies scaling in zoological pharmacology. J Zoo Wildl Med. 2008, 39:517–526.

Lim JI, et al. The role of gravity in gentamicin induced toxic effects in a rabbit model. Arch Ophthalmol. 1994, 112:1363–1367.

McElroy DE, Ravis WR, Clark CH. Pharmacokinetics of oxytetracycline hydrochloride in rabbits. Amer J Vet Res. 1987, 48:1261–1263.

Morris TH. Antibiotic therapeutics in laboratory animals. Lab Anim. 2006, 29:16–36.

Paul-Murphy J. Critical care of the rabbit. Vet Clin Exot Anim. 2007, 10:437–461.

Pledger T, et al. Penicillin treatment schedule determination and associated tissue residues in the rabbit. J Appl Rabbit Res. 1990, 13:199–207.

Porter WP, et al. Absence of therapeutic blood concentrations of tetracycline in rats after administration in drinking water. Lab Anim Sci. 1985, 35:71–75.

Rosenthal KL. Therapeutic contraindications in exotic pets. Sem Av Exot Pet Med. 2004, 13:44–48.

Sharpnack DD, et al. Quinolone arthropathy in juvenile New Zealand White rabbits. Lab Anim Sci. 1994, 44:436–442.

Summa MEL, et al. Efficacy of oral ivermectin against Trichosomoides crassicanda in naturally infected laboratory rats. Lab Anim Sci. 1992, 42:620–622.

ANESTHESIA

This section describes anesthetics commonly available in veterinary clinics or laboratory animal facilities. Anesthetics or other drugs used frequently outside the United States but not yet licensed for use in the country (e.g., Hypnorm®—fentanyl plus fluanisone) are noted briefly. Refinement of anesthetic techniques in laboratory animal practice has resulted in a plethora of commercially available species- and size-specific anesthetic equipment for rabbits and rodents, including induction chambers, face masks, platforms to facilitate endotracheal intubation, nonrebreathing anesthetic circuits, downdraft tables, rodent ventilators, heating mats, and other small mammal monitoring equipment.

Many factors affect the response of rabbits and rodents to anesthetics. Such factors include sex, age, species, strain, weight, percent body fat, health and nutritional status, ingesta content, time of day, genetic background, type of bedding, environmental temperature during recovery, cardiovascular and respiratory system effects, and respiratory and metabolic rates. The large, ingesta-filled ceca of rabbits and guinea pigs may result in overdosing due to an overestimation of the true body weight. For nocturnal species, drug-induced sleeping times will be longer in the afternoon, when hepatic metabolic activity is at low ebb.

Cedar and pine bedding emit volatile oils such as pinenes that, over time, activate hepatic cytochrome P450 metabolizing enzymes. This may lead to increased rates of metabolism for drugs that are transformed by these systems, such as various anesthetics and analgesics, and as a result, reduced efficacy and sleeping times when these agents are given to animals housed on these beddings. Kiln drying of softwood shavings at high temperatures may eliminate many of these volatile oils; however, this type of bedding is best avoided for any experimental studies that depend on hepatic drug metabolism.

Most anesthetics cause a dose-dependent depression of physiologic homeostasis, including cardiovascular, respiratory, and thermoregulation systems. The physiologic changes can vary considerably with different anesthetics. Interpretation and appropriate response to the various parameters measured require experience and training with the anesthetic regimen and the species being anesthetized. The level of consciousness, antinociception (analgesia), and functioning of the cardiovascular (including fluid balance), respiratory, and thermoregulation systems are used to assess the adequacy of the anesthetic regimen.

Loss of consciousness occurs at a light plane of anesthesia and is sufficient for purposes of restraint or minor noninvasive procedures. Consciousness is lost before antinociception occurs, and at a light anesthetic plane, can be regained by painful stimuli.

Lack of response to painful stimuli (antinociception) occurs at a surgical stage of anesthesia. Prior to surgery, adequate antinociception should be ascertained by the presence or absence of various reflexes (described below). Individual animal responses vary widely, and a single reflex response may not be adequate for assessing the surgical plane of anesthesia or the level of analgesia.

Preoperative Procedures

Animals in poor clinical condition require stabilization prior to anesthesia and surgery. Obesity and old age, which are common in pet species, will increase anesthetic risk. Candidates for anesthesia and surgical procedures should, if possible, be free from respiratory disease. Withholding food from rabbits and rodents is not necessary as they are unable to vomit. In larger species, such as chinchillas, guinea pigs, and rabbits, food may be withheld for 4–6 hours to reduce the volume of the gastrointestinal tract. Food should not be withheld from small rodents for more than 2–3 hours because of the possibility of hypoglycemia and dehydration, as these species typically will not drink if they do not eat. Potable water should always be available to small mammal patients up to the time of anesthetic induction. Preoperative administration of warm, subcutaneous fluids, such as lactated Ringer's solution, at 10 mL/kg may be beneficial in debilitated small rodents.

Glycopyrrolate or atropine sulfate may be administered subcutaneously 30 minutes before anesthesia to reduce salivary and bronchial secretions, and decrease vagal tone. Glycopyrrolate does not cross the blood-brain barrier and is more effective blocking drug-induced bradycardia in rabbits and rodents, compared with atropine. Some rabbits and rodents elaborate plasma atropinesterase, which hydrolyzes and inactivates atropine. Glycopyrrolate may be preferred for this reason, but if atropine is to be used, the dose may need to be increased or administered at more frequent intervals to achieve the desired effect. The level of atropinesterase activity further depends on season of year and the sex, strain, age, and weight of rabbit or rodent.

Anesthetic Administration

Because many small mammal pets have subclinical respiratory disease that results in hypoventilation and mild respiratory compromise, preoxygenation with 100% O_2 for 3–5 minutes prior to anesthetic induction may be useful to minimize anesthetic-induced apnea, which may further exacerbate any underlying hypoxemia and result in sudden death. Preoxygenation may also help to reduce breath-holding and subsequent apnea often seen in rabbits induced with gas anesthetics such as isoflurane.

Rabbits and rodents should be restrained gently but firmly during induction and induced as quickly as possible. In rabbits and guinea pigs, in particular, sudden death has been reported during gas anesthesia induction when animals are highly excited or are permitted to struggle. It is hypothesized that sudden catecholamine release from the adrenal glands during excitement and struggling may lead to coronary vessel constriction, acute cardiac ischemia, and sudden death.

Induction of inhalant anesthesia in rodents is facilitated by use of an induction chamber, with an appropriate scavenging system to minimize exposure of personnel to waste gases. The induction chamber should be as small as possible to adequately accommodate the animal with minimal dead space. Clear plastic containers with lids and rubber gasket seals

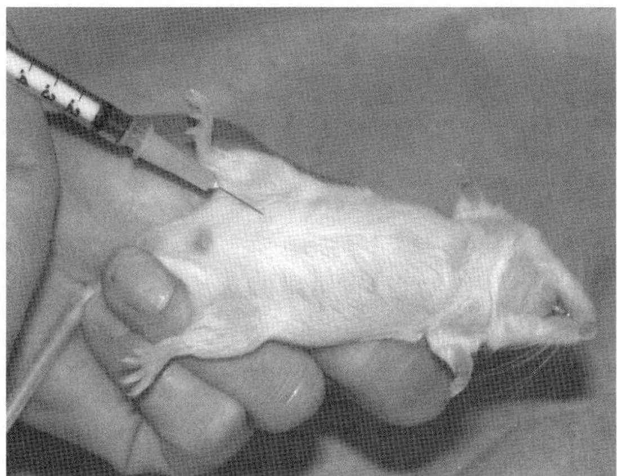

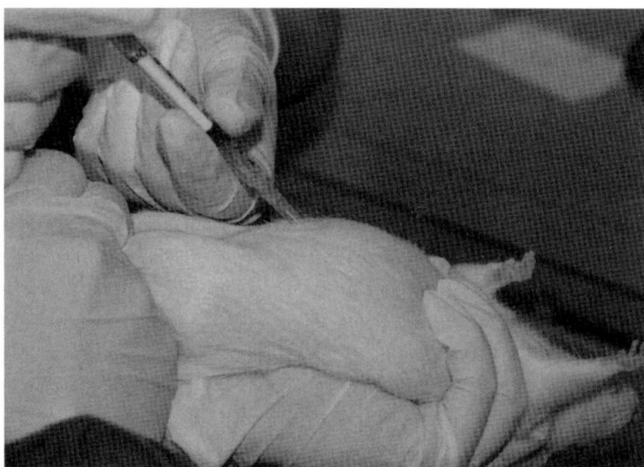

FIGURE 3.20. Technique for intraperitoneal injection into a mouse (left) and rat (right).

may be modified for this purpose. Once induced, the animal is quickly removed from the chamber, and either intubated or placed on a face mask and attached to a nonrebreathing anesthetic circuit for maintenance. Rabbits may be induced by face mask using the towel wrap for restraint (see Figure 2.9). A downdraft table or other appropriate scavenging system should be used, especially if the animal is maintained on a face mask.

Injectable anesthetics may be given under the skin folds on the back of the neck (SC), deeply into the hindlimb or epaxial muscles (IM), or into the peritoneal cavity (IP). Intramuscular (IM) injections should be avoided in small rodents because of the potential for pain upon injection, subsequent sloughing of skin and muscle due to drug-induced necrosis, and the possibility of self-mutilation when acidic or irritating agents are injected. Intraperitoneal (IP) injections are given by sharp puncture at a 60° angle with an appropriate-sized needle in the lower left abdominal quadrant while firmly restraining the animal in a head-down position (Figure 3.20).

Ketamine is preferably given SC or IP to small rodents because of muscle irritation upon intramuscular injection. Aspirating the syringe before injection will help to ensure that the anesthetic is administered into the peritoneal cavity and not into organs or blood vessels. Because of their large cecum, it has been estimated that 20% of IP injections in guinea pigs inadvertently penetrate abdominal organs. Prolonged induction and recovery times may be indicative of injection of the anesthetic into an organ. Dosages and body weights should be determined accurately to avoid fatalities in these small mammal species.

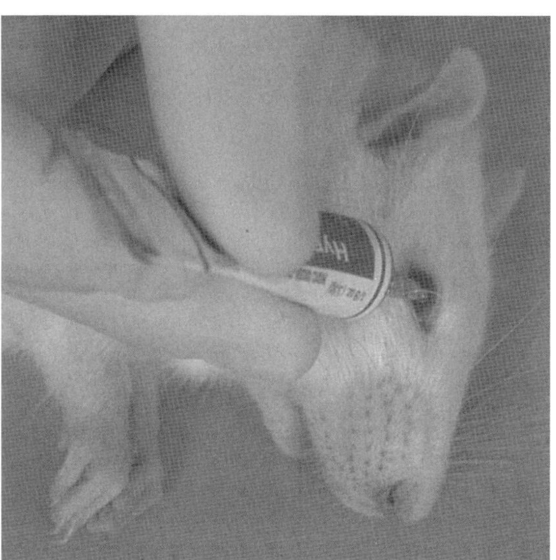

FIGURE 3.21. Sterile ophthalmic lubricant being placed in the eye of an anesthetized rat.

Because of the large eye size, rodent and rabbit palpebrae may not close completely during anesthesia. Sterile, nonmedicated ophthalmic drops or ointment should be used on all patients to minimize corneal drying (Figure 3.21). Patients should be positioned carefully to avoid direct contact of the cornea with the heating pad or blanket (Figure 3.22).

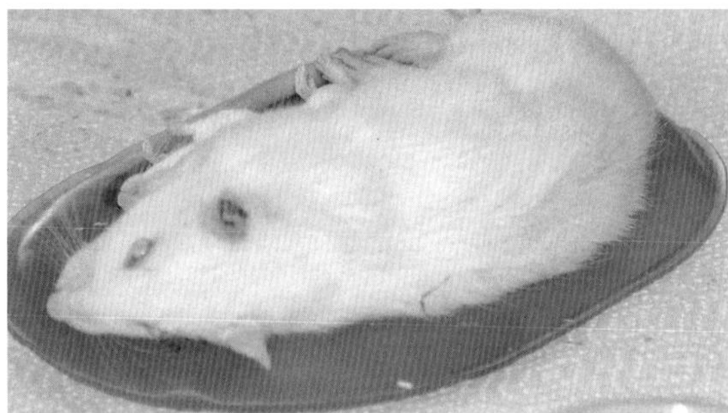

FIGURE 3.22. Microwavable gel pack for maintaining rodent body heat during anesthesia.

Oxygen should be given by face mask during injectable anesthesia to counteract drug-induced hypoxemia and possible corneal injury.

Endotracheal Intubation

Rabbits and rodents rarely regurgitate and are anesthetized frequently without endotracheal intubation for a multitude of surgical procedures, including most dentistries, lumpectomies, and routine spay and neuter procedures. However, for surgical procedures involving thoracotomies, those disrupting respiratory neuromuscular signaling, or when required for research purposes, endotracheal intubation may be advisable. Animals should be induced and intubated after cough and swallowing reflexes are abolished. For rabbits, propofol administered via an IV catheter at a dose of 7.5 mg/kg (administer 50% of calculated dose by slow bolus and top up with additional propofol to effect) may assist with initial induction and relaxation in preparation for intubation. Relaxation of the jaw musculature signifies that the animal is anesthetized sufficiently to begin intubation. The mouths of rabbits and rodents do not open widely and visualization of the larynx is difficult. Topical anesthetic (e.g., lidocaine) should not be sprayed into the oral cavity of small rodents because of the danger of asphyxiation, irritation, and toxicity; however, it can be applied with cotton swabs to the soft palate and pharynx. Topical anesthesia to prevent laryngospasm in rabbits should be used cautiously before intubation because the anesthetic suppresses the convenient forward motion of the glottis during swallowing.

Intubation is not easy to accomplish in any of these species. Care must be taken to obtain customized equipment, practice and master the technique, and avoid traumatizing the sensitive oral and respiratory structures. The large fleshy tongue of these species, large teeth, deep, narrow oral cavity, and small mouth complicate the process. The palatal ostium in the guinea pig further obscures the epiglottis. For rabbits, commercially available 2.0–3.5 uncuffed endotracheal tubes cut to a suitable length to minimize dead space will be useful for most adult animals. Animals should be lightly anesthetized in sternal recumbency with hyperextension of the neck before attempting the procedure. There are many different intubation techniques described, which may involve either a blind procedure that relies on the sound of airflow as the tube is passed into the trachea or direct visualization of the larynx with a specialized laryngoscope, rigid endoscope, or otoscopic cone with a side opening. The anatomy and technique can be reviewed and practiced on dead animals. Care should be taken not to bend the head too far dorsally because cervical vertebral fracture may occur. Endotracheal tubes for rodents may be custom-made from appropriately sized and modifed IV catheters.

More than two to three attempts at intubation may result in epiglottal hemorrhage and trauma. Respiratory secretions accumulating during anesthesia may be removed by suction or cotton swabs. Rabbits have a highly vascularized submucosal plexus within the trachea. Movement of the head with the endotracheal tube in place or prolonged surgeries in intubated animals may result in postprocedural tracheal edema, fibrosis, and stenosis in rabbits. This is manifested clinically within 2–10 days following the procedure by tachypnea, inactivity, reduced food consumption, respiratory stridor, and cyanosis. Severely affected animals may die.

Use of inflatable pediatric laryngeal mask airways (size 0–1) has also been described in rabbits. These airways are significantly easier to place than endotracheal tubes; however, they may result in more waste gas emissions and may also lead to postprocedural pharyngeal trauma and bleeding.

Anesthetic Overdose

Anesthetic overdose is indicated by diaphragmatic breathing, gasping, loss of various reflexes, and cyanosis. Severe cases may result in death. If the respiratory rate can be determined, a decrease to less than 40% of the normal rate indicates impending respiratory failure. Assuming a patent airway is present, artificial respiration, respiratory stimulants, or anesthetic antagonists can be used. Such drugs include doxapram (2–10 mg/kg IM or IV every 15–20 min), naloxone (0.01–0.1 mg/kg IP, IM, or IV), nalorphine (1–5 mg/kg IV), levallorphan (0.45 mg/kg IV), yohimbine to reverse xylazine (0.2–1 mg/kg IM or IV), or atipamezole to reverse medetomidine (SC or IV administered at the same volume as medetomidine). Warmed, 37 °C (98.6 °F) isotonic saline can be given by IV or IP routes.

Gentle manual cardiopulmonary resuscitation via compression of the sternum 50–100 times per minute or blowing with a Pasteur pipette bulb or tightly fitting face mask into the animal's nose may stimulate respiration, as may gently swinging the animal repeatedly or tipping the animal from horizontal to head down. Pressing the end of the nose between the nostrils with a blunt probe, pen, or the edge of a fingernail may stimulate the animal to take a breath. Oxygen should be supplied, if it is not already being given.

Supportive Care

It is critical that anesthetized rabbits and rodents be kept warm, well hydrated, and well oxygenated from induction through recovery. Hypothermia decreases drug metabolism and elimination and may prolong anesthesia, sedation, and recovery. Because body heat loss and metabolic rate can be related to a surface area to body weight ratio, loss of heat or decreased rate of metabolism of a drug is more rapid in mice than in rabbits. Commercially available circulating warm water blankets, warm air blankets (such as the Bair Hugger®), and thermal pads designed with rectal temperature probes for feedback are available for small animals. Electrical heating pads, microwavable heat pads, water bags or bottles, and lamps should be used with extreme caution to prevent overheating, dehydration, or thermal burns. Animals should be insulated from stainless steel surfaces and covered with a light-weight drape, stockinette, or bubble-wrap whenever possible, taking care not to impede respiration. During recovery, oxygen-supplying intensive care units are helpful, and experimental animals can be grouped together for additional warmth, when possible. Environmental temperatures of 30–35 °C (86–95 °F) for rodents and 25 °C (77 °F) for rabbits are appropriate.

Intraoperative monitoring of anesthetized animals may be accomplished using measures of arterial blood oxygen saturation (pulse oximetry) (Figure 3.23), body temperature, capnometry (for intubated animals), indirect or direct blood pressure (Figure 3.24), and electrocardiography. Respiratory alert monitors designed for larger small animal species may not detect the small volume of gas emitted during respiratory excursions of rabbits and rodents.

Intraoperative fluids, preferably warmed to body temperature, such as 0.9% saline, 4% glucose, or lactated Ringer's solution, can be given IV, SC, IP, or intraosseously (IO) at a rate of 5–10 mL/kg/hr. Commercially available fluid warmers can be used with IV extension sets, or tubing can be passed through a container of warm water. Intravenous catheters can easily be placed in rabbits (auricular, cephalic, or lateral saphenous veins) and rats (tail vein) and can often be placed in the cephalic or lateral saphenous vein of other rodents (Figures 3.25 and 3.26). With practice, intraosseous catheter placement is also possible and can be used when needed. Syringe drivers or syringe infusion pumps (e.g., Springfusor® syringe infusion pump) are useful for administering fluids to very small patients (Figure 3.27). Postoperative maintenance fluids are given at 40–80 mL/kg/day until it is certain that the animal is eating and drinking sufficiently.

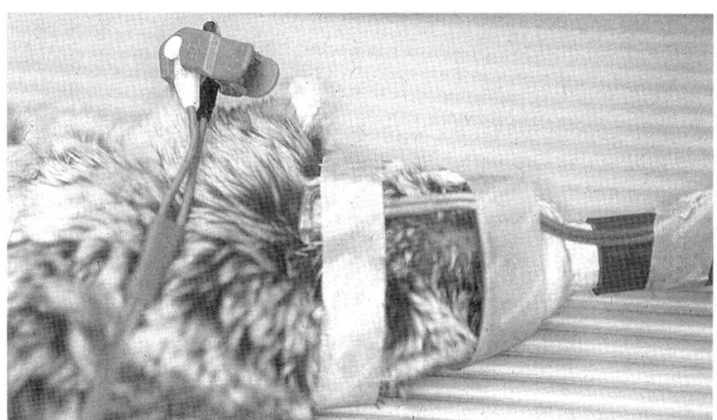

FIGURE 3.23. Chinchilla anesthetized by isoflurane in oxygen, delivered by a face mask. A pulse oximeter clamp is placed on the forelimb to monitor arterial blood oxygen saturation and a Doppler flow probe is taped over the jugular vein, giving an audible heart rate.

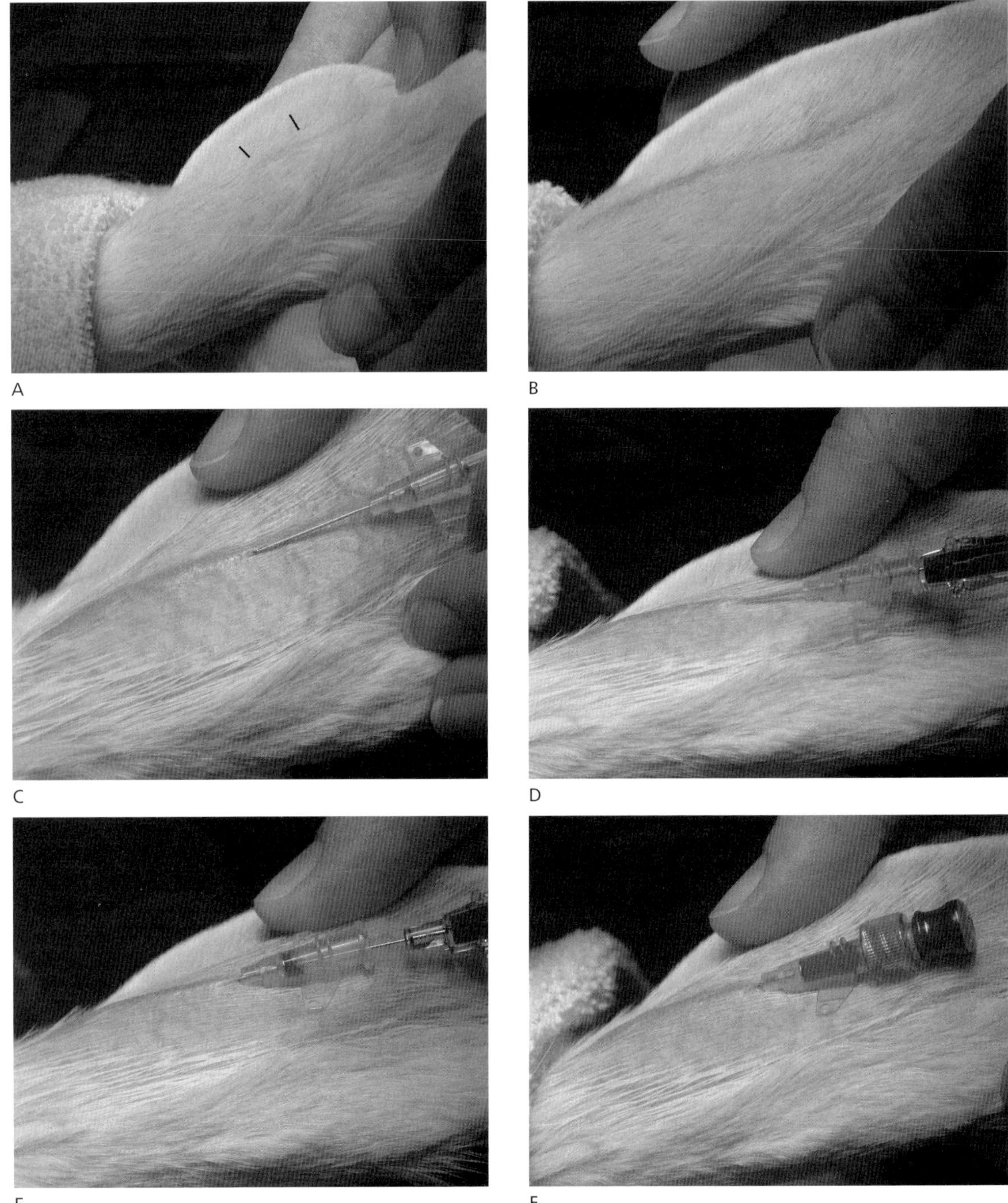

FIGURE 3.24. Sequence of events to catheterize the central auricular artery of the rabbit for direct blood pressure monitoring. Prior to plucking, the ear artery is not visible (A) (arrows). After plucking the hair, the artery is readily visualized (B). Following surgical preparation of the catheter site, a 25g IV catheter may be introduced into the vessel and the stylet removed (C, D, E). The catheter is capped and flushed (F).

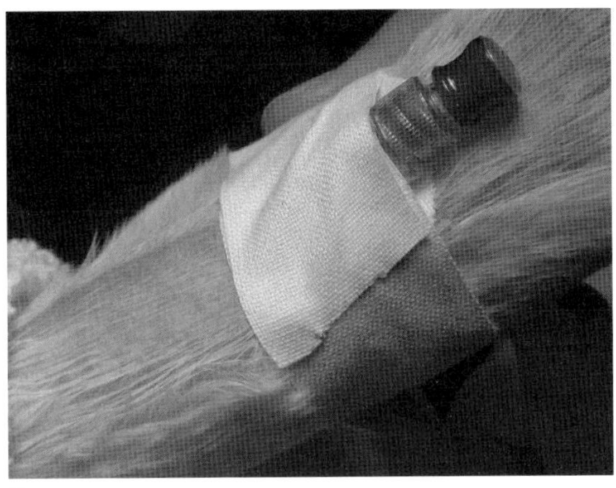

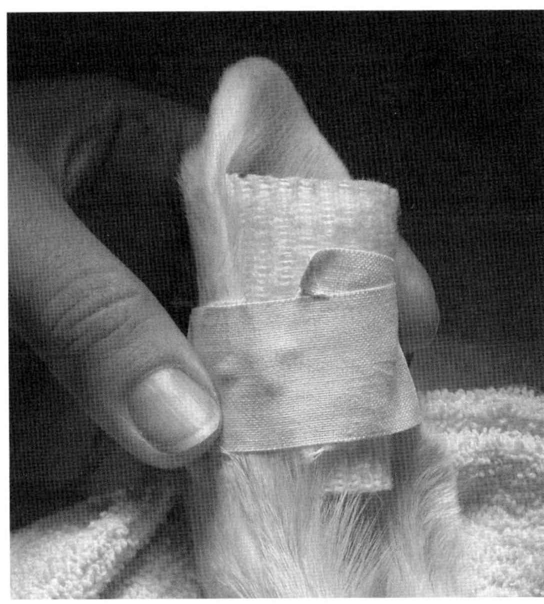

G H

FIGURE 3.24. *(continued)* To secure it, the catheter is taped into place and a roll of cotton gauze is taped to the inside of the ear for stabilization of the catheter (G, H).

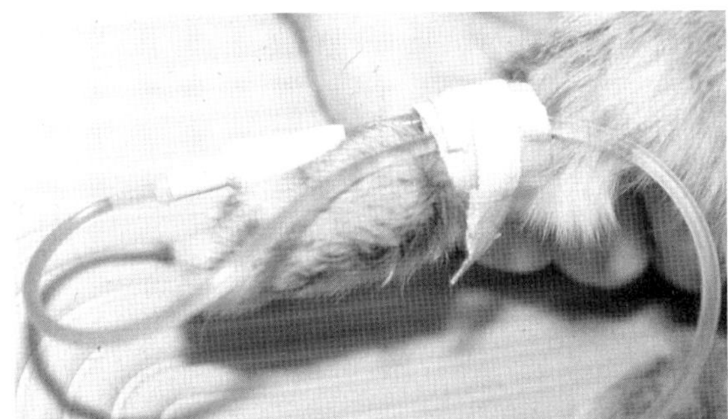

FIGURE 3.25. A cephalic catheter may be placed in the rabbit for fluid administration.

Breathing may be compromised in chinchillas, guinea pigs, and rabbits placed in dorsal recumbency, because of the weight of the large abdominal contents pressing on the relatively small thorax, especially in obese animals. Elevating the head and thorax will help prevent respiratory compromise. Administration of oxygen during anesthesia with injectable agents, especially ketamine and xylazine, is critical to avoid hypoxemia, which may predispose animals to corneal lesions and other problems. Cyanosis and pulse oximeter SpO_2 readings of <65% are often observed in spontaneously breathing rats anesthetized with injectable agents (Figure 3.28).

Respiratory stimulants (e.g., doxapram) may be indicated in some circumstances, and appropriate analgesia must always be provided. Antibiotics may be given to rats and mice when asepsis is not possible or is compromised. Antibiotics should be used sparingly, if at all, in guinea pigs, hamsters, gerbils, chinchillas, and rabbits. Wounds should be attended to regularly and bedding changed as needed to keep the surgical site clean.

Postsurgical feeding and hydration are critically important, and warmed 4% glucose solution SC, palatable high caloric food supplements such as Ensure® or Boost®, or warmed oatmeal or baby pablum can be provided in addition to pelleted feeds and good-quality vegetables where indicated (Figure 3.29). Provision of food and water on the cage floor, rather than in overhead containers, will facilitate access. Postsurgical deaths frequently result from anesthetic overdose, hypothermia, hypoxemia, fluid loss, or acidosis.

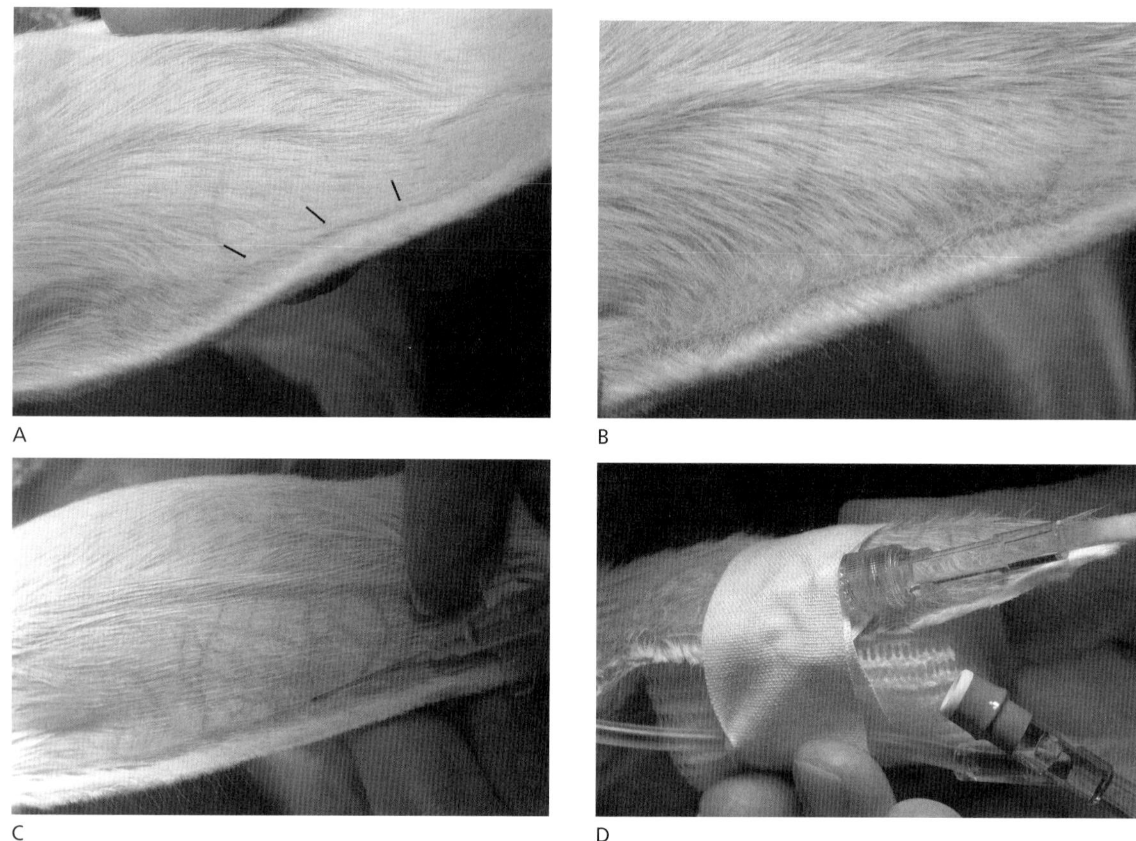

FIGURE 3.26. The marginal ear vein is a convenient site to catheterize for fluid delivery in rabbits. The vein is barely visible prior to plucking (A) (arrows). Catheter placement and support is similar to that described for the auricular artery (B, C, D).

Topical and Local Anesthesia

Lidocaine, bupivacaine, and other topical anesthetics may be used in rabbits and rodents as in other small animals. The vasoconstrictor epinephrine (1:200,000) may be used with topical anesthesia to prolong the local analgesia, which may last up to 4 hours for bupivacaine. Lidocaine at 0.5–1.0% may be used for epidural anesthesia in rabbits. Epidural lidocaine administration to rabbits results in mesenteric venodilation. The total volume of any local anesthetic must be carefully calculated to avoid systemic toxicity in small mammal species, and it may induce sudden cardiovascular collapse if given accidentally by IV injection.

EMLA® or Maxilene® cream (with active ingredients of prilocaine/lidocaine and lidocaine, respectively) can be used to desensitize skin for procedures such as venipuncture or ear notching.

Anesthesia in Rabbits

Concerns regarding anesthesia in rabbits include the following: (1) rabbits may be easily stressed and in some cases the physiologic response and catecholamine release are marked (as described); (2) if inadequately restrained, rabbits may struggle during face mask induction and luxate or fracture lumbar vertebrae; (3) preexisting respiratory disease, such as that caused by infection with *Pasteurella multocida*, a small, easily occluded trachea, a capacious cecum, and considerable variation between individuals complicate induction and may cause varied responses to anesthetics; (4) unpredictable responses to atropine

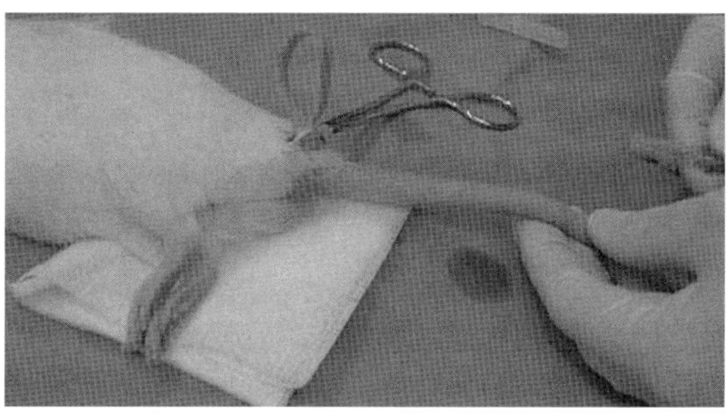

A

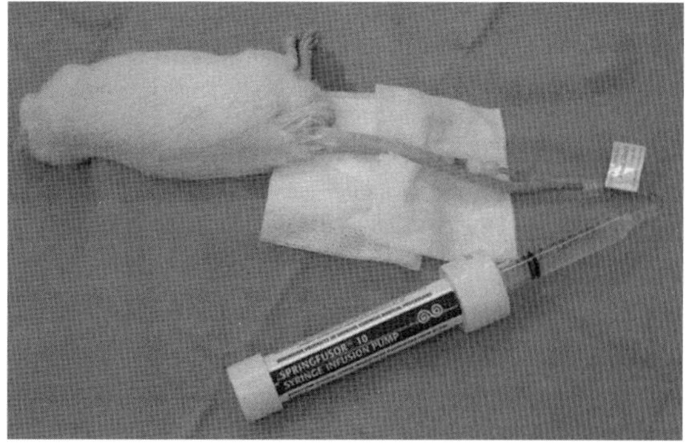

B

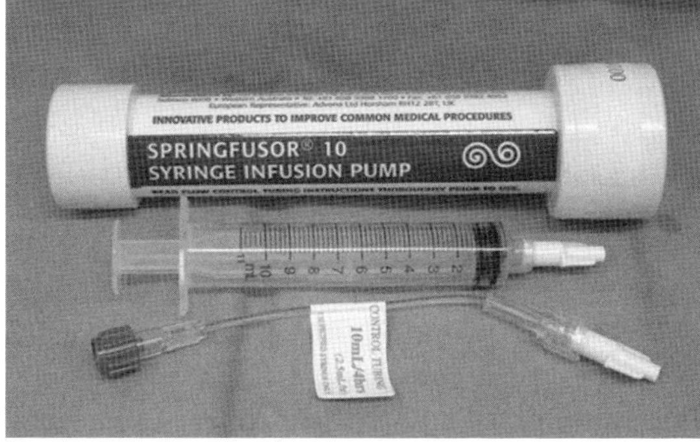

C

FIGURE 3.27. Fluids may be administered intravenously to rats using the lateral tail vein. A tourniquet applied to the base of the tail facilitates visualization of the vessel (A). A Springfusor® syringe infusion pump is a convenient means of providing ongoing IV fluids to small patients (B, C) (see text).

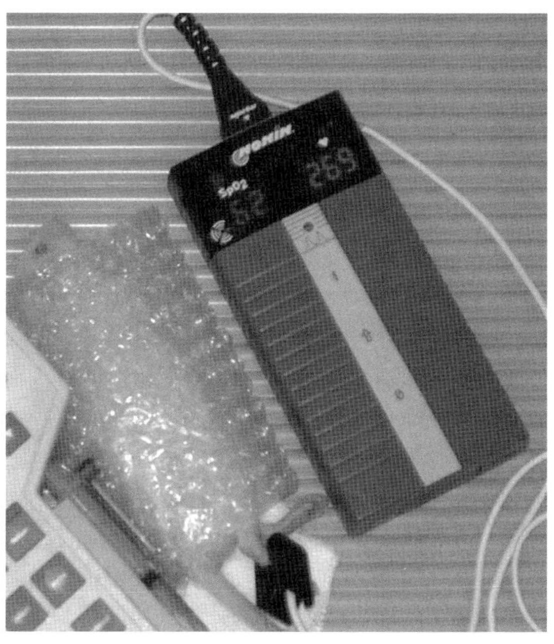

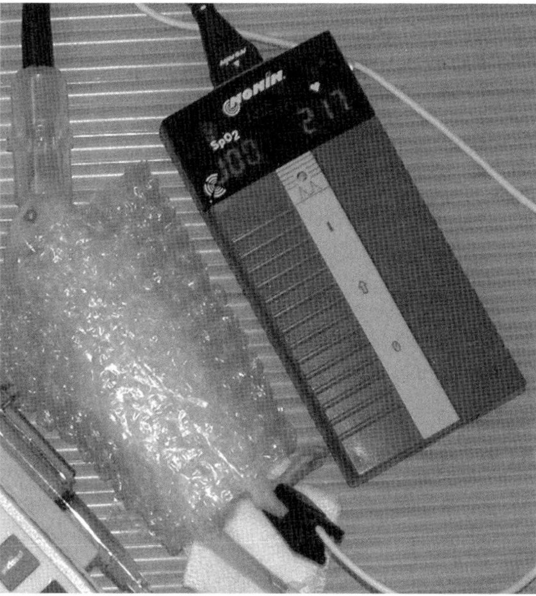

FIGURE 3.28. When possible, oxygen supplementation should be provided to small rodents anesthetized with injectable agents to prevent hypoxemia. The rat depicted in this image has been anesthetized with a ketamine/xylazine combination. Pulse oximeter values are shown before (left) and after (right) oxygen supplementation by face mask. Arterial oxygen saturation levels less than 90% are considered to reflect hypoxia in an anesthetized patient.

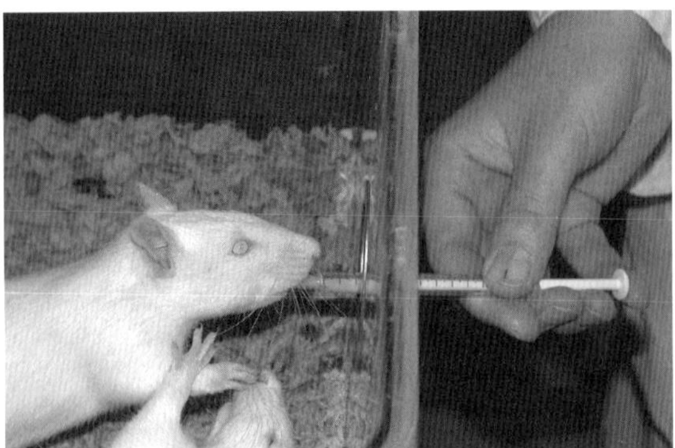

FIGURE 3.29. Rat licking Ensure® from a syringe.

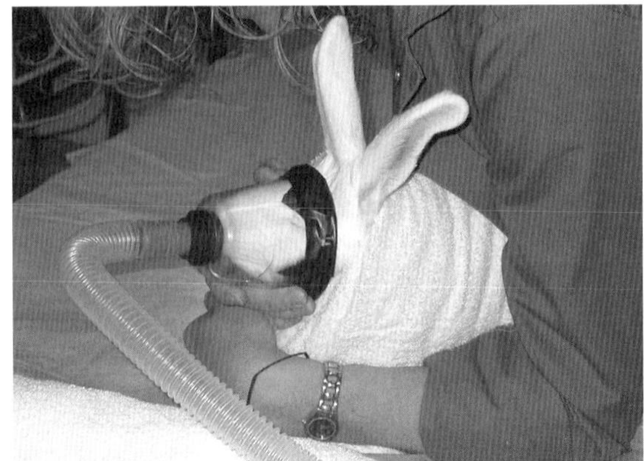

FIGURE 3.30. Face mask induction of a rabbit. The animal is firmly restrained in a towel wrap to minimize struggling.

because of plasma atropinesterase; and (5) dehydration, hypothermia, and postoperative intestinal stasis and inappetence all can make anesthetizing a rabbit a challenge.

With some care and preplanning, most rabbits are anesthetized safely and without difficulty. While endotracheal intubation requires practice, as most techniques do, anesthesia usually presents few real problems, provided animals are not excited or permitted to struggle during induction.

Inhalant Anesthetics in Rabbits

Inhalant anesthetics are very useful in rabbits, assuming appropriate concentrations are delivered and precautions are followed concerning body warmth and hydration. Preanesthetic medication with a tranquilizer or sedative and analgesic, whenever possible, will help minimize stress. Induction can then be accomplished more easily by face mask (Figure 3.30). Induction can also be carried out with appropriate dosages of ketamine plus a sedative, such as acepromazine, diazepam or midazolam, xylazine, or medetomidine, or by IV propofol. See Table 3.13 for suggested drugs and dosages.

Rabbits have a respiratory rate of approximately 30–60 breaths/minute and a tidal volume of 4–6 mL/kg, which is small compared with cats at 10–15 mL/kg. Inhalant anesthetics are administered to rabbits via a nonrebreathing circuit using a contoured face mask, laryngeal mask airway, or an endotracheal tube. Suggested levels for isoflurane are 5% for induction and 2–3% for maintenance, and for sevoflurane are 6–8% for induction and 3–6% for maintenance, with appropriate oxygen flow rate depending on the size of rabbit and whether or not it is intubated.

Endotracheal Intubation

If using a laryngoscope for intubation, a Wisconsin laryngoscope blade size 1 is appropriate if the body weight is more than 3 kg and size 0 if the weight is less than 3 kg. A 40 mm laryngoscope is suitable for an adult rabbit. The laryngoscope blade is "walked" over the tongue to the soft palate, followed by the stylet (5 French polypropylene urinary catheter) in the tube (infant Cole endotracheal tube of 2–3 mm OD in 1–3 kg rabbits and 3–4 mm OD in heavier rabbits). The laryngeal opening may be desensitized with 0.25 mL of 1% lidocaine applied with a cotton swab or aerosol. The glottis is a delta-shaped orifice deep to the bibbed edge of the epiglottis. The stylet in the tube is then introduced into the larynx, or the stylet is removed before passage into the larynx, which rebounds when the tube touches the glottis. The tube is gently rotated as it advances into the trachea, and the stylet, if present, is removed.

By extending the rabbit's neck without lifting the forefeet from the table, the tube may be passed blindly into the trachea. Proper placement is indicated by clouding of the tube lumen on expiration, by palpation of one rigid tube in the throat (tube within trachea only), and by hearing breathing sounds through the tube (Figure 3.31). The blind technique requires practice and has several variants,

Table 3.13. Suggested drugs and dosages for rabbit preanesthetic medication. (Caution: Most uses and dosages are extralabel.)

Drug(s)	Dosage	Route	Comments
Acepromazine	1–2 mg/kg	IM	Light to moderate sedation
Acepromazine +hydromorphone	0.1 mg/kg +0.2 mg/kg	IM IM	Premedication; acepromazine may prolong recovery
Acepromazine +butorphanol	0.1 mg/kg +0.4 mg/kg	IM IM	Premedication; acepromazine may prolong recovery
Midazolam	0.5–2 mg/kg	IM	Light to moderate sedation
Midazolam +hydromorphone	0.2–0.5 mg/kg +0.2 mg/kg	IM IM	Premedication
Midazolam +butorphanol	0.2–0.5 mg/kg +0.4 mg/kg	IM IM	Premedication
Midazolam +ketamine	0.3 mg/kg +5–15 mg/kg	IM IM	Produces premedication to light anesthesia
Xylazine	2–5 mg/kg	IM	Light to moderate sedation, some analgesia
Medetomidine	0.1–0.5 mg/kg	IM; SC	Light to heavy sedation
Diazepam	5–10 mg/kg	IM	Light to moderate sedation
Hypnorm®	0.2–0.5 mL/kg	IM	Light to heavy sedation

References:
Benson KG, Paul-Murphy J. Clinical pathology of the domestic rabbit. Vet Clin Exot Anim. 1999, 2:539–551.
Flecknell P. Laboratory Animal Anesthesia, 2nd ed. London: Academic Press, 1996.
Morrisey JK, Carpenter JW. Formulary. In: Ferrets, Rabbits and Rodents: Clinical Medicine and Surgery, 2nd ed. Quesenberry KE, Carpenter JW (eds.). St Louis: Saunders, 2004, 436–444.

but once mastered is performed easily in most rabbits.

Laryngeal Mask Airway

The laryngeal mask airway (LMA) is an alternative to a face mask or endotracheal tube and consists of an airway tube, a mask, and a mask inflation link. The mask is inserted over the larynx and forms a junction between the upper airway and the trachea. Insertion of the mask requires some practice to protect it from the rabbit's teeth and to advance it to the correct position, but once in place it provides the ability for positive pressure ventilation (Figure 3.32).

Injectable Anesthetics in Rabbits

Injectable anesthetic procedures for rabbits (and rodents) are usually effective, inexpensive, convenient, and simple; however, potential problems with their use include associated respiratory depression, interindividual variation in depth of anesthesia and analgesia, and difficulty in calculating depth of anesthesia as determined by the various indicator reflexes. The best indicators of depth of anesthesia, in order of decreasing reliability, are ear pinch, pedal, corneal (water drop), and palpebral reflexes. The pinna or ear pinch is a sensitive indicator in rabbits and persists longer than do the other reflexes.

CLINICAL PROCEDURES

Most injectable regimens are based on the dissociative anesthetic drug ketamine, plus one or more drugs with muscle relaxing, sedative, and analgesic properties. Drugs added to or administered with ketamine include acepromazine, xylazine or medetomidine, or diazepam or midazolam. Butorphanol may also be added for analgesia. Other combinations are based on tiletamine and zolazepam (tiletamine at doses of approximately 32 mg/kg or greater is nephrotoxic in rabbits), fentanyl and droperidol, or fentanyl and fluanisone. Supplemental oxygen should always be provided during injectable anesthesia.

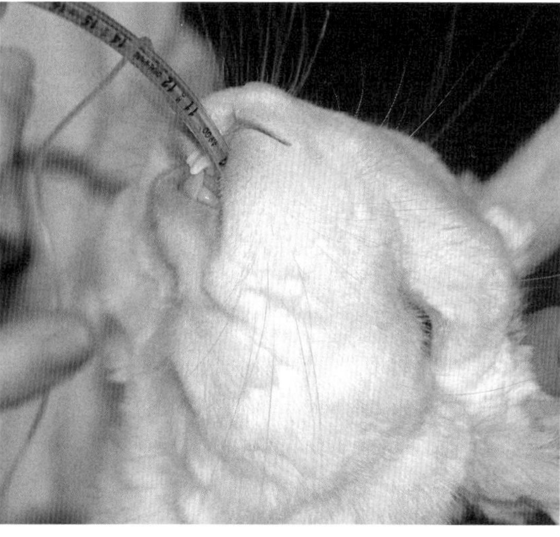

FIGURE 3.31. Blind endotracheal intubation in a rabbit.

Ketamine

Ketamine HCl is a dissociative anesthetic with wide application in rabbits and rodents. Ketamine HCl solution is buffered to a pH of 3.5–5.5 and local muscle irritation occurs on injection. Ketamine given alone at any dosage (e.g., 20–45 mg/kg IM) produces variable analgesia (less for visceral and skeletal applications) and poor muscle relaxation in rabbits and rodents. Analgesia may be satisfactory in the abdominal skin but incomplete in the throat. Ketamine may induce cardiovascular stimulation, muscle rigidity, salivation, electroencephalographic changes, and serum chemistry alterations. The popularity of ketamine for use in rabbits and rodents is based on mixtures or sequential administration in various combinations with acepromazine, xylazine or medetomidine, diazepam or midazolam, inhalant anesthetics, butorphanol, and other drugs. These combinations may improve muscle relaxation and sedation, augment analgesia, and prolong surgical anesthesia.

Ketamine and Xylazine

Xylazine is an alpha-2 adrenergic agonist tranquilizer and potent sedative. Xylazine can be combined with ketamine or administered separately. Ketamine and xylazine are usually combined in a syringe and given IM at 20–50 mg/kg ketamine with 2 mg/kg xylazine, but lower doses of both drugs, especially of xylazine, may be used. Higher dosages of ketamine may be necessary to reach surgical anesthesia, and lower dosages of xylazine may be used to reduce the meta-

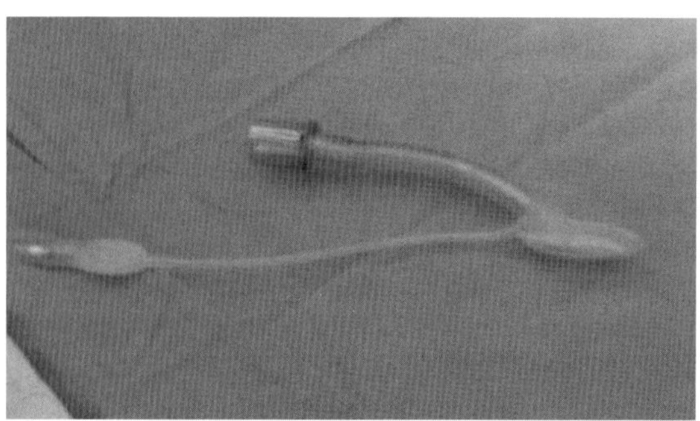

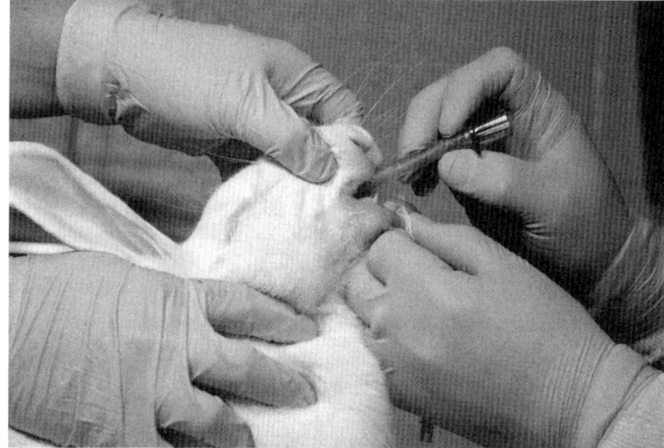

FIGURE 3.32. Laryngeal mask airway (left) and restraint for LMA placement in the rabbit (right). Courtesy of A.J. Wang.

bolic alkalosis and decrease the arterial oxygen saturation, sensitivity to noise, and profound secondary hypotension that characterize the pharmacologic actions of xylazine. Xylazine also contributes to analgesia and muscle relaxation. The combination may be given by IV infusion as ketamine 1 mg/min with xylazine at 0.1 mg/min or by intranasal instillation of ketamine (10 mg/kg) with 3 mg/kg xylazine diluted with 0.9% saline. Induction for these combinations is approximately 10 minutes, and surgical anesthesia lasts from 10 to 75 minutes (average 30–45 minutes). Supplemental oxygen should always be provided. Recovery from sedation without reversal may take 6 hours. The effects of xylazine may be reversed with an injection of 0.2 mg/kg yohimbine IV or 0.001 mg/kg atipamezole, SC, IV, or IP. A ketamine/xylazine combination given at 50 mg/kg and 5 mg/kg, respectively, has caused severe acidosis, anuria, respiratory depression, and death in rabbits.

Ketamine, Xylazine, and Acepromazine
Ketamine, xylazine, and acepromazine may be used in a three-way mixture (i.e., 35 mg/kg ketamine, 3 mg/kg xylazine, 0.75 mg/kg acepromazine IM) to provide a significantly longer duration of anesthesia (99 ± 20 min) than for ketamine/xylazine alone. Side effects include depressed respiratory rate, heart rate, and especially blood pressure (may be critical in a hypovolemic patient). Individual practitioners working with healthy, well-hydrated rabbits may find this combination and the side effects acceptable, especially if intravenous fluids are provided intraoperatively. Ketamine may be given with acepromazine (1–2 mg/kg IM) alone, without xylazine, for deep sedation, but this combination is not suitable for general anesthesia.

Ketamine and Diazepam
Ketamine at 60–80 mg/kg IM can be preceded by 30 minutes with the benzodiazepine tranquilizer diazepam at 5–10 mg/kg IM to provide anesthesia in the rabbit. The drugs should not be mixed, and diazepam does not potentiate the analgesic effects of ketamine.

Ketamine and Midazolam
Midazolam is a water-soluble benzodiazepine that produces sedation, muscle relaxation, and some respiratory and vascular depression. Midazolam and ketamine may be administered intranasally to rabbits in a saline-diluted mixture of 1.0 mg/kg midazolam and 25 mg/kg ketamine. Anesthetic activity persists for approximately 50 minutes.

Ketamine, Medetomidine, and Diazepam
Medetomidine is an alpha-2 adrenergic agonist with sedative and analgesic properties. Medetomidine given at 0.5 mg/kg IM with ketamine (20 mg/kg IM) and diazepam (0.75–1.5 mg/kg SC) provides 7–16 minutes of induction time and 30–60 minutes of surgical anesthesia. Ketamine (25 mg/kg IM) and medetomidine (0.5 mg/kg IM) may also be given without diazepam for surgical anesthesia. Medetomidine should be reversed with atipamezole postoperatively to enhance recovery.

Ketamine, Xylazine, and Butorphanol
A combination of ketamine 35 mg/kg, xylazine 5 mg/kg, and butorphanol 0.1 mg/kg IM can increase anesthesia time over ketamine/xylazine alone and ensure longer, more predictable analgesia. Less autonomic depression occurs than that associated with a ketamine/xylazine/acepromazine combination.

Propofol
Propofol is an excellent induction agent for rabbits prior to intubation. Recommended IV induction doses range from 5 to 15 mg/kg (bolus), but 7.5–8.45 mg/kg is considered the minimum required for intubation. As for other species, rabbits may become apneic after administration of propofol boluses.

Light anesthesia follows for approximately 2 minutes at 5 mg/kg, 4 minutes at 10 mg/kg, and 9 minutes at 15 mg/kg IV. The slow drip dose is 0.2–0.8 mg/kg/min for sedation and 0.8–1.3 mg/kg/min for anesthetic maintenance. Premedication with acepromazine (2 mg/kg IM), medetomidine (0.25 mg/kg IM), and atropine (0.5 mg/kg IM) may facilitate propofol injections and provide analgesia and muscle relaxation, and this combination reduces the propofol dose to 4 mg/kg IV. Supplementary analgesics should be given if a painful procedure is to be performed, as propofol provides no analgesia. Recovery takes 2–5 minutes and depends on animal weight and not on bolus dose.

Although propofol is safe for rabbits when used and stored properly, it does cause attenuation of the vagal component of heart rate that is under baroreceptor control as well as a 25–30% decrease in cardiac output. Long-term anesthesia with propofol may result in atelectasis, hypoxemia, and hypostatic congestion. Respiratory arrest may occur in rabbits with propofol doses of 20 mg/kg. Propofol does not impair fertility, induces little variation in arterial blood pressures, and does not undergo enterohepatic circulation.

The drug is conjugated in the liver and predominantly (60–90%) eliminated via the kidney, with approximately 2% passing in the feces. The drug can be administered to rabbits via the lateral ear vein.

Anesthesia in Guinea Pigs

A guinea pig has a normal respiratory rate between 40 and 130 respirations/minute and an approximate tidal volume of 3.8 mL/kg body weight. The body weight of guinea pigs may be overestimated by the large cecum. The pedal reflex is not always a reliable indicator of a surgical plane of anesthesia in guinea pigs. Postoperative adjuncts should include hydration with warmed saline or other fluids, provision of a warm, quiet environment, and special efforts to stimulate postoperative feeding.

Inhalant Anesthetics in Guinea Pigs and Chinchillas

Isoflurane

Guinea pigs and chinchillas can be induced using an induction chamber (Figure 3.33), by face mask, or by injection, and maintained on 2–3% isoflurane in oxygen. A small feline anesthetic mask with a latex glove or balloon taped over the opening to construct a diaphragm with an appropriate-sized opening can be used if a commercial guinea pig mask is not available.

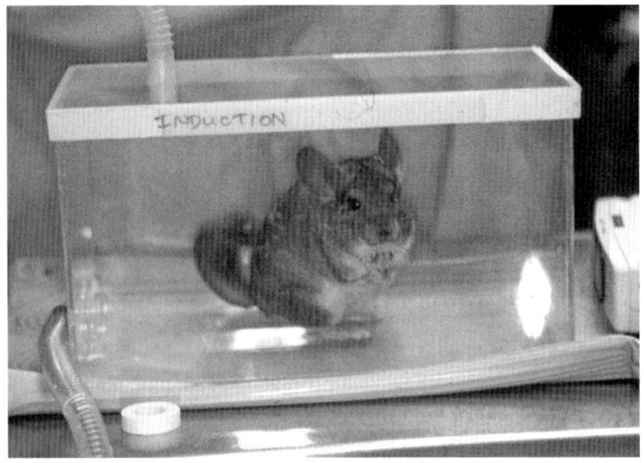

FIGURE 3.33. Chamber induction of a chinchilla.

Endotracheal Intubation

In guinea pigs, only the rostral 1/3 of the tongue is free and mobile, and a food bolus is often held between the tongue and the hard palate. Before the guinea pig can be intubated, the bolus must be scooped out. For intubation, the guinea pig is placed in dorsal recumbency, and adhesive tape is used to hold the upper jaw to the table surface. The tongue obscures the larynx in guinea pigs. The mouth is cleaned with organic iodide antiseptic, and an 8 cm, 1.5–2.5 mm OD tube with stylet is passed over a laryngoscope placed to the left of the upper incisors parallel to the floor of the mouth. The tube is introduced to the epiglottis, which is angled upward. Actual insertion into the trachea is conducted blindly during inspiration. The tube is passed gently into the trachea, and if used, a respirator can be set at 25 strokes/minute to deliver 1.5 mL/100 g of air/stroke. A mouth gag is placed in the mouth, and the tube is taped to the gag and around the snout.

Injectable Anesthetics in Guinea Pigs

It is difficult to achieve surgical anesthesia using injectable agents in the guinea pig, with the exception of Hypnorm® (not available in the United States) combined with a benzodiazepine (e.g., midazolam). In addition, intramuscular injections may produce muscle necrosis and self-mutilation, and intraperitoneal injections are inconsistently absorbed. For these reasons, inhalational anesthesia is recommended for major procedures in guinea pigs.

Sodium Pentobarbital

Sodium pentobarbital (1% solution) administered IP is difficult to dose appropriately because of the indefinite injection site, differential absorption, varying dispersion of the drug in the peritoneal cavity, and narrow therapeutic window between the anesthetic dose and the dose inducing respiratory depression and death. Sodium pentobarbital may be given IP at 25–35 mg/kg body weight. This dose will provide approximately 30–100 minutes of surgical anesthesia. A combination with chlorpromazine at 25 mg/kg will extend the anesthesia to 50 or more minutes. Diazepam (8 mg/kg) and pentobarbital (20 mg/kg) given IP may produce surgical anesthesia after 13 minutes. Sodium pentobarbital provides no intraoperative analgesia and frequently results in prolonged anesthetic recoveries, hypoventilation, hypothermia, and hypoxemia.

Ketamine and Xylazine

Ketamine (40–60 mg/kg) and xylazine (2–5 mg/kg) given IP provide approximately 30 minutes of anesthesia; however, analgesia may not be sufficient for major surgery in some animals and may require the addition of butorphanol. Guinea pigs evinced pain on injection, but the hindlimb paddling seen under pentobarbital anesthesia has not been reported for this combination and muscle relaxation is also good. IM injection of this combination may produce muscle necrosis and self-mutilation and SC or IP injection may be more suitable.

Acute, fatal gastric distention has been reported after anesthesia of 44- to 49-day pregnant guinea pigs with ketamine at 20 mg/kg and xylazine at 2 mg/kg IM. During the procedure, one external jugular vein was cannulated. Food had not been withheld preoperatively.

Ketamine and Diazepam

This combination may be given with ketamine at 25–100 mg/kg IM and diazepam at 0.1–2.5 mg/kg IM. Pain will occur on injection and the combination provides no analgesia; however, the resulting immobilization may be useful for such procedures as trimming overgrown premolar teeth.

Ketamine and Acepromazine

Ketamine dosages in guinea pigs at 25–55 mg/kg combined with acepromazine at 0.75–3 mg/kg IM, IP, or SC are useful for restraint. This combination provides no analgesia and is not suitable for surgical procedures.

Anesthesia in Hamsters

Hamsters have a respiratory rate of approximately 35–135 respirations/minute, a tidal volume of approximately 0.8 mL, and a minute volume of approximately 64 mL. Depth of anesthesia in hamsters may be determined using righting reflex, pedal withdrawal, and muscle tone, and by pinching abdominal skin with mosquito forceps. The pedal withdrawal reflex is elicited by pinching the interdigital webbing with fingers or forceps for up to 1 second per site.

Inhalant Anesthetics in Hamsters

After induction in a chamber, or by injection, hamsters can be maintained on isoflurane in O_2 at 2–3%, using a tight-fitting rodent face mask or face mask created from a modified 60 mL syringe barrel.

Injectable Anesthetics in Hamsters

Telazol® and Xylazine

Telazol® (tiletamine/zolazepam) at 30 mg/kg combined with xylazine at 10 mg/kg given IP produces approximately 30 minutes of surgical anesthesia. Intramuscular injections of Telazol® alone reportedly caused inconsistent anesthesia and muscle necrosis.

Ketamine and Xylazine

Hamsters may be anesthetized with 50–100 mg/kg ketamine combined with xylazine at 5 mg/kg IP. This dose provided approximately 28 minutes of surgical anesthesia in the extremities and 36 minutes in the abdomen. Intramuscular injection of ketamine causes extensive muscle necrosis in hamsters.

Ketamine and Acepromazine

Ketamine may be given at 100 mg/kg IP with acepromazine at 1–4 mg/kg IM for deep sedation.

Ketamine and Diazepam

Ketamine is given at 100 mg/kg IP with diazepam at 0.5 mg/kg IM or 5.0 mg/kg IP. This combination provides no intraoperative analgesia.

Hypnorm®

Hypnorm® (fentanyl/fluanisone; not available in the United States) combined with either diazepam or midazolam, given IP, provides excellent surgical anesthesia and analgesia lasting about 20–40 minutes. The respiratory depressant effects of the drug can be partially reversed with nalbuphine or butorphanol, while maintaining good postoperative analgesia.

Sodium Pentobarbital

Sodium pentobarbital administered intraperitoneally to hamsters at 60–90 mg/kg produces surgical anesthesia lasting 30–45 minutes. This drug provides no intraoperative analgesia and has a narrow therapeutic margin of safety.

Anesthesia in Gerbils

The respiratory rate of gerbils is approximately 90 respirations/minute.

As with the other small rodents, after induction in a chamber, or by injection, gerbils can be maintained on isoflurane at 2–3%, using a tight-fitting rodent face mask.

Injectable Anesthetics in Gerbils

Ketamine Combinations

Ketamine (75 mg/kg) and medetomidine (0.5 mg/kg) combined and given SC or IP produces a moderate surgical plane of anesthesia in gerbils. Medetomidine can be reversed using atipamezole (1 mg/kg SC or IP). Ketamine (50 mg/kg) and diazepam (5–10 mg/kg) or xylazine (2 mg/kg) given IP will produce immobilization but not anesthesia, and these combinations are not suitable for surgery. Acepromazine may cause seizures in gerbils and is not recommended.

Fentanyl

A combination of fentanyl (0.05 mg/kg SC) and metomidate (50 mg/kg SC) reliably produces general anesthesia in gerbils. Hypnorm® (fentanyl/fluanisone) and a benzodiazepine is reported to be less effective in gerbils than in other rodents, producing only light anesthesia.

Sodium Pentobarbital

Sodium pentobarbital administered intraperitoneally at 60 mg/kg body weight to a maximum dose of 6 mg will lightly anesthetize a gerbil for 30–45 minutes. Dosages required for surgical anesthesia (80 mg/kg IP) often result in death.

Anesthesia in Mice

The mouse has an average respiratory rate of 60–220 respirations/minute and an approximate tidal volume of 0.15 mL. Intravenous injections are made using a 28–30 g needle into the lateral tail vein, after restraining the mouse in an appropriate homemade or commercially available device. Warming the tail dilates the vessels and facilitates needle entry. Care should be taken not to aspirate blood or inject air emboli.

Inhalant Anesthetics in Mice

As with other small rodents, use of an induction chamber facilitates inhalation anesthesia in mice, after which they can be maintained on isoflurane at 2–3%, using a tight-fitting rodent face mask. Manifolds with multiple ports are commercially available that allow several mice to be anesthetized simultaneously, which may be convenient when batching surgeries for some research projects. Mice may be intubated for research purposes (Figure 3.34).

Injectable Anesthetics in Mice

The response to injectable anesthetic agents is highly dependent on the strain or stock of mouse used. When in doubt, a small pilot study is recommended to optimize the dose levels.

Ketamine Combinations

Ketamine (75 mg/kg) and medetomidine (1.0 mg/kg) given IP produce moderate surgical anesthesia in most strains of mice but may not be suitable for laparotomy. Ketamine (80–100 mg/kg) and xylazine (10 mg/kg) may provide up to 30 minutes of surgical anesthesia, depending on the strain. Ketamine (100 mg/kg) and acepromazine (5 mg/kg) or diazepam (5 mg/kg) or midazolam (5 mg/kg) may produce immobilization or light anesthesia in some strains.

Fentanyl

Fentanyl (0.06 mg/kg) and metomidate (60 mg/kg) combined and given SC will produce surgical anesthesia in some mice. Hypnorm® combined with midazolam or diazepam provides surgical anesthesia lasting 30–40 minutes in mice, and anesthesia can be partially reversed with nalbuphine, buprenorphine, or butorphanol.

Propofol

In mice, propofol given IV at 26 mg/kg leads to 4–6 minutes of anesthesia. The LD_{50} of propofol in mice is approximately 53 mg/kg.

Tribromoethanol Solutions

Tribromoethanol solutions of tert-amyl alcohol and 2,2,2-tribromoethanol have been used for short-term

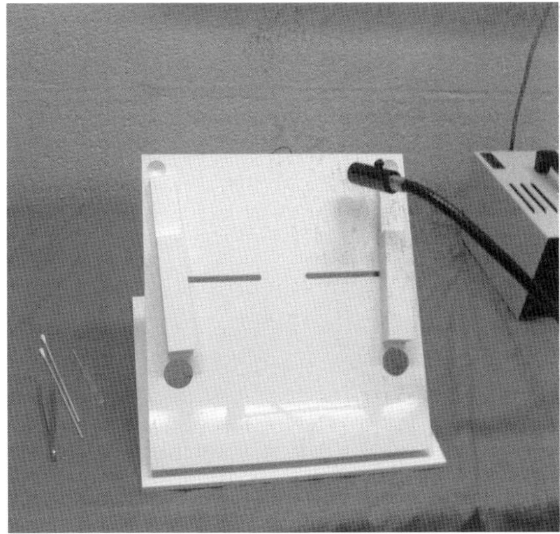

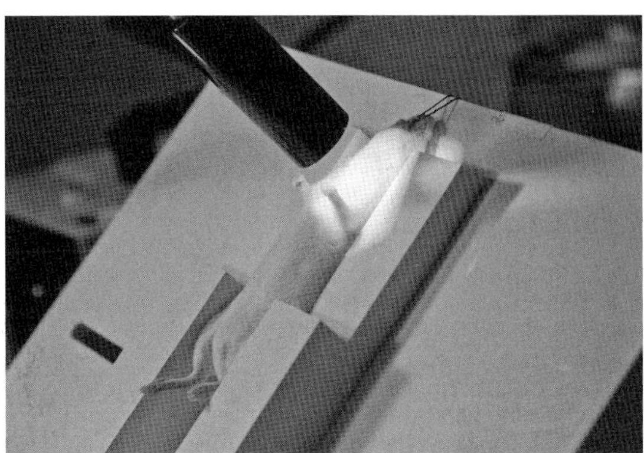

FIGURE 3.34. Mice and rats may be intubated for research purposes. The technique is facilitated with commercially available intubation bases and a bright light source (left). Visualization of the oropharynx is accomplished by shining the light source on the cervical region (right). Courtesy of A.J. Wang.

imaging or surgical procedures in mice, rats, and gerbils. The mixture is popular in research settings because it is not a controlled substance and can be prepared from readily purchased nonpharmaceutical-grade chemicals. When used, the chemical mixture should only be administered on a single occasion in any animal because of the risk for adhesions and ileus with repeated IP use. Because of this, some institutions only permit the mixture to be used during acute terminal procedures in rodents. It was once manufactured specifically for use as an anesthetic by Winthrop Laboratories under the trade name Avertin®, but this product is no longer available. Tribromoethanol is an irritant, especially at high doses, high concentrations, or with repeated use. Tribromoethanol degrades in the presence of heat or light to produce toxic byproducts, and these degraded solutions can be both nephrotoxic and hepatotoxic. Administration of degraded tribromoethanol solutions has been associated with death, often 24 hours after surgery.

Sodium Pentobarbital

As for other species, sodium pentobarbital provides little to no analgesia and has a narrow therapeutic margin of safety in mice. Sodium pentobarbital diluted with normal saline to 6 mg/mL and injected IP at 40–80 mg/kg body weight may provide 20–40 minutes of surgical anesthesia in mice. A combination of chlorpromazine (25–50 mg/kg) and sodium pentobarbital (40–60 mg/kg) IP may augment anesthesia times.

Male mice and fasted animals are more susceptible to the pharmacologic effects of pentobarbital.

Anesthesia in Rats

The respiratory rate of rats is 70–115 breaths/minute, and the tidal volume is 0.6–2.0 mL.

Inhalant Anesthetics in Rats

Use of an induction chamber with 5% isoflurane facilitates inhalation anesthesia in rats, after which they can be maintained at 2–3%, with an oxygen flow at 0.5–1 L/min using a tight-fitting rodent face mask. As for mice, anesthesia machine manifolds with multiple ports are commercially available that allow several rats to be anesthetized at a time, which may be useful for some research projects. Lack of withdrawal following a toe or tail pinch is the most reliable indicator of appropriate anesthetic depth in rats.

Injectable Anesthetics in Rats

Ketamine Combinations

Ketamine (75 mg/kg) and xylazine (10 mg/kg) or medetomidine (0.5 mg/kg) mixed together and given SC or IP provides surgical anesthesia in most strains of rats. Light anesthesia can be accomplished with ketamine (75 mg/kg) combined and given IP with acepromazine (2.3 mg/kg), diazepam (5 mg/kg), or midazolam (5 mg/kg). Xylazine and medetomidine mixtures cause profound hypotension and hypoxemia and supplemental oxygen should always be given. Both drugs can be reversed with atipamezole (1 mg/kg SC).

Fentanyl

Fentanyl (300 ug/kg) and medetomidine (300 ug/kg) mixed and given IP produces approximately 60 minutes of surgical anesthesia in rats. Recovery can be facilitated by reversal of fentanyl with either nalbuphine (1.0 mg/kg SC, IP) or butorphanol (2 mg/kg SC, IP), and reversal of medetomidine with atipamezole (1 mg/kg SC, IP). Hypnorm® combined with diazepam or midazolam provides surgical anesthesia with excellent muscle relaxation lasting approximately 20–40 minutes. The fentanyl component can be reversed as described above.

Sodium Pentobarbital

As for other species, the drug poses a considerable risk for anesthesia, as the anesthetic dose of pentobarbital in rats (30–50 mg/kg) is close to the LD_{50} (60 mg/kg), and rats vary greatly in their individual response to the drug. Pentobarbital has poor analgesic properties in rats and induces profound hypothermia, hypoxemia, and excitement on induction.

Sodium pentobarbital administered IP at 10–20 mg/kg in young rats and 30–50 mg/kg in older rats (males require doses approximately 5 mg/kg higher) produces anesthesia in 5–10 minutes. At 40 mg/kg, light surgical anesthesia is obtained with moderate to severe respiratory and cardiovascular depression.

Propofol

In small rodents, propofol may have effects similar to those seen in other species. Induction is stress-free and relaxation may be maintained for up to 3 hours (1–2 mL/kg IV for induction, then constant infusion at 4–6 mL/kg/hr to effect). In rats, 60–95% of injected propofol is eliminated in the urine, and 13–31% in the feces. Doses of 5 mg/kg (IV) produce approximately 2–4 minutes of sleeping time, and doses of 25–30 mg/kg produce 15–32 minutes of anesthesia. In rats, no enterohepatic circulation occurs. The LD_{50} of propofol rats is 42 mg/kg.

Inactin

Inactin is a thiobarbiturate useful for prolonged anesthesia in the rat and male hamster, although proximal renal tubular reabsorption and effects on renin activity occur in rats, and hyperglycemia accompanies its use in hamsters. The drug provides smooth induction and 3–4 hours of anesthesia when given IP to rats at 80–100 mg/kg. Analgesic activity is variable and IV administration provides less variable response than does IP administration. Induction inhalant anesthesia simplifies the injection.

Other Anesthetics

Many useful drugs are, for various reasons, not licensed for use in the United States. Two such combination products used with success in rabbits and rodents are Althesin® and Hypnorm®.

Alphaxalone/Alphadolone (Althesin®)

The combination of these two steroidal (pregnanediones) anesthetics provides fast, smooth induction when administered IV, and repeated doses to prolong sleeping time have little effect on total recovery time. The drugs are metabolized rapidly and are effective for long-term anesthesia if injected repeatedly IV. The solubilizing agent used may cause histamine release, IM and IP routes produce varied anesthetic effects (the large volume needed precludes IM use in small animals), the combination cannot be used with barbiturates, and, in rabbits and rats, the combination provides insufficient analgesia. The dosage is 8–12 mg/kg IV for mice, rabbits, and rats, to 40 mg/kg IP for guinea pigs, and 80–120 mg/kg IP for hamsters and gerbils. Clinical use of these agents requires experience because results may be uncertain and uneven.

Fentanyl/Fluanisone (Hypnorm®)

This combination of a potent narcotic analgesic (fentanyl) and a neuroleptic tranquilizer-sedative (fluanisone) can be given IM, IP, SC, or IV with midazolam to anesthetize rabbits and rodents.

In addition to providing excellent analgesia, the combination suppresses excitement and provides muscle relaxation. Respiratory depression, poor muscle relaxation (when used without midazolam), hypotension, and bradycardia may occur. The dosage is approximately 0.1 mL/30 g IP for the mouse to 0.5 mL/kg IM or IP for other small rodents and rabbits to 1 mL/kg IM for guinea pigs. The drug is usually combined with 2 mg/kg IP diazepam or midazolam.

A convenient anesthesia cocktail can be made for injection of fentanyl/fluanisone (Hypnorm®) and midazolam (5 mg/mL) as follows: 1 part Hypnorm® + 2 parts sterile water for injection + 1 part midazolam (mixed in this order to prevent precipitation). Administer 1.0 mL/100 g (mouse), or 0.27 mL/100 g (rat) IP. The effects can be reversed by naloxone (0.1 mg/kg IV) (narcotic antagonist) or buprenorphine (0.1 mg/kg IV) (partial opioid agonist/antagonist).

Endotracheal Intubation in Small Rodents

The trachea can be entered through a tracheostomy or by deep tissue (bright light) illumination of the oropharynx. The standard method, however, is to pass a tube through the mouth and into the glottis. Direct visualization of the pharynx and laryngeal areas is important. The anesthetized rodent is placed in dorsal recumbency with the head extended and the upper jaw taped to the table top. The tongue is pulled sideways and upward, and an otoscope cone with a slit in one side or a 0.4 mm 10 × 25 mm curved spatula is placed over the base of the tongue. Alternatively, a penlight placed over the external surface of the neck will permit direct visualization of the trachea during tongue retraction.

Elevation of the tongue reveals the glottis, which can be wiped with 1% lidocaine on a cotton swab. The tube (16 g catheter of 1.0–1.5 mm OD in hamster or mouse, 2.0–2.5 mm OD in rat) should be shortened to reduce dead space and is passed (rotating) into the trachea on inspiration. The end of the tube should be blunted to reduce laryngeal trauma. Proper placement is determined by movement of a hair held over the end of the tube. If used, a respirator is set at 1.5 mL/100 g body weight to deliver 25–80 strokes per minute.

Expanded and ongoing use of mice in biomedical research has spawned an explosion of devices available to facilitate this research. Among these are platforms specially designed to facilitate endotracheal intubation in mice. Techniques described for intubating other small rodents may also be applied to mice.

References

Aeschbacher G, Webb AT. Propofol in rabbits. 1. Determination of an induction dose. Lab Anim Sci. 1993, 43:324–335.

———. Propofol in rabbits. 2. Long-term anesthesia. Lab Anim Sci. 1993, 43:328–335.

Bechtold SV, Abrutyn D. An improved method of endotracheal intubation in rabbits. Lab Anim Sci. 1991, 41:630–631.

Benson KG, Paul-Murphy J. Clinical pathology of the domestic rabbit. Vet Clin Exot Anim. 1999, 2:539–551.

Brammer A, West CD, Allen SL. A comparison of propofol with other injectable anaesthetics in a rat model for measuring cardiovascular parameters. Lab Anim. 1993, 27:250–257.

Brown JN, Thorne PR, Nuttall AL. Blood pressure and other physiological responses in awake and anesthetized guinea pigs. Lab Anim Sci. 1989, 39:142–148.

Carpenter JW. Caring for rabbits. Vet Med. 1995, 90:340–364.

Conlon KC, et al. Atraumatic endotracheal intubation in small rabbits. Lab Anim Sci. 1990, 40:221–222.

Cunliffe-Beamer TI, Freeman IC, Myers DD. Barbiturate sleeptime in mice exposed to autoclaved or unautoclaved wood bedding. Lab Anim Sci. 1981, 32:672–675.

Curl JL, Peters LL. Ketamine hydrochloride and xylazine hydrochloride anaesthesia in the golden hamster (Mesocricetus auratus). Lab Anim. 1983, 17:290–293.

Dawson DL, Scott-Conner C. Adjunctive use of local anesthetic infiltration during guinea pig laparotomy. Lab Anim. 1988, 17:35–36.

Field KJ, White WJ, Lang CM. Anaesthetic effects of chloral hydrate, pentobarbitone and urethane in adult male rats. Lab Anim. 1993, 27:258–269.

Flecknell PA. Laboratory Animal Anaesthesia, 2nd ed. London: Academic Press, 1996.

Flecknell PA, Roughan JV, Hedenqvist P. Induction of anaesthesia with sevoflurane and isoflurane in the rabbit. Lab Anim. 1993, 33:41–46.

Forsythe DB, et al. Evaluation of Telazol/xylazine as an anesthetic combination for use in Syrian hamsters. Lab Anim Sci. 1992, 42:497–502.

Gaertner DJ, Boschert KR, Schoeb TR. Muscle necrosis in Syrian hamsters resulting from intramuscular injections of ketamine and xylazine. Lab Anim Sci. 1987, 37:80–83.

Gillett CS. Selected Drug Dosages and Clinical Reference Data. In: The Biology of the Laboratory Rabbit, 2nd ed. Manning PJ, Ringler DH, Newcomer CE (eds.). San Diego: Academic Press, 1994.

Gilroy BA, Varga JS. Use of ketamine-diazepam and ketamine-xylazine combinations in guinea pigs. Vet Med Small Anim Clin. 1980, 75:508–509.

Hobbs BA, et al. Comparison of several combinations for anesthesia in rabbits. Amer J Vet Res. 1991, 52:669–674.

Hogan QH, et al. Mechanism of mesenteric venodilation after epidural lidocaine in rabbits. Anesthesiol. 1994, 81:939–945.

Imai A, Eislele PH, Steffey EP. A new airway device for small laboratory animals. Lab Anim. 2005, 39:111–115.

Kazakos GM, et al. Use of the laryngeal mask airway in rabbits: placement and efficacy. Lab Anim. 2007, 36:29–34.

Keller GL, Bauman DH, Abbott L. Yohimbine antagonism of ketamine and xylazine anesthesia in rabbits. Lab Anim. 1988, 17(3):28–30.

Ko JCH, et al. A comparison of medetomidine-propofol and medetomidine-midazolam-propofol anesthesia in rabbits. Lab Anim Sci. 1992, 42:503–507.

Kujime K, Natelson BH. A method for endotracheal intubation of guinea pigs (Cavia porcellus). Lab Anim Sci. 1981, 31:715–716.

Lieggi CC, Artwohl JE, Leszczynski JK, et al. Efficacy and safety of stored and newly prepared tribromoethanol in ICR mice. Contemp Top Lab Anim Sci. 2005, 44(1):17–22.

Lieggi CC, Fortman JD, Kleps RA, et al. An evaluation of preparation methods and storage conditions of tribromoethanol. Contemp Top Lab Anim Sci. 2005, 44(1):11–16.

Lipman NS, Marini RP, Erdman SE. A comparison of ketamine/xylazine and ketamine/xylazine/acepromazine anesthesia in the rabbit. Lab Anim Sci. 1990, 40:395–398.

Lipman NS, Phillips PA, Newcomer CE. Reversal of ketamine/xylazine anesthesia in the rabbit with yohimbine. Lab Anim Sci. 1987, 37:474–477.

Lovell DP. Variation in pentobarbitone sleeping time in mice. 1. Strain and sex differences. Lab Anim. 1986, 20:85–90.

———. Variation in pentobarbitone sleeping time in mice. 2. Variables affecting test results. Lab Anim. 1986, 20:91–96.

———. Variation in barbiturate sleeping time in mice. 3. Strain X environment interaction. Lab Anim. 1986, 20:307–312.

Macrae DJ, Guerreiro D. A simple laryngoscopic technique for the endotracheal intubation of rabbits. Lab Anim. 1989, 23:59–61.

Marini RP, et al. Ketamine/xylazine/butorphanol: a new anesthetic combination for rabbits. Lab Anim Sci. 1991, 42:57–62.

Meyer RE, Fish RE. A review of tribromoethanol anesthesia for production of genetically engineered mice and rats. Lab Anim. 2005, 34(10):47–52.

Morrisey JK, Carpenter JW. Formulary. In: Ferrets, Rabbits and Rodents, Clinical Medicine and Surgery, 2nd ed. Quesenberry KE, Carpenter JW (eds.). St Louis: Saunders, 2004; 436–444.

Nevalainen T., et al. Evaluation of anaesthetic potency of medetomidine-ketamine combination in rats, guinea pigs and rabbits. Acta Vet Scand. 1989, 85:139–143.

Olson ME, Vizzutti D, Morck DW, et al. The parasympatholytic effects of atropine sulfate and glycopyrrolate in rats and rabbits. Can J Vet Res. 1994, 58(4):254–258.

Palmore WP. A fatal response to xylazine and ketamine in a group of rabbits. Vet Res Commun. 1990, 14:91–98.

Papaioannou VE, Fox JG. Efficacy of tribromoethanol anesthesia in mice. Lab Anim Sci. 1993, 43(2):189–192.

Phaneuf LR, Barker S, Groleau MA, et al. Tracheal injury following endotracheal intubation and anesthesia in rabbits. J Amer Assoc Lab Anim Sci. 2006, 45:67–72.

Popilskis SJ, et al. Comparison of xylazine with tiletamine-zolazepam (Telazol) and xylazine-ketamine anesthesia in rabbits. Lab Anim Sci. 1991, 41:51–53.

Radde GR, Hinson A, Crenshaw D, et al. Evaluation of anesthetic regimens in guinea pigs. Lab Anim. 1996, 30:220–227.

Reid WD, et al. An effective combination of anaesthetics for 6-h experimentation in the golden Syrian hamster. Lab Anim. 1989, 23:156–162.

Robertson SA, Eberhart S. Efficacy of the intranasal route for administration of anesthetic agents to adult rabbits. Lab Anim Sci. 1994, 44:159–165.

Russell GB, Graybeal JM. Differences in anesthetic potency between Sprague-Dawley and Long-Evans rats for isoflurane but not nitrous oxide. Pharmacol. 1995, 50:162–167.

Smith JC, Bolon B. Comparison of three commercially available activated charcoal canisters for passive scavenging of waste isoflurane during conventional rodent anesthesia. Contemp Top Lab Anim Sci. 2003, 42(2):10–15.

Smith JC, et al. Endotracheal tubes versus laryngeal mask airways in rabbit inhalation anesthesia: ease of use and waste gas emissions. Contemp Top Lab Anim Sci. 2004, 43:22–25.

Smith W. Responses of laboratory animals to some injectable anaesthetics. Lab Anim. 1993, 27:30–39.

Turner MA, Thomas P, Sheridan DJ. An improved method for direct laryngeal intubation in the guinea pig. Lab Anim. 1992, 26:25–28.

Turner PV, Albassam MA. Susceptibility of rats to corneal lesions after injectable anesthesia. Comp Med. 2005, 55(2):182–189.

Wixson SK. Anesthesia and Analgesia. In: The Biology of the Laboratory Rabbit, 2nd ed. Manning PJ, Ringler DH, Newcomer CE (eds.). San Diego: Academic Press, 1994.

Wixson SK, et al. A comparison of pentobarbital fentanyl-droperidol, ketamine-xylazine and ketamine-diazepam anesthesia in adult male rats. Lab Anim Sci. 1987, 37:726–730.

Wyatt JD, Scott RAW, Richardson ME. The effects of prolonged ketamine-xylazine intravenous infusion on arterial blood pH, blood gases, mean arterial blood pressure, heart and respiratory rates, rectal temperature and reflexes in the rabbit. Lab Anim Sci. 1989, 39:411–416.

Yamamoto Y, et al. Airway management with the laryngeal tube in rabbits. Lab Anim. 2007, 36:33–35.

Yasaki S, Dyck PJ. A simple method for rat endotracheal intubation. Lab Anim Sci. 1991, 41(6):620–622.

ANALGESIA

Principles of appropriate pain management go hand-in-hand with successful anesthetic techniques. For both human and veterinary medicine, the key to successful analgesic therapy remains preemptive treatment. This avoids the physiologic phenomenon known as "wind-up," in which chronic, unrelieved pain induces a hyperalgesic state that is much more difficult to relieve. Knowledge and understanding of animal pain have increased dramatically in recent years, and the use of analgesics in laboratory rabbits and rodents is considered a moral imperative and ethical responsibility of the clinician and researcher. Analgesics are an adjunct to complete perioperative care of the patient and do not substitute for good surgical technique, accompanied by competent nursing care.

Analgesics are selected for potency and duration effect and also with an eye to their potential side effects. For research animals, consideration should also be given to their potential for interference with the research project. Some analgesic side effects to consider include heightened activity, pica, sensitivity to noise, cardiovascular or respiratory system depression, reduced water or food consumption, interactions with other drugs, and alterations in basal physiologic characteristics.

Analgesics should always be given for procedures or conditions that might be considered painful when conducted in humans. As a rule of thumb, the duration of analgesia supplied should be 6–12 hours for minor or superficial surgery (e.g., skin biopsy), 24–48 hours for major surgery (e.g., ovariohysterectomy), and up to 3 or 4 days for major orthopedic or intrathoracic surgical procedures. While these generalizations may be useful for periprocedural planning, individual animals should always be monitored closely for evidence of pain behaviors and treated accordingly.

Pain may be very difficult to detect in rabbits and rodents because they are prey species and instinctively hide behaviors that may be detrimental to their overall survival if noted by potential predators. Manifestations of pain in rabbits and rodents include decreased food and water intake, weight loss, piloerection, listlessness, salivation, chromodacryorrhea, chewing, licking, tooth grinding, hunched posture, vocalization, self-mutilation, or aggression. Decreased water intake is especially significant because fluid loss often accompanies anesthesia and surgery. Postoperative patients with pain may require supplemental hydration. Physiologic parameters such as heart rate, blood pressure, respiratory rate, glucose level, and levels of certain hormones may be increased in painful animals.

The general classes of drugs used to relieve pain include nonsteroidal antiinflammatory drugs (NSAIDs), opiates and opioids (synthetic narcotic derivatives), and locally acting agents (e.g., topical and local anesthetics, as described in the previous section). NSAIDs are generally short-acting drugs, but they provide significant antiinflammatory and analgesic action, for example, ketoprofen and meloxicam. Opiates and opioids provide a short to moderate duration of action and mild to moderate analgesia with the exception of opiates, which provide high levels of analgesia, for example, morphine, oxymorphone, and fentanyl. The choice of agent is dependent on the procedure, but in general, a combination of agents with different noncompetitive pharmacologic actions provides the best analgesic coverage.

Analgesic dosages compiled from a variety of sources are listed in Tables 3.14 and 3.15.

Table 3.14. Suggested analgesic dosages for rabbits, guinea pigs, and chinchillas. (Caution: Most uses and dosages are extralabel.)

Drug	Rabbit (mg/kg)	Guinea Pig (mg/kg)	Chinchilla (mg/kg)
NSAIDS			
Acetylsalicylic acid	10–100 PO q8–24h	50–100 PO q4h PO	87 PO
Carprofen	1–2.2 PO q12h	1–2 PO q12–24h	4 PO q24h
Flunixin	1.1 SC,IM q12h	2.5–5.0 SC q12–24h	1–3 SC q12h
Ibuprofen	2–7.5 PO q12–24h	10 PO q4h	
Ketoprofen	1 IM q12–24h	1 SC q12–24h	1 SC q12–24h
Meloxicam	0.1–0.5 PO,SC q12–24h	0.1–0.3 PO,SC q24h	0.1–0.3 PO,SC q24h
Piroxicam	0.2 PO tid	6 PO q24h	
Tramadol	10 PO q24h		
Opioids			
Buprenorphine	0.01–0.05 SC,IM,IV q6–12h	0.05 SC, q8–12h	0.05 SC, q8–12h
Butorphanol	0.1–1.0 SC,IM,IV q4–6h	0.4–2.0 SC q4h	0.2–2.0 IM q4h
Meperidine	5–10 SC,IM q2–3h	2–10 SC,IM q2–3h	10–20 SC,IM q6h
Morphine	2–5 SC,IM q2–4h	2–5 SC q4h	2–5 SC; q2–4h
Hydromorphone	0.1–0.2 SC,IM,IV q6–8h		
Oxymorphone	0.05–0.20 SC,IM q6–12h	0.2–0.5 SC q6–12h	
Fentanyl patch (Duragesic)	0.5 patch per 3 kg rabbit × 72 h		
Meloxicam	0.2 PO,SC q24h		
Local Anesthetics			
Bupivicaine	<1.5 infiltrated SC		
Lidocaine	<2 infiltrated SC		

References:

Dobromylskyj P, et al. Management of Postoperative and Other Acute Pain. In: Pain Management in Animals. Flecknell PA, Waterman-Pearson A (eds.). London: Saunders, 2000; 81–145.

Johnston MS. Clinical approaches to analgesia in ferrets and rabbits. Sem Av Exot Pet Med. 2005, 14:229–235.

Morrisey JK, Carpenter JW. Formulary. In: Ferrets, Rabbits and Rodents: Clinical Medicine and Surgery, 2nd ed. Quesenberry KE, Carpenter JW (eds.). St Louis: Saunders, 2004; 436–444.

Pollock C. Postoperative management of the exotic animal patient. Vet Clin Exot Anim. 2002; 5:183–212.

Table 3.15. Suggested analgesic dosages for hamsters, gerbils, mice, and rats. (Caution: Most uses and dosages are extralabel. All dosages listed are mg/kg.)

Drug	Hamster	Gerbil	Mouse	Rat
NSAIDS				
Acetylsalicylic acid	240 PO q24h	100 PO	100–120 PO q4h	100–120 PO q4h
Carprofen	5 SC q24h	5 SC q24h	5 SC,PO q24h	5 SC,PO q24h
Flunixin	2.5 SC q12–24h	2.5 SC,IM; q12h	2.5 SC q12–24h	2.5 SC q12–24h
Ibuprofen			7–15 PO q4h	10–30 PO q4h
Ketoprophen	5 SC	5 SC	5 SC	5 SC
Meloxicam			1–2 PO,SC	1.0 PO,SC; q24h
Piroxicam	3 PO; q24h	3 PO; q24h	3 PO; q24h	3 PO; q24h
Opioids				
Buprenorphine	0.1–0.5 SC q8h	0.01–0.2, SC, IM; bid-tid	0.05–2.5 SC q6–12h	0.02–0.50 SC,IM,IP,IV q6–12h OR 0.10–0.25 PO q8–12h
Butorphanol	1–5 SC q4h	1–5 SC; q2–4h	1–5 SC q4h	1–2 SC q4h
Meperidine	20 SC q2–3h		10–20 SC q2–3h	10–20 SC q2–3h
Morphine	2–5 SC q2–4h	2–5 SC; q2–4h	2–5 SC q2–4h	2–5 SC; q2–4h
Oxymorphone	0.2–0.5 SC q6–12h	0.2–0.5 SC,IM; q6–12h	0.2–0.5 SC q6–12h	0.2–0.5 SC q6–12h

References:
Dobromylskyj P, et al. Management of Postoperative and Other Acute Pain. In: Pain Management in Animals. Flecknell PA, Waterman-Pearson A (eds.). London: Saunders, 2000; 81–145.
Hawkins MG. The use of analgesics in birds, reptiles, and small exotic mammals. J Exot Pet Med. 2006, 15:177–192.
Morrisey JK, Carpenter JW. Formulary. In: Ferrets, Rabbits and Rodents: Clinical Medicine and Surgery, 2nd ed. Quesenberry KE, Carpenter JW (eds.). St Louis: Saunders, 2004; 436–444.
Pollock C. Postoperative management of the exotic animal patient. Vet Clin Exot Anim. 2002, 5:183–212.

Opiates and Opioids

Opiates and opioids commonly used in rabbits and rodents include buprenorphine, butorphanol, fentanyl, meperidine, morphine, nalbuphine, oxymorphone, and pentazocine.

Buprenorphine hydrochloride is a partial opiate agonist used primarily for its analgesic effects. It can also be used to reverse the depressant effects of mu-opiates, such as fentanyl or morphine, while still providing postprocedural analgesia. Because of its slow onset of action, the drug should be given early in the procedure. Side effects include mild respiratory depression that is not readily reversed by naloxone, and pica, which is particularly evident in rats at higher doses. Buprenorphine may increase postoperative activity, decrease food intake leading to body weight loss, and alter circadian rhythm. The increased activity caused by this analgesic may disguise the behavioral effects of pain itself. Adequate water consumption is a good indicator of the intended analgesic effect of the drug. Buprenorphine is useful because of its extended duration of action, which may be 6–8 hours.

Butorphanol tartrate is an agonist/antagonist opioid analgesic and can also be used to reverse the effects of mu-opiates and still provide analgesia. It has minimal cardiovascular effects and produces mild respiratory depression. Butorphanol tartrate causes decreased food intake. The duration of effect is 2–4 hours with a half-life in rabbits of 3.16 hours after SC injection, and the drug is more suitable for acute rather than chronic pain. Butorphanol significantly reduces the minimum alveolar concentration of isoflurane in rabbits such that lower inhalant levels are needed to maintain general anesthesia, improving the safety of the anesthetic procedure when both agents are used together.

Fentanyl is a mu-opiate with a rapid onset of action, and it produces profound analgesia, sedation, and respiratory depression. The duration of action is very short, only 30–60 minutes. A slow-release transdermal patch, lasting up to 48 hours, is also available and has been used in rabbits. The patch must be protected from oral ingestion and must be placed on clipped skin 24 hours prior to induction of a painful procedure.

Meperidine hydrochloride is a short-acting opioid analgesic with a rapid onset of action. It may cause depressant effects on the heart, respiratory depression and decreased gastric motility, and may also cause histamine release when given IV. The drug is irritating given SC and the duration of effect is 2–3 hours.

Morphine is a mu-opiate agonist and produces marked sedation in addition to analgesia. The duration of effect is approximately 4 hours.

Nalbuphine is a mixed agonist/antagonist used as an analgesic and also to reverse effects of mu-opioids. The duration of effect is approximately 4 hours.

Oxymorphone is considered a more potent opiate than its parent compound, morphine. The duration of effect is 2–4 hours. Respiratory depression and bradycardia may occur with its use and adverse effects can be reversed with naloxone.

Pentazocine is a mixed opioid agonist/antagonist. It has a rapid onset of action and will reverse the effects of mu-opioids. The duration of effect is 3–4 hours.

Naloxone is a pure antagonist to the opiate/opioid agonist-antagonists listed above. A dose of 0.01–0.1 mg/kg reverses sedative and depressant effects of these analgesics. Naloxone has a duration of action of 45–90 minutes and may need to be readministered, if the duration of action of the original opiate or opioid exceeds this time period.

Tramadol is a synthetic opioid that has become popular for treatment of mild to severe chronic pain. It is not a controlled substance, it can be given orally, and it is relatively inexpensive compared to other opioids. Tramadol is highly unpalatable and a strong flavoring agent should be used to maximize acceptance of the drug.

Nonsteroidal Antiinflammatory Drugs (NSAIDS)

NSAIDs (e.g., aspirin, acetaminophen, ibuprofen, flunixin, ketoprofen, carprophen, meloxicam) are useful analgesics for mild to moderate pain, when inflammation is present, or in situations where opioids are contraindicated. Flunixin meglumine is not recommended for use in rabbits because of uncertain analgesic properties when used in that species. For some of these compounds, oral formulations are not available, and tablets must be crushed and mixed with flavored syrup and given slowly through a syringe at the corner of the mouth. One exception is the liquid suspension formulation of meloxicam, which can readily be given by mouth and has the added benefit of lasting up to 24 hours.

References

Allen DG, Pringle JK, Smith DA, et al. Handbook of Veterinary Drugs, 2nd ed. Philadelphia: Lippincott Williams and Wilkins, 1998.

Dobromylskyj P, et al. Management of Postoperative and Other Acute Pain. In: Pain Management in Animals. Flecknell PA, Waterman-Pearson A (eds.). London: Saunders, 2000, 81–145.

Fiat JW, Sanford J, Smith MW. The assessment and control of the severity of scientific procedures on laboratory animals. Lab Anim. 1990, 24:97–130.

Flecknell P, Waterman-Pearson A (eds.). Pain Management in Animals. London: Saunders, 2000.

Foley PL, et al. Evaluation of fentanyl transdermal patches in rabbits: blood concentrations and physiologic response. Comp Med. 2001, 51:239–244.

Hawkins MG. The use of analgesics in birds, reptiles, and small exotic mammals. J Exot Pet Med. 2006, 15:177–192.

Johnston MS. Clinical approaches to analgesia in ferrets and rabbits. Sem Av Exot Pet Med. 2005, 14:229–235.

Kamp EH, Jones RCW, Tillman SR, et al. Quantitative assessment and characterization of visceral nociception and hyperalgesia in mice. Am J Physiol. 2003, 284:G434–G444.

Liles JH, Flecknell PA. The effects of buprenorphine, nalbuphine and butorphanol alone or following halothane anesthesia on food and water consumption and locomotor movement in rats. Lab Anim. 1992, 26:180–189.
Meyers D. Tramadol. Sem Av Exot Pet Med. 2005, 14:284–287.
Morrisey JK, Carpenter JW. Formulary. In: Ferrets, Rabbits and Rodents: Clinical Medicine and Surgery, 2nd ed. Quesenberry KE, Carpenter JW (eds.). St Louis: Saunders, 2004; 436–444.
Pollock C. Postoperative management of the exotic animal patient. Vet Clin Exot Anim. 2002, 5:183–212.
Portnoy LG, Hustead DR. Pharmacokinetics of butorphanol tartrate in rabbits. Amer J Vet Res. 1992, 53:541–543.
Roughan JV, Flecknell PA. Buprenorphine: A reappraisal of its antinociceptive effects and therapeutic use in alleviating post-operative pain in animals. Lab Anim. 2002, 36:322–343.
Stasiak KL, Maul D, French E, et al. Species-specific assessment of pain in laboratory animals. Contemp Top Lab Anim Sci. 2003, 42(4):13–20.
Thompson AC, et al. Analgesic efficacy of orally administered buprenorphine in rats: methodologic considerations. Comp Med. 2004, 54:293–300.
Turner PV, Chen HC, Taylor WM. Pharmacokinetics of meloxicam in rabbits after single and repeat oral dosing. Comp Med. 2006, 56(1):63–67.
Turner PV, Kerr C, Healy A, et al. Effect of meloxicam and butorphanol on reduction of the minimum alveolar concentration of isoflurane in rabbits. Amer J Vet Res. 2006, 67(5):770–774.
Wright-Williams SL, Courade JP, Richardson CA, et al. Effects of vasectomy surgery and meloxicam treatment on faecal corticosterone levels and behaviour in two strains of laboratory mouse. Pain. 2007, 130(1–2):108–118.
Yashpal K, Katz J, Coderre TJ. Effects of preemptive or postinjury intrathecal local anesthesia on persistent nociceptive responses in rats. Anesthesiol. 1996, 84:1119–1128.

SURGERY

Many indications for and general admonitions regarding surgery of rabbits and rodents exist. Rodents are small, which necessitates special instruments and skills. They lose body heat and fluids rapidly, and surgical anesthesia is not always easily obtained, especially for long procedures. Preoperative stabilization, asepsis, hemostasis, corneal protection, pain relief, prevention of hypothermia, and postoperative care remain essential concerns and responsibilities. Fluid replacement should be provided with isotonic fluids before and during the procedure. Apparently small blood losses may have serious consequences, for example, 20% of total blood volumes are as follows: mouse 0.4–0.6 mL (8–12 drops); gerbil 1.0–2.0 mL; hamster 1.0–2.4 mL; rat 4–6 mL; guinea pig 8–16 mL; chinchilla 6–10 mL; and rabbit 65 mL. Because rabbits and rodents do not vomit, withholding feed prior to surgery may not be necessary, as it may lead to postoperative ketoacidosis. For rabbits, guinea pigs, and chinchillas, 4–6 hours of food withdrawal will reduce ingesta content and provide a more accurate body weight for drug dose calculations. Water should be given up to the time of surgery. A sterile nonmedicated ophthalmic ointment should always be placed on the corneas to prevent drying and ulceration.

Instruments used for surgery in small animals are suitable for use in rabbits. Additional instruments that may be useful for routine rabbit and rodent surgery include (1) magnification loupes; (2) radiosurgical or electrosurgical equipment for hemostasis; (3) automatic skin stapling devices and metal skin clips (9 and 12 mm); (4) sterile cotton-tipped applicators and small pieces of gauze; and (5) other small or microsurgical instruments including iris scissors, small retractors, metal spoons, scalpels, hemostats, burrs, and various small tissue and hemostatic forceps and clips.

Surgery in the Rabbit

Surgery in rabbits is often undertaken, both in clinical practice and for experimental purposes. Several procedures are common, including surgery of the genital system, urolith removal, abscess removal and wound repair, ocular procedures, and fracture fixation.

Operative site preparation should be done gently. Care must be taken when clipping fur to prevent abrading or lacerating the thin skin. Rabbit fur is fine and dense, which can make preoperative clipping especially difficult. The hair should be clean and dry, and a clean, sharp no. 40 clipper blade held flat against the skin, as the skin is stretched taut. Clipping itself should be done slowly and carefully to avoid injury. Excessive use of alcohol or wetting of the fur contributes to hypothermia and should be avoided, as should vigorous scrubbing of the fragile skin.

Positioning with head and neck extended helps keep the airway open. Obstruction can occur if the neck is flexed or twisted, even with an endotracheal tube in place. Rabbits are especially susceptible to the complications of dehydration (blood and fluid loss), core temperature depression, hypovolemic shock, ileus, renal and respiratory depression, and postsurgical anorexia. Supportive care should be provided during anesthesia, as discussed previously in the "Anesthesia" section. An intravenous catheter can be placed in the cephalic, lateral saphenous, jugular, or marginal ear veins or an intraosseous catheter placed for administration of warm replacement fluids at 5–10 mL/kg/hr and to provide cardiovascular support and emergency IV access. A catheter placed in the auricular artery may be used for direct blood pressure monitoring (see Figure 3.24).

Gentle intraoperative tissue handling will reduce postoperative inflammation and associated pain. The skin should be closed with a subcuticular pattern, if possible, and the knot buried. Skin sutures may be tolerated if not placed too tightly; however, rabbits often remove skin sutures during normal grooming. Skin staples are more difficult, but not impossible, for rabbits to remove. If used, these should be removed within 7–10 days of surgery. Although convenient for the surgeon, sterile cyanoacrylate skin adhesive should be used with caution in small mammal species, as it induces a strong exothermic reaction that can produce significant skin necrosis, which may impair wound healing. Use of Elizabethan collars is discouraged unless absolutely necessary, as they are not well tolerated and can result in anorexia and further complications. Preoperative acclimation to the collar may help to increase tolerance if collar use is deemed absolutely necessary.

Postoperative maintenance fluids should be given at 40–80 mL/kg/day until it is certain the rabbit is eating and drinking sufficiently. If necessary, nutritional support can be provided by syringe-feeding or placement of a nasogastric tube (see "Other Special Techniques" below). Palatable food should be offered in an easily accessible manner to encourage early return to eating and to reduce the risk of postoperative ileus.

Laparotomy

Before the abdominal wall is incised, the urinary bladder should be emptied by applying gentle manual pressure dorsocaudally on the lower abdomen or by catheterization. Care must be taken, as this thin-walled structure is easily traumatized. A midline incision through the linea alba is appropriate for most abdominal procedures. The urinary bladder and the large thin-walled cecum, which often lie directly beneath the incision, must be avoided on entry.

Rabbits are prone to abdominal adhesion formation and are used as experimental models of postsurgical adhesions in humans. Any foreign material, such as glove talc, lint from cotton swabs, or suture material, may induce adhesion formation. Absorbable, small diameter (4-0 or 5-0), synthetic suture material on an atraumatic needle will help minimize this problem, as will gentle tissue handling and frequent moistening of the viscera with saline. Use of the calcium channel blocker verapamil hydrochloride, 200 ug/kg PO every 8 hr for nine doses, has reduced adhesion formation experimentally and can be used in cases where adhesions are more likely, such as surgery on the bowel, ruptured pyometra, or abdominal abscess. Oral ibuprofen may also help minimize adhesions. Metal hemostatic clips are useful, as they cause minimal tissue reaction, are less likely to tear friable tissue, and reduce surgical time. Catgut and silk are not recommended as routinely used suture materials in rabbits or rodents because of the marked inflammatory response that they induce, which may result in adhesions.

The peritoneum and muscle layers are usually closed in a single layer, using 3-0 or 4-0 synthetic suture material in a simple continuous or simple interrupted pattern. Care must be taken to oppose, but not crush, the abdominal wall, as tight sutures and ischemia of the peritoneum have been associated with adhesions. The skin should be closed using a subcuticular pattern, taking care to bury the knots. One or two stay skin sutures may be necessary to oppose the skin edges; these likely will be removed by the rabbit overnight but may prevent access to the underlying knot and suture material in the immediate postoperative period. Wound contraction begins the second day postincision and contracts to 40% of the original area by 7 days postsurgically.

Ovariohysterectomy

Ovariohysterectomy of pet rabbits is a routine procedure in many veterinary practices and is indicated for both prevention and treatment of a number of disorders. If performed between 5 and 6 months of age, the procedure not only prevents unwanted pregnancy but will prevent uterine adenocarcinoma later in life and may prevent aggression, territorial behavior, and marking. Ovariohysterectomy may also be performed as a treatment for pyometra, reproductive tract neoplasias or other diseases, and to terminate an unwanted pregnancy.

The reproductive tract of rabbits consists of a long, distensible vagina that leads to a bicornuate uterus, with each horn having its own cervix; there is no uterine body. A marked constriction in diameter delineates each uterine horn from the long, convoluted, friable oviducts. The ovaries are often surrounded by fat and may be difficult to see. The broad ligaments are fat laden and friable, especially in older does. The extremely long gastrointestinal tract of this herbivore completely fills the abdominal cavity and results in constant pressure on the abdominal wall, which must be taken into consideration when incising into and closing the body cavity.

Expression of the urinary bladder should be done gently to avoid trauma or rupture, and is best done with the rabbit held upright, to allow the urine to drain out of the vestibule. Expression of the urinary bladder in dorsal recumbency may allow the urine to pool in the cranial vagina, which may leak into the surgical site upon removal of the uterine horns. With the animal in dorsal recumbency, the surgical site is prepared from vulva to midthorax. A 3–5 cm midline incision is made midway between the pubis and umbilicus. The abdominal muscle wall is lifted away from the underlying viscera prior to incising the linea alba, to avoid incising the underlying thin-walled cecum and urinary bladder, which are often pressing against the body wall. Incidentally, pinworms, if present, may be seen clearly through the cecal wall. Intraabdominal fat may obscure vessels, and it increases friability of tissues. The uterus lies dorsal to and often is concealed by the urinary bladder, which should be retracted caudally. After exteriorizing the uterus, the ovaries are located at the end of each long, curled oviduct. The ovarian pedicles are fatty and friable, and care must be taken during manipulation and when applying hemostats to prevent tearing. Often there is only room to apply one hemostat. A spay hook should not be used for exposing the ovaries. Ligatures or metal vascular clips are placed and the stumps transected and inspected for bleeding prior to releasing them. Larger vessels of the broad ligament are ligated or cauterized prior to transection. Smaller vessels may be clamped and torn with hemostats. The uterine horns may be transfixed and transected either cranial or caudal to the cervices. Care must be taken to avoid incorporating the ureters. If the uterus is transected caudal to the cervices, the flaccid vagina should be oversewn to prevent leakage of urine into the abdomen. Abdominal wall closure is routine.

Cystotomy

Cystotomy is performed in the rabbit to treat urolithiasis or neoplasia or to thoroughly flush crystals from the urinary bladder to correct urine scalding, if flushing via a urethral catheter has failed. The urinary bladder wall may become grossly thickened due to irritation or infection. Urolithiasis frequently recurs, as the pathogenesis is not completely understood. Associated cystitis should be treated based on culture and sensitivity of urine and a piece of urinary bladder wall.

A urethral catheter is preplaced to assist with flushing. After routine preparation and incision of the abdominal wall from pubis to umbilicus, the urinary bladder is exteriorized and the surrounding abdomen is packed with moist gauze. Urine is removed from the bladder by cystocentesis. Stay sutures of 3-0 synthetic material are placed at either end of the intended incision and the bladder wall incised, taking care to avoid the ureters and major blood vessels. The urolith or neoplasm is removed, and the urinary bladder and ureters are thoroughly explored, prior to lavaging with copious amounts of warm saline. Saline is flushed through the urethral catheter to dislodge any crystals or calculi, and to ensure patency. The bladder wall is closed with a single-layer inverting pattern that does not penetrate the lumen. Abdominal wall closure is routine. Fluids and urethral catheterization may need to be continued for several days postoperatively until the rabbit is urinating freely on its own.

Gastrotomy

Gastrotomy in the rabbit is indicated for removal of foreign bodies, treatment of neoplasia, and trichobezoar removal when other therapeutic methods, including hydration, massage, motility stimulation, and alfalfa hay or pineapple juice feeding, have not been succesful. Rabbits should be stabilized before surgery with parenteral fluids containing glucose and analgesics for 1–3 days, if possible. The abdominal wall is surgically prepared from pubis to midthorax, and a midline incision made, taking care not to damage the underlying organs. Stay sutures are placed in the greater curvature of the stomach, and the surrounding abdomen packed with moist laparotomy pads to minimize contamination. An avascular area of the stomach wall is incised between the greater and lesser curvature. The gastric content is removed using forceps or a spoon, the stomach lavaged with warm saline, and the mucosa examined for ulceration. The pylorus is palpated and probed to confirm patency and the duodenum is closely examined for viability. Necrotic areas are resected, if necessary. The stomach is closed in a two-layer inverting suture using 3-0 synthetic monofilament. After lavaging the abdominal cavity with warm saline, closure is routine. Good postoperative nursing care, including fluids, analgesics, supplemental feeding, gut-motility enhancers, and visits from the owner, will hasten recovery.

Other Soft Tissue Surgery

Orchidectomy

Rabbits are castrated to avoid pregnancies; stop urine spraying; reduce aggression; treat orchitis, trauma, or neoplasia; or as part of an experimental study. Rabbits have large, elongated testes, which descend into the scrotal sacs at approximately 2–3 months of age. Inguinal canals remain open throughout the animal's life, and testes move freely between abdomen and scrotal sacs. Intestinal herniation, however, is rare in intact animals because large epididymal fat pads block the passages. Herniation is rare also in castrated rabbits even if the tunics are left open, despite the open passage. Despite this, closed castration, or closure of the inguinal canal after open castration, is recommended.

The surgical approach may be scrotal or prescrotal. The rabbit is placed in dorsal recumbency, and the scrotal sacs, caudal abdomen, and medial thighs surgically prepared. Gentle abdominal pressure can be applied to push the testicles into the scrotal sacs, if they have been retracted.

The scrotal approach involves making two incisions, one over each scrotal sac. The testicle is stabilized between thumb and forefinger, ensuring that it doesn't inadvertently get pushed back into the abdomen, and a 1 cm incision is made through just the skin, for a closed technique, or through both the skin and the parietal vaginal tunic for an open castration. In a closed castration, the tightly adherent skin is dissected away from the tunic to free up the testicle, and a hemostat applied to the tunic-encased spermatic cord. A transfixing ligature is placed, and the tunic and cord transected distal to the suture and removed (Figure 3.35). In an open castration, the testicle is exteriorized through the incision in the parietal vaginal tunic, and the spermatic vessels ligated. The gubernaculum is left attached to the lumen of the vaginal tunic, and tension applied to the testicle, which everts the tunic and allows a transfixing ligature to be placed around the tunic as close as possible to the inguinal opening, after which the tunic is transected, in essence removing the same tissues as in the closed technique. The scrotum is closed with 5-0 nonabsorbable skin sutures, which are usually left alone by the rabbit for long enough for the skin to seal.

One incision is made for the prescrotal, or antescrotal, approach on the ventral midline just cranial to the scrotal sacs. The testicles are pushed cranially into the incision and removed via either an open or closed technique. A subcuticular skin closure is used.

Castrated bucks should be kept isolated and quiet overnight. Castrated rabbits maintain mounting activity for a month or more, but other aggressive and sexual activities diminish rapidly. Castrated bucks should be kept away from intact does for at least 3–4 weeks after surgery.

Abscess Removal

Rabbit abscesses are thick-walled and the pus is caseous. Surgical resection of the entire abscess is preferred to lancing and draining, which are often unsuccesful. Recurrence is common if the entire abscess capsule is not removed. Abscesses on the

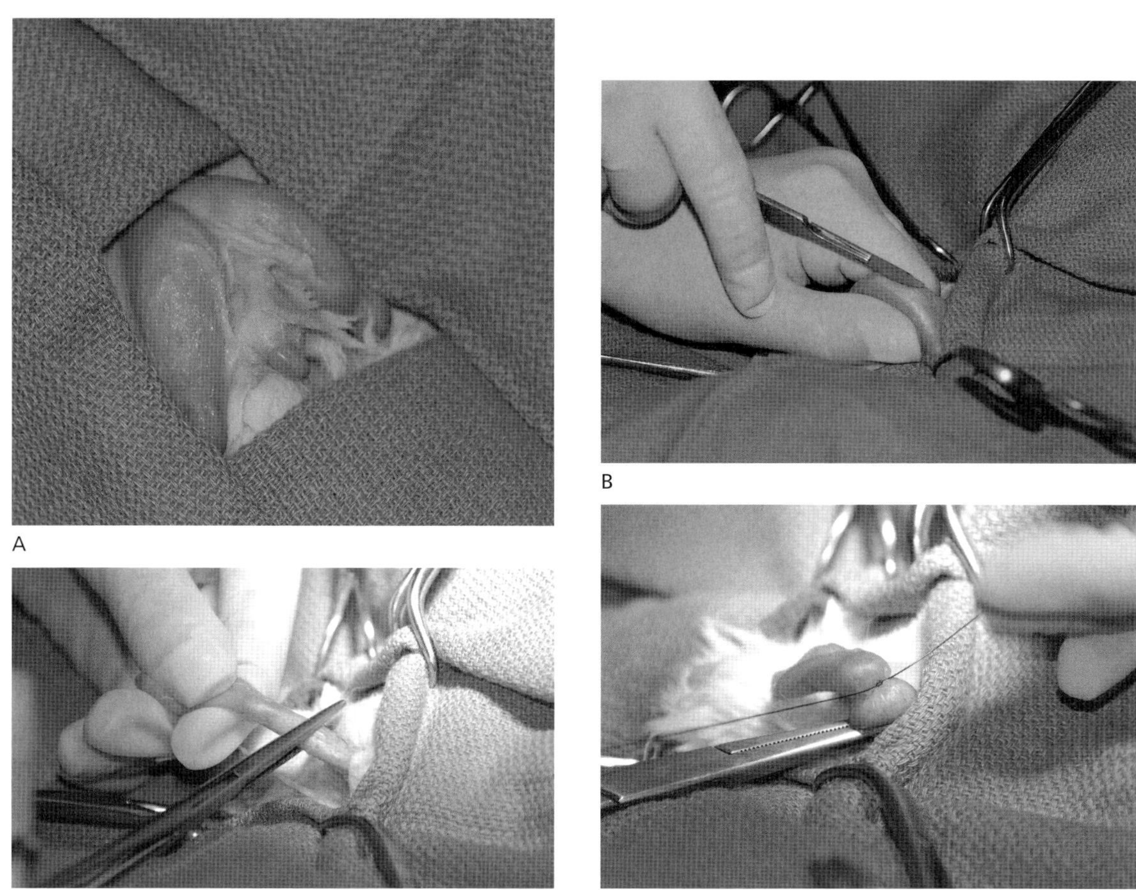

FIGURE 3.35. Technique for closed castration of the rabbit. A: the surgical site is prepped and draped for surgery. B: The skin is incised over the testicle. C: The testicle is exteriorized and the spermatic cord and vessels within the vaginal tunic are clamped. D: The spermatic cord and vessels are ligated, the testicle is removed, and the stump is evaluated for bleeding prior to replacement within the scrotum.

head should be radiographed to determine if there is bony involvement. Abscesses are commonly associated with dental disease, and total resection of these lesions is often not possible, carrying a guarded prognosis, especially if there is an associated osteomyelitis. Destruction of the abscess capsule can be achieved chemically by flushing with hydrogen peroxide, mechanically by dissection, or by radiosurgery. The surgery site can be left open and flushed daily or packed with antibiotic-impregnated polymethylmethacrylate beads and closed.

Enucleation

Indications for enucleation include lack of response to medical treatment for a number of intraocular disorders, corneal perforation, neoplasia, and retrobulbar abscess. Skull radiographs may be necessary to detect bony lesions. Periodic buphthalmos can be associated with an intrathoracic mass, which can be confirmed with thoracic radiographs.

In rabbits, a transconjunctival approach is performed most commonly. The globe is dissected free from the conjunctiva through a circumferential bulbar conjunctival incision at the limbus. Sharp and blunt dissection is used to free the globe from the extraocular muscles, and a ligature or hemostatic clip is applied to the optic nerve and associated blood vessels prior to transection. After removal of the nictitating membrane and lacrimal gland, the eyelid margins are removed and sutured together.

The transpalpebral or en bloc approach involves suturing the eyelids together, incising the eyelid skin circumferentially, and dissecting as close to the bony orbit as possible, removing all structures. The optic nerve and vessels are ligated or a hemostatic clip applied. Skin edges are sutured together to close the orbit.

With either technique, antibiotic-impregnated polymethylmethacrylate beads may be implanted into the orbit to preserve normal contour and provide high levels of antibiotic locally.

Entropion

Entropion in rabbits is characterized by inward curling of the lid resulting in persistent conjunctivitis with discharge and blepharospasm. Corneal opacity, neovascularization, and ulceration may be additional signs. Surgical correction of entropion should be preceded and followed by topical and possibly systemic administration of antibiotics (e.g., trimethoprim/sulfa or enrofloxacin). Elliptical portions of affected lids are elevated and incised 2 mm from the entropic margin, as would be done in a dog or cat. Direct pressure on the incision line controls bleeding, and skin closure is with a simple interrupted pattern using 4-0 to 6-0 synthetic polymer sutures (e.g., nylon or polypropylene). Orbital lesions should regress within 14 days of surgery.

Conjunctival Hyperplasia

At least two conditions in rabbits involving the conjunctiva or nictitating membrane can be corrected by minor surgical procedures. A general, circumorbital ingrowth of a thickened, vascular, conjunctival fold over the cornea (conjunctival overgrowth or pseudopterigium) can be removed using fine forceps and scissors. Direct pressure applied for a few minutes controls hemorrhage.

Glandular or lymphoid hyperplasia of the nictitating membrane may produce a pea-sized lump in the region of the medial canthus. The mass is removed by incision into the lid surface lying against the eyeball; the cartilage is avoided. Fine absorbable sutures (5-0 or 6-0) are used to close the wound, and bleeding is generally minimal.

Orthopedic Procedures

Fractures of long bones are caused by inadvertent drops, improper restraint, dog or cat bites, limbs caught in cage wire, or territorial fighting between two does. Bones that are broken most often in rabbits are the tibia, femur, radius, and humerus (Figure 3.36). Fractures in rabbits are usually closed and can be repaired as in cats; however, rabbit bones with thin cortices are fragile and light, and "thumping" can break down fixation devices. Internal fixation for midshaft fractures in otherwise healthy patients is achieved by open reduction and pinning with small Steinmann pins or Kirchner wire(s). Tissue glue applied intermittently is useful for bone union. A continuous line will interfere with cortical bone union. Skin sutures or clips are removed in 1–2 weeks, and pins in 4–6 weeks. Closed pinning techniques can produce good results in small animals.

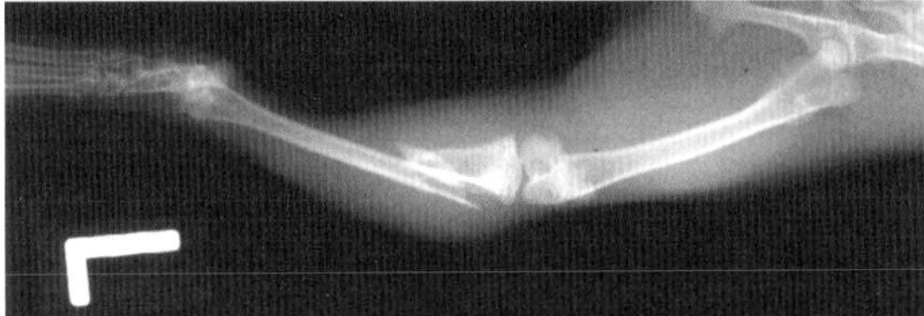

FIGURE 3.36. Lateral survey radiograph of a closed tibial and fibular fracture in a rabbit.

Surgery in Rodents

Commonly performed surgeries in rodents include reproductive tract surgeries, abscess removal, lumpectomy and removal of mammary tumors, and urolith removal, as well as a large number of procedures performed for experimental purposes. Like rabbits, guinea pigs and chinchillas are prone to developing ileus and adhesions following abdominal surgery. With all rodents, careful attention to perioperative support, including provision of supplemental heat, replacement fluids, pain control, nutritional support, and gentle handling, is critical to facilitate recovery and healing in these delicate creatures.

Orchidectomy

Pet rodents are castrated to minimize fighting between males, to minimize odor, or as population control when males are housed with females. If improperly performed, bowel evisceration, strangulation, or herniation may result, with death of the pet as a possible sequela. Improperly performed guinea pig castration has resulted in at least two cases of disciplinary action by veterinary licensing bodies in recent years, one in Canada, and one in the UK. A thorough appreciation of the reproductive tract anatomy of rodents is essential to prevent postoperative complications.

Rodents do not possess a discrete scrotum like the dog or cat; instead the testicles are present within two separate scrotal swellings or sacs. The scrotal sacs are visible externally as a pair of swellings on either side of the penis. The tunica vaginalis lines each scrotal sac and is derived from an outpouching of parietal peritoneum, which communicates directly with the peritoneal cavity through the inguinal canal. Each scrotal sac contains the large testicle, with its associated vascular supply, and a large fat body associated with the epididymis that usually extends into the inguinal canal. Unlike the dog or cat, this inguinal canal remains open throughout life, and in rodents and rabbits, the testicles may be withdrawn through this canal into the abdominal cavity. The diameter of the inguinal canal is so large that an incision into the tunica vaginalis is, in essence, an incision into the abdominal cavity. This is an extremely important consideration when performing an orchidectomy in these animals since failure to close the inguinal canal could result in serious postoperative complications.

Another anatomical consideration is the close proximity of the contaminated prepuce and anus to the surgical sites. Placing a cotton-tipped wooden applicator stick into the anal opening of larger rodents helps prevent passage of fecal pellets into the surgical field (Figure 3.37). In addition, the long prepuce of chinchillas can be secured cranially to the ventral abdomen with atraumatic tape to keep it out of the sterile field.

Closed, open, and abdominal castration techniques have been used in rodents. The closed technique is similar to that described for the rabbit. After surgical preparation and ensuring the testicles are in the scrotal sacs, the testicle is stabilized between thumb and forefinger and a 1 cm incision is made into each scrotal sac, taking care not to incise the tunica vaginalis. The testicle encased in the tunica vaginalis is dissected free, so that the tunica-encased cord is exposed. After crushing with a hemostat, a transfixing ligature is placed through the cord, and the testicle and tunica vaginalis are transected distal to the ligature. The skin incision is closed with skin sutures or sterile tissue glue, taking care not to get any glue on the skin surface, which may incite the animal to chew at the area. This technique eliminates any opening into the abdominal cavity, and the transfixing ligature provides added security against slippage of the ligature. However, dissection of the tightly adherent skin from the tunica vaginalis can be time consuming.

With an open technique, which involves incising through the skin and tunica vaginalis, care must be taken to prevent postoperative herniation of viscera into the scrotal sac. One method is to leave behind the epididymal fat pad to block the inguinal opening, prior to suturing the skin. However, herniation of the bowel or bladder may still occur following this technique. A superior method involves ligating the spermatic vessels but leaving the gubernaculum attached to the tunica vaginalis. By applying tension to the testicle, the attached tunic can be stretched taut and easily dissected free from the surrounding skin, after which a transfixing ligature is placed as close to the inguinal opening as possible, taking care not to incorporate any vessels or viscera. Skin is closed as for the closed technique (Figure 3.37). An alternate technique in rats involves making a single 1 cm midline incision at the distal scrotal tip, pushing the testicles caudally, and cutting each tunic. Each testicle and epididymis is exteriorized, and the cord is ligated. The skin is closed with 9 mm clips, taking care not to clip the anus shut.

In the less commonly used abdominal technique, a ventral midline incision is made over the caudal abdomen, the testicles are pushed from the inguinal canal into the surgical site, spermatic cord is ligated, and testicles removed, followed by routine closure of the abdominal wall, using a subcuticular pattern.

Ovariohysterectomy

Indications for ovariohysterectomy include prevention of pregnancy and mammary gland tumors and treatment of dystocia, pyometra, and cystic ovaries. The reproductive anatomy of female rodents resembles that of the dog and cat, except in rats, which have two cervices. After surgical preparation, a ventral midline incision is made, taking care not to lacerate underlying viscera. The uterine horns are located and traced cranially to the ovaries. The

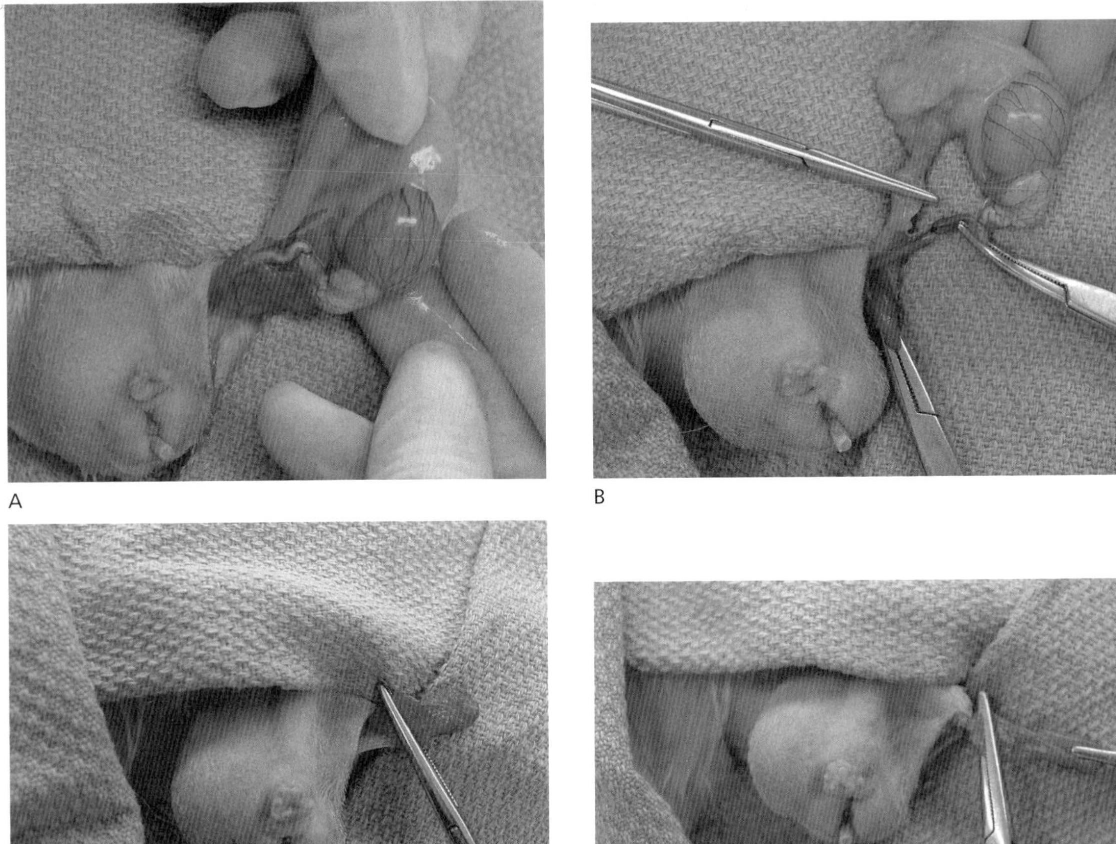

FIGURE 3.37. Open technique for guinea pig castration. A: After incising the skin and tunic, the testicle and fat pad are exteriorized. B: The tunic is teased away from the testicle by tearing the gubernaculum (bottom clamp), and the spermatic cord and any vessels in the fat pad are clamped and ligated. C: The ligated stumps are allowed to retract back into the abdomen and the tunic is clamped as proximally as possible, taking care not to entrap stumps. D: A transfixing ligature is placed at the proximal end of the tunic, effectively closing the inguinal canal. The excess tunic is then trimmed away, and the skin closed with sutures or tissue glue. A cotton applicator with the stick cut short is placed in the anus to prevent fecal pellets from contaminating the site. Courtesy of Dennilyn Parker.

ovarian pedicles are ligated, as are any large vessels in the broad ligament. The uterus is ligated caudal to the cervix. The abdominal wall is closed using appropriately sized synthetic suture material in a simple continuous or simple interrupted pattern, followed by a subcuticular closure of the skin or careful use of tissue glue.

Ovariectomy

Ovariectomy of rodents may be performed for experimental purposes. The rodent is placed in sternal recumbency, and the skin is clipped over the lumbar spine and flanks. A transverse flank incision is made on each side 0.5–1 cm caudal to the last rib and ventral to the epaxial muscles. Alternatively a single 1–1.5 cm dorsal midline incision is made and shifted to either side of the flank over this area. Subcutaneous tissues and abdominal wall muscles are separated, and the peritoneum punctured approximately 5 mm off midline to reveal and permit extraction, ligation, and transection of the fat-imbedded ovary through the flank incision. The oviduct may also be removed at the same time; bleeding rarely occurs following this procedure. Metal clips or 4-0 or 5-0 sutures can be used to close the body wall and should be removed within 7 days of surgery. Tight skin sutures should be avoided to reduce irritation and subsequent chewing at the incision. Because guinea pigs may have ovarian cysts on the oviduct, cycling may continue despite the ovariectomy.

Abscess Removal

Rodent abscesses are often circumscribed by dense fibrous capsules and generally contain thick, purulent material, often due to a mixture of aerobic and anaerobic bacteria. If not amenable to surgical removal in toto, abscesses should be lanced, flushed and left open to drain, or implanted with antibiotic-impregnated polymethylmethacrylate beads and closed. Culture and sensitivity of the abscess capsule for both aerobic and anaerobic organisms should be done to guide systemic antibiotic choice, keeping in mind that many antibiotics are toxic in some rodents. Submandibular abscesses in guinea pigs may be due to infection of lymph nodes with *Streptococcus zooepidemicus,* and septicemia may result if these are opened and drained. Surgical resection may be challenging due to close association with the vagal nerve, jugular vein, and carotid arteries. Treatment may be restricted to systemic antibiotics and hot compresses.

Lumpectomy

Skin and subcutaneous lumps are common in rodents. Benign mammary tumors in rats may be very large and are generally easily removed, although larger tumors often become necrotic and highly vascularized. Prior to surgery, the surgeon should ensure that there is adequate skin to close the incision. The rat is anesthetized, and the encapsulated tumor is removed through a cutaneous incision. Ligation of connecting blood vessels is necessary. Mammary tumors in mice and many other skin tumors, such as fibrosarcomas, are locally invasive and may be difficult to completely remove. Sebaceous adenomas in guinea pigs can become quite large and are filled with caseous sebum, which should not be confused with pus. Guinea pigs have a moderate amount of loose skin over the dorsum, which facilitates excision. Skin sutures may be placed in areas inaccessible to the rodent's teeth.

Cystotomy

The primary indication for cystotomy in rodents is to remove urinary calculi. Calculi may be present in the urethra, urinary bladder, ureters, or renal pelvices (Figure 3.38). Signs of calculi and cystitis include hematuria, urine dribbling, anorexia, and evidence of pain and distress. A radiograph may confirm the presence of urinary calculi. A kidney may be enlarged because of hydronephrosis or renal calculi.

The surgical procedure is similar to that in rabbits, although preplacement of a urethral catheter may not always be possible. Urine culture and sensitivity and culture of a piece of the urinary bladder wall should be performed to determine if antibiotic therapy is indicated. Urinary calculi often recur.

Fracture Repair

Fractures of long bones are caused by being dropped, being bitten by dogs or cats, or catching limbs in cage wire. Bones most often broken are the tibia, femur, radius, and humerus (Figures 3.39 and 3.40). Adjuncts to fracture repair may be fluid therapy for shock and quiet housing to reduce stress.

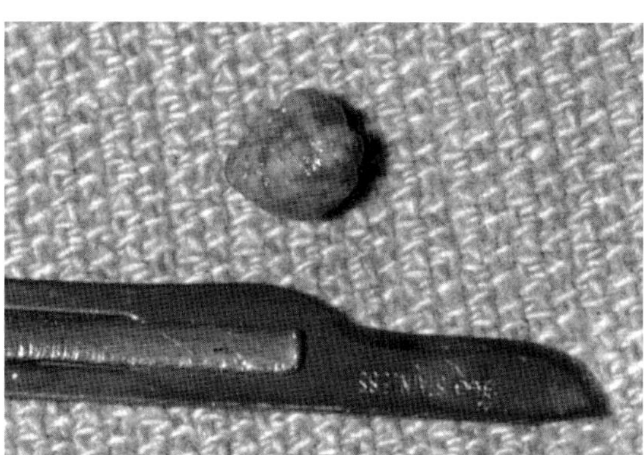

FIGURE 3.38. Urolith removed from a pet hamster via cystotomy.

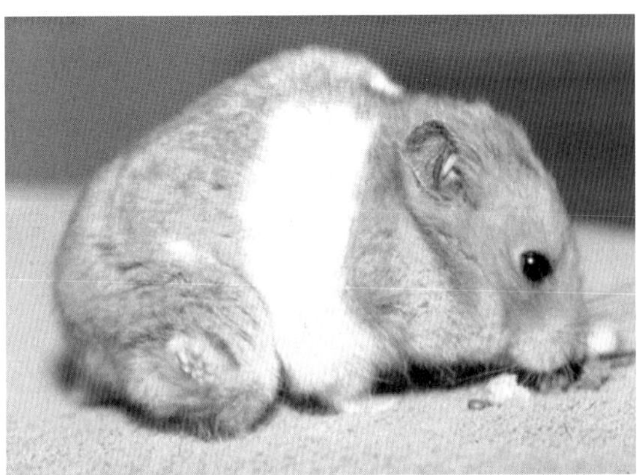

FIGURE 3.39. Hamster with fractured femur.

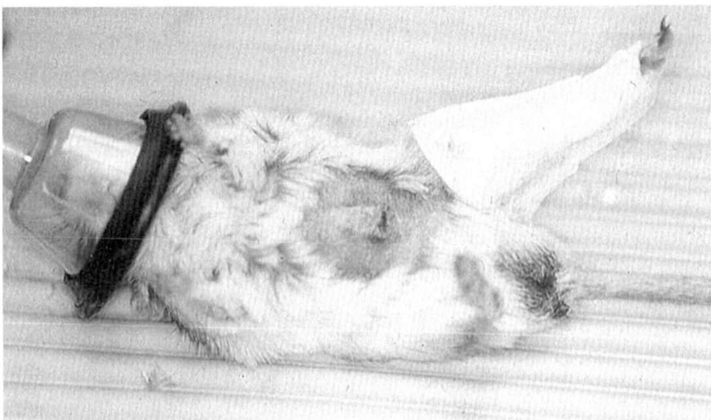

FIGURE 3.40. Male gerbil with tibial fracture repaired by external fixation. The ventral marking gland is visible on the abdomen and is developing a neoplastic growth at its caudal end.

Nonscreen radiographic film techniques may be needed to reveal fractures in small bones, and anesthesia must be adequate to relax muscles and allow reduction of the fragments. An anatomic characteristic other than small size that increases the challenge of fracture repair in small rodents is the enclosure of femurs and humeri in the trunk mass or the abdominal skin. Internal fixation for midshaft fractures in otherwise healthy patients is achieved by open reduction and pinning with small polypropylene rods with or without glue, Steinmann pins, or Kirchner wire(s). In very small animals, a hypodermic needle may be used as an intramedullary pin. Plastic pins may be fixed by passing a metal pin through both cortices and the pin. Skin sutures or clips are removed in 1–2 weeks, and pins in 4–6 weeks. Closed pinning techniques produce good results in small animals. An Elizabethan collar may be useful to prevent the animal from chewing at the affected area (Figure 3.41).

External fixation devices, including taping the affected limb to the body wall and splinting with rolled film or small sticks, are often unsuccessful because of self-mutilation. Traction casts, consisting of a taped foot drawn through a plastic syringe cover, may be succesful, although the usual outcome is chewing and self-mutilation. The foot is bound to a piece of adhesive tape, the broken limb pulled almost through the tube, and the tape wrapped to the distal end of the tube. Padding in or around the tube openings may be necessary. Casts and splints are more practical for forelegs rather than for rear legs. An additional treatment option that is often preferred is to provide nothing more than cage rest and allow the limb to heal with the possible complication of malunion.

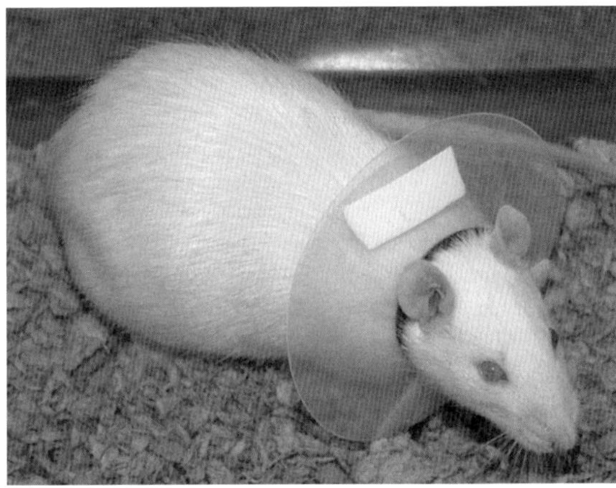

FIGURE 3.41. Elizabethan collar fitted for a rat.

DENTAL PROCEDURES IN RABBITS AND RODENTS

All teeth of rabbits, guinea pigs, and chinchillas are open-rooted (continually growing), while in hamsters, gerbils, rats, and mice only the incisors grow continually. Rabbits have two pairs of maxillary incisors (one behind the other) and one pair of mandibular incisors. The cheek teeth of rabbits, guinea pigs, and chinchillas are arranged in parallel rows, and the maxillary dental arch is wider than the mandibular arch, similar to horses (see Table 3.16 for dental formulas). Tooth overgrowth is common in all species (Figures 3.42–3.47).

Dental procedures are challenging due to the small size and gape of the oral cavity. Access to the incisors poses little problem; however, recognition of their normal length and appearance is critical to avoid unnecessary trimming, which could harm the animal and interfere with food apprehension. Access to premolars and molars is more difficult, and care must be taken to guard against trauma to the cheeks, gums, and tongue while performing dental work. Dental specula and cheek dilators are commercially available for pet rabbits and rodents and will assist with visualization of the cheek teeth (Figure 3.48). Inappropriate conformation and diet composition may be responsible for overgrowth of teeth and associated conditions seen in captive rabbits and rodents.

Incisor trims may be accomplished using a low-speed hand drill or burr in an anesthetized animal.

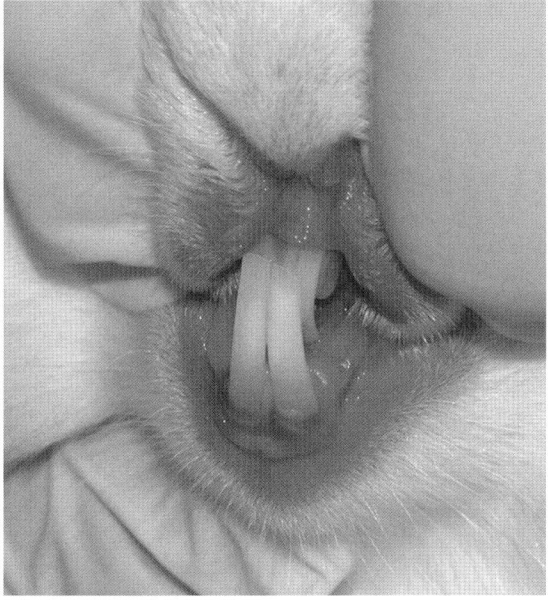

FIGURE 3.42. Incisor malocclusion in a rabbit.

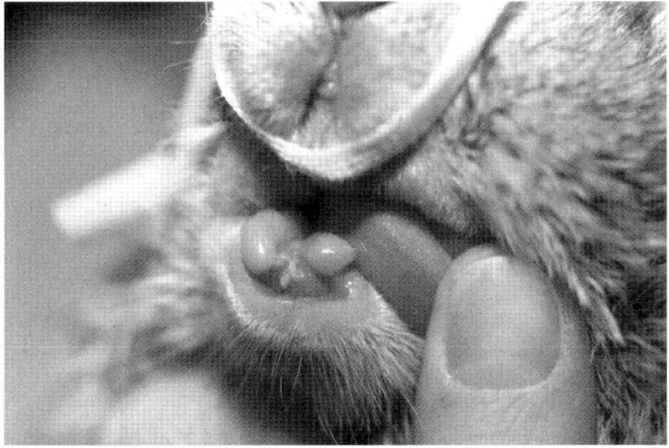

FIGURE 3.43. This rabbit is missing the lower incisors. The four upper incisors may require regular trimming to prevent overgrowth.

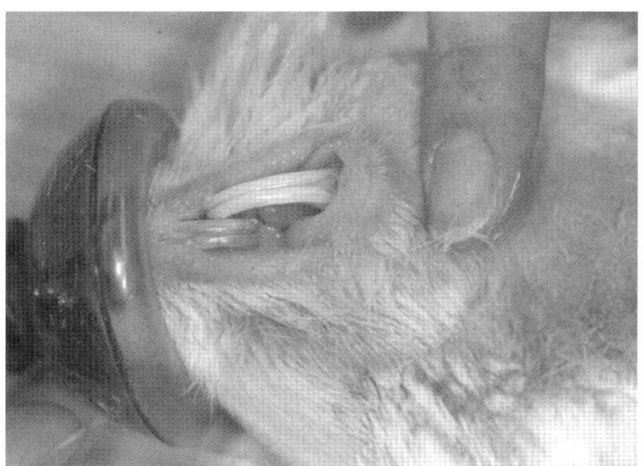

FIGURE 3.44. Incisor malocclusion in a guinea pig. A moist dermatitis is also present in the cervical region ("slobbers") due to excess salivation.

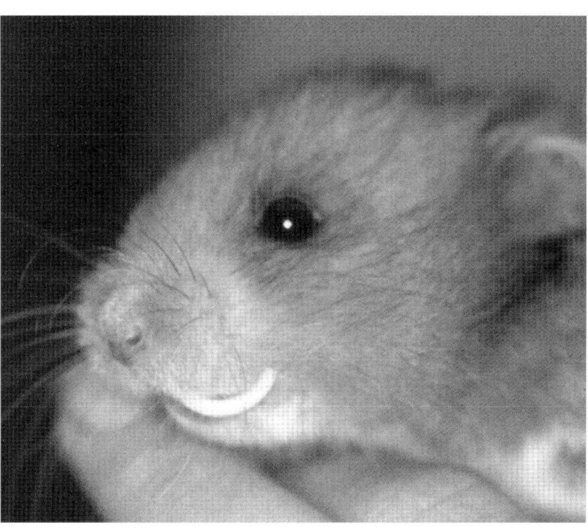

FIGURE 3.45. A hamster with unilateral overgrowth of an upper incisor.

Care should be taken to maintain the normal ratio of upper:lower incisor length. Trimming of points on the cheek teeth may be done in a similar manner with care taken not to lacerate the tongue or buccal mucosa. Clipping or sawing the teeth in conscious animals predisposes to rough edges, vertical fractures with pulp exposure, and tooth root abscesses, and may be painful and stressful for the rabbit and for the client.

The open-rooted teeth of rabbits, particularly the incisors, may be removed as a cure for malocclusion

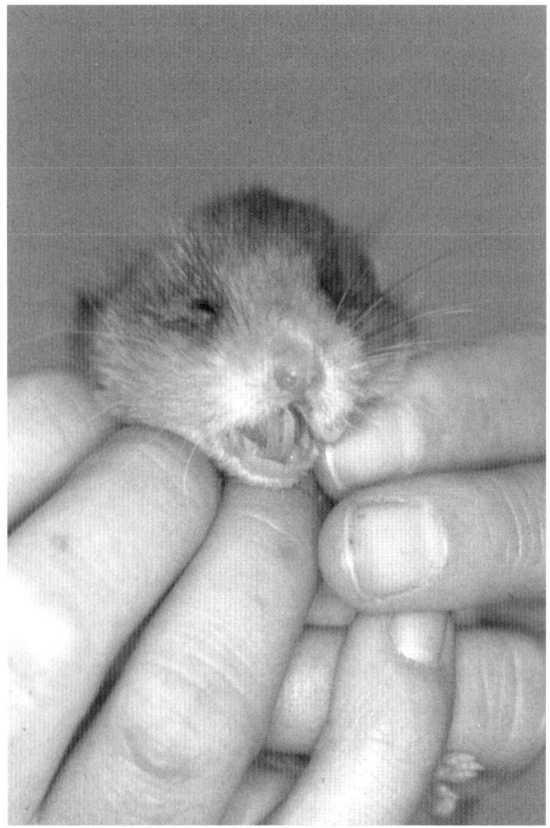

FIGURE 3.46. Incisor overgrowth in a pet hamster.

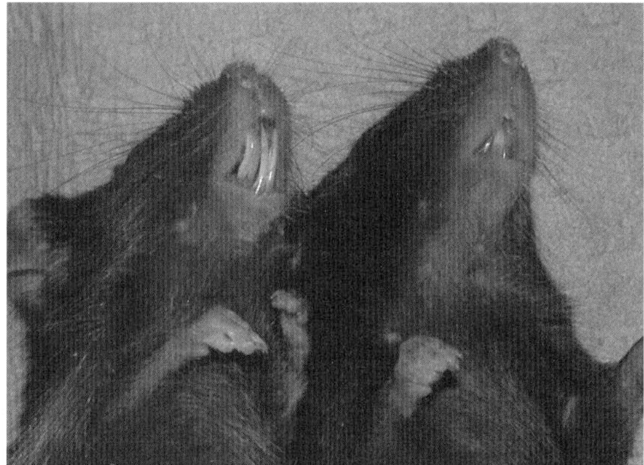

FIGURE 3.47. Mice with incisor overgrowth.

Table 3.16. Dental formulas of rabbits and rodents.

		Incisors	Canines	Premolars	Molars
Rabbit	2×	$\frac{2}{1}$	$\frac{0}{0}$	$\frac{3}{2}$	$\frac{3}{3}$
Guinea pig	2×	$\frac{1}{1}$	$\frac{0}{0}$	$\frac{1}{1}$	$\frac{3}{3}$
Chinchilla	2×	$\frac{1}{1}$	$\frac{0}{0}$	$\frac{1}{1}$	$\frac{3}{3}$
Hamster	2×	$\frac{1}{1}$	$\frac{0}{0}$	$\frac{0}{0}$	$\frac{3}{3}$
Gerbil	2×	$\frac{1}{1}$	$\frac{0}{0}$	$\frac{0}{0}$	$\frac{3}{3}$
Rat	2×	$\frac{1}{1}$	$\frac{0}{0}$	$\frac{0}{0}$	$\frac{3}{3}$

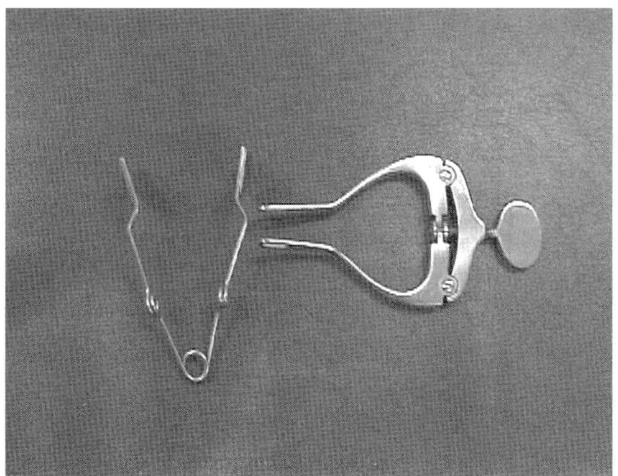

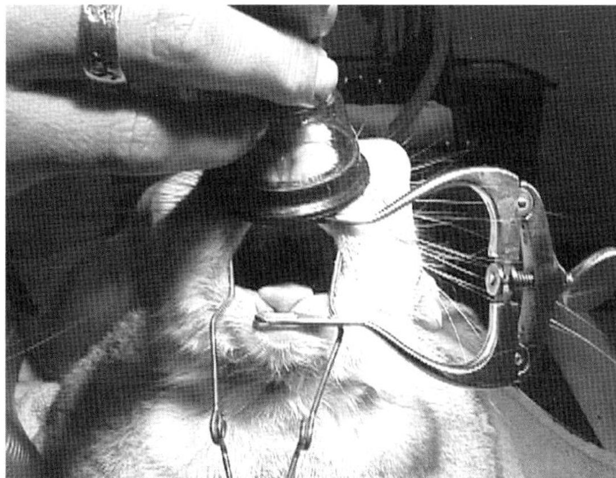

FIGURE 3.48. Incisor speculum and cheek dilator for rabbits (left). Visualization of the dental cavity of an anesthetized rabbit with depicted instruments in place (right).

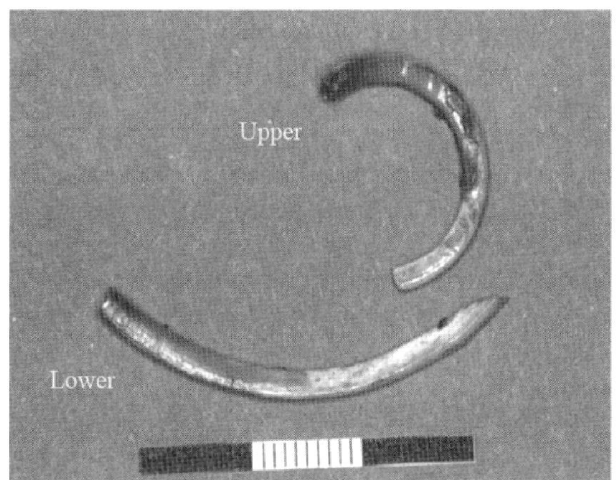

FIGURE 3.49. Incisors extracted from a mature rabbit. The peg teeth are not shown but should also be extracted to avoid overgrowth.

and the associated overgrowth, particularly when tooth trimming may be required at very frequent intervals. Opposing teeth must also be removed. To extract an incisor tooth, the patient is anesthetized, radiographed to determine condition and location of roots, and given an antibiotic (e.g., enrofloxacin) if abscessation is suspected.

Periodontal ligaments, especially those on medial surfaces of the incisors, are broken down using a small elevator, root tip pick, or bent 18-gauge needle. The loosened teeth are then pushed into the alveolus to break any remaining ligaments, before removal using gentle pressure with an extractor or forceps and pulling along the curvature of the teeth. Lower incisors are removed first (Figure 3.49). The smaller, upper caudal incisors have straight roots that can be removed easily but may break. If roots are broken (the root is soft and hollow), the remaining tooth root will generate and erupt as a tooth in 6–8 weeks. Cheek tooth removal is more difficult, and an extra-oral buccotomy must be attempted, assuming one can do such a procedure on a fragile skull. Open sockets are flushed with an antiseptic, or roots may be cultured if an abscess is suspected, and the rabbit given antibiotics for several days.

References

Arnbjer J. Pseudopterygium in a pygmy rabbit. Vet Med Small Anim Clin 1979, 74:737–738.

Bennett RA. Soft Tissue Surgery. In: Ferrets, Rabbits and Rodents, Clinical Medicine and Surgery, 2nd ed. Quesenberry KE, Carpenter JW (eds.). St Louis: Saunders, 2004; 316–328.

Brown SA. Surgical removal of incisors in the rabbit. J Small Exotic Anim Med. 1992, 1:150–153.

Capello V. Clinical technique: treatment of periapical infections in pet rabbis and rodents. J Exot Pet Med. 2008, 17:124–131.

Capello V, Cauduro A. Clinical technique: application of computed tomography for diagnosis of dental disease in the rabbit, guinea pig and chinchilla. J Exot Pet Med. 2008, 17:93–101.

Emily P. Problems peculiar to continually erupting teeth. J Small Exot Anim Med. 1991, 1:56–59.

Gillett NA, Brooks DL, Tillman PC. Medical and surgical management of gastric obstruction from a hairball in the rabbit. J Am Vet Med Assoc. 1983, 183:1176–1178.

Harcourt-Brown F. Textbook of Rabbit Medicine. Oxford: Butterworth Heinemann, 2002.
Jenkins JR. Soft Tissue Surgery. In: Ferrets, Rabbits and Rodents, Clinical Medicine and Surgery, 2nd ed. Quesenberry KE, Carpenter JW (eds.). St Louis: Saunders, 2004; 221–230.
Kaplan H, Timmons E. The Rabbit: A Model for the Principles of Mammalian Physiology and Surgery. New York: Academic Press, 1979.
Lumley JSP, et al. Essentials of Experimental Surgery. London: Butterworth & Co, 1990.
Meredith A, Redrobe S. BSAVA Manual of Exotic Pets, 4th ed. Gloucester, UK: British Small Animal Veterinary Association, 2002.
Niles J, Williams J. Suture materials and patterns. In Pract. 1999, 21:308–320.
Olson ME, Bruce J. Ovariectomy, ovariohysterectomy and orchidectomy in rodents and rabbits. Can Vet J. 1986, 27:523–527.
RCVS Disciplinary Committee: Disciplinary committee orders name to be removed from the register. Vet Rec. 2000, 146:174.
Redrobe S. Soft tissue surgery of rabbits and rodents. Sem Av Exot Pet Med. 2002, 11(4):231–245.
Reiter AM. Pathophysiology of dental disease in the rabbit, guinea pig and chinchilla. J Exot Pet Med. 2008, 17(2):70–77.
Rich GA. Rabbit orthopedic surgery. Vet Clin Exot Anim. 2002, 5:157–168.
Richardson C, Flecknell P. Routine neutering of rabbits and rodents. In Pract. 2006, 28:70–79.
Rickards DA, Hinko PJ, Morse EM. Orthopedic procedures for laboratory animals and exotic pets. J Am Vet Med Assoc. 1972, 161:728–732.
Steinleintner A, Lambert H, Kazensky C, et al. Reduction of primary postoperative adhesion formation under calcium channel blockade in the rabbit. J Surg Res. 1990, 48:42–45.
Swindle MM, Shealy PM. Common Surgical Procedures in Rodents and Rabbits. In: Handbook of Rodent and Rabbit Medicine. Laber-Kaird K, Swindle MM, Flecknell PA (eds.). Oxford: Pergamon, 1996.

SEROLOGIC TESTING FOR COLONY HEALTH SURVEILLANCE

Serology is the primary method for monitoring the disease status of specific pathogen free (SPF) rodent and rabbit colonies. Viral infections in conventionally housed rodents are common and may influence health and experimental results, especially mouse hepatitis virus and parvovirus infections, which are among the most common diseases of laboratory mice in North America. The detection of rodents carrying antiviral antibodies, and possibly the virus itself, is an important consideration in disease prevention in rodent colonies whether bred for research or for the pet trade. Viral agents are typically monitored by a combination of pathogen detection systems (PCR, histopathology, viral culture) and serodiagnosis. Adventitial bacterial diseases may also cause significant complications in research colonies. Many of the more common pathogenic organisms, such as *Salmonella* spp and *Bordetella* spp in all species and *Pasteurella multocida* in rabbits, have been eliminated by selective breeding or embryo rederivation. The presence of these agents is typically monitored by culture and serology. *Helicobacter* spp are commonly detected in research colonies and can be diagnosed by histopathology, culture, PCR, or serology. Parasitic diseases such as mites in mice, hamsters, and rabbits, or pinworms in all species may be occasionally diagnosed in a laboratory setting, typically by direct observation of the adult or ova.

Use of barrier housing, quarantine, health screening for incoming animals, and routine health surveillance of sentinel or experimental animals are strategies used to maintain and monitor colony pathogen status and are similar to those implemented for large groups of agricultural animals (i.e., a "herd health approach"). The scope and characteristics of a health monitoring program are unique for each facility, and include consideration of size of the program, types of research, presence of immunodeficient animals, source of animals, types of housing, and many other factors. A detailed discussion of program development is outside the scope of this review. Several publications review the rationale and recommendations for development of a program for monitoring and surveillance of diseases in rabbit and rodent colonies.

Sentinel Testing Procedures

Commercial laboratories that provide the majority of rodent serology testing do so primariy for the research community. Several of these labs also offer services to clinical practitioners, which might be

Table 3.17. Summary of common rabbit and rodent diagnostic serology tests.

Virus	Species Tested	Primary Test	Secondary Test	Prevalence
PVM	M, R, H, Gp, (Rb)	E	IFA, Path	Moderate to minimal lung lesions
Reo-3	M, R, H, Gp	E	IFA	Low to moderate
TMEV	M, R	E	IFA	Low to moderate. Also called TO or GDVII
KRV	R	HI	IFA, Path	Common—abortions and resorptions
H-1	R	E	IFA	Rare
K	M	E	IFA	Rare—need for testing in question
MVM	M	E	HAI	Common—orphan parvo viruses cross-react in diagnostic tests
Polyoma	M, (H)	E	IFA	Very rare
Sendai	M, R, H, Gp	E	IFA, Path	Very common—lung lesions
MHV	M	E	IFA, Path	Common—many strains of virus, gut syncytia
SDAV-RCV	R	E	IFA, Path	Common—many strains of virus, salivary and Harderian gland lesions
SV-5	H, Gp	E	IFA	Low to moderate—significance unknown
EDIM	M	E	IFA, Path	Low to moderate
Adenoviruses	M, H, (R)	E	IFA, Path	Common in hamsters and conventional mice
Ectromelia	M	E	Path, IFA	Uncommon—may cause high mortality
LCM	M, H, Gp, R	E	IFA	Uncommon—zoonotic disease
LDHV	M	LDH plasma enzyme assay		Incidence uncertain—colorimetric assay. No clinical signs
Mouse Thymic Virus	M	E	IFA, Path	Rare thymic necrosis in neonates
Cytomegalo-viruses	Gp, R, M	IFA, Path		Common in guinea pigs—causes lesions in salivary glands
Mycoplasma pulmonis	R, M	E	Culture, Path	Common in conventional colonies—readily cultured
CAR Bacillus	R, Rb, M, Gp, H	E	Path, IFA	Common—silver stain of respiratory epithelium
Tyzzer's Disease (*Clostridium piliforme*)	M, R, H, Gp Gb, Rb	E	Path, IFA	Common
Encephalitozoon cuniculi	Rb, Gp, H, M, R	E	Path, IFA	Common

M = mouse, R = rat, H = hamster, Gp = guinea pig, Rb = rabbit, Gb = gerbil, IFA = immunofluorescence, HAI = hemagglutination inhibition, E = ELISA = enzyme-linked immunosorbent assay, Path = histopathology helpful, in parenthesis—indicates the test is not commonly performed.

useful for diseases such as *Encephalitozoon* spp infection of rabbits or LCMV infections of hamsters or mice. Laboratories have traditionally used enzyme-linked immunosorbent assays (ELISA) as a screening tool to measure antibodies to organisms associated with clinical or subclinical disease in rodents. Positive results are typically confirmed by most laboratories using a more specific technique, such as indirect fluorescent antibody or Western blot analysis. Multiplex fluorescent immunoassay (MFI) is a type of liquid phase bead-based ELISA assay that makes use of flow cytometric technology. This technique permits screening of multiple antibodies with one serum sample. Because only 0.2 uL of undiluted serum can be used to test reactivity against a large number of pathogens, this technique is highly suitable for screening rodent samples and has been developed by major rodent serologic diagnostic laboratories in North America.

Polymerase chain reaction (PCR) testing is also available for many diseases of laboratory and pet rodents. Many of the PCR assays can be run using fecal samples. Clinicians should remember that the PCR test will only indicate infection when the agent is being shed, which may be a short period of time for acute infections that result in complete recovery. This is typically the period before serum antibody response has occurred, and it is feasible to use PCR to screen for active pathogen replication and serology to evaluate recovered or persistent infection. Table 3.17 summarizes the more common serologic tests suggested for screening sera from various species.

Collection, processing, dilution, and storage of rodent sera intended for serologic testing must follow an established protocol if results are to be meaningful. Collection tubes must be clean and hemolysis, excessive tissue products, and bacterial growth must be avoided. For small rodents, blood may be collected and processed without dilution. A dilution technique can also be used as follows. One-half mL of blood is collected into 1.0 mL of isotonic phosphate-buffered saline. For larger animals (greater than 100 g), 1.0 mL of blood is collected into 2.0 mL of saline. Assuming a 50% packed cell volume, the final serum concentration will be 1:5. Serum may also be diluted after centrifugation. The saline:blood mixture is allowed to clot for 30 minutes and is then ringed, covered, and refrigerated. Sera are separated and heat-activated in a water bath at 56 °C (133 °F) for 30 minutes. A minimum of 0.2 mL of diluted serum is required for virus serology screening panels. The clinician should consult with the laboratory performing diagnostic evaluations to determine the preferred method for sample preparations for serology or PCR.

References

Baker DG. Natural pathogens of laboratory mice, rats, and rabbits and their effects on research. Clin Microbiol Rev. 1998, 11(2):231–266.

Compton SR, Holmberger FR, Paturzo FX, et al. Efficacy of three microbiological monitoring methods in a ventilated cage rack. Comp Med. 2004, 54:382–392.

Compton SR, Riley LR. Detection of infectious agents in laboratory rodents: traditional and molecular techniques. Comp Med. 2001, 51(2):113–119.

Jenkins JR. Rabbit diagnostic testing. J Exot Pet Med. 2008, 17:4–15.

———. Rodent diagnostic testing. J Exot Pet Med. 2008, 17:16–25.

Koszdin KL, Digiacomo RF. Outbreak: detection and investigation. Contemp Top Lab Anim Sci. 2002, 41(3):18–27.

Laber-Laird K, Proctor M. An example of a rodent health monitoring program. Lab Anim. 1993, 22(8):24–32.

LaRegina MC, Lonigro J. Serologic screening of murine pathogens: basic concepts and guidelines. Lab Anim. 1988, 17(8):40–47.

Lennox AM. Equipment for exotic mammal and reptile diagnostics and surgery. J Exot Pet Med. 2006, 15:98–105.

Miller L. Orphan parvovirus: an enigmatic plague for rodent research. Lab Anim. 1993, 22(8):33–34.

Rehg JE, Toth LA. Rodent quarantine programs: purpose, principles, and practice. Lab Anim Sci. 1998, 48:438–447.

Reimers TJ, Lamb SV. Radioimmunoassay of hormones in laboratory animals for diagnostics and research. Lab Anim. 1991, 20(5):32–38.

Shek WR. Role of housing modalities on management and surveillance strategies for adventitious agents of rodents. ILAR J. 2008, 49:316–325.

Thibert P. Control of microbial contamination in the use of laboratory rodents. Lab Anim Sci. 1980, 30:339–351.

Various. ILAR J. 2008, vol. 49(3): Detection and Management of Microbial Contamination in Laboratory Rodents. (The entire issue is devoted to this subject.)

Wagner JE, Besch-Williford CL, Steffen EK. Health surveillance of laboratory rodents. Lab Anim. 1991, 20(5):40–45.

Williams C, et al. Microbiological evaluation of a newly constructed animal facility. Contemp Top Lab Anim Sci. 2005, 44:7–11.

OTHER SPECIAL TECHNIQUES

Administration of Substances

Oral

The method of administering a substance by mouth depends on whether one animal or many animals are being treated, and whether the animal is a pet or part of an experimental study. Rabbits and rodents may voluntarily accept oral medications if they are available in a palatable, liquid form, which may require mixing with flavored syrup, or the assistance of a compounding pharmacy. Force-feeding by syringe requires firm restraint, gentle insertion of a 1–3 mL syringe partway into the oral cavity, slow injection, and careful cleaning of the face area afterward for patient comfort. Use of a small syringe allows for placement within the oral cavity and is generally more succesful than using a 5 mL or larger syringe, even if refilling must be done more often.

In experimental studies, where accurate administration of a dose is critical, direct delivery of the substance into an animal's esophagus or stomach may be required. In rabbits a premeasured, lubricated, no. 8 to 10 French infant feeding tube or soft catheter can be passed through a speculum, such as an open-ended 3 mL syringe barrel, to prevent chewing. Placement of the tube can be verified by aspiration (if air comes back freely, the tube is likely in the lungs), injecting air into the tube while listening for gurgling over the stomach, and palpating the cervical area for the presence of both the trachea and the feeding tube.

Placement of a nasogastric or esophagostomy tube can also be done if repeated administrations are necessary, or with anorexic pet rabbits that require nutritional supplementation. Nasogastric tube placement requires topical anesthesia in the nostril and is not technically difficult to perform. The small tube diameter allows only liquids to pass, the tube may interfere with nasal breathing, and rabbits may dislodge the tube from their nose during grooming (Figure 3.50). Elizabethan collars can be placed but add to animal discomfort. Esophagostomy tube placement requires general anesthesia; however, postoperative animal comfort is greater, breathing is not compromised, and tubes are rarely pulled out. The larger diameter allows food with more substance to be given. Placement is performed similar to that for a cat.

Curved, ball-ended metal or plastic feeding needles are commercially available for oral dosing of rabbits and rodents (Figure 3.51). Rodents are restrained firmly in an upright position. The lubricated needle is gently passed over the midline of the tongue and used as leverage to extend the neck of the rodent until its nose is pointing toward the ceiling. Gravity and the swallowing reflex will facilitate passage into the esophagus—force should never be used as esophageal rupture may occur (Figure 3.52 and 3.53). If the needle does not pass easily, it should be removed and repositioned. Respiratory distress may occur if the needle inadvertently enters the trachea.

Administration of pills or capsules is challenging. Most guinea pigs will willingly take flavored vitamin C tablets, or the tablet can be pushed back behind the fleshy cheek invaginations, which stimulates a chewing response. Small tablets may be hidden in

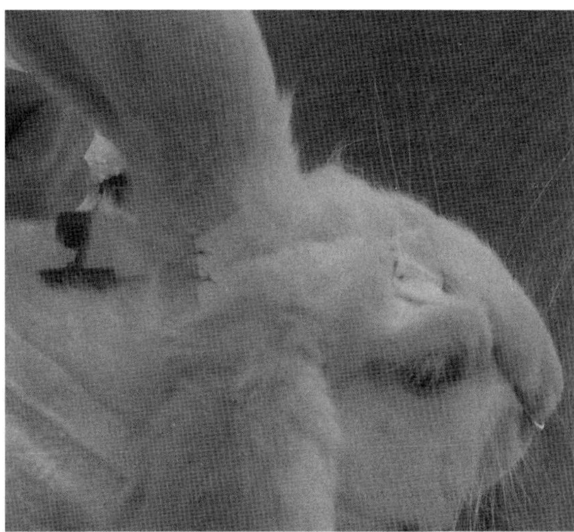

FIGURE 3.50. Nasogastric tube in a rabbit. For chronic administration of fluid or food, the tube has been secured in place and affixed to the skin of the head.

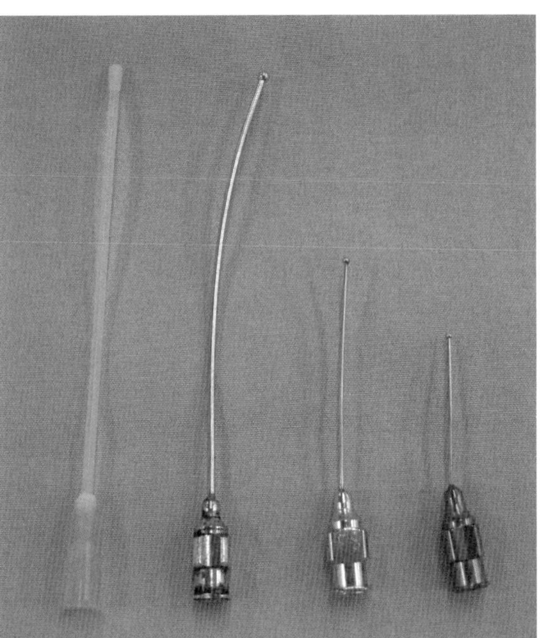

FIGURE 3.51. Plastic and metal ball-tipped gavage needles for rodents.

pieces of food, such as raisins, or crushed and mixed with Ensure® or some other palatable liquid.

Parenteral

Substances can be delivered subcutaneously, intraperitoneally, intravenously, intraosseously, and by nebulization. Intramuscular injections can be given to most rabbits; however, they occasionally result in muscle necrosis and self-mutilation in smaller rodents, so they must be given with care. The intraosseous route may be used for fluid or blood administration if intravenous cannulation is not possible.

Nasolacrimal Duct Flushing in Rabbits

Flushing of the nasolacrimal ducts is performed both as a therapeutic measure and to collect material for diagnostic tests, such as bacterial culture and sensitivity. In most rabbits it can be accomplished using topical anesthetic and restraint in a towel wrap (see Figure 2.9). After allowing sufficient time for the anesthetic to take effect, a 22- to 25-gauge intravenous catheter (without stylet), or the largest size possible, is introduced into the single punctum by pulling the lower lid laterally and directing the catheter medially, and sliding it several mm into the

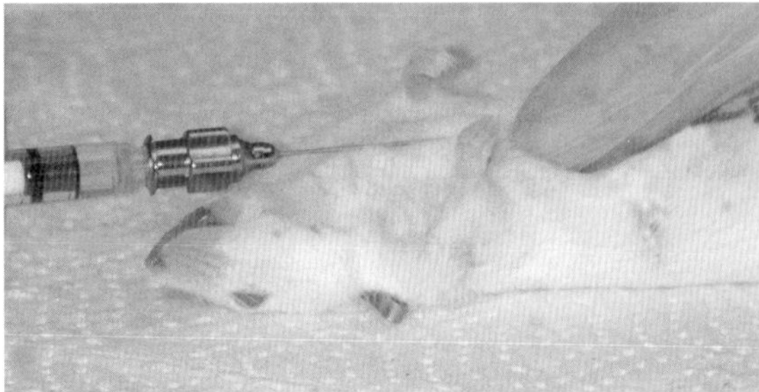

A

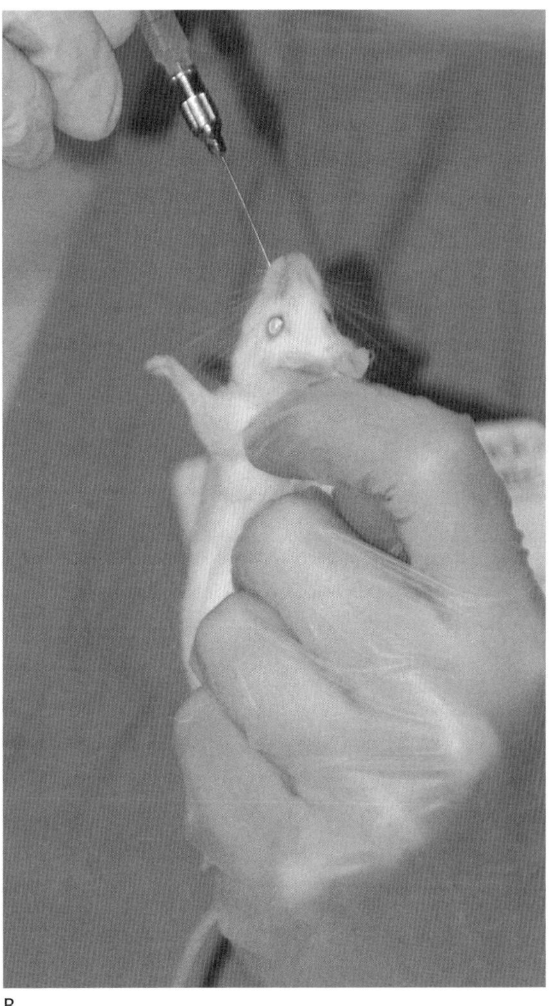

B

FIGURE 3.52. The length of gavage needle to be inserted should always be measured externally on the animal to minimize the likelihood of injury (A). For intragastric gavage, the end of the needle should extend to the xiphoid. The animal must be restrained firmly to minimize struggling and prevent injury (B).

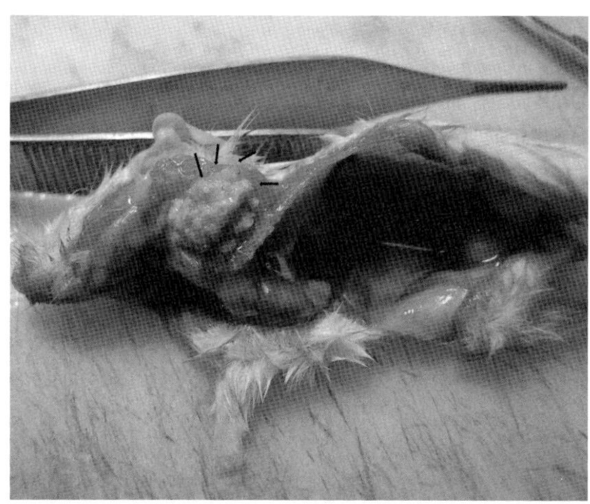

FIGURE 3.53. Esophageal rupture (arrows) may occur as depicted in this mouse if the animal is permitted to struggle during oral gavage, if too great a volume of material is gavaged, or if force is used to place the gavage needle. The gavage needle should pass readily into the stomach. Courtesy of David Hobson.

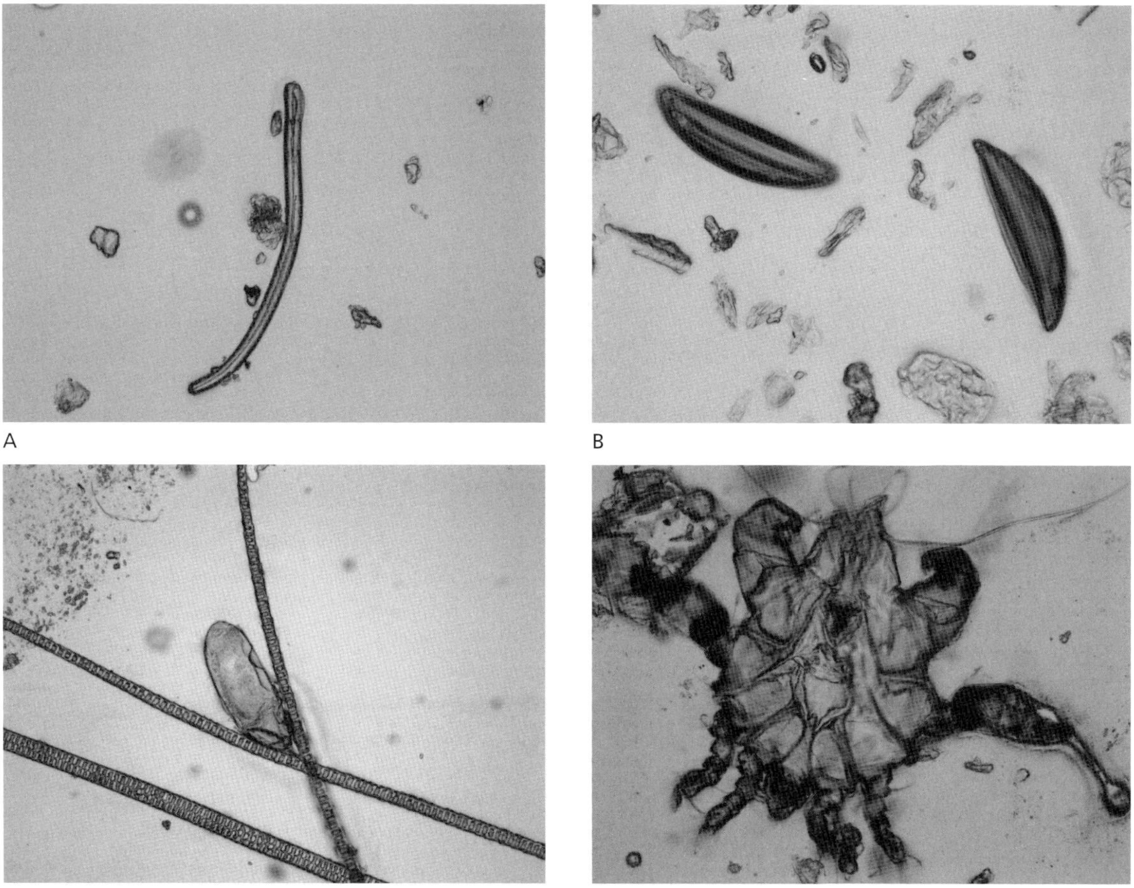

A

B

C

D

FIGURE 3.54. Photomicrograph demonstrating characteristic appearance of cellophane tape with attached (A) *Syphacia* spp larval form, (B) *Syphacia* spp ova, (C) fur mite egg, and (D) fur mite picked up by tape.

large slit-like opening at the fornix. If resistance to fluid instillation is met after the catheter has entered the duct, it has likely come up against the 90° turn the duct makes before continuing down the nose. The catheter should be withdrawn 1–2 mm to allow fluid to travel freely around this corner. Five to ten mL of warm sterile saline is flushed through the duct to dislodge caseous material, and a sterile Petri dish or other suitable container can be used to collect the material as it exits the nose. Acetylcysteine can be added to the saline to break down obstructive debris. A small amount of ophthalmic ointment containing an antibiotic, such as gentamicin, can be instilled after the saline flush. Care must be taken not to apply too much pressure to obstructed ducts, as rupture of the duct and subsequent abscess formation may occur (see Figure 3.16). If flushing cannot relieve the obstruction, twice daily warm compresses and massage over the rostrum for several days can be performed before attempting the flush again. Appropriate topical and systemic antibiotics and antiinflammatory agents should be used in conjunction with flushing.

Other Techniques

The "cellophane tape test" is frequently used to detect the presence of pinworm eggs in rodents. For this technique, a piece of clear tape is pressed gently against the anus. The tape is affixed to a slide and examined under a microscope for the presence of larvae or ova (Figure 3.54). Only pinworm eggs from *Syphacia* spp can be detected with this method. The same technique can be used to identify fur mites and their ova.

Many other techniques are used in practice and in research that are beyond the scope of this text. Milk collection, bile duct cannulation, bronchoalveolar lavage, and others are included in the references.

References

Bihun C, Bauck L. Basic Anatomy, Physiology, Husbandry and Clinical Techniques. In: Ferrets, Rabbits, and Rodents: Clinical Medicine and Surgery, 2nd ed. Quesenberry KE, Carpenter JW (eds.). St. Louis: Saunders, 2004; 286–298.

Mader DR. Basic Approach to Veterinary Care. In: Ferrets, Rabbits, and Rodents: Clinical Medicine and Surgery, 2nd ed. Quesenberry KE, Carpenter JW (eds.). St. Louis: Saunders, 2004; 147–154.

Wagner F, Fehr M. Common ophthalmic problems in pet rabbits. J Exot Pet Med. 2007, 16:158–167.

EUTHANASIA

Euthanasia (from the Greek words for "easy death") in veterinary medicine refers to humane killing of an animal. Euthanatize is the preferred verb form, but euthanize is also acceptable.

Implied in humane killing is a rapid transition from consciousness to unconsciousness and a death that is painless, quick, quiet, and free of fear and distress.

Euthanasia should be carried out by trained personnel using methods, substances, and facilities reviewed and approved under institutional policy and governmental regulations, and in accordance with regional social, ethical, or religious conventions.

In general, animals should not be killed while crowded or while directly in the presence of other animals not being killed. The method of euthanasia will vary with the age of the animal, the species, number, and the intended postmortem use of the animal or its tissues. Agents and procedures specifically contraindicated in the most current version of the American Veterinary Medical Association's euthanasia guidelines (www.avma.org) should not be used for euthanasia.

Additional and significant concerns with euthanasia include adverse stress on human participants (operator effects and esthetics), considerations regarding distress or appearance of distress, and effects of the method of euthanasia on postmortem evaluation and intended uses of the animal or its parts.

Those administering euthanasia agents to animals must be aware of potential signs of distress. For small mammal species, these may include distress vocalizations, struggling, attempts at escape, panting, salivation, and urination and defecation. Regardless of the technique used, it is critical to verify animal death following euthanasia. Methods of verifying death include cardiac auscultation for lack of heartbeat, exsanguinations, use of a physical method following a chemical or gaseous method of euthanasia, or thoracotomy via diaphragm transection.

The method of euthanasia selected must be compatible with animal welfare and the goals of the research study. Euthanasia agents may induce various biological and chemical changes, and knowledge of these changes is essential. Sodium pentobarbital may induce congestion of alveolar capillaries, congestive splenomegaly, damage to serosal cells of the liver and pancreas, increased plasma glucose and triglycerides, and increases in certain brain chemicals. Carbon dioxide euthanasia often results in multifocal pulmonary petechiation, perivascular edema of lungs, and occasionally, rupture of small intrathoracic capillaries with subsequent localized hemorrhage. Prolonged exposure to CO_2 (i.e., slow-fill chamber method) may also result in marked serum chemistry alterations and hemolysis of blood samples, which may be important for clinical pathology evaluations. Among physical methods, cervical dislocation leads to trauma and marked cervical hemorrhage, while decapitation often leads to reflex inhalation of blood into bronchioles and alveolar spaces.

Euthanasia of Rabbits

Sodium pentobarbital is an excellent agent for rabbit euthanasia if the drug is administered IV, generally by catheter or butterfly needle into a marginal ear vein. The solution is very irritating if administered perivascularly. The rabbit may be tranquilized beforehand with acepromazine SC at 2 mg/kg. A terminal gasp may occur in the unconscious rabbit, which may be unnerving if the owner is present. This is less likely to occur if the animal is sedated prior to barbiturate administration. Intraperitoneal injection can also be used, but longer times are involved than with IV administration, and there is some concern about peritoneal irritation by this route because of acidity of the barbiturate solution. Sodium pentobarbital is regulated in both Canada and the United States (Schedule II in the U.S.), and accurate controls and usage records must be maintained.

Inhalant anesthetics are cost-effective euthanasia agents for rabbits that weigh less than 7 kg. Inhalants must be vented from the site, and operator exposure must be prevented with the use of an appropriate scavenge system or filter. Animals that are not sedated or well restrained may struggle and breath hold during induction, which may be distressing for the observer. Potassium chloride may be administered IV or intracardially to animals that are deeply anesthetized to ensure loss of heart function. For inhalant euthanasia of rabbits, the 2007 AVMA guidelines recommend, in order of preference, halothane, enflurane, isoflurane, sevoflurane, methoxyflurane, and desflurane.

Carbon dioxide may be used for small rabbits but should only be used as compressed gas in cylinders. The chamber used should be as small as necessary to hold the rabbit. If the rabbit is placed in the chamber, the flow rate of CO_2 should displace at least 20% of chamber volume per minute. Because CO_2 is heavier than air, the chamber should open from the top. If the euthanizing chamber is incompletely filled with gas, animals may avoid the agent by climbing to the top. The time required to euthanatize immature animals with CO_2 is longer than for adults. The rabbit may struggle and undergo induction excitement as the chamber fills, which may be esthetically unpleasant for the observer. Carbon dioxide leaves no tissue residue and has limited effects on cellular architecture. Great care must be taken to ensure the CO_2-exposed animal is dead, especially a neonatal animal. Little information is available regarding aversion to CO_2 in rabbits; however, there is enough information available in other small mammal species with this agent to suggest that it may be noxious to rabbits as well. Care must be taken with large CO_2 chambers to ensure that there is good ventilation to minimize operator exposure to large volumes of CO_2 while bending over to remove the animal from the chamber.

Cervical dislocation or decapitation is considered a conditionally acceptable method only in rabbits that weigh less than 1 kg. The rabbit's head is held in one hand and the hind limbs in the other hand. The rabbit is stretched and the neck twisted dorsally to separate the first cervical vertebra from the skull. Electrical activity in the brain may continue for a few seconds. Cervical dislocation must be conducted by trained persons and for justifiable reasons, for example, if no chemicals can be used. Blood may be inhaled into the tracheal opening and create the impression in naive observers that the rabbit had a hemorrhagic disease.

Other methods that may be conditionally acceptable in rabbits but only used with great care involve carbon monoxide exposure or stunning by a single, sharp blow to the central skull bones. A nonpenetrating captive bolt system (Zephyr stun gun) is increasingly being used for stunning commercial rabbits at abattoirs in parts of the United States and Ontario.

Materials or methods that should not be used include chloral hydrate, nitrogen or argon gases, captive bolt, electrocution, or cervical dislocation or decapitation on rabbits that weigh more than 1 kg. Rabbits and rodents are sometimes exsanguinated to obtain hyperimmune antisera. Because of anxiety associated with hypovolemia, exsanguination should be done only on deeply sedated or anesthetized animals.

Euthanasia of Small Rodents

Inhalant agents recommended for euthanizing small rodents are halothane, enflurane, isoflurane, sevoflurane, methoxyflurane, and desflurane, in that order, given in air or oxygen and used in well-vented areas. Neonatal rodents are resistant to hypoxic death and other agents or methods may be preferred for this age group. Rodents being euthanatized in chambers should be of the same species, should not be crowded or layered, and should not be wetted with the anesthetic. The chamber should be cleaned before use to minimize odors that may signal distress, and the animals should be restrained if likely to hurt themselves or others during the process.

Carbon dioxide used in a slow-filled, nonprecharged chamber is an effective and inexpensive euthanasia agent for small rodents. The animal should be placed in as small a chamber as necessary to hold it. The flow of CO_2 should be gradually increased to minimize distress. For example, an appropriate flow rate is approximately 20% of the chamber volume per minute, or 6 psi. The animals should be left in the chamber for 4–5 minutes until respiration has ceased. Following this, the animal should be removed and the absence of respiration confirmed, prior to disposal. Use of a second method to confirm death increases operator confidence that the animal has been euthanatized. Rats die approximately six times as rapidly in a prefilled chamber than in a fixed–flow rate chamber but may undergo more rapid excitement during induction. There is continued controversy regarding whether CO_2 inhalation is aversive to small rodents and whether this is a humane killing method for rodents, and this is an area of active and ongoing research. The acceptability of CO_2 as a euthanasia agent of small rodents must be evaluated as new data becomes available.

Neonatal rodents are resistant to the hypoxia-inducing effects of CO_2 and alternative methods are recommended (e.g., injection with chemical agents, cervical dislocation, or decapitation). If dead rodents or rabbits are to be used to feed other animals (snakes, carnivores, and raptors), euthanasia with CO_2 is recommended to increase palatability and to avoid secondary poisoning with a euthanasia agent.

For small rodents, IV injections may be difficult; thus, the intraperitoneal approach is used commonly for chemical agents. Concentrated barbiturate solutions specifically intended for euthanasia are available, but there is concern that these agents may be irritating when given by the IP route. The recommended dosage for euthanasia with sodium pentobarbital is 150–200 mg/kg. Care must be taken to ensure that the heart has stopped prior to disposal. Sodium pentobarbital administered IV or IP is an excellent euthanasia agent; however, rodents should be placed in small cages to reduce excitement and injury during anesthetic induction prior to death. Barbiturates are controlled substances and are not available to all animal care personnel.

Cervical dislocation or decapitation may be used with convincing justification and by trained personnel. To euthanatize small rodents by cervical dislocation, the animal is grasped on the neck at the base of the skull or a rod is placed over the neck at the skull base and the tail is pulled. Dislocation usually occurs in the posterior cervical or thoracic spine.

Microwave irradiation is used by neurobiologists to fix brain chemicals as they occur in vivo. No other method of euthanasia does this as well. Specially designed instruments that focus high-power microwaves directly on the head are required. Only small rodents can be euthanized this way, and the instruments are expensive. Kitchen microwave ovens are not suitable.

Rapid freezing by immersion in liquid nitrogen is not acceptable for killing animals unless they are first deeply anesthetized. Another acceptable euthanasia method is carbon monoxide exposure, but this must occur in a well-ventilated area to ensure operator safety.

Methods not recommended for use in rodents in the United States include nitrogen or argon gas inhalation, cervical dislocation, and decapitation of animals that are larger than rats.

References

AVMA Guidelines on Euthanasia. 2007. http://www.avma.org/issues/animal_welfare/euthanasia.pdf, accessed February 10, 2009.

Artwohl J, et al. Report of the ACLAM task force on rodent euthanasia. L Amer Assoc Lab Anim Sci. 2006, 45(1):98–105.

Bhathena SJ. Comparison of effects of decapitations and anesthesia on metabolic and hormonal parameters in Sprague-Dawley rats. Life Sci. 1992, 50:1649–1655.

Blackshaw JN, et al. The behaviour of chickens, mice and rats during euthanasia with chloroform, carbon dioxide and ether. Lab Anim. 1988, 22:67–75.

Bosland MC. Is decapitation a humane method of euthanasia in rodents? A critical review. Contemp Top Lab Anim Sci. 1995, 34(2):46–48.

Clarification Concerning the Use of Carbon Dioxide. http://grants.nih.gov/grants/guide/notice-files/NOT-OD-02-062.htmL, accessed February 10, 2009.

Close B, et al. Recommendations for euthanasia of experimental animals: Part 1. Lab Anim. 1996, 30:293–316.

Den RF. Pain perception in decapitated rat brain. Life Sci. 1991, 49:1399–1402.

Fawell JK, Thomson C, Cooke L. Respiratory artifact produced by carbon dioxide and pentobarbitone sodium euthanasia in rats. Lab Anim. 1972, 6:321–326.

Feldman DB, Gupta BN. Histopathologic changes in laboratory animals resulting from various methods of euthanasia. Lab Anim Sci. 1976, 26:218–221.

Hackbarth H, Kuppers N, Bohnet W. Euthanasia of rats with carbon dioxide—animal welfare aspects. Lab Anim. 2000, 34:91–96.

Hewett TA, et al. A comparison of euthanasia methods in rats, using carbon dioxide in prefilled and fixed flow rate filled chambers. Lab Anim Sci. 1993, 43:579–582.

Holson RR. Euthanasia by decapitation: evidence that this technique produces prompt, painless unconsciousness in laboratory rodents. Neurotoxicol Teratol. 1992, 14:253–257.

Mikesk JA, Klemm WR. EEG evaluation of humaneness of asphyxia and decapitation euthanasia of the laboratory rat. Lab Anim Sci. 1975, 25:175–179.

OMAFRA. Zephyr Rabbit Stun Gun. 2005. http://www.omafra.gov.on.ca/english/food/inspection/animalhealthandwelfare/Zephyr_Stungun.htm. Accessed February 19, 2009.

Pecaut MJ, Smith AL, Jones TC, et al. Modification of immunologic and hematologic variables by method of CO2 euthanasia. Comp Med. 2000, 50(6):595–602.

Prien T, et al. Haemolysis and artifactual lung damage induced by a euthanasia agent. Lab Anim. 1988, 22:170–172.

Chapter 4

Clinical Signs and Differential Diagnoses

The clinical signs commonly encountered in rabbits and rodents are associated with a variety of conditions involving all major systems, including the integumentary, gastrointestinal, cardiopulmonary, genitourinary, nervous, musculoskeletal, and endocrine systems. The content of this chapter, arranged by species, provides differential diagnoses for various commonly observed clinical signs. These diagnostic alternatives are based on published literature as well as the authors' experiences and are not meant to be exhaustive but rather to cover the most common diseases seen. Additional information, where needed, may be extrapolated from other species or gleaned from the references. Detailed information concerning specific diagnoses may be found through the index, in the species-categorized references in chapter 5, or in the general reference works listed in chapters 1 and 2. Diagnosis based on clinical signs alone can be presumptuous, and confirmation by taking a thorough history, conducting a clinical examination, and adjusting the assessment based on the results of further diagnostic testing may be necessary. A summary of zoonotic conditions affecting rabbits and rodents may be found in Table 4.25 at the end of this chapter. Good hygiene practices including routine hand washing or sanitation after handling any animal should always be promoted in the clinic, institution, home, and commercial settings to minimize the risk of disease transmission between animals and their human caregivers.

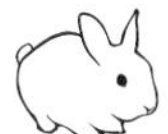

THE RABBIT

Skin Conditions

As for many small mammal species, rabbits are prized for their soft fur and beautiful coat. Skin problems are readily observed by owners, and although they rarely cause serious disease or death, they are one of the most common presenting signs in clinical practice. A list of infectious and noninfectious differential diagnoses may be found in Table 4.1.

Alopecia

Hair loss or thinning in rabbits may be caused by hormonally induced hair pulling for nests in pregnant or pseudopregnant does, hair chewing related to boredom or stereotypy, overgrooming of self or another (barbering), dietary insufficiency (e.g., fiber deficiency), or ectoparasitism, most commonly *Cheyletiella parasitovorax* infection (back or face). Hair may be inadvertently pulled out more readily with maloccluded or broken incisors, reinforcing the concept that the teeth should always be examined. Demodectic and sarcoptic mites are typically associated with pruritus and dermatitis. Less common conditions are mechanical hair loss from rubbing on the cage or feeder, dermatophyte infection, and hair pulling by other house pets or humans. Seasonal molting may also produce hair coat irregularities and thinning, although molting is rarely a cause of alopecia. Hereditary causes of hairlessness, including genetically furless strains, exist. Alopecia may develop after several weeks of antiviral or anticancer therapy in rabbits and has been reported following treatment with ribavirin and doxycycline.

Swellings and Masses

Single or multiple subcutaneous masses in rabbits are commonly due to abscesses caused by *Pasteurella multocida* or *Staphylococcus aureus* infection, although other bacteria such as *Yersinia pestis* (cutaneous plague, in areas where the bacteria are endemic), *Fusobacterium necrophorum* (Schmorl's disease),

Table 4.1. Common presenting skin conditions and differential diagnoses in rabbits.

Condition	Differential Diagnoses
Alopecia	Noninfectious
	Pregnancy/pseudopregnancy
	Fighting/trauma
	Mechanical, e.g., cage bars, hopper
	Exfoliative dermatosis (Dutch)
	Seasonal molting
	Behavioral stereotypy (barbering)
	Hereditary hairlessness
	Drug therapy, e.g., antivirals, anticancer therapies
	Dietary deficiency, e.g., low fiber
	Infectious
	Ectoparasites, e.g., *Cheyletiella* spp
	Dermatophytosis, e.g., *Trichophyton* spp
Swellings/Masses	Noninfectious
	Trauma/hemorrhage
	Cyst
	Neoplasia (fibroma, lymphoma, papilloma)
	Myiasis, e.g., *Cuterebra* spp
	Mammary gland dysplasia (secondary to pituitary adenoma)
	Infectious
	Abscesses, e.g., *Pasteurella* spp,
	Staphylococcus spp, *Fusobacterium* spp (Schmorl's disease or necrobacillosis)
	Myxomatosis
	Plague (cutaneous bubos, following *Yersinia pestis* infection; rare)
	Mastitis
Dermatitis	Noninfectious
	Sebaceous adenitis
	Exfoliative dermatitis, e.g., thymoma
	Chemical/electrical burn
	Toxicoses
	Pododermatitis
	Urine scalding
	Ehlers-Danlos syndrome
	Dietary deficiency, e.g., zinc
	Fly or tick bites
	Myiasis
	Infectious
	Viral, e.g., myxomatosis
	Bacterial, e.g., *Streptococcus* spp, *Staphylococcus* spp, *Pseudomonas* spp (wet dewlap disease/moist dermatitis), *Treponema cuniculi* (rabbit syphilis)
	Yeast infections, e.g., *Malassezia* dermatitis
	Dermatophytosis, e.g., *Trichophyton* spp, *Microsporum* spp
	Parasitic, e.g., fleas, *Psoroptes cuniculi* (ear mites), pediculosis, scabies, *Notoedres* spp, *Cheyletiella* spp, *Demodex cuniculi*

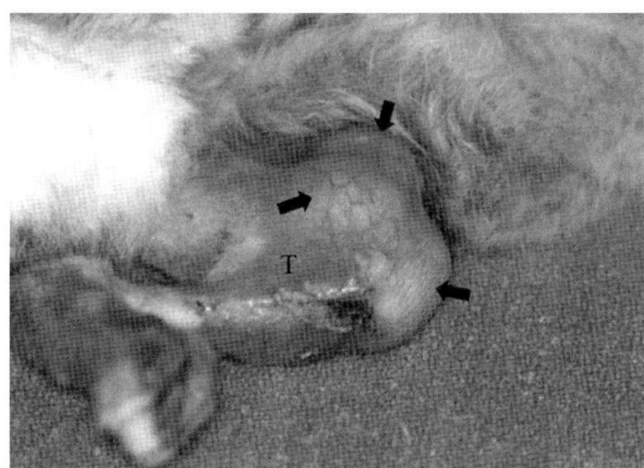

FIGURE 4.1. Subcutaneous swellings (arrows) around the site of fracture repair of the tibia (T) in a rabbit caused by *Pasteurella multocida*–induced abscessation.

and *Pseudomonas aeruginosa* (wet dewlap disease) may be sporadically involved (Figure 4.1). Mammary gland dysplasia has been reported secondary to pituitary adenoma in the rabbit. Neoplasia (fibromas, osteosarcomas, myxomas, epitheliotropic lymphoma, papillomas), hematomas, cysts, nonspecific granulomas, myiasis from subcutaneous *Cuterebra* spp larval encystment, diseased mammary glands (e.g., mastitis), and *Coenurus serialis* (*Taenia* spp) cysts are other causes of cutaneous swellings and masses.

Dermatitis

Inflammation of the skin, variably indicated by erythema, alopecia, scaliness, crusting, seborrhea, or ulceration, can be caused by any of several noninfectious causes and infectious agents. Chemical or electrical burns and toxicoses should always be considered in rabbits that roam freely in the house, highlighting the importance of close supervision of rabbits during exercise, and this is an important question to ask when taking the history. Similarly, a thorough history may rule out the possibility of dietary deficiencies. The ear mite, *Psoroptes cuniculi*, causes crust formation and reddening of the ear canal, the inner aspect of the pinna, and in rare circumstances the moist areas of the dewlap or perineum. The mite itself is seen readily under a microscope or by using a hand lens. The fur mite, *Cheyletiella parasitovorax* (walking dandruff), may cause scaly dandruff accumulations deep in the hair coat and occasionally causes hair loss and an oily dermatitis on the face or back. This differs for sarcoptid mites, which are found rarely on the face, ears, and limbs. *Demodex cuniculi* infection has been reported less commonly in rabbits as well as *Malassezia*-induced dermatitis. Another common dermatopathy is decubital ulcer formation with pododermatitis (sore hocks). Some rabbits develop a dry necrosis on the plantar surface of one or both hind feet following housing on wire or housing in excessively wet or soiled conditions. This problem may be exacerbated by self-mutilation with secondary bacterial contamination.

Less common causes of dermatopathies include bites by flies; fleas, typically dog or cat fleas such as *Ctenocephalides felis* or *C. canis*; lice such as *Hemodipsus ventricosus*, which may induce anemia; and tick bites (*Hemaphysis leporipalustrus*) in rabbits housed outdoors. Sebaceous adenitis, urine scalding (especially in obese rabbits), an immune-mediated exfoliative dermatosis of Dutch rabbits, thymoma-induced scaling, and Ehlers-Danlos syndrome have also been reported in rabbits.

Bacterial dermatopathies can be caused by a number of organisms. Infection with *Pseudomonas aeruginosa* (wet dewlap disease) may be seen in rabbits that play with their water bottles or that are housed in damp unhygienic environments. The condition is characterized by a greenish-blue discoloration of the fur and a distinctive odor. Purulent discharge from rhinitis and conjunctivitis due to *Pasteurella multocida* often causes dermatitis of the surrounding skin. Other bacteria infecting the skin include *Staphylococcus aureus*, *Fusobacterium necrophorum* (typically infecting wounds), *Actinomyces pyogenes*, and *Treponema cuniculi* infections of the genitalia and nose. Any moist, ulcerative dermatitis condition can be secondarily infested with maggots (myiasis), particularly in rabbits housed outside. Other causes of dermatopathies in rabbits include dermatophytosis, predominantly from *Trichophyton mentagrophytes* infection. A significant proportion of rabbits may carry this agent subclinically.

Gastrointestinal Conditions

Anorexia

Anorectic rabbits, defined as those animals that have consumed 25% or less of their normal daily ration

Table 4.2. Common presenting gastrointestinal conditions and differential diagnoses in rabbits.

Condition	Differential Diagnoses
Anorexia	Noninfectious Dental disease (malocclusion, ptyalism) Gastric stasis Sudden dietary change Insufficient water supply Change in husbandry practices (environmental stress) Moldy feed Oral foreign body Gastric/intestinal obstruction Intestinal accident Gastric ulcers Oral papillomatosis Pain Neoplasia Postanesthetic anorexia Loss of olfactory sense (secondary to rhinitis) Secondary to hepatic lipidosis Infectious Secondary to disease—see below
Diarrhea	Noninfectious Dietary indiscretion (carbohydrate overload) Mucoid enteropathy Food allergy Low-fiber diet Inappropriate use of antibiotics (*C. difficile* overgrowth) Hepatic lipidosis (pregnancy toxemia) Aflatoxicosis Infectious Viral enteritis, e.g., rotavirus, coronavirus (higher morbidity and mortality) Bacterial enterocolitis, e.g., *Clostridium spiroforme* (typhlocolitis), *Clostridium piliforme* (Tyzzer's disease), *Lawsonia* spp (proliferative enteritis), *E. coli* (both EPEC and EHEC serotypes), *Salmonella* spp Protozoal infection, e.g., coccidiosis (*Eimeria* spp), cryptosporidiosis Hepatitis, e.g., coccidiosis (*Eimeria stiedae*), listeriosis (does), tularemia, staphylococcosis Parasitic infection (rarely induces diarrhea), e.g., pinworms (*Passalurus ambiguus*; perianal itching), heavy tapeworm larval infestation (abdominal distension)
Constipation	Noninfectious Obesity Inappropriate diet (low fiber) Lack of exercise Dysautonomia/cecal impaction Anorectal papilloma (nonviral)
Pendulous Abdomen	Noninfectious Pregnancy Obesity Uterine adenocarcinoma Hydrometra Cardiac disease with ascites GI disorders Infectious Hepatic coccidiosis Pyometra Metritis

for 3 or more consecutive days or with complete cessation of food ingestion for 1 or more days, commonly present to practitioners and should be considered a medical emergency and treated aggressively. Rabbits that remain off feed for prolonged periods of a week or more may develop an irreversible fatal fasting condition with a very poor prognosis. Rabbits that are off feed will generally not drink, and fluid assessment and replenishment are appropriate in most cases while trying to determine the underlying cause of anorexia. The most common etiologies of this condition relate to dental disease (often accompanied by ptyalism with a resultant moist chin or dewlap), gastric stasis usually caused by inappropriate low-fiber diets, sudden dietary or management changes, pain from any cause (often accompanied by bruxism), and systemic disease of any nature. Other potential causes of anorexia in rabbits include recovery from anesthesia, environmental stress such as increased ambient temperature, insufficient water supply, dehydration from any cause, unpalatable or moldy feed, changed feeding or watering devices, gastric ulceration, gastrointestinal accident such as intussusception or obstruction, loss of olfactory senses secondary to rhinitis, neoplasia, and acidotic or ketotic conditions secondary to hepatic lipidosis.

Although large trichobezoars may be found in the stomachs of anorectic rabbits, current thinking is that this hair accumulates secondary to gastric or enteric stasis and that large hair masses rarely are responsible for primary gastric obstructions.

Diarrhea

A specific cause of diarrhea in a rabbit is often difficult to determine. Weanling animals are particularly susceptible, because the simultaneous change in diet (from high fat and protein in milk to a more fiber-based diet) and concomitant digestive system maturation, stresses of transport, social group changes, and waning of maternal antibodies converge to enhance susceptibility to opportunistic pathogens. Fluid assessment and replacement and an assessment of overall hygiene practices are appropriate in all circumstances. In most instances, the definitive diagnosis is multifactorial and complex, involving two or more introduced or resident microorganisms, changes in the intestinal milieu, alterations in management practices, and elaboration of bacterial enterotoxins. Specific examples of such relationships include colibacillosis and coccidial co-infection, clostridial enterotoxemia preceded by Tyzzer's disease (*Clostridium piliforme* infection) or *Lawsonia intracellularis* infection, or rotavirus infection and clostridial enterotoxin elaboration following carbohydrate overload and bacterial overgrowth.

Noninfectious causes of diarrhea include dietary indiscretion (carbohydrate overload or low-fiber diets), aflatoxins in the feed, food allergy, antibiotic-induced dysbiosis with overgrowth of *C. difficile* and enterotoxin production, mucoid enteropathy, and hepatic lipidosis secondary to pregnancy toxemia or obesity.

Specific infectious causes of diarrhea to consider include rotaviral and coronaviral infections in kits and weanlings, coliform infections in rabbits of all ages, *Clostridium spiroforme* typhlocolitis, *Lawsonia intracellularis* ileitis, and *Clostridium piliforme* typhlitis. Protozoal overgrowth by coccidia is very common, while *Cryptosporidium parvum* infections are less common. Endoparasite infestation rarely results in diarrhea. Pinworm infestation (*Passalurus ambiguus*) is common in pet rabbits yet is usually subclinical or presents with mild perianal irritation.

Hepatitis may also present clinically as diarrhea or as abdominal distension and runting in young animals. Common causes of hepatitis include hepatic coccidiosis and hepatitis secondary to systemic bacterial infection, for example, *Staphylococcus* spp, *Listeria moncytogenes*, and *Francisella tularensis*.

Constipation

Obesity, inappropriate diets with high carbohydrate and low fiber content, and lack of exercise are the most common causes of constipation in rabbits. Cases of dysautononia with cecal impaction and degeneration of autonomic neurons are rare and untreatable. Anorectal papillomas are not related to virally induced oral papillomas, which are seen in up to 30% of pet rabbits, but because they are friable masses, they may induce mild rectal bleeding if they become ulcerated, leading to obstipation, and associated constipation. Signs resolve readily with surgical removal of the masses.

Pendulous Abdomen

Intestinal disorders with gas and fluid accumulation, hepatic coccidiosis, metritis, pyometra, uterine adenocarcinomas, hydrometra, pregnancy, cardiac disease with ascites accumulation, and obesity all may cause an enlarged abdomen in rabbits.

Cardiopulmonary Conditions

Nasal Discharge

Serous or mucopurulent rhinitis with sneezing is classically associated with *Pasteurella multocida* infection (snuffles) (Table 4.3). Discharge may also be seen on the forelegs, as animals attempt to groom themselves. *Staphylococcus aureus*, *Bordetella bronchiseptica*, and *Neisseria* spp may also be upper respiratory pathogens in rabbits. Dental disease may result in nasal discharge, especially with overgrowth of molar tooth roots. A nasal discharge may accompany heat stress, allergies to hay or feed dust, nasal foreign bodies, neoplasia fungal abscesses, myxomatosis, and rabbit pox. Myxomatosis is a deadly but rare viral condition of rabbits in most

Table 4.3. Common presenting cardiopulmonary conditions and differential diagnoses in rabbits.

Condition	Differential Diagnoses
Nasal Discharge/ Rhinitis/Sneezing	Noninfectious
	Dental disease (molar roots)
	Allergy (dust, hay)
	Increased temperature
	Nasal foreign body
	Neoplasia
	Infectious
	Pasteurella multocida
	Other bacterial infections, e.g., *Staphylococcus aureus, Bordetella bronchiseptica, Neisseria* spp
	Fungal infection, e.g., *Aspergillus* spp
	Rabbit pox
	Myxomatosis
Dyspnea	Noninfectious
	Primary cardiac disease (pulmonary edema, pleural effusion)
	Anesthetic-induced myocardial necrosis
	Stress
	Toxic, e.g., avocado leaf ingestion
	Foreign body
	Aspiration
	Chylothorax
	Tracheal stenosis
	Neoplasia, e.g., lymphoma, thymoma, pulmonary metastases of uterine adenocarcinoma
	Infectious
	Bacterial pneumonia, e.g., *Pasteurella multocida, Staphylococcus aureus, Klebsiella pneumomiae, Bordetella bronchiseptica*
	Viral infection, e.g., rabbit hemorrhagic disease (calicivirus), rabbit herpesvirus infection

areas of the world except California, Australia, and parts of Europe and Brazil, where it has become enzootic with less serious manifestations in certain wild rabbit species. Affected animals may initially present with serous or mucous nasal discharge but rapidly develop other signs such as subcutaneous edema and swellings, fever, and depression, suggestive of severe systemic illness.

Dyspnea

Labored breathing is often associated with chronic pneumonia caused by *Pasteurella multocida*. Other bacterial infections, caused by agents such as *S. aureus*, *B. bronchiseptica*, and *Klebsiella pneumonia*, may contribute to the disease pathogenesis. Dyspnea may also occur with various viral infections, such as calicivirus (rabbit hemorrhagic disease) or rabbit herpesvirus infection. Tracheal foreign body, aspiration, and toxicity secondary to avocado leaf ingestion with resultant pulmonary edema have also been reported. Tracheal stenosis may occur in rabbits following endotracheal intubation, leading to stertorous respiration. In addition, administration of alpha-2 agonists for anesthesia has resulted in myocardial necrosis, pulmonary edema with resultant dyspnea, and death, likely due to profound hypoxemia. These injectable anesthetic agents can be used safely in rabbits if supplemental oxygen is provided. Dyspnea with sudden death may occur in stressed rabbits and is thought to be due to coronary artery vasoconstriction following sudden catecholamine release. As pet rabbits receive better care and live to older ages, primary heart disease is an increasingly common diagnosis. Dyspnea may result from pulmonary edema or pleural effusions secondary to heart failure, most commonly due to dilated cardiomyopathy. Neoplasia that results in chylothorax (e.g., thymoma) and mediastinal masses interfering with respiration (e.g., lymphosarcoma) or that reduce pulmonary capacity (e.g., metastatic uterine adenocarcinoma) may also result in dyspnea. Pneumonia and cardiac disease in rabbits usually result in sudden death, but careful ante mortem examination may reveal cyanosis (blue discoloration) of the iris, mucosa, and ears (especially in albino animals), weight loss, depression, and respiratory difficulties.

Endocrine Conditions

Endocrine disease is extremely uncommon in rabbits. Pseudopregnancy may occur following a sterile or unsuccessful mating; however, this is a normal condition that resolves spontaneously between 2 and 3 weeks postbreeding. Diabetes mellitus has been reported in New Zealand white rabbits, as has mammary dysplasia secondary to a prolactin-secreting pituitary adenoma.

Yellow Fat

The occasional presence of distinctive yellow fat in rabbits is caused by a homozygous recessive condition that results in a failure to metabolize xanthophylls. The accumulation of xanthophylls has no deleterious effect on rabbits.

Nervous and Musculoskeletal Conditions

Signs of neuromuscular disease are commonly seen in pet rabbits (Table 4.4). A complete neurologic exam is recommended to localize the lesion; however, signs may be difficult to interpret as not every animal may respond as expected because of stress or species-specific variation (e.g., rabbits lack a menace reflex). Note that the rabbit has no cauda equina and the spinal cord extends the length of the vertebral canal.

Head Tilt/Torticollis

Head tilt or wry neck (Figure 4.2) is due in many cases to an otitis media/interna caused by bacteria (usually *Pasteurella multocida*) extending from the pharynx via the eustachian tubes. At times, no specific inner ear lesions are detected radiographically and other potential causes may include trauma, toxin ingestion (e.g., lead paint ingestion), cerebral larval migrans following exposure to embryonated *Baylisascaris* spp eggs, toxoplasmosis, encephalitozoonosis, or neoplasia. Extension of an ear mite infection from the external ear to the inner ear is rare, and in any case such an invasion would be complicated by bacterial infection.

Seizure and Depression

Encephalopathies with resultant seizures or depression may result from bacterial infections or abscesses

Table 4.4. Common presenting nervous and musculoskeletal conditions and differential diagnoses in rabbits.

Condition	Differential Diagnoses
Head Tilt/Torticollis	Noninfectious
	Trauma
	Cerebral larval migrans, e.g., *Baylisascaris* spp
	Cerebrovascular accident
	Peripheral vestibular disease
	Toxins, e.g., lead (paint)
	Neoplasia, e.g., pituitary adenoma
	Infectious
	Otitis media/interna secondary to bacterial infection, e.g., *Pasteurella multocida, Staphylococcus aureus*
	Brain abscess
	Severe otitis externa, e.g., *Psoroptes cuniculi*
	Toxoplasmosis
	Encephalitozoonosis
Seizures	Noninfectious
	Pregnancy toxemia
	Cerebral larval migrans
	Heat stroke
	Toxins, e.g., lead (paint)
	Hypoxia
	Hypovitaminosis A
	Severe systemic disease, e.g., rabbit hemorrhagic disease, terminal sepsis
	Idiopathic epilepsy
	Neoplasia
	Infectious
	Bacterial encephalitis/meningitis/abscess, e.g., *Pasteurella multocida, Listeria monocytogenes, Staphylococcus aureus, Streptococcus* spp
	Encephalitozoonosis
	Viral infection, e.g., herpesvirus encephalitis, rabies virus
Paresis/Paralysis	Noninfectious
	Trauma (leg/muscle)
	Vertebral fracture
	Scoliosis
	Splayleg (congenital or acquired)
	Spondylosis/spondylitis
	Osteoarthritis
	Spinal neoplasia
	Severe anemia, e.g., secondary to blood loss
	Severe inanition
	Intervertebral disk disease
	Hypovitaminosis E/selenium deficiency
	Hypovitaminosis A
	Toxicity, e.g., lead, insecticide
	Cerebrovascular accident
	Infectious
	Spinal abscess
	Encephalitozoonosis
	Toxoplasmosis
	Rabies virus
	Bacterial encephalitis

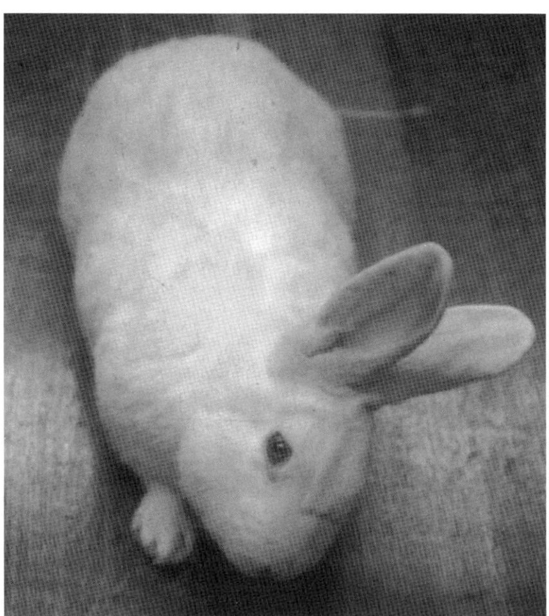

FIGURE 4.2. Torticollis is a common presenting sign in rabbits and may be caused by several etiologies.

(e.g., *P. multocida*, *L. monocytogenes*, *S. aureus*), herpesvirus infections (rabbit-specific herpesviruses as well as human herpes simplex viruses), encephalitozoonosis, and cerebral migration by *Baylisascaris* spp larvae. Severe systemic disease of any form may result in depression or seizures, for example, terminal septicemia and pregnancy toxemia. Other less common causes of seizures include various toxins, hypoxia, heat stroke, neoplasia, idiopathic epilepsy of blue-eyed white rabbits, and vitamin A deficiency. Rabies virus infections of rabbits have been reported in animals with access to the outdoors, generally following raccoon attacks, but are very uncommon.

Incoordination, Paresis, and Paralysis

Incoordination, weakness, and paralysis are commonly caused by vertebral or limb injury. If rabbits are dropped, allowed to thrash about during restraint, or become excited in a cage, they may fracture the lower spine and damage the spinal cord, because of their high muscle to bone ratio. The degree and duration of the resulting paresis or paralysis and loss of bladder and sphincter control depend on the severity and location of the cord lesion. Hindlimb paralysis with loss of deep pain sensation always carries a poor prognosis. Other causes of incoordination and paresis include muscular dystrophy secondary to nutritional deficiencies (vitamin A, E, or selenium), cerebrospinal nematodiasis, cerebrovascular accident, encephalitozoonosis, otitis interna, bacterial encephalitis, insecticide poisoning, pregnancy toxemia, anemia secondary to blood loss, severe inanition, heat exhaustion, spinal abscess or neoplasia, spondylosis or spondylitis, and osteoarthritis. Rare conditions include rabies virus infection, magnesium deficiency, congenital splayleg, and several other rare inherited musculoskeletal conditions. Splayleg, or the inability to adduct one or more limbs secondary to developmental deformities of the joints and muscles, has also been attributed to the presence of a smooth flooring surface during postnatal development.

Ocular Conditions

Conjunctivitis and Dacryocystitis

Conjunctivitis and dacryocystitis with or without corneal damage caused by *P. multocida* infection occur commonly and may be associated with a mucopurulent discharge. Dacryocystitis may also arise secondary to blockage of the lacrimal duct by dental abscesses or maxillary tooth root elongation. Other bacteria, *Chlamydophila* spp, dust or other foreign matter in the eye, trauma, dystrichiasis, trichiasis (especially in French Rex), and rabbit pox also may cause an ocular discharge and irritation of the conjunctiva. Corneal ulceration secondary to trauma is a common sequela of bacterial conjunctivitis. Exudate and infection from the conjunctiva may spread over the face and under the chin. If *Pseudomonas* spp infection is involved, fur adjacent to the lesion may be stained blue-green.

Blepharitis

Dry, crusty scabs adhering to the orbital skin and mucous membranes may be caused by *Treponema cuniculi*, the agent of rabbit venereal spirochetosis. Accompanying lesions may occur on the genitalia and nose. *P. multocida and S. aureus* infection also may induce blepharoconjunctivitis. Myxomatosis is confined geographically to the West Coast of the United States, Europe, Australia, and some other areas. The disease may involve generalized or nodular swelling of the eyelids, along with a thick mucous discharge. Other eyelid conditions seen occasionally include ectropion and entropion, and trauma associated with fighting.

Exopthalmos

Bulging of a rabbit's eye unilaterally or bilaterally may occur with retrobulbar abscess, as a self-limiting sequela to indwelling external jugular catheters or cervical restraint, or with buphthalmos, which is described further in chapter 5. Other reported causes of unilateral exophthalmos include the presence of *Taenia serialis* coenurus, orbital neoplasia, cellulitis, retrobulbar fat prolapse, and salivary mucocele. Bilateral periodic exophthalmos has been associated with mediastinal masses such as thymoma or lymphoma. Primary ocular neoplasms are rare in rabbits.

Other Conditions

Cyclopia, lens or optic disc coloboma, corneal dystrophy, heritable cataracts, cataracts and uveitis following *Encephalitozoon* spp infection in dwarf breeds (phacoclastic uveitis), conjunctival overgrowth (pseudopterygium), persistent hyperplastic primary vitreous, corneal dermoids, lipid keratopathy, and deep glandular hyperplasia of the nictitating membrane (cherry eye) are ophthalmic problems seen less commonly. Entropion and ectropion have been reported and can be surgically corrected.

Genitourinary Conditions

Increased water intake and urination by rabbits accompany lactation, heat stress, febrile disease, dry feed, salty diets, renal disease, and enteritis (Table 4.5). Potable water must be provided to rabbits at all times. Absorption of calcium by rabbits is not as well controlled by vitamin D, parathyroid hormone, and estrogen as for other species. Serum calcium levels in rabbits are directly proportional to calcium levels in the diet and may fluctuate widely. The result is that 50% or more of ingested dietary calcium is excreted in the urine and the end-product may be somewhat thick, cream-colored, or contain mineral debris and porphyrin (reddish) pigments.

Hematuria

Normal rabbit urine can be pale yellow to red-orange to brown, may vary from clear to opaque, and can resemble pus or blood. Many cases of "bloody" urine turn out to be normal porphyrin-pigmented urine. In addition, blood in the urine must be distinguished from blood originating from the reproductive tract. If the urine contains blood, then bacterial cystitis, bladder polyps, pyelonephritis, renal infarcts, urolithiasis, disseminated intravascular coagulation (DIC), and leptospirosis should be considered. Hemorrhage or bloody discharge from the reproductive tract may occur with ruptured endometrial aneurysms, ulcerated uterine adenocarcinoma, pyometra, or abortion.

Other Renal Conditions

Chronic renal failure with increased drinking and urination, secondary to inappropriate diet and an elevated Ca:P ratio, is common in older rabbits. Inappropriate vitamin D supplementation with dystrophic mineralization of the kidney can also occur. Acute renal failure following gentamicin, NSAID, or Telazol® administration has been reported in rabbits. Less common causes of renal disease include various congenital abnormalities (e.g., cyst, hydroneprosis, and renal agenesis) and fatty infiltration of the kidney in obese animals. Renal tumors are relatively common, including lymphoma and embryonal nephroma (Wilm's tumor).

Vaginal Discharge

The source and nature of a suspected discharge should be determined to distinguish it from normal urine, which may be red-tinged due to porphyrin secretion, and pasty due to its high mineral content. Uterine adenocarcinomas and uterine venous aneurysms may result in a bloody discharge. Purulent discharge may be caused by *P. multocida* or *S. aureus* infection. A sanguinous discharge may be associated with abortion. Prolapsed vagina and uterus have both been reported.

Infertility

Infertility in rabbits is difficult to diagnose. Factors that may contribute to a real or apparent infertility in animals of either sex are immaturity or senescence of the buck or doe, heat stress, caloric or other nutritional imbalances, such as low-protein diets, hypovitaminosis A, D, or E, or hypervitaminosis A, which are common. Other conditions contributing to infer-

Table 4.5. Common presenting genitourinary conditions and differential diagnoses in rabbits.

Condition	Differential Diagnoses
Renal Conditions	Noninfectious
	Urolithiasis
	Chronic renal failure
	Hypervitaminosis D (dystrophic mineralization)
	Hydronephrosis
	Renal agenesis
	Toxicoses, e.g., gentamycin, Telazol®, NSAIDs, dietary mycotoxins
	Renal cysts
	Bladder polyps
	Fatty infiltration (pregnancy toxemia)
	Neoplasia, e.g., lymphoma, embryonal nephroma (Wilm's tumor)
	Infectious
	Pyelonephritis/nephritis/cystitis secondary to bacterial infection, e.g., *Pasteurella multocida, Staphylococcus aureus, E. coli*
	Renal abscess
	Encephalitozoonosis
Uterine Conditions	Noninfectious
	Cystic endometrial hyperplasia
	Pregnancy toxemia
	Infertility, e.g., inadequate protein, hypovitaminosis A, D, E, or hypervitaminosis A
	Abortion, e.g., stress, hyperthermia, trauma
	Uterine torsion
	Uterine/vaginal prolapse
	Endometrial venous aneurysms
	Hydrometra
	Neoplasia, e.g., uterine adenocarcinoma
	Infectious
	Pyometra/metritis following bacterial infection, e.g., *Pasteurella multocida, Staphylococcus aureus*
	Listeriosis (abortion)
	Vulvitis, e.g., *Treponema cuniculi*
Mammary Gland Conditions	Noninfectious
	Mammary gland hyperplasia/dysplasia
	Agalactia
	Neoplasia
	Infectious
	Mastitis, e.g., *S. aureus*
Male Reproductive Conditions	Noninfectious
	Intestinal herniation and strangulation postcastration
	Trauma
	Interbuck fighting with testicular evisceration
	Neoplasia
	Infectious
	Orchitis and epididymitis following *P. multocida, Brucella* spp, or *T. cuniculi* infection

tility include overcrowding, overuse of bucks for breeding, autumnal breeding depression, an incompatible mate, estrogenic stimulation, uterine infection (*Chlamydophila* spp, *Listeria* spp, *S. aureus, Moraxella* spp, *P. multocida, Brucella* spp, *Salmonella* spp), uterine venous aneurysms or neoplasia, orchitis, venereal spirochetosis, excessive noise, and retained placentas.

Prenatal Mortality

Resorption, abortion, and stillbirths occur at different times of gestation; however, the causes of fetal loss may be similar. The more common causes of fetal loss are metritis due to listeriosis and pasteurellosis, excessively large litters, pregnancy toxemia, inadequate caloric intake, and other nutritional imbalances (see above). Less frequent causes of prenatal mortality include arsanilic acid poisoning, DDT poisoning, congenital abnormalities, heat stress, systemic disease, overcrowding, and nitrate toxicity.

Postnatal Mortality of Kits

There are a number of noninfectious causes of perinatal mortality of kits. Maternal inexperience, handling of kits or disturbing the nest, inadvertent cannibalism during consumption of the placenta, insufficient nest material, outside disturbances, deformed, chilled, or injured young, thirst, aspiration pneumonia, caloric deficiency, vitamin A excess in the doe, young animals that have fallen out of the nest, and agalactia can all lead to neonatal neglect or death. Agalactia can result from gastric stasis, malocclusion, anorexia, mastitis, or restricted access to water.

Death of young rabbits can also be caused by enterotoxemia (*E. coli*), trampling, enteropathies, peracute *Pasteurella multocida* septicemia, starvation or dehydration, pyloric stenosis, and ingestion of quaternary ammonium residues. Young may die after suckling a doe with staphylococcal mastitis.

Sudden Death

Death of mature rabbits with few or no preceding signs is a common problem. This situation may occur with acute stress, acute or chronic bacterial pneumonia and disease (especially pasteurellosis), heat stress, enterotoxemia, coliform infections, underlying heart disease, dehydration, electrocution (from electrical cord chewing), intoxications, and ketoacidosis (pregnancy toxemia). The death of does when the litter is a few weeks old is most likely a result of toxemia caused by *Clostridium* spp or the consequence of retained placenta(s).

References

Abitol MM, Driscoll SG, Ober WB. Placental lesion in experimental toxemia in the rabbit. Am J Obstet Gynecol. 1976, 125:942–948.

Adams CE, Singh MM. Semen characteristics and fertility of rabbits subjected to exhaustive use. Lab Anim. 1981, 15:157–161.

Andrew SE. Corneal diseases of rabbits. Vet Clin Exot Anim. 2007, 5:341–356.

Arnbjer J. Pseudopterygium in a pygmy rabbit. Vet Med Small Anim Clin. 1979, 74:737–738.

Artwohl JE, Seps SL, Cera LM. Sudden death in rabbits. Lab Anim. 1988, 17:19–20.

Baird CR. Biology of Cuterebra lepuscule Townsend (Diptera: Cuterebridae) in cottontail rabbits in Idaho. J Wildl Dis. 1983, 19:214–218.

Baum I. What's your diagnosis? Hematuria in a rabbit. Lab Anim. 1982, 21:16–18.

Baxter JS. Posterior paralysis in the rabbit. J Small Anim Pract. 1975, 16:267–271.

Bellhorn RW. Laboratory Animal Ophthalmology. In: Veterinary Ophthalmology, 2nd ed. Gelatt KN (ed.). Philadelphia: Lea & Febiger, 1991; 656–679.

Bishop CR. Reproduction of rabbits and rodents. Vet Clin Exot Anim. 2002, 5:507–535.

Bray MV, et al. Endometrial venous aneurysms in three New Zealand white rabbits. Lab Anim Sci. 1991, 42:360–362.

———. Hydrometra in a New Zealand white rabbit. Lab Anim Sci. 1991, 41:628–629.

Canny CJ, Gamble CS. Fungal diseases of rabbits. Vet Clin Exot Anim. 2003, 6:429–433.

Cema Z, et al. Spontaneous and experimental infections of domestic rabbits by Sarcocystis cunilculi Brumpt, 1913. Folia Parasit (PRAHA). 1981, 28:313–318.

Confer AW, Ward BC, Hines FA. Arsanilic acid toxicity in rabbits. Lab Anim Sci. 1980, 30:234–236.

Cosgrove M, Wiggins JP, Rothenbacher H. Sarcocystis spp. in the Eastern cottontail (Sylvilagus floridanus). J Wildl Dis. 1982, 18:37–40.

Crossley DA. Oral biology and disorders of lagomorphs. Vet Clin Exot Anim. 2003, 6:629–659.

Crowell-Davis SL. Behavior problems in pet rabbits. J Exot Pet Med. 2007, 16:38–44.

Dade AW, et al. An epizootic of cerebral nematodiasis in rabbits due to Ascaris columnaris. Lab Anim Sci. 1975, 25:65–69.

Davidson MG. Ophthalmology of exotic pets. Comp Cont Educ. 1985, 7:724–730, 735–737.

Deeb BJ, DiGiacomo RF. Cerebral larva migrans caused by Baylisascaris sp in pet rabbits. J Am Vet Med Assoc. 1994, 205:1744–1747.

DiGiacomo RF, Deeb BJ, Anderson RJ. Hypervitaminosis A and reproductive disorders in rabbits. Lab Anim Sci. 1992, 42:250–254.

Dubey JP, et al. Fatal toxoplasmosis in domestic rabbits in the USA. Vet Parasitol. 1992, 44:305–309.

Fisher PG. Exotic mammal renal disease: causes and clinical presentation. Vet Clin Exot Anim. 2006, 9:33–67.

———. Exotic mammal renal disease: diagnosis and treatment. Vet Clin Exot Anim. 2006, 9:69–96.

Fox JG, et al. Congenital entropion in a litter of rabbits. Lab Anim Sci. 1979, 29:509–511.

Frame SR, Mehdi NA, Turek JJ. Naturally occurring mucocutaneous histoplasmosis in a rabbit. J Comp Pathol. 1989, 10:351–354.

Garibaldi BA, et al. Hematuria in rabbits. Lab Anim Sci. 1987, 37:769–772.

Garibaldi BA, Fox JG, Musto DRT. Atypical moist dermatitis in rabbits. Lab Anim Sci. 1990, 40:652–653.

Garibaldi BA, Moyer C, Fox JG. Diagnostic exercise: mandibular swelling in a rabbit. Lab Anim Sci. 1990, 40:77–78.

Gillette CS, et al. Alopecia associated with ribavirin administration in rabbits. Lab Anim Sci. 1990, 40:207–208.

Giordano C, Weigt A, Vercelli A, et al. Immunohistochemical identification of Encephalitozoon cuniculi in phacoclastic uveitis in four rabbits. Vet Opthalmol. 2005, 8:271–275.

Harvey RG, et al. A connective tissue defect in two rabbits similar to the Ehlers-Danlos syndrome. Vet Rec. 1990, 126:130–132.

———. Demodex cuniculi in dwarf rabbits (Oryctolagus cuniculus). J Small Anim Pract. 1990, 31:204–207.

Heatley JJ, Smith AN. Spontaneous neoplasms of lagomorphs. Vet Clin Exot Anim. 2004, 7:561–577.

Hedenqvist P, Roughan J, Orr H, et al. Assessment of ketamine/medetomidine anesthesia in the New Zealand white rabbit. Vet Anesth Analg. 2001, 28:18–25.

Hellmann W. Effects of fever and hyperthermia on the embryonic development of rabbits. Vet Rec. 1979, 104:389–390.

Hill PB, Lo A, Eden CAN, et al. Survey of the prevalence, diagnosis, and treatment of dermatological conditions in small animals in general practice. Vet Rec. 2006, 158:533–539.

Hobbs BA, Parker RF. Uterine torsion associated with either hydrometra or endometritis in two rabbits. Lab Anim Sci. 1990, 40: 535–536.

Jacobson HA, McGinnes BS, Catts EP. Bot fly myiasis of the cottontail rabbit, Sylvilagus floridanus mallurus in Virginia with some biology of the parasite, Cuterebra buccata. J Wildl Dis. 1978, 14:56–66.

Jones SMP, Carrington SD. Pasteurella dacryocystitis in rabbits. Vet Rec. 1988, 122:514–515.

Kazacos KR, Kazacos EA. Diagnostic exercise: neuromuscular condition in rabbits. Lab Anim Sci. 1988, 38:187–189.

Kouchi M, Ueda Y, Horie H, et al. Ocular lesions in Watanabe heritable hyperlipidemic rabbits. Vet Ophth. 2006, 9:145–148.

Krogstad AP, Simpson JE, Korte SW. Viral diseases of the rabbit. Vet Clin Exot Anim. 2005, 8:123–138.

Kuristyn I, Naumann S, Kaup FJ. Torticollis in rabbits: etiology, pathology, diagnosis and therapy. Berliner and Munchener, Tieraerztliche Wochenschrift. 1986, 99:14–19.

Langford MP, et al. Conjunctivitis in rabbits caused by enterovirus type 70 (EV 70). Invest Ophthalmol Vis Sci. 1986, 27:915–920.

Leland MM, Hubbard GB, Dubey JP. Clinical toxoplasmosis in domestic rabbits. Lab Anim Sci. 1992, 42:318–319.

Lopushinsky T. Myiasis of nesting cottontail rabbits. J Wildl Dis. 1970, 6:98–100.

Martin MW, Darke PG, Else RW. Congestive heart failure with artrial fibrillation in a rabbit. Vet Rec. 1987, 121:570–571.

McNitt JI. Effect of frequency of service of male rabbits on fertility. J Appl Rabbit Res. 1981, 4:18–20.

Mendlowski B. Neuromuscular lesions in restrained rabbits. Vet Pathol. 1975, 12:378–386.

Millichamp NJ, Collins BR. Blepharoconjunctivitis associated with Staphylococcus aureus in a rabbit. J Am Vet Med Assoc. 1986, 189:1153–1154.

Moore CP, Dubielzig R, Glaza SM. Anterior corneal dystrophy of American Dutch belted rabbits: biomicroscopic and histopathologic findings. Vet Pathol. 1987, 24:28–33.

Morrell JM. Hydrometra in the rabbit. Vet Rec. 1989, 125:325.

Munger RJ, Langevin N, Podval J. Spontaneous cataracts in laboratory rabbits. Vet Ophth. 2002, 5:177–181.

Mykytowycz R, Fullagar PJ. Effect of social environment on reproduction in the rabbit, Oryctolagus cuniculus (L.). J Reprod Fertil Suppl. 1973, 19:503–522.

Nettles VF, et al. An epizootic of cerebral nematodiasis in cottontail rabbits. J Am Vet Med Assoc. 1975, 167:600–604.

Ngatia TA, et al. Arteriosclerosis and related lesions in rabbits. J Comp Pathol. 1989, 101:279–286.

O'Donoghue PN, Whatley BF. Pseudomonas aeruginosa in rabbit fur. Lab Anim. 1971, 5:251–255.

O'Reilly A, McCowan C, Hardman C, et al. Taenia serialis causing exophthalmos in a pet rabbit. Vet Ophth. 2002, 5:227–230.

Owiny J, Vandewoude S, Painter TJ, et al. Hip dysplasia in rabbits: association with nest box flooring. Comp Med. 2001, 51(1):85–88.

Pariault R. Cardiovascular physiology and diseases of the rabbit. Vet Clin Exot Anim. 2009, 12:135–144.

Patton NM, Cheeke PR. Etiology and treatment of young doe syndrome. J Appl Rabbit Res. 1980, 3:23–24.

Phaneuf LR, Barker S, Groleau MA, et al. Tracheal injury following endotracheal intubation and anesthesia in rabbits. J Amer Assoc Lab Anim Sci. 2006, 45:67–72.

Port CD, Dodd DC. Two cases of corneal epithelial dystrophy in rabbits. Lab Anim Sci. 1983, 33:587–588.

Redrobe S. Calcium metabolism in rabbits. Sem Av Exot Pet Med. 2002, 11:94–101.

Reusch B. Rabbit gastroenterology. Vet Clin Exot Anim. 2005, 8:351–375.

Ryan T. Obstetrics in rabbits. J Small Anim Exotic Med. 1991, 1:26–27.

Shaw NA, et al. Zinc deficiency in female rabbits. Lab Anim. 1974, 8:1–7.

Shell LG, Saunders G. Arteriosclerosis in a rabbit. J Am Vet Med Assoc. 1989, 194:679–680.

Vernau, KM, Grahn, BH, Clarke-Scott, HA, et al. Thymoma in a geriatric rabbit with hypercalcemia and periodic exophthalmos. J Am Vet Med Assoc. 1995, 206:820–822.

Volopich S, Gruber A, Hassan J, et al. Malignant B-cell lymphoma of the Harder's gland in a rabbit. Vet Ophth. 2005, 8:259–263.

Wagner F, Fehr M. Common ophthalmic problems in pet rabbits. J Exot Pet Med. 2007, 16:158–167.

Ward GS, Crumrine MH, Mattloch JR. Inflammatory exostosis and abscessation associated with Fusobacterium nucleatum in a rabbit. Lab Anim Sci. 1981, 31:280–281.

Watson GL, Evans MG. Listeriosis in a rabbit. Vet Pathol. 1985, 22:191–193.

Weisbroth SW, Wang R, Scher S. Immune and pathologic consequences of spontaneous Cuterebra myiasis in domestic rabbits (Oryctolagus cuniculus). Lab Anim Sci. 1973, 23: 241–247.

Williams CSF, Gibson RB. Sore dewlap: Pseudomonas aeruginosa on rabbit fur and skin. Vet Med Small Anim Clin. 1975, 70:954–955.

Yamini B, Stein S. Abortion, stillbirth, neonatal death, and nutritional myodegeneration in a rabbit breeding colony. J Am Vet Med Assoc. 1989, 194:561–562.

Zimmerman TE, et al. Soft tissue mineralization in rabbits fed a diet containing excess vitamin D. Lab Anim Sci. 1990, 40:212–215.

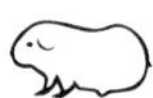

THE GUINEA PIG

Skin Conditions

Alopecia

A number of causes for hair loss exist in the guinea pig including hereditary hairlessness in breeds that have become popular in recent years (e.g., Skinny pigs) (Table 4.6). Hair loss, thinning, or failure of hair to grow may occur in intensively bred sows, particularly in the last trimester of pregnancy when metabolic demands are considerable. Sows that are repeatedly bred lose increasing amounts of hair with successive pregnancies and lactations. Hair loss or growth depression are seen also in young pigs near weaning age, in older sows with cystic rete ovarii, and in animals that consume protein-deficient feed (usually less than 15% crude protein) or other nutritionally deficient diets, such as those with inadequate vitamin C or zinc levels. Guinea pigs often barber one another and younger animals approaching sexual maturity may fight, resulting in hair loss and bite wounds. Abrasion on rough surfaces, such as feeders, fungal infections (*Trichophyton mentagrophytes*), and certain drug therapies may also result in hair loss.

Swellings and Masses

Subcutaneous abscesses are common in guinea pigs. *Streptococcus zooepidemicus* (cervical lymphadenopathy or "lumps") and *Staphylococcus aureus* (bumblefoot or chronic pododermatitis with little pus accumulation) infection are common (Figure 4.3). *S. aureus*–induced mastitis also is seen. *Streptobacillus moniliformis* and *Yersinia pseudotuberculosis* also occasionally induce abscesses. Neoplasia is rare in guinea pigs but epithelial tumors seen include trichofolliculoma and mammary adenocarcinoma as well

Table 4.6. Common presenting skin conditions and differential diagnoses in guinea pigs and chinchillas.*

Condition	Differential Diagnoses
Alopecia	Noninfectious
	Fighting/trauma*
	Mechanical, e.g., feeder*
	Behavioral stereotypy (barbering)*
	Hereditary hairlessness (Skinny pig and other naked varieties)
	Cystic rete ovarii (endocrinopathy)
	Late pregnancy
	Drug therapy, e.g., anticancer therapies
	Nutritional deficiencies, e.g., zinc, hypovitaminosis C
	Infectious
	Dermatophytosis,* e.g., *Trichophyton* spp
Swellings/Masses	Noninfectious
	Trauma/hemorrhage*
	Neoplasia (fibrosarcoma, lymphoma, mammary adenocarcinoma, trichofolliculoma, cavian leukemia with lymphadenopathy)
	Infectious
	Cervical lymphadenitis (*Streptococcus zooepidemicus*)
	Abscesses,* e.g., *Staphylococcus* spp, *Yersinia pseudotuberculosis*
	Mastitis
Dermatitis	Noninfectious
	Fighting/bite wounds*
	Contact allergy
	Pododermatitis
	Nutritional deficiencies, e.g., hypovitaminosis C
	Urine scalding*
	Infectious
	Bacterial,* e.g., *Streptococcus* spp, *Staphylococcus* spp
	Yeast, e.g., *Malassezia* dermatitis
	Dermatophytosis, e.g., *Trichophyton* spp
	Parasitic, e.g., fleas (*Ctenocephalides felis*), fur mites (*Chirodiscoides caviae, Demodex caviae*), sarcoptic mange (*Trixacarus caviae*), pediculosis (*Gyropus ovalis, Gliricola porcelli*), myiasis

*Denotes conditions that may also occur in chinchillas.

as fibrosarcoma, lymphoma, and a retrovirus-induced cavian leukemia with associated lymphadenopathy. Long-haired guinea pigs often develop a large mat of hair gummed together with waxy secretions from the supracaudal perianal gland at the base of the spine, which is occasionally mistaken for a tumor. The gland is testosterone-sensitive and occasionally hypertrophies in intact males.

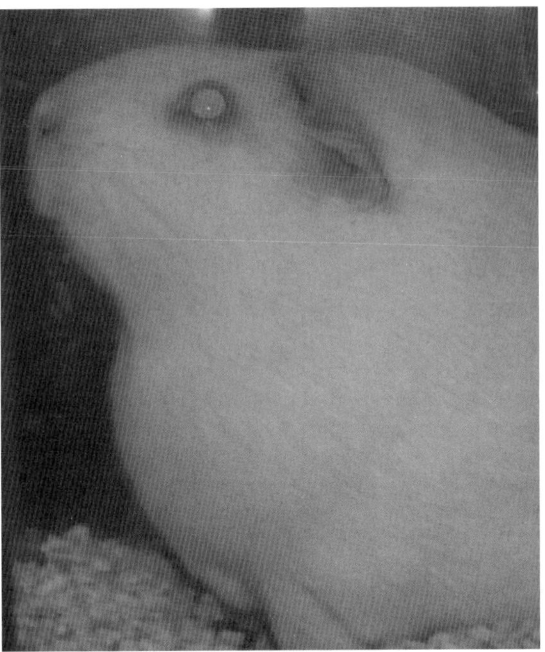

FIGURE 4.3. Cervical swelling in a guinea pig caused by cervical lymphadenitis.

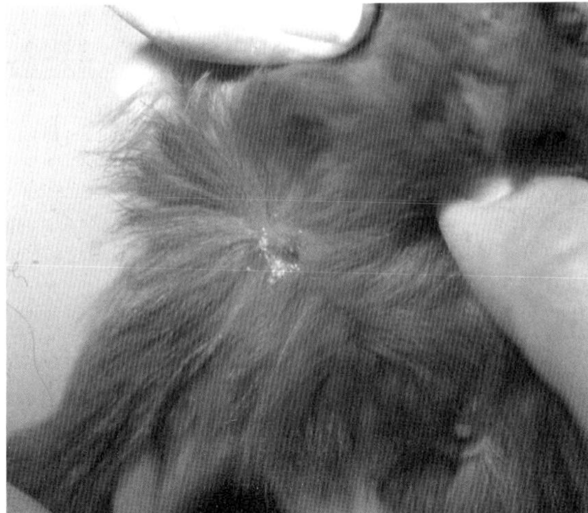

FIGURE 4.4. Lice eggs (nits) may be seen deep in the hair coat around the nipple of this young guinea pig.

Rough Hair Coat

Abyssinian guinea pigs normally have a rough hair coat characterized by several rosettes or whorls of hair. Generalized roughness of hair coat is also associated with illness, leaky water bottles, damp and dirty cages, and hypovitaminosis C.

Dermatitis

Bite wounds, usually on the ears, dorsum, or rump, may lead to superficial ulceration of the skin with secondary bacterial contamination. *Trixacarus caviae* mite infestation (sarcoptic mange) is intensely pruritic for most guinea pigs and is characterized by frantic scratching episodes culminating in seizure-like activity. Other causes of dermatitis include fungal and yeast infections, pediculosis, and cutaneous acariasis. The rabbit ear mite *Psoroptes cuniculi* may infect guinea pigs when these species are co-housed. Subclinical dermatophyte infection is common and may induce patchy scaling lesions on the face and back. Mites (*Chirodiscoides* spp) tend to affect the trunk, as do bacterial infections, whereas lice are found primarily on the head and neck (Figure 4.4). Lesions of ectoparasitism are usually exacerbated by scratching, as occurs with *T. caviae* and louse infestation. Preputial dermatitis has been reported in boars and urine scalding is seen in both sexes housed in wet conditions or with renal disease. Guinea pigs are messy eaters and drinkers and cages must be changed regularly to keep the animals clean and dry. Myiasis (fly strike) may occur in guinea pigs housed indoors under unsanitary conditions that permit moist, ulcerative dermatitis to occur. The infestation may go undetected for some time in longer-haired breeds because of hair matting. Pododermatitis may result when guinea pigs are housed on wire flooring (Figure 4.5). A moist dermatitis may result when animals have overgrown cheek teeth with resultant entrapment of the tongue and interference with swallowing ("slobbers"—see below) (Figure 4.6).

Gastrointestinal Conditions

Anorexia

Healthy guinea pigs are generally enthusiastic at mealtime and anorexia may be a sign of a serious underlying systemic condition (Table 4.7). Overgrowth of molars may result in sharp points that cause discomfort or mucosal laceration during chewing. Guinea pigs may salivate ("slobbers") in cases of malocclusion, particularly if their tongue

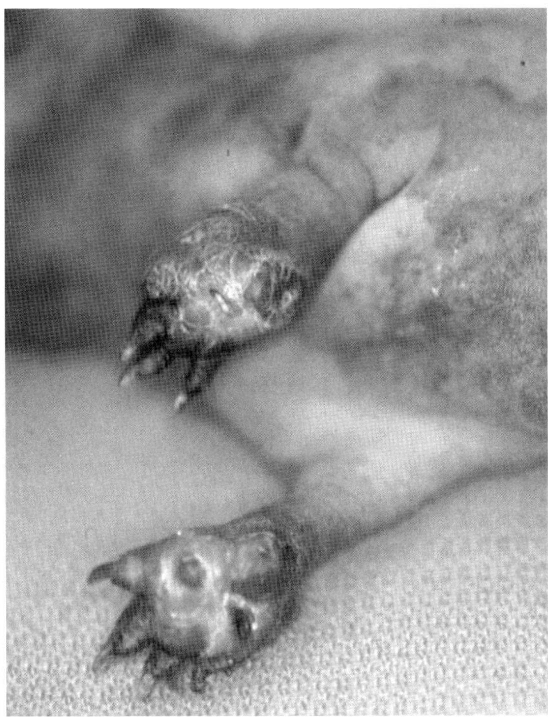

FIGURE 4.5. Bilateral pododermatitis in a Skinny pig that was housed in a cage with a wire bottom. Courtesy of Marina Brash.

becomes entrapped between overgrown molars in the lower dental arcade, when their teeth are sore and loose as occurs with hypovitaminosis C, and following heat stress. Sudden dietary changes, changes in management practices, or insufficient access to clean, fresh water may also induce anorexia, as can pregnancy toxemia. Gastric dilatation with severe abdominal distension is an acute emergency in guinea pigs, sometimes occurring secondary to rapid dietary changes, and requires immediate deflation by stomach tube or surgical correction to prevent volvulus sequel (Figure 4.7).

Diarrhea

When an enteropathy does occur in a guinea pig, the disease is generally rapidly fatal with few clinical signs. Supportive fluids and supplemental heat can be offered, but the prognosis is generally poor. Infectious causes of diarrhea include Tyzzer's disease (*Clostridium piliforme* infection), coliform infections, salmonellosis, yersiniosis, a coronaviral

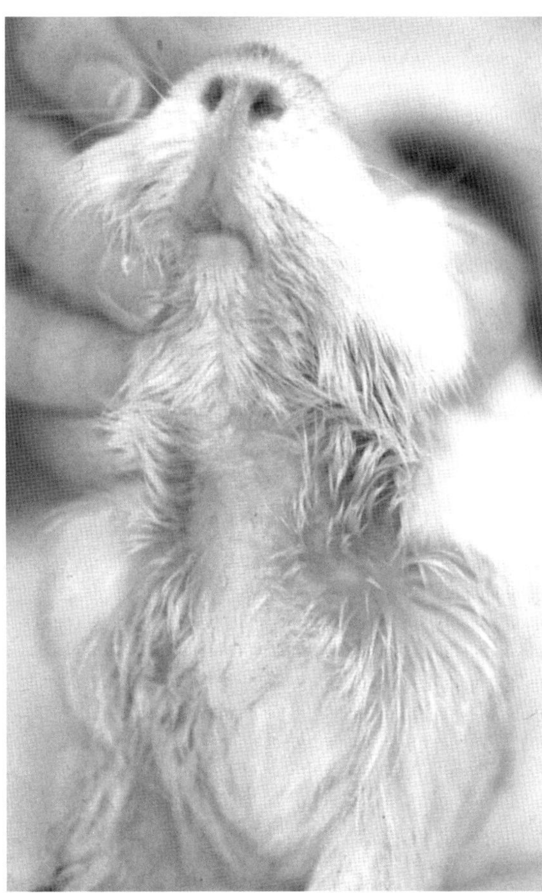

FIGURE 4.6. Moist cervical dermatitis or "slobbers" in a guinea pig with incisor and cheek teeth malocclusion.

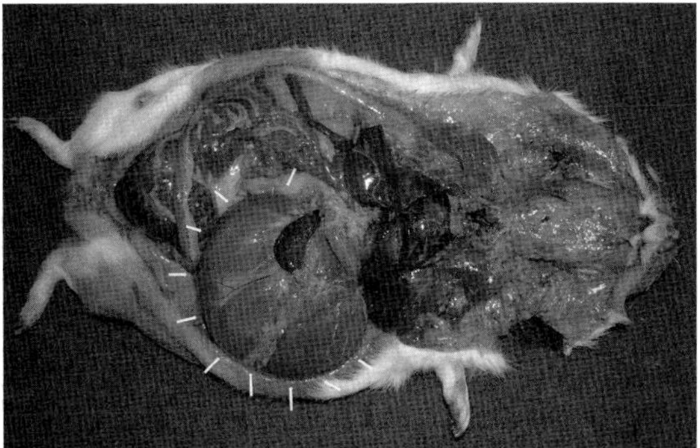

FIGURE 4.7. Massive gastric dilatation in a guinea pig (arrows), diagnosed at necropsy.

Table 4.7. Common presenting gastrointestinal conditions and differential diagnoses in guinea pigs and chinchillas.*

Condition	Differential Diagnoses
Anorexia	Noninfectious
	Dental disease (malocclusion, ptyalism)*
	Hypovitaminosis C (scurvy)
	Sudden dietary change
	Pregnancy toxemia
	Insufficient water supply
	Change in husbandry practices (environmental stress)
	Gastric dilatation*
	Intestinal accident
	Pain*
	Gastric foreign body with peritonitis
	Neoplasia
	Infectious
	Secondary to disease—see below
Diarrhea	Noninfectious
	Dietary indiscretion (carbohydrate overload)
	Low-fiber diet
	Inappropriate use of antibiotics (*C. difficile* overgrowth)
	Intestinal amyloidosis
	Infectious
	Viral enteritis, e.g., coronavirus
	Bacterial enterocolitis, e.g., *Clostridium piliforme* (Tyzzer's disease), *E. coli*, *Salmonella* spp, *Yersinia* spp
	Protozoal infection, e.g., coccidiosis (*Eimeria caviae*), cryptosporidiosis, and giardiasis*
Constipation	Noninfectious
	Obesity*
	Inappropriate diet* (low fiber)
	Lack of exercise*
	Colonic atony and fecal impaction (aged boars)

*Denotes conditions that may also occur in chinchillas.

wasting syndrome with diarrhea in young pigs, and other clostridial infections, for example, *C. difficile* and *C. perfringens*. Rapidly fatal acute enteritis and typhlitis may result from narrow spectrum antibiotic administration, which eliminates the normal bacterial flora and induces bacterial overgrowth and dysbiosis. Nematode infections are rare in guinea pigs and are typically subclinical. Cryptosporidiosis and giardiasis may cause diarrhea, poor weight gain, and potentially death in young guinea pigs. Noninfectious causes of diarrhea and ileus are common in guinea pigs and include dietary indiscretion (carbohydrate overload), diets low in fiber, and intestinal amyloidosis secondary to chronic inflammation. Once established, there is no cure for this last condition.

Constipation

Fecal impaction may occur in intact boars, generally greater than 2.5 years of age, secondary to colonic atony, and is treated by regular, gentle manual evacuation of the colon. Following scent marking, intact older males may accumulate shavings, fecal debris, genital secretions, and other material around the anus, forming a dense mat of material known as a scrotal plug, which may make it difficult for them to defecate. Boars should be examined on a regular basis to ensure there is no accumulation of debris around their anus. Obesity, inappropriate diet, and lack of exercise may all contribute to constipation.

Cardiopulmonary Conditions

Heart disease is rarely seen in guinea pigs. Rhabdomyomatosis, a congenital condition involving storage of glycogen within myofibers, which appears grossly as pale streaking of the heart surface, can be extensive but does not appear to contribute to symptomatic cardiac disease. Similarly, fatty infiltration of the myocardium can be quite extensive but is interpreted as an incidental finding.

Rhinitis, Dyspnea, and Other Pulmonary Conditions

Oculonasal discharge frequently accompanies respiratory disease in guinea pigs (Table 4.8). Bacterial

Table 4.8. Common presenting cardiopulmonary conditions and differential diagnoses in guinea pigs and chinchillas.*

Condition	Differential Diagnoses
Nasal Discharge/ Rhinitis/Sneezing	Noninfectious Dental disease* (molar roots) Allergy (dust, hay) Increased temperature* Nasal foreign body* Neoplasia* Infectious *Bordetella bronchiseptica** Other bacterial infections,* e.g., *Staphylococcus aureus, Pasteurella multocida, Streptococcus* spp, *Pseudomonas* spp
Dyspnea	Noninfectious Stress* Gastric torsion Pregnancy toxemia Foreign body Aspiration pneumonia Neoplasia,* e.g., lymphoma with pleural effusion, pulmonary adenoma Infectious Bacterial pneumonia,* e.g., *Bordetella bronchiseptica, Streptococcus* spp, *Pasteurella multocida, Staphylococcus aureus, Klebsiella pneumoniae* Viral infection, e.g., adenovirus, parainfluenza virus, cytomegalovirus

*Denotes conditions that may also occur in chinchillas

organisms that are commonly involved in respiratory disease in guinea pigs include *Bordetella bronchiseptica*, *Streptococcus pneumoniae*, and *Streptococcus zooepidemicus*. Organisms less frequently involved include *Klebsiella pneumoniae*, *Pasteurella multocida*, *Pseudomonas aeruginosa*, and *Staphylococcus aureus*. Systemic infections with parainfluenza virus, adenovirus, and, rarely, cytomegalovirus may result in mild rhinitis and cervical lymphadenopathy. Acute, fatal pneumonia has been reported infrequently following adenoviral infection in young animals. Noninfectious conditions causing respiratory distress are heat stress, sudden fear or excitement with massive catecholamine release, allergy, tooth root elongation (malocclusion), diaphragmatic hernia, nasal foreign body, pregnancy toxemia, gastric torsion, and some forms of neoplasia, such as lymphoma with pleural effusion.

Endocrine Conditions

Diabetes mellitus has been reported sporadically in guinea pigs. This condition presents as in other animals with polyuria, polydipsia, glycosuria, and ketosis. Moderate to marked fatty infiltration of the pancreas occurs frequently with increasing age but is not linked to increased susceptibility to diabetes mellitus.

Nervous and Musculoskeletal Conditions

Head Tilt or Torticollis

Head tilt is uncommon in guinea pigs but may be caused by otitis media/interna induced by a bacterial infection (Table 4.9). Encephalopathies that lead to head tilt, such as toxoplasmosis and brain abscesses, are seen rarely.

Incoordination and Seizures

A common cause of incoordination or paralysis is nerve, bone, or soft tissue injury from a fall. Guinea pigs have fragile skeletons and must be handled carefully. Pregnancy toxemia, other toxicities, heat stroke, enterotoxemia, streptococcal meningitis, and various muscular disorders (e.g., dystrophies) are other causes of incoordination and, rarely, seizures. Severe sarcoptic mange caused by *T. caviae* may induce intense pruritus such that infested guinea pigs appear to be seizuring. Rabies virus infection is extremely uncommon in guinea pigs in North America but has been reported in guinea pigs with outdoor access.

Paresis or Paralysis

Hypovitaminosis C, characterized by subperiosteal hemorrhage and swollen and painful joints, is a common cause of immobility. Affected animals may squeal when restrained and have concurrent poor hair coats and anorexia. Systemic diseases, such as *Bordetella bronchiseptica* infection, streptococcosis with secondary polyserositis, and salmonellosis also may result in reluctance to move. Osteoarthritis, severe pododermatitis with secondary osteomyelitis, spinal fracture, and various diet-related myopathies are other possible causes of paresis and paralysis. Back injury with edema and hemorrhage around the spinal cord may result in temporary paralysis. Osteodystrophy fibrosa or nutritional secondary hyperparathyroidism has been reported in guinea pigs fed diets high in calcium, for example, alfalfa-based diets. Guinea pigs, especially if housed in large round or square cages, may run in circles when excited. Stampeding guinea pigs, circling or not, often will leap from an open cage regardless of the height above the floor, resulting in trauma and fractures. Rectangular cages and objects or barriers within the cage discourage circling.

Ocular Conditions

Conjunctivitis in guinea pigs is commonly due to a bacterial infection in a marginally scorbutic animal. Animals present with swollen lids with a moderate serous or mucopurulent discharge. Bacteria involved may include *Bordetella bronchiseptica*, *Streptococcus* spp, *Staphylococcus aureus*, or *Pasteurella* spp. *Chlamydophila psittaci* infection causes inclusion body conjunctivitis in young animals. This infection is generally self-limiting, lasting 3 weeks, but may also recur on a cyclical basis in some animals. Chlamydiosis presents as mild chemosis and conjunctivitis with a serous or mucopurulent discharge. Panophthalmitis may be caused by the bacteria noted, including *Streptococcus zooepidemicus*.

Cataracts are seen as an autosomal dominant condition in some guinea pig strains and may be associated with diabetes mellitus or with a deficiency of

Table 4.9. Common presenting nervous and musculoskeletal conditions and differential diagnoses in guinea pigs and chinchillas.*

Condition	Differential Diagnoses
Head Tilt/Torticollis	Noninfectious
	Trauma*
	Toxoplasmosis
	Cerebrovascular accident
	Toxins, e.g., lead (paint)
	Infectious
	Otitis media/interna secondary to bacterial infection,* e.g., *Bordetella bronchiseptica*, *Streptococcus* spp, other Gram-negative bacteria
	Brain abscess*
Seizures	Noninfectious
	Pregnancy toxemia
	Heat stroke*
	Toxins, e.g., lead (paint)
	Hypoxia*
	Severe systemic disease*
	Severe sarcoptic mange infestation
	Neoplasia*
	Trauma*
	Infectious
	Bacterial encephalitis/meningitis/abscess,* e.g., *Streptococcus pneumoniae*, *Pasteurella multocida*, *Staphylococcus aureus*
	Rabies virus
Paresis/Paralysis	Noninfectious
	Trauma* (leg/muscle)
	Heavily pregnant sows
	Hypovitaminosis C (swollen joints, fractures, periarticular hemorrhage)
	Dietary deficiencies,* e.g., hypovitaminosis E
	Pododermatitis with osteomyelitis
	Osteoarthritis
	Severe inanition*
	Toxicity, e.g., lead (paint)
	Infectious
	Polyserositis/arthritis,* e.g., streptococcal infection
	Spinal abscess*
	Toxoplasmosis
	Rabies virus

*Denotes conditions that may also occur in chinchillas.

L-tryptophan. Long-term open lids, as may occur during anesthesia, can lead to corneal, anterior chamber, and lens dessication, and sterile ophthalmic lubricant should always be used in addition to oxygen supplementation by face mask or nasal tube, if injectable anesthetics are used.

"Pea eye" involves the unilateral or bilateral formation of hyperplastic nodules of the lacrimal or zygomatic glands, which may be located on the inferior conjunctival surface. Removal of the nodules is not advised unless the masses are so large as to cause exposure keratitis.

Other ocular conditions reported in guinea pigs include osseous choristoma (ectopic mineralization of the ciliary body), lymphosarcoma with conjunctival involvement, and conjunctival dermoid.

Genitourinary Conditions

Renal Conditions

Urolithiasis is common in both male and female guinea pigs (Table 4.10). Normal guinea pig urine is thick, pale yellow, and cloudy. Calculi can occur at any site along the urinary tract and are usually composed of calcium salts, for example, phosphate, carbonate, or struvite. Ureteral calculi are virtually impossible to remove due to the small diameter of the guinea pig ureters. Urethral calculi in males may sometimes be retropulsed into the bladder prior to cystotomy; in females, they may pass spontaneously. Bacterial cystitis occurs more commonly in older sows and may be caused by *Streptococcus* spp, *S. aureus*, or *E. coli* infection.

Chronic renal failure is common in older guinea pigs of both sexes. The disease is likely multifactorial and may involve inappropriate diets, fatty infiltration of the kidney following pregnancy toxemia, dystrophic mineralization following inappropriate vitamin D supplementation, or other toxicities. Renal cysts and neoplasia are uncommon.

Infertility

Real or apparent infertility or decreased production in guinea pigs may be related to age at the time of breeding, stress from management changes, estrogens in the feed, bedding or other debris adhering to the genitalia (scrotal plugs), increased ambient temperature, nutritional deficiency, metritis, environmental stress, mate aggression or incompatibility, or discomfort secondary to preputial dermatitis.

Prenatal Mortality

Dystocia is common in sows because of the large size of the precocious offspring. Sows bred after mineralization of the fibrocartilaginous joint that forms the pubic symphysis will also have difficulty birthing. Uterine torsion, obesity, and uterine inertia may all contribute to dystocia. Abortions and stillbirths in guinea pigs occur with nutritional deficiencies, bacterial metritis or orchitis, stress, hyperthermia, trauma, and pregnancy toxemia.

Litter Desertion or Death

Neonatal guinea pigs are precocious, and maternal attention other than nursing and licking is not necessary for survival, although the mother should remain with the young, if at all possible, for at least the first 2 weeks. Factors that reduce maternal attention include mastitis, maternal inexperience, and environmental disturbances, such as noise or active cagemates. Young that weigh less than 60g at birth usually die within a few days.

Other Conditions

Cystic rete ovarii occur commonly in aged sows (Figure 4.8). Uterine leiomyoma is frequently seen in conjunction with these cysts. Mammary gland tumors occur with equal frequency in boars as in sows. As in rabbits, the inguinal canal remains open

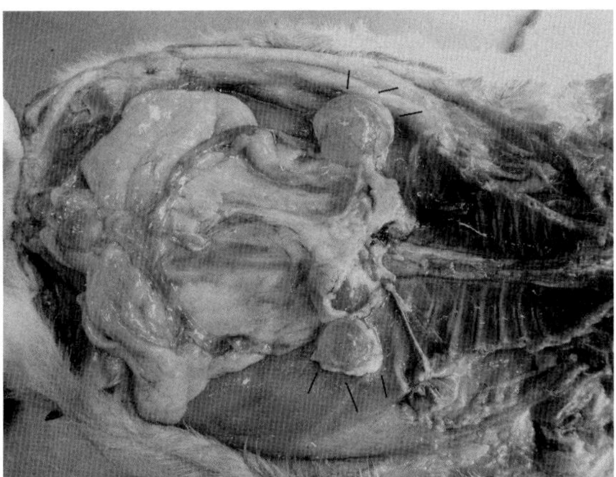

FIGURE 4.8. Bilateral cystic rete ovarii (arrows) in an aged sow.

Table 4.10. Common presenting genitourinary conditions and differential diagnoses in guinea pigs and chinchillas.*

Condition	Differential Diagnoses
Renal Conditions	Noninfectious Urolithiasis Chronic renal failure* Hypervitaminosis D (dystrophic mineralization) Fatty infiltration due to pregnancy toxemia Hydronephrosis* Toxicoses, e.g., gentamycin, NSAIDs Renal cysts Neoplasia,* e.g., lymphoma Infectious Pyelonephritis/nephritis/cystitis secondary to bacterial infection,* e.g., *Streptococcus* spp, *S. aureus, E. coli, Yersinia* spp Renal abscess* Coccidiosis, e.g., *Klossiella cobayae*
Uterine/Ovarian Conditions	Noninfectious Cystic endometrial hyperplasia* Cystic rete ovarii Dystocia, e.g., oversized pups, inability of pubic symphysis to separate, uterine torsion, obesity, uterine inertia Pregnancy toxemia Infertility,* e.g., inadequate protein, hypovitaminosis A, D, E, or hypervitaminosis A, behavioral problems Abortion,* e.g., stress, hyperthermia, trauma Neoplasia,* e.g., uterine leiomyoma* Infectious Pyometra/metritis following bacterial infection,* e.g., *Bordetella bronchiseptica, Streptococcus* spp, *E. coli, S. aureus*
Mammary Gland Conditions	Noninfectious Mammary gland hyperplasia/dysplasia Agalactia* Neoplasia* Infectious Mastitis,* e.g., *S. aureus, Klebsiella* spp, *E. coli, Pasteurella* spp
Male Reproductive Conditions	Noninfectious Intestinal herniation and strangulation postcastration Scrotal plugs Trauma Neoplasia Infectious Orchitis and epididymitis* following *B. bronchiseptica* and *Streptococcus* spp infection

*Denotes conditions that may also occur in chinchillas.

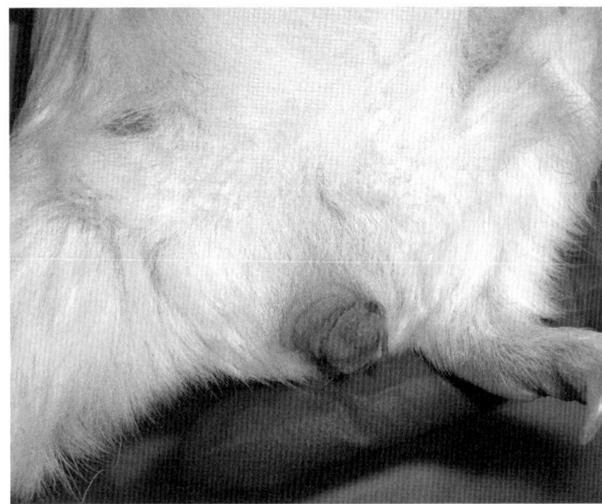

FIGURE 4.9. Prolapsed vagina in a guinea pig.

in boars throughout life, and intestinal herniation and strangulation may occur if the rings are not closed at neutering. Uterine prolapse may occur rarely (Figure 4.9).

Sudden Death

Death with few or no preceding signs may be caused by sudden stress or fear, chilling of pups or overheating animals of any age, septicemia or toxemia (salmonellosis, typhlitis, enteritis, pregnancy toxemia, antibiotic toxicity), pneumonia, gastric volvulus, dystocia, or dehydration.

References

Aidred P, Hill AC, Young C. The isolation of Streptobacillus moniliformis from the cervical abscesses of guinea pigs. Lab Anim. 1974, 8:275–277.

Allgoewer I, Ewringmann A, Pfleghaar S. Lymphosarcoma with conjunctival manifestation in a guinea pig. Vet Ophth. 1999, 2:117–119.

Belihorn RW. Laboratory Animal Ophthalmology. In: Veterinary Ophthalmology, 2nd ed. Gelatt KN (ed.). Philadelphia: Lea & Febiger, 1991; 656–679.

Bishop CR. Reproductive medicine of rabbits and rodents. Vet Clin Exot Anim. 2002, 5:507–535.

Cullen CL, Grahn BH, Wolfer J. Diagnostic ophthalmology. Can Vet J. 2000, 41:502–503.

Deeb BJ, DiGiacomo RF, Wang SP. Guinea pig inclusion conjunctivitis (GPIC) in a commercial colony. Lab Anim. 1989, 23:103–106.

Donnelly TM, Brown CJ. Guinea pig and chinchilla care and husbandry. Vet Clin Exot Anim. 2004, 7:351–373.

Fisher PG. Exotic mammal renal disease: causes and clinical presentation. Vet Clin Exot Anim. 2006, 9:33–67.

———. Exotic mammal renal disease: diagnosis and treatment. Vet Clin Exot Anim. 2006, 9:69–96.

Green LE, Morgan KL. Toxoplasma abortion in a guinea pig. Vet Rec. 1991, 29:266–267.

Greenacre CB. Spontaneous tumors of small mammals. Vet Clin Exot Anim. 2004, 7:627–651.

Harmsen R, Sittig N. The effect of testosterone on the development of the perianal glands of the guinea pig Cavia porcellus. J Exper Zool. 2005, 186:269–272.

Hawkins MG, Graham JE. Emergency and critical care of rodents. Vet Clin Exot Anim. 2007, 10:501–531.

Heatley JJ. Cardiovascular anatomy, physiology, and diseases of rodents and small exotic mammals. Vet Clin Exot Anim. 2009, 12:99–113.

Jaax GP, et al. Coronavirus-like virons associated with a wasting syndrome in guinea pigs. Lab Anim Sci. 1990, 40:375–378.

Kashuba C, et al. Small mammal virology. Vet Clin Exot Anim. 2005, 8:107–122.

Legendre LFJ. Oral disorders of exotic rodents. Vet Clin Exot Anim. 2003, 6:601–628.

Marshall KL. Fungal diseases in small mammals: therapeutic trends and zoonotic considerations. Vet Clin Exot Anim. 2003, 6:415–427.

Ocholi RA, et al. An epizootic infection of Citrobacter freundii in a guinea pig colony: short communication. Lab Anim. 1988, 22:335–336.

Okewole PA, et al. Abortion in guinea pigs. Vet Rec. 1989, 124:248.

Pollock C. Fungal diseases of laboratory rodents. Vet Clin Exot Anim. 2003, 6:401–413.

Rehg JE, Yarbrough BA, Pakes SP. Toxicity of cecal filtrates from guinea pigs with penicillin-associated colitis. Lab Anim Sci. 1980, 30:524–531.

Spink RR. Urolithiasis in a guinea pig (Cavia porcellus). Vet Med Small Anim Clin. 1978, 73:501–502.

Tzipori S, et al. Diarrhea due to Cryptosporidium infection in artificially reared lambs. J Comp Med. 1981, 14:100–105.

Van Herck H, et al. Dermal cryptococcosis in a guinea pig. Lab Anim. 1988, 22:91.

Wappler O, Allgoewer I, Schaeffer EH. Conjunctival dermoid in two guinea pigs: a case report. Vet Ophth. 2002, 5:245–248.

Wood M. Cystitis in female guinea pigs. Lab Anim. 1981, 15:141–143.

Yeatts JWG. Rabbit mite infestation [letter]. Vet Rec. 1994, 134:359–360.

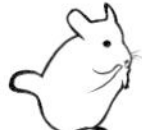

THE CHINCHILLA

Chinchillas and guinea pigs are similar species in many respects and share propensities for developing certain diseases. Conditions seen in both guinea pigs and chinchillas have been indicated in the preceding tables for guinea pigs, and the text comments for these conditions apply to chinchillas equally. This section will only cover conditions specific to chinchillas.

Skin Conditions

The dense hair coat of chinchillas is not permissive to ectoparasite infestation; however, dermatophytosis is quite common, either as clinical or subclinical disease, and subcutaneous abscesses may also occur. Fur chewing may be seen as a behavioral vice, and seborrhea and matted hair coats may result if chinchillas are not given regular access to a dust bath. Fur slip is a condition unique to chinchillas and presents as clumps of hair that fall out or are left in one's hand when chinchillas are stressed and simultaneously grasped superficially, for example, during a clinical examination. This is an escape mechanism, allowing the animal to avoid the perceived threat. Depending on the stage of the hair cycle that follicles are in when fur slip occurs, it may be months before the coat regrows completely. Chinchillas should not be scruffed for restraint, for this reason, but should be firmly held around the body.

Gastrointestinal Conditions

Malocclusion from molar crown elongation occurs in chinchillas and may result in anorexia if animals are unable to close their mouth or chew. Ptyalism may also be an indication of dental disease in chinchillas and animals may not show clinical signs until the disease is advanced, resulting in a poor prognosis.

Gastric stasis, ileus, and enteritis are also seen frequently in chinchillas from similar conditions to those reported for guinea pigs. Dense mats of ingested hair may rarely lead to gastric obstruction.

Cardiopulmonary Conditions

Because of their dense fur coats and inability to sweat, chinchillas are particularly susceptible to heat stroke and sudden collapse with rapid death. Cardiomyopathy has been reported in chinchillas. Bacterial pneumonias occur with equal frequency in chinchillas and are usually of Gram-negative origin, for example, *Bordetella* spp, *Klebsiella* spp, *Pasteurella* spp, and so forth.

Endocrine Conditions

Endocrine disease is uncommon in chinchillas. Diabetes mellitus has been reported sporadically.

Nervous and Musculoskeletal Conditions

Chinchillas are able to formulate adequate amounts of vitamin C from their diet and do not develop scurvy, as do guinea pigs. They are a more athletic, faster moving animal than guinea pigs and tend not to experience as many traumatic injuries after falls, although tibial fractures have been reported secondary to inadvertent dropping. Because of their very large tympanic bullae, head tilt following bacterial otitis media/interna infection is more common in chinchillas, and the infectious agents are the same as for guinea pigs. *Pseudomonas aeruginosa* may also cause otitis interna in chinchillas. Pododermatitis is not a significant disease entity in chinchillas. Chinchillas are very susceptible to encephalitis following listeriosis. This condition may also result in enteritis and diarrhea and is often rapidly fatal. Fatal cerebrospinal nematodiasis caused by *Baylisascaris procyonis* larvae can occur if chinchilla feed or bedding becomes contaminated with raccoon feces.

Ocular Conditions

Asteroid hyalosis and cataract may be seen in older animals. Exophthalmos caused by orbital *Taenia* coenurus is reported in the chinchilla.

Genitourinary Conditions

Urolithiasis is uncommon in chinchillas, although chronic renal failure may occur. Like guinea pigs, chinchilla young are fully developed at birth (precocious); however, the pups tend to be smaller at birth and dystocia is uncommon in chinchillas. Fur ring with secondary paraphimosis occurs in boars. The circumferential ring of hair can be lubricated and slipped off the end of the penis or cut away to reduce the constriction. Penile prolapses may also occur, although the etiology is unknown. The penis should be kept clean and lubricated and the prognosis is generally good for spontaneous resolution. The chinchilla does not have a true scrotum; rather, they have pouches that support the caudal epididymis. This normal anatomical arrangement should not be mistaken for cryptorchidism.

Sudden Death

Sudden death without clinical signs in chinchillas is caused most commmonly by heat stroke, peracute systemic disease, for example, pneumonia or listeriosis, sudden stress or fright, cardiac disease, or enterotoxemia.

References

Bishop CR. Reproductive medicine of rabbits and rodents. Vet Clin Exot Anim. 2002, 5:507–535.

Crossley DA. Dental disease in chinchillas in the UK. J Small Anim Pract. 2001, 42:12–19.

Donnelly TM, Brown CJ. Guinea pig and chinchilla care and husbandry. Vet Clin Exot Anim. 2004, 7:351–373.

Fisher PG. Exotic mammal renal disease: causes and clinical presentation. Vet Clin Exot Anim. 2006, 9:33–67.

———. Exotic mammal renal disease: diagnosis and treatment. Vet Clin Exot Anim. 2006, 9:69–96.

Fritsche R, Simova-Curd S, Clauss M, et al. Hyperthyroidism in connection with suspected diabetes mellitus in a chinchilla (Chinchilla laniger). Vet Rec. 2008, 163:454–456.

González Pereyra ML, Carvalho EC, Tissera JL, et al. An outbreak of acute aflatoxicosis on a chinchilla (Chinchilla lanigera) farm in Argentina. J Vet Diagn Invest. 2008, 20(6):853–856.

Greenacre CB. Spontaneous tumors of small mammals. Vet Clin Exot Anim. 2004, 7:627–651.

Hawkins MG, Graham JE. Emergency and critical care of rodents. Vet Clin Exot Anim. 2007, 10:501–531.

Heatley JJ. Cardiovascular anatomy, physiology, and diseases of rodents and small exotic mammals. Vet Clin Exot Anim. 2009, 12:99–113.

Holmberg BJ, Hollingsworth SR, Osofsky A, et al. Taenia coenurus in the orbit of a chinchilla. Vet Ophth. 2007, 10:53–59.

Kashuba C, et al. Small mammal virology. Vet Clin Exot Anim. 2005, 8:107–122.

Kern TJ. Rabbit and rodent ophthalmology. Sem Av Exot Pet Med. 1997, 6:138–145.

Legendre LFJ. Malocclusions in guinea pigs, chinchillas and rabbits. Can Vet J. 2002, 43:385–390.

———. Oral disorders of exotic rodents. Vet Clin Exot Anim. 2003, 6:601–628.

Marshall KL. Fungal diseases in small mammals: therapeutic trends and zoonotic considerations. Vet Clin Exot Anim. 2003, 6:415–427.

Pollock C. Fungal diseases of laboratory rodents. Vet Clin Exot Anim. 2003, 6:401–413.

Sanford SA. Cerebrospinal nematodiasis caused by Baylisascaris procyonis in chinchillas. J Vet Diagn Invest. 1991, 3:77–79.

Schaeffer DO, Donnelly TM. Disease Problems of Guinea Pigs and Chinchillas. In: Ferrets, Rabbits, and Rodents: Clinical Medicine and Surgery, 2nd ed. Quesenberry KE, Carpenter JW (eds.). Philadelphia: Saunders, 2004.

Wilkerson MJ, Melendy A, Stauber E. An outbreak of listeriosis in a breeding colony of chinchillas. J Vet Diagn Invest. 1997, 9:320–323.

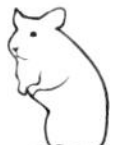

THE HAMSTER

Skin Conditions

Alopecia

Low-protein diets (less than 16% crude protein) may contribute to alopecia in hamsters, and the nutritional information should be reviewed carefully when purchasing food (Table 4.11). Aged, immunologically compromised hamsters may develop demodecosis with alopecia, scaliness, and pustules over the rump and back. Less commonly, hamsters may also develop dermatophytosis, hereditary hairlessness, hair loss associated with an endocrine neoplasm or chronic renal disease, epitheliotropic lymphoma (Figure 4.10), or mechanical loss from constant rubbing on a cage or feeder. Male hamsters housed together may cannibalize the flank glands of one another. Loss of facial hair occurs occasionally around the vibrissae, likely due to mechanical reasons.

Swellings and Masses

Normal structures in hamsters often thought erroneously to be abnormal swellings are the pendulous testes, distended cheek pouches, and the paired flank glands. Note that the flank glands are found on the sides of Syrian hamsters but are on the ventrum of

Table 4.11. Common presenting skin conditions and differential diagnoses in hamsters.

Condition	Differential Diagnoses
Alopecia	Noninfectious
	Fighting/trauma
	Hereditary hairlessness
	Mechanical, e.g., feeder
	Nutritional deficiencies, e.g., zinc, protein
	Endocrine-associated, e.g., Cushing's disease
	Contact allergy
	Neoplasia, e.g., lymphoma
	Infectious
	Dermatophytosis, e.g., *Trichophyton* spp
	Demodecosis, e.g., *D. aurati, D. criceti*
Swellings/Masses	Noninfectious
	Trauma/hemorrhage
	Impacted cheek pouches
	Neoplasia (flank gland tumors, melanoma, basal cell tumors, fibrosarcoma, lymphoma, mammary adenocarcinoma)
	Infectious
	Abscesses, e.g., *Staphylococcus* spp, *Proteus* spp
	Granulomas
	Mastitis
Dermatitis	Noninfectious
	Fighting/bite wounds
	Nutritional deficiencies, e.g., low protein
	Wet or abrasive bedding
	Endocrinopathy (e.g., hyperadrenocorticism)
	Infectious
	Bacterial, e.g., *Staphylococcus* spp
	Dermatophytosis, e.g., *Trichophyton* spp
	Parasitic, e.g., mites (*Notoedres* spp, *Demodex* spp)

dwarf hamsters, similar to the gerbil ventral marking gland. Pathologic processes causing palpable swellings include abscesses, various neoplasms such as flank gland tumors (Figure 4.11), melanoma, lymphoma, and mastocytoma, mastitis, impacted cheek pouches, and, rarely, granulomas in the skin and lymph nodes caused by *Mycobacterium* spp. Fighting, with secondary abscesses, is common, and females tend to be more aggressive than males. Impacted cheek pouches are readily treated by everting them under anesthesia and gently cleaning out the inspissated material. Cutaneous epitheliomas and transmissible lymphomas are thought to be due to hamster polyomavirus infection.

Rough Hair Coat

Hamsters in cages with leaking water bottles and soiled bedding; with polyuria, endocrine dysfunction, or diarrhea; and those housed with incompatible cagemates may have rough hair coats. A rough hair coat is a nonspecific sign of fighting, inadequate diet or management, or disease.

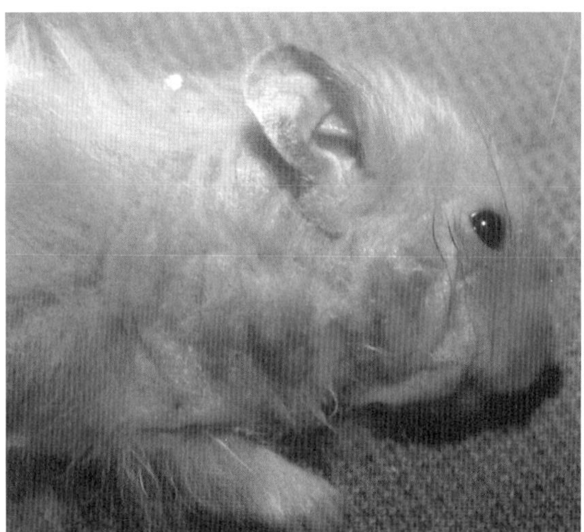

FIGURE 4.10. Cutaneous lymphosarcoma in a hamster. The condition causes irregular thickening, crusting, and ulceration of the skin.

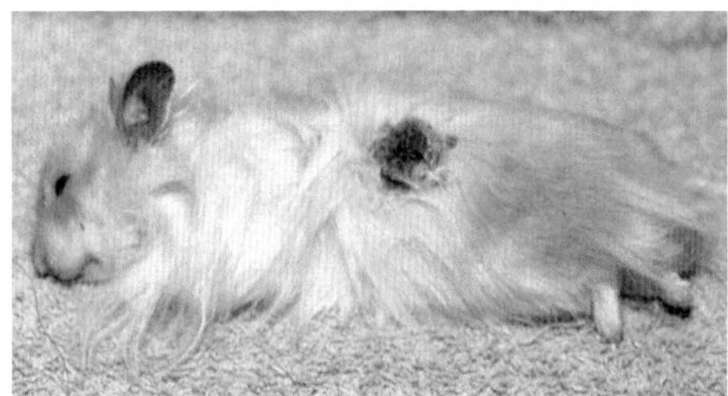

FIGURE 4.11. Flank gland tumor in a male hamster.

Dermatitis

Inflammation of the skin is most often seen in association with bite wounds and secondary infection with bacteria such as *S. aureus, P. pneumotropica*, or *Streptococcus* spp. Other possible causes of dermatitis include demodectic mange; *Notoedres* spp infection, which produces crusty lesions around the ear, nose, feet, and perianal area; and dermatophytosis. Demodectic mange may also induce a greasy, matted coat and occurs most often in immunocompromised older animals with concurrent disease. Abrasion of the skin by wood shavings has also been reported.

Gastrointestinal Conditions

Anorexia

As for other rodents, the incisors of hamsters continue to grow throughout life. If malocclusion results, animals may not be able to prehend food properly, and anorexia with or without excess salivation may result (Table 4.12). Dental deformities and domed calvaria have been reported in young hamsters following in utero infection of the dam with hamster parvovirus. Other causes of anorexia or inappetence include systemic disease, lack of access to clean potable water, intestinal accidents such as intussusception with heavy cestode burden, pain from any source, or neoplasia. Multicentric lymphoma is commonly seen as hamsters age and may induce inappetence and weight loss.

Diarrhea

The vague term "wet tail" is the common synonym for the diarrheal complex that may occur in hamsters. Proliferative enteritis is common in young animals and is caused by *Lawsonia intracellularis* infection, which confers a thickened, corrugated appearance to the intestinal serosa. Diarrhea in hamsters may also result from coliform and clostridial infection, salmonellosis, Tyzzer's disease (*Clostridium piliforme* infection), intestinal or hepatic amyloidosis, protozoal overgrowth of *Giardia* spp or *Spironucleus* spp, or cecal dysbiosis following narrow spectrum antibiotic administration with development of secondary clostridial enterotoxemia. Treatment of *Salmonella* spp infections in any small mammal pet is controversial because the condition is zoonotic and treatment may lead to a carrier state with bacterial shedding into the environment. Sequelae to diarrhea may include intestinal obstructions, intussusception, or rectal prolapse (a dark red tubular protrusion from the anus) (Figure 4.12). Reduction of the prolapsed rectum is frequently unsuccessful unless the underlying etiology is resolved.

Constipation

Constipation in hamsters may be related to *Rodentolepis nana* and *Hymenolepis diminuta* cestode infestations in the small intestine, obesity, lack of adequate fiber in the diet, lack of exercise, or

Table 4.12. Common presenting gastrointestinal conditions and differential diagnoses in hamsters.

Condition	Differential Diagnoses
Anorexia	Noninfectious
	Dental disease (malocclusion, deformities)
	Insufficient water supply
	Intestinal accident
	Amyloidosis
	Pain
	Neoplasia
	Infectious
	Secondary to disease—see below
Diarrhea	Noninfectious
	Dietary indiscretion (carbohydrate overload)
	Low-fiber diet
	Inappropriate use of antibiotics (*C. difficile* overgrowth)
	Intestinal amyloidosis
	Infectious
	Bacterial enterocolitis, e.g., *Lawsonia intracellularis*, *Clostridium piliforme* (Tyzzer's disease), *C. perfringens*, *C. difficile*, *E. coli*, *Salmonella* spp
	Protozoal infection, e.g., giardiasis, spironucleosis
Constipation	Noninfectious
	Obesity
	Inappropriate diet (low fiber)
	Lack of exercise
	Infectious
	Cestode impaction, e.g., *Rodentolepis* spp, *Hymenolepis* spp

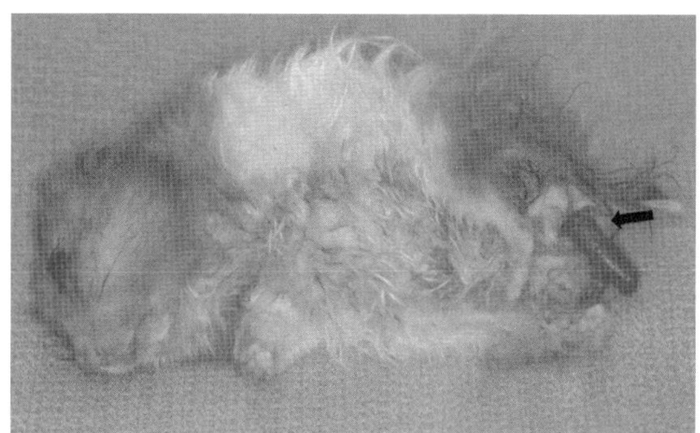

FIGURE 4.12. Prolapsed rectum in a hamster (arrow).

bedding ingestion with subsequent impaction. In general, cestode infestation is innocuous and subclinical in hamsters. Both *R. nana* and *H. diminuta* are zoonotic and *R. nana* may be transmitted directly to humans, without an intermediate host.

Oxyuriasis is common, usually involving species that affect other rodents (i.e., *Syphacia* spp); however, heavy burdens may be maintained with no apparent clinical signs.

Cardiopulmonary Conditions

Nasal Discharge

Nasal discharge is uncommon in hamsters but may be induced by irritation from volatile oils found in nonautoclaved softwood bedding (Table 4.13).

Table 4.13. Common presenting cardiopulmonary conditions and differential diagnoses in hamsters.

Condition	Differential Diagnoses
Nasal Discharge/ Rhinitis/Sneezing	Noninfectious
	Irritation (volatile oils from softwood bedding)
	Nasal polyps
	Infectious
	Bacterial infection, e.g., *Pasteurella pneumotropica, Staphylococcus aureus, Streptococcus* spp
Dyspnea	Noninfectious
	Heat stress
	Primary cardiac disease (cardiomyopathy, atrial thrombosis)
	Systemic disease
	Aspiration pneumonia
	Neoplasia, e.g., lymphoma with pleural effusion, pulmonary adenoma
	Infectious
	Bacterial pneumonia, e.g., *Bordetella bronchiseptica, Streptococcus* spp, *Pasteurella pneumotropica, Staphylococcus aureus, Klebsiella pneumomiae*
	Viral infection, e.g., Sendai virus

Neoplasms other than nasal polyps are rare in hamsters, as is bacterial rhinitis.

Dyspnea

Both cardiomyopathy and atrial thrombosis are common in aging hamsters. Typical signs of disease include cyanosis, weight loss, reduced activity, and rapid, shallow breathing. Cardiomyopathy is a progressive, autosomal recessive condition in some strains of Syrian hamsters. Treatment of cardiomyopathy is symptomatic, and drug doses may be extrapolated from other small animal species, with careful monitoring. Left atrial thrombosis occurs more commonly in female hamsters and at an earlier age than in males. The disease appears to be related to androgen levels, as neutered males have an increased susceptibility to developing the disease compared with intact males.

Respiratory disease is also common in hamsters, and most frequently induced by bacterial infections, such as *Streptococcus* spp, *Pasteurella pneumotropica, Bordetella* spp, or *Klebsiella pneumoniae*. Viral rhinitis and pneumonia secondary to Sendai virus infection tend to be subclinical and mild but may predispose animals to more serious secondary bacterial infections. Heat stress, severe systemic disease of any cause, aspiration of bedding or food, and neoplasia may also induce dyspnea in hamsters.

Endocrine Conditions

Adrenocortical disease is one of the most common conditions of hamsters, typically affecting older males, and may result from either primary hyperadrenocorticism (adrenocortical hyperplasia or adenoma) or secondary hyperadrenocorticism following ACTH release from a pituitary tumor. The clinical signs are typical, including bilaterally symmetrical flank alopecia, hyperpigmentation, comedones, polyuria, and polydipsia. Hamsters secrete both cortisol and corticosterone, so serum cortisol results may not be diagnostic. The diagnosis is typically based on clinical signs, and defining an appropriate medical treatment regime is difficult.

Diabetes mellitus is seen commonly in certain strains of the Chinese hamster and presents as weight loss, polyuria, polydipsia, and glycosuria. Treatment is supportive with weight management, reduction of carbohydrate treats, and insulin.

Both thyroid gland tumors and hypothyroidism are reported in Syrian hamsters.

Nervous and Musculoskeletal Conditions

Trauma and musculoskeletal injury are common in hamsters, due to fighting, falls, and overenthusiastic restraint (Table 4.14). Hamsters are frequently osteoporotic because of inappropriate diets and should be restrained gently. Hamsters are an important source of lymphocytic choriomeningitis virus (LCMV) infection in humans. The condition is generally subclinical in hamsters but may be transmitted to human handlers during routine handling. Appropriate hygiene should always be undertaken after handling hamsters. Other nervous and musculoskeletal conditions are rare.

Ocular Conditions

Bacteria, bedding dust, bite wounds, and LCMV infection can cause conjunctival reaction or infection

Table 4.14. Common presenting nervous and musculoskeletal conditions and differential diagnoses in hamsters.

Condition	Differential Diagnoses
Head Tilt/ Torticollis	Noninfectious
	Trauma
	Cerebrovascular accident
	Toxins, e.g., lead (paint)
	Neoplasia
	Infectious
	Otitis media/interna secondary to bacterial infection, e.g., *Pasteurella pneumotropica, Staphylococcus aureus*
	Brain abscess
Seizures	Noninfectious
	Heat stroke
	Hypoxia
	Idiopathic seizure
	Severe systemic disease
	Neoplasia
	Infectious
	Bacterial encephalitis/meningitis/abscess, e.g., *Streptococcus* spp
Paresis/Paralysis	Noninfectious
	Trauma (leg/muscle)
	Compression (overrestraint)
	Fractures, e.g., osteoporosis
	Osteoarthritis
	Severe anemia, e.g., tumor
	Severe inanition
	Infectious
	Spinal abscess

in hamsters. A hamster-specific cytomegalovirus has been reported to induce sialodacryoadenitis. Tooth root infections can extend into the orbit forming a retrobulbar abscess, and trauma to the eyeball may lead to corneal opacity or rupture of the globe. Proptosis may be induced in hamsters iatrogenically during restraint because of their shallow orbits. The eye can be enucleated or sometimes can be carefully cleaned and replaced, using sterile lubricant, under anesthesia.

Genitourinary Conditions

Renal Conditions

Chronic renal failure is common in aging hamsters and is often caused by an idiopathic condition (nephrosclerosis) or renal amyloidosis (Table 4.15). Clinical signs include weight loss, anorexia, ascites, polyuria, and polydipsia. Treatment is supportive and the prognosis is grave. Multiple renal, hepatic, or biliary cysts are occasionally noted at necropsy in

Table 4.15. Common presenting genitourinary conditions and differential diagnoses in hamsters.

Condition	Differential Diagnoses
Renal Conditions	Noninfectious Chronic renal failure (nephrosclerosis) Hydronephrosis Amyloidosis Polycystic disease Neoplasia, e.g., lymphoma Infectious Pyelonephritis/nephritis/cystitis secondary to bacterial infection, e.g., *Staphylococcus aureus, E. coli* Renal abscess
Uterine/Ovarian Conditions	Noninfectious Cystic endometrial hyperplasia Infertility, e.g., inadequate protein or fat, inappropriate light cycle, senescence, immaturity, mate incompatibility, low ambient temperature Abortion, e.g., stress, hyperthermia, trauma Neoplasia, e.g., granulosa cell tumor, uterine adenocarcinoma Infectious Pyometra/metritis following bacterial infection, e.g., *Pasteurella multocida, Staphylococcus aureus*
Mammary Gland Conditions	Noninfectious Neoplasia Infectious Mastitis, e.g., *S. aureus*
Male Reproductive Conditions	Noninfectious Trauma Neoplasia Infectious Orchitis and epididymitis following fighting injury and bacterial infection

older Syrian hamsters. Cysts are thin-walled and filled with clear fluid. They are likely congenital in nature and are considered incidental.

Reproductive Conditions

Female hamsters normally produce a copious stringy discharge postovulation, which has a distinctive smell. This should not be mistaken for pyometra, which is rare in hamsters. Ovarian thecal or granulosa cell tumors occur with relatively high frequency, and uterine adenocarcinoma is common in certain lines of dwarf hamsters. Mammary conditions including mastitis and mammary adenocarcinoma are seen sporadically in hamsters. Treatment for most reproductive conditions is ovariohysterectomy.

Infertility

Actual or apparent infertility in hamsters may be due to immaturity (younger than 5 weeks) or senescence (older than 15 months), low-protein or low-fat diets, cold ambient temperatures, prolonged darkness with or without single, short light exposures every 24 hours (reversible), normal winter breeding quiescence, pair incompatibility, inadequate nest, or using anestrus females just removed from an all-female group. Virgin hamsters older than 6–7 months exhibit a high degree of infertility on first breeding.

Prenatal Mortality

Nutritional deficiencies (caloric or protein), systemic disease, large fetal loads, and environmental stress may lead to fetal loss. Maternal destruction of neonates or sucklings, usually accompanied by cannibalism, is common among hamsters, especially in group-housed hamsters with a strong sense of territory. Cannibalism can be precipitated by handling the young (when younger than 10 days) or the nest, disturbing the mother, leaving the male in the cage beyond 1 week postpartum, not providing adequate nesting material or privacy, agalactia or mastitis, noise, changing the husbandry routine, the presence of sick or deformed young, or insufficient feed or water. There is little difference in maternal behaviors between primiparous and multiparous dams.

Sudden Death

Death after nonspecific signs or without preceding signs may be due to such geriatric conditions as atrial thrombosis, amyloidosis (more common in females), cardiomyopathy, renal disease, and neoplasia. Other fatal conditions include trauma, inadequate access to water, enteric disease, chilling or overheating, and antibiotic-induced intestinal dysbiosis. Rare conditions resulting in sudden death include salmonellosis, tularemia, streptococcal infection, and pregnancy ketosis. Hamsters may estivate if the ambient temperature drops below 15 °C and may appear comatose or dead. This should not be mistaken for sudden death and animals may be revived with judicious rewarming.

References

Budman LA, D'Amico TA. Heart lesions in a white hamster. Lab Anim. 1994, 23:17–18.

Chesterman FC, Pomerance A. Cirrhosis and liver tumors in a closed colony of golden hamsters. Br J Cancer. 1965, 19:802–811.

Cunnane SC, Bloom SR. Intussusception in the Syrian golden hamster. B J Nutr. 1990, 63:231–237.

Davis AJ, Jenkins S. Cryptosporidiosis and proliferative ileitis in a hamster. Vet Pathol. 1986, 23:632–633.

Griffin HE, et al. Hamster limb loss. Lab Anim. 1989, 18:19–20.

Heatley JJ. Cardiovascular anatomy, physiology, and diseases of rodents and small exotic mammals. Vet Clin Exot Anim. 2009, 12:99–113.

Karbe E. Disseminated mycobacteriosis in the golden hamster. Zentrabl Veterinarmed [B]. 1987, 34:391–394.

Kummeneje K, Nesbakken T, Mikkelsen T. Streptococcus agalactiae infection in a hamster. Acta Vet Scand. 1975, 16:554–556.

Lesher RJ, Jeszenka EV, Swan ME. Enteritis caused by Pasteurella pneumotropica infection in hamsters. J Clin Microbiol. 1985, 22:448.

Lisk RD, Langenber KK, Buntin JD. Blocked sexual receptivity in grouped female golden hamsters: independence from ovarian function and continuous group maintenance. Biol Reprod. 1980, 22:237–242.

Marques DM, Valenstein ES. Individual differences in aggressiveness of female hamsters: response to intact and castrated males and to females. Anim Behav. 1977, 25:131–139.

McMartin DN. Morphologic lesions in aging Syrian hamsters. J Gerontol. 1979, 34:502–511.

Meshorer A. Leg lesions in hamsters caused by wood shavings. Lab Anim Sci. 1976, 26:827–829.

Nelson WB. Fatal hairball in a long-haired hamster. Vet Med Small Anim Clin. 1975, 70:1193.

Pollock WB. Prolapse of invaginated colon through the anus in golden hamsters (Mesocricetus auratus). Lab Anim Sci. 1975, 25:334–336.

Pour P, et al. Spontaneous tumors and common diseases in two colonies of Syrian hamsters. I. Incidence and sites. J Nat Cancer Inst. 1976, 56:931–935.

Rudeen PK, Reiter RJ. Influence of a skeleton photoperiod on reproductive organ atrophy in the male golden hamster. J Reprod Fertil. 1980, 60:279–283.

Saunders GK, Scott DW. Cutaneous lymphoma resembling mycosis funguides in the Syrian hamster (Mesocricetus auratus). Lab Anim Sci. 1988, 38:616–617.

Schmidt RE, Reavill DR. Cardiovascular disease in hamsters: review and retrospective study. J Exot Pet Med. 2007, 16:49–51.

Srivastrava KK. Impaction of the cheek pouch in a Syrian (golden) hamster. Contemp Top Lab Anim Sci. 1992, 31:26–27.

Wise DA. Aggression in the female golden hamster: effects of reproductive state and social isolation. Horm Behav. 1974, 5:235–250.

Yoon CH, Peterson JS, Corrow D. Spontaneous seizures: a new mutation in Syrian golden hamsters. J Hered. 1976, 67:115–116.

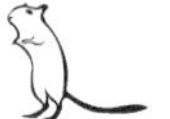

THE GERBIL

Skin Conditions

Alopecia

Mechanical irritation with a resulting bald nose may occur if there are rough points on the feeder or cage and barbering will occur if animals are overcrowded (Table 4.16). Endocrine-associated bilaterally symmetrical alopecia is relatively common in older gerbils and often is secondary to cystic ovaries or hyperadrenocorticism. Fighting, trauma, poor diets, and high relative humidity are also associated with hair loss. Degloving injuries of the tail (tail slip) may occur when the tip is grasped. This is treated with amputation proximal to the injury.

Swellings and Masses

Tail and perianal abscesses may occur from fighting if animals are overcrowded. Cutaneous neoplasia occurs with high incidence in gerbils. The most common tumor is associated with the ventral marking gland and may be a benign adenoma or malignant adenocarcinoma (see Figure 3.40). In either case, complete resection is generally curative. Other tumors include squamous cell carcinoma, melanoma, mastocytoma, epitheliotropic lymphoma, basal cell carcinoma, and aural cholesteatoma. This last tumor is only found in gerbils and humans. Mammary tumors have not been reported in gerbils.

Dermatitis

Ectoparasite infestations are uncommon but can be treated with amitraz or ivermectin when they occur. Focal ulcerative dermatitis may be seen with *Demodex meroni* infestation and fur mites (*Acarus farris* and *Liponyssoides sanguineus*). Nasal dermatitis (sore nose) is common, with or without conjunctivitis and forepaw dermatitis, particularly in group-housed animals stressed by overcrowding, dirty bedding, and high intracage humidity (Figure 4.13). This condition is thought to be due to hypersecretion of porphyrin-containing secretions from the Harderian gland, with accumulation of the irritating material around the nares and eyes. The condition can lead to self-trauma and frequently focal ulceration with secondary staphylococcal infection. Improving general management and husbandry, reducing overcrowding, and providing gerbils with a sand bath at regular intervals may all assist with clearing this condition.

Gastrointestinal Conditions

Major gastrointestinal conditions of gerbils are very similar to those seen in hamsters (refer to Table 4.12). Gerbils are exquisitely sensitive to *Clostridium*

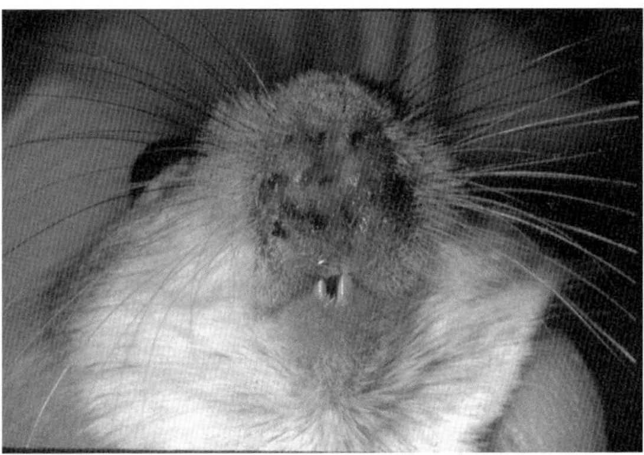

FIGURE 4.13. Nasal dermatitis in a gerbil.

Table 4.16. Common presenting skin conditions and differential diagnoses in gerbils.

Condition	Differential Diagnoses
Alopecia	Noninfectious
	Fighting/trauma
	Mechanical, e.g., food hopper
	Nutritional deficiencies, e.g., protein
	High relative humidity (>50%)
	Endocrine-associated, e.g., Cushing's disease, ovarian cysts
	Infectious
	Dermatophytosis, e.g., *Trichophyton* spp
	Demodecosis, e.g., *D. aurati, D. criceti*
Swellings/ Masses	Noninfectious
	Trauma/hemorrhage
	Neoplasia, e.g., ventral marking gland tumor, melanoma, aural cholesteatoma, basal cell carcinoma, squamous cell carcinoma, epitheliotropic lymphoma
	Infectious
	Abscesses, e.g., *Staphylococcus* spp, *Proteus* spp
	Mastitis
Dermatitis	Noninfectious
	Fighting/bite wounds
	Nutritional deficiencies, e.g., low protein
	Tail slip
	Coarse bedding
	Lack of dust bath (nasal dermatitis)
	Infectious
	Bacterial, e.g., *Staphylococcus* spp
	Infection of the ventral marking gland
	Dermatophytosis, e.g., *Trichophyton* spp
	Parasitic, e.g., mites (*Acarus* spp, *Demodex* spp)

piliforme infection and will often be found dead peracutely following infection. *Citrobacter rodentium* has also been associated with massive outbreaks of diarrhea and mortality in colonies of gerbils. Gerbils may occasionally be infested with an intestinal pinworm, *Dentostomella translucida*, or other species of rodent pinworms (*Syphacia* spp); however, these infestations tend to be subclinical, even with relatively heavy burdens. Obesity and hypercholesterolemia are common in gerbils fed all seed diets, particularly sunflower seeds. Owners should be advised to purchase an appropriate high-quality pelleted diet and to only feed seeds as an occasional treat.

Cardiopulmonary Conditions

Myocardial degeneration may occur spontaneously in gerbils. A serous nasal discharge may be associated with heat stress, allergy, or, rarely, respiratory infection. Pneumonia is seen infrequently in pet or laboratory gerbils and tends to be due to Gram-negative bacterial infection. Pulmonary edema or pleural effusion from mediastinal masses or diaphragmatic hernia also may cause dyspnea.

Endocrine Conditions

Diabetes mellitus has been reported as a sequela to obesity in gerbils. Clinical signs are typical of those seen in other small animal species and include polydipsia, polyuria, glycosuria, and hyperglycemia. Dietary management with weight loss has been described for treatment. Hyperadrenocorticism secondary to adrenal gland or pituitary tumors is rarely reported in gerbils and may be associated with symmetrical alopecia, polydipsia, and polyuria. Cystic ovaries occur commonly in older females and can induce abdominal distension, dyspnea, and endocrine-associated alopecia. Ovariohysterectomy is curative.

Nervous and Musculoskeletal Conditions

Gerbils routinely stomp their feet rapidly to communicate or signal danger to other gerbils. This should not be misinterpreted as seizure activity or ataxia.

Head Tilt

Otitis interna or encephalitis may cause a head tilt, although gerbils have a seeming resistance to otitis media. Such resistance may be associated with an effective ear drainage system. Keratin plugs produced by aural cholesteatomas may also induce head tilt.

Incoordination and Seizures

Epileptiform seizures in gerbils are hypnotic, cataleptic, or convulsive episodes with a variable threshold for onset. These seizures, initiated by handling, startling, sudden loud noises, or environmental change, occur in approximately 20–30% of the gerbil population, although the incidence of this genetically influenced trait ranges from near zero to very high. Gerbils are also highly susceptible to cerebrovascular accidents because of their unique cerebral circulation. Anesthetized animals should always be supplemented with oxygen until fully recovered to minimize hypoxemia and central ischemic events.

Ocular Conditions

Gerbils may develop primary conjunctivitis, dacryoadenitis usually associated with *Pasteurella pneumotropica*, other ocular disease following *Staphylococcus* spp infections, or ocular disorders secondary to debilitating systemic disease. Ocular disorders in gerbils often are associated with inflammation, enlargement of the globe or prolapse of the retroorbital Harderian glands. Dust and irritating volatile oils from softwood bedding can also cause increased lacrimation. Gerbils often secrete red porphyrin-containing tears in response to nonspecific stressors (chromodacryorrhea).

Genitourinary Conditions

Renal Conditions

Chronic renal failure (interstitial nephritis, tubular nephrosis, glomerulonephropathy) occurs commonly in gerbils older than 1 year of age and is likely related to long-term feeding of inappropriate diets. Gerbils are also susceptible to systemic amyloidosis and may present with nonspecific signs of weight loss, inappetence, and poor hair coat. Pyelonephritis secondary to *Citrobacter rodentium* infection, renal cysts, and hydronephrosis has been uncommonly reported. General treatment for renal disease of noninfectious origin is supportive with attempts to reduce protein and phosphorus in the diet.

Infertility

Gerbils are considered monogamous animals, and the loss of a mate may abrogate mating interest in the survivor. Gerbils have a high incidence of reproductive disorders, especially ovarian or periovarian cysts or neoplasms. Females with large ovarian cysts may be presumed pregnant because of cystic abdominal enlargement. Other causes of infertility in the gerbil include pair incompatibility, sexual immaturity or senescence (older than 18 months), overcrowding, pesticide or other toxin ingestion or absorption, nutritional deficiencies, environmental disturbances, very low temperatures, and various systemic diseases.

Prenatal Mortality

Abortions and stillbirths are difficult to detect because the fetal remains are often buried or consumed. Prenatal deaths may be induced by nutritional deficiencies, systemic or genital disease, trauma, or stress.

Litter Desertion or Death

Approximately 20% of young gerbils do not survive to weaning because of lack of maternal care, lactation failure, suffocation, crushing, or inability to reach or operate feeders or waterers. Maternal neglect or lactation failure may also result from wire-floored or transparent caging, lack of nesting material, lack of water, small litters (1–2 pups), environmental disturbances, presence of an aggressive male, or abnormal or injured young. Loss of an imperfect or threatened litter results in the dam's return to estrus. One of the most common causes of cannibalism among rodents is food or water deprivation.

Sudden Death

Chilling or overheating, septicemia, renal failure, Tyzzer's disease, amyloidosis, starvation or dehydration, neoplasia, and trauma all may cause sudden death in gerbils.

References

Bresnahan JF, et al. Nasal dermatitis in the Mongolian gerbil. Lab Anim Sci. 1983, 33:258–263.

Farrar PL, et al. Experimental nasal dermatitis in the Mongolian gerbil: effect of bilateral harderian gland adenectomy on development of facial lesions. Lab Anim Sci. 1988, 38:72–76.

Heatley JJ. Cardiovascular anatomy, physiology, and diseases of rodents and small exotic mammals. Vet Clin Exot Anim. 2009, 12:99–113.

Loskota WJ, Lomas P, Rich ST. The gerbil as a model for the study of epilepsies. Seizure patterns and ontogenesis. Epilepsia. 1974, 15:109–119.

Robbins MEC. Seizure resistance in albino gerbils. Lab Anim. 1976, 10:233–235.

Ross CR, et al. Experimental transmission of Syphacia muris among rats, mice, hamsters and gerbils. Lab Anim Sci. 1980, 30:35–37.

Vincent AL, Rodrick GE, Sodeman WA, Jr. The pathology of the Mongolian gerbil (Meriones unguiculatus): a review. Lab Anim Sci. 1979, 29:645–651.

White MR. Ovarian cysts in an aged gerbil. Lab Anim. 1990, 19:20–22.

Wightman SR, Mann PC, Wagner JE. Dihydrostreptomycin toxicity in the Mongolian gerbil (Meriones unguiculatus). Lab Anim Sci. 1980, 30:71–75.

Wightman SR, Pilitt PA, Wagner JE. Dentostomella translucida in the Mongolian gerbil (Meriones unguiculatus). Lab Anim Sci. 1978, 28:290–296.

Yahr P, et al. Effects of castration on aggression between male Mongolian gerbils. Behav Biol. 1977, 19:189–205.

Yahr P, Kessler S. Suppression of reproduction in water-deprived Mongolian gerbils (Meriones unguiculatus). Biol Reprod. 1975, 12:249–254.

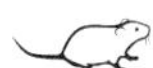

THE MOUSE

Skin Conditions

Alopecia

Barbering is a common observation among cages of mice, particularly among adult breeding mice (Table 4.17). The muzzle and other areas of the body are shaved closely by cagemates in strain-specific patterns. The behavior is learned and is not necessarily performed by the most dominant animal in the cage. When seen, it is usually a sign of overcrowding, social problems requiring regrouping, or a need for increased cage complexity. Although usually only superficial hair chewing occurs, occasionally the skin is abraded, which may represent a site of entry for bacteria, leading to abscess or ulcer formation. Hair thinning or loss in mice is frequently associated with acariasis (*Myobia musculi, Myocoptes musculinus*, and *Radfordia affinis*), and in some strains, infestation may result in intense pruritus with overgrooming and self-traumatization. Treatment is with ivermectin or selamectin, although caution should be exercised when using either of these agents with breeding mice because of the potential for teratogenesis and neonatal toxicity. Another cause of hair loss is abrasion on feeders or cage tops. Dermatophytosis (*T. mentagrophytes*) is often subclinical or may cause focal hair loss with well-demarcated patches of crusting. Treatment is with oral griseofulvin or either of enilconazole or ketoconazole as a wash. Hereditary hairless and nude (athymic) strains of mice are used in some research applications. Older mice may develop rough hair coats and seborrhea.

Swellings and Masses

Abscesses from fighting wounds are common in most mouse strains, are seen more frequently in males, and are most frequently associated with secondary *Staphylococcus aureus* infection (Figure 4.14). In some cases, serotypes of this bacterium are

Table 4.17. Common presenting skin conditions and differential diagnoses in mice.

Condition	Differential Diagnoses
Alopecia	Noninfectious
	Barbering
	Fighting/trauma
	Hereditary hairlessness
	Mechanical, e.g., feeder
	Nutritional deficiencies, e.g., zinc, protein
	Infectious
	Dermatophytosis, e.g., *Trichophyton* spp
	Fur mite infestation, e.g., *Myobia musculi, Myocoptes musculinus, Radfordia affinis*
Swellings/Masses	Noninfectious
	Trauma/hemorrhage
	Neoplasia (lymphoma, mammary adenocarcinoma)
	Infectious
	Abscesses, e.g., *Staphylococcus* spp, *Proteus* spp
	Granulomas
	Mastitis
Dermatitis	Noninfectious
	Fighting/bite wounds
	Hypersensitivity
	Gangrenous necrosis from nesting material fibers
	Nutritional deficiencies, e.g., low protein or fat
	Ringtail (low humidity or temperature)
	Infectious
	Bacterial, e.g., *Staphylococcus* spp
	Dermatophytosis, e.g., *Trichophyton* spp
	Parasitic, e.g., fur mites (*Myobia musculi, Myocoptes musculinus, Radfordia affinis*), lice (*Polyplax serrata*)
	Viral, e.g., mousepox

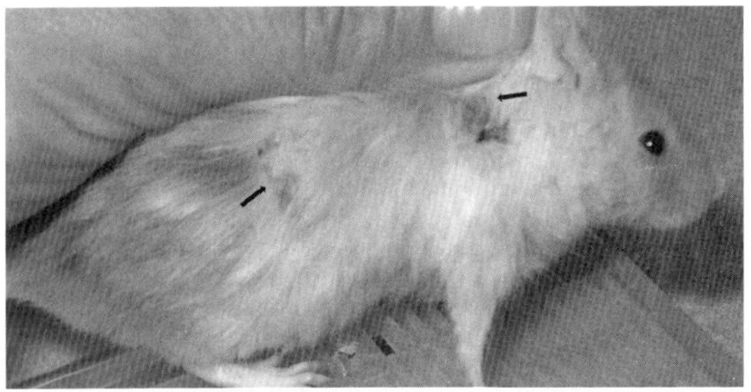

FIGURE 4.14. Multifocal areas of superficial ulceration and crusting in a pet mouse (arrows). The cause for the condition was unknown. Courtesy of Irene Phillips.

similar to those found on the skin of human handlers, suggesting that anthropozoonotic transmission of the bacterium may occur. Cutaneous neoplasia is rare but squamous cell carcinoma has been reported. Retrovirus-induced mammary adenocarcinoma occurs with relatively high frequency in older females, and because of the broad distribution of mammary tissue, masses may be found anywhere from the back of the tail, along the sides and ventrum, to the back of the neck. Metastases occur late in the process and lumpectomy with ovariohysterectomy is often curative. Multicentric lymphoma may present

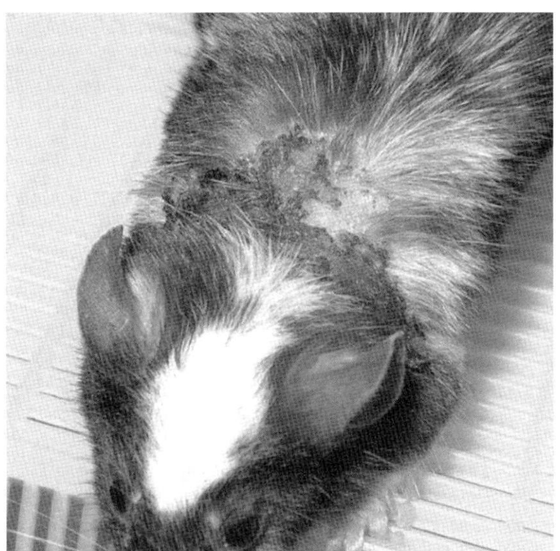

FIGURE 4.15. Severe ulcerative dermatitis on the shoulders and back of a mouse, likely due to a hypersensitivity reaction. Courtesy of Irene Phillips.

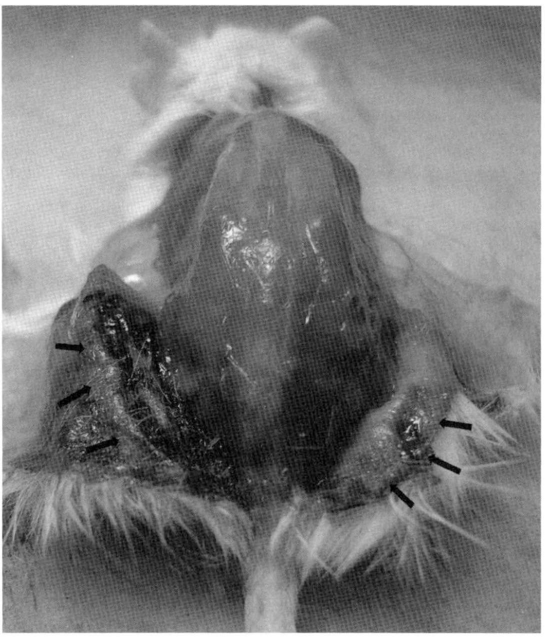

FIGURE 4.16. Necropsy photo of severe bilateral posterior cellulitis (arrows) that had presented clinically as posterior paresis in a male mouse, induced by fighting. Courtesy of David Hobson.

as masses within the cervical, axillary, or inguinal areas.

Low environmental humidity (<20%) can cause ringtail, in which one or more annular constrictions develop on the tail in association with edema, necrosis, and sloughing of the distal tissue.

Dermatitis

Acariasis, pediculosis (*Polyplax serrata*), and bite wounds are common causes of dermatitis. Severe lice infestations may lead to anemia in younger animals. Allergies to fur mite antigens, exacerbated by self-traumatization, present as highly pruritic lesions on the back, neck, head, and shoulders. These lesions range from simple alopecia to small scabs to extensive superficial ulcerative dermatitis, particularly in mice with a C57BL/6 background (black mice) (Figure 4.15). C57BL/6 mice may also develop an idiopathic ulcerative dermatitis, the cause of which remains uncertain. A necrotic dermatitis caused by an autoimmune vasculitis has been reported in a number of strains and may present as necrosis of the tips of the ears and tail. Bite wounds, common among group-housed male mice, are usually seen on the rump, preputial area, and tail (Figure 4.16). Mice should be picked up regularly and examined thoroughly for signs of fighting and incompatibility. Biting of the preputial or scrotal areas may cause localized preputial and scrotal infections, peritonitis, and even spinal meningitis. Adhesions may develop between the intestines and the scrotal wall. Other causes of dermatitis in mice include mousepox, dietary deficiencies, and dermatophytosis. Infection with ectromelia virus (mousepox), a reportable disease in the United States, may lead to dry gangrene and amputation of the distal extremities, if mice are allowed to survive. Gangrenous necrosis of the distal extremities has also been reported in suckling mice when fibers of cotton nesting material used for enrichment become wrapped around their limbs. Swelling and dry gangrene of the tail are sometimes seen in infant mice and rats exposed to low humidity or low temperatures. The tail is used for thermoregulation in rats and mice and either of these environmental conditions may lead to shunting of blood away from the tail with subsequent ischemic necrosis. The condition presents as annular swellings around the tail vertebrae, lending it the common name of ringtail. Mild forms of the condition are reversible by adjusting environmental conditions if caught early in the process.

Gastrointestinal Conditions

Anorexia

Anorexia occurs frequently in mice and the cause may be difficult to pinpoint. Animals without access to fresh water will not eat. Mice should be monitored closely when new waterers are introduced to ensure that they are able to access and drink from them. Other causes of anorexia include malocclusion of the incisors with consequent difficulty prehending food, pain, neoplasia, and systemic disease (Table 4.18).

Diarrhea

Diarrhea in unweaned mice is often attributable to rotavirus (EDIM), reovirus, or coronavirus (MHV) infection. Rotavirus infection may be self-limiting; however, coronavirus infection is often lethal unless endemic in a colony. The feces are usually yellow and sticky, matting the neonatal hair. Tyzzer's disease; salmonellosis; *Citrobacter rodentium*, *Helicobacter* spp, *E. coli*, or *Enterococcus* spp

Table 4.18. Common presenting gastrointestinal conditions and differential diagnoses in mice.

Condition	Differential Diagnoses
Anorexia	Noninfectious
	Dental disease (malocclusion, deformities)
	Insufficient water supply
	Intestinal accident
	Amyloidosis
	Pain
	Neoplasia
	Infectious
	Secondary to disease—see below
Diarrhea	Noninfectious
	Dietary indiscretion (carbohydrate overload)
	Infectious
	Viral enterocolitis, e.g., coronavirus (mouse hepatitis virus), rotavirus (epizootic diarrhea of infant mice), reovirus
	Bacterial enterocolitis, e.g., *Citrobacter rodentium, Lawsonia intracellularis, E. coli*, *Salmonella* spp, *Enterococcus* spp, *Helicobacter* spp, *Clostridium piliforme*
	Protozoal infection, e.g., coccidiosis, giardiasis, spironucleosis
Constipation	Noninfectious
	Obesity
	Inappropriate diet (low fiber)
	Lack of exercise
Rectal Prolapse	Estrogenic stimulation
	Oxyuriasis, e.g., *Aspiculuris tetraptera*, *Syphacia obvelata*
	Chronic bacterial infection, e.g., *Helicobacter* spp, *Citrobacter rodentium*

infection; coccidiosis; giardiasis; spironucleosis; and various dietary factors all may cause diarrhea in mice. Pinworm infestation is common; however, the condition rarely causes clinical signs, even with a high parasite burden. Similarly, mice may be infected with cestodes (*Rodentolepis* spp and *Hymenolepis* spp) but clinical signs are rare.

Prolapsed Rectum

The rectum of mice is weakly anchored by the mesocolon and prone to prolapse with straining. Rectal prolapse may be seen with any condition inducing diarrhea, for example, MHV, *Helicobacter* spp, or *Citrobacter* spp infection, following perianal irritation caused by oxyurid infestation, or with estrogenic stimulation.

Cardiopulmonary Conditions

Myocardial degeneration and fibrosis are seen relatively commonly at necropsy in older mice; however, clinical disease is rarely noted. Significant epicardial and myocardial mineralization are also seen commonly in some strains of mice, for example, DBA, without apparent clinical effect, and the etiopathogenesis of this condition is unknown.

Nasal Discharge

Rhinitis may be induced in mice by dust or volatile oils present in softwood bedding (Table 4.19). Bacterial and viral infections often initiate as rhinitis with sneezing and conjunctivitis and may progress to lower respiratory infections and pneumonia depending on the immunocompetence of the mouse and whether there is secondary bacterial infection.

Sendai virus, *Mycoplasma pulmonis*, and *Pasteurella pneumotropica* infections are common causes of rhinitis. Less common respiratory pathogens include *Klebsiella pneumoniae*, *Corynebacterium kutscheri*, coronavirus infection, and ectromelia virus infection. Pulmonary adenomas are seen commonly in aging mice.

Endocrine Conditions

Spontaneous diabetes mellitus has been reported in obese mice fed high carbohydrate diets, but other spontaneous endocrine conditions are highly unusual.

Table 4.19. Common presenting cardiopulmonary conditions and differential diagnoses in mice.

Condition	Differential Diagnoses
Nasal Discharge/ Rhinitis/Sneezing	Noninfectious
	Irritation (dust, volatile oils from softwood bedding)
	Infectious
	Bacterial infection, e.g., *Pasteurella pneumotropica, Staphylococcus aureus, Streptococcus* spp
	Viral infection, e.g., Sendai virus
Dyspnea	Noninfectious
	Heat stress
	Primary cardiac disease (cardiomyopathy)
	Systemic disease
	Aspiration pneumonia
	Neoplasia, e.g., lymphoma, pulmonary adenoma
	Infectious
	Bacterial pneumonia, e.g., *Mycoplasma pulmonis*, CARB, *Streptococcus* spp, *Pasteurella pneumotropica, Staphylococcus aureus, Klebsiella pneumoniae*
	Viral infection, e.g., Sendai virus

Nervous and Musculoskeletal Conditions

Otitis media/interna is commonly seen in mice and may be due to infection with *Pasteurella pneumotropica*, *Streptococcus* spp, or other bacterial agents. Idiopathic vasculitis affecting cerebral arteries may also induce otitis interna and incoordination. Bacterial encephalitis and central neoplasia are uncommon; however, trauma from falls may lead to incoordination and seizures, and audiogenic seizures may occur in some strains of mice when exposed to sudden, loud noises. Mice can be carriers of LCMV but rarely show clinical signs of disease. Virus may be shed in the urine of asymptomatic mice.

Ocular Conditions

Conjunctivitis occurs commonly in mice and is generally attributable to infection with Sendai virus, *Pasteurella pneumotropica, P. aeruginosa, Streptococcus* spp, or *Mycoplasma pulmonis* infection. Irritation from dusty bedding or volatile oils from softwood bedding, high environmental ammonia levels, and lacrimal gland inflammation may also result in the condition.

Panophthalmitis

Pasteurella pneumotropica is the most common bacterial cause of orbital inflammation in mice, but *Pseudomonas* spp and LCMV infection may occur also.

Cataracts

Cataracts in mice may be caused by prolonged dessication of the globe, as may occur with surgery, genetic predisposition, and as a consequence of uveitis.

Corneal dystrophy is very common in mice and may appear as opacities on the corneal surface. Retinal degeneration commonly develops in albino strains as they age and is caused by exposure to excessive light levels. Microphthalmia is an inherited characteristic and seen frequently in some strains of mice.

Genitourinary Conditions

Renal Conditions

Renal disease is relatively common in mice and may be associated with infectious causes, such as bacterial cystitis and pyelonephritis in breeding females, usually secondary to *E. coli* or *Staphylococcus aureus* infection or chronic renal failure in aged rodents of both sexes (Table 4.20). Renal amyloidosis also occurs in older mice and may contribute to renal failure. Renal abscessation occurs sporadically, likely following bacteremia episodes, and renal cysts are generally congenital and incidental in nature. Hydronephrosis may be uni- or bilateral and may be congenital or acquired. Hydronephrosis with hydroureter may occur in aging males due to an ejaculatory plug lodged in the urethra. These animals present with abdominal distension and anorexia and generally have a poor prognosis.

Reproductive Conditions

Infertility

Reduced fertility or abortion in mice may be caused by chemicals; estrogenic stimulation, for example, phytoestrogens in the diets; inappropriate light cycles; immaturity or senescence; overcrowding; noise; metritis due to *Pasteurella pneumotropica, Mycoplasma pulmonis, Klebsiella oxytoca*, or *Streptobacillus moniliformis* infections; inbreeding; dichlorvos (used sometimes to treat fur mite infestations); low temperature; and nutritional restriction. Hydrometra due to imperforate hymen will also result in infertility, and breeding pairs producing these offspring should be culled, as the condition is heritable (Figure 4.17). Cystic endometrial hyperplasia and neoplasms such as uterine stromal polyp, leiomyoma, and granulosa cell tumor may occur in older females. Mammary adenocarcinoma is relatively common in mice, and the tumors are caused by retroviral infection (mouse mammary tumor virus). They are generally slow to metastasize. Bacterial orchitis, epididymitis, and preputial gland infection are not uncommon in male mice. Seminal vesicle impaction with massive abdominal distension may be seen in aged males, in addition to testicular tumors.

Litter Desertion or Death

Mouse litters are abandoned or destroyed if nests are inadequate, the litter is small, the pups are injured or abnormal, the dam is malnourished resulting in agalactia, the nest or young are disturbed or

Table 4.20. Common presenting genitourinary conditions and differential diagnoses in mice.

Condition	Differential Diagnoses
Renal Conditions	Noninfectious
	Chronic renal failure
	Hydronephrosis
	Urethral obstruction, e.g, ejaculatory plug
	Amyloidosis
	Renal cyst
	Neoplasia, e.g., lymphoma
	Infectious
	Pyelonephritis/nephritis/cystitis secondary to bacterial infection, e.g., *Staphylococcus aureus, E. coli*
	Renal abscess
Uterine/Ovarian Conditions	Noninfectious
	Cystic endometrial hyperplasia
	Hydrometra (imperforate hymen)
	Infertility, e.g., inadequate protein or fat, inappropriate light cycle, senescence, immaturity, low ambient temperature
	Abortion, e.g., stress, hyperthermia, trauma
	Neoplasia, e.g., uterine stromal polyp, leiomyoma, granulosa cell tumor, teratoma
	Infectious
	Pyometra/metritis following bacterial infection, e.g., *Pasteurella multocida, Staphylococcus aureus*
Mammary Gland Conditions	Noninfectious
	Neoplasia
	Infectious
	Mastitis, e.g., *S. aureus*
Male Reproductive Conditions	Noninfectious
	Trauma
	Seminal vesicle impaction
	Neoplasia
	Infectious
	Preputial gland abscess
	Orchitis and epididymitis following fighting injury and bacterial infection

handled, or the young become dehydrated or cold because of inadequate nest material, humidity, or temperature. A variety of environmental disturbances, such as high-pitched sound associated with cage washers and steam hoses, will cause maternal distress and litter abandonment. One of the most common causes of death in suckling mice is an epizootic MHV infection. Other pathogens, such as salmonella or rotavirus, can also affect maternal and litter health.

Uterine prolapse is uncommon but may follow dystocia or abortions of large fetuses.

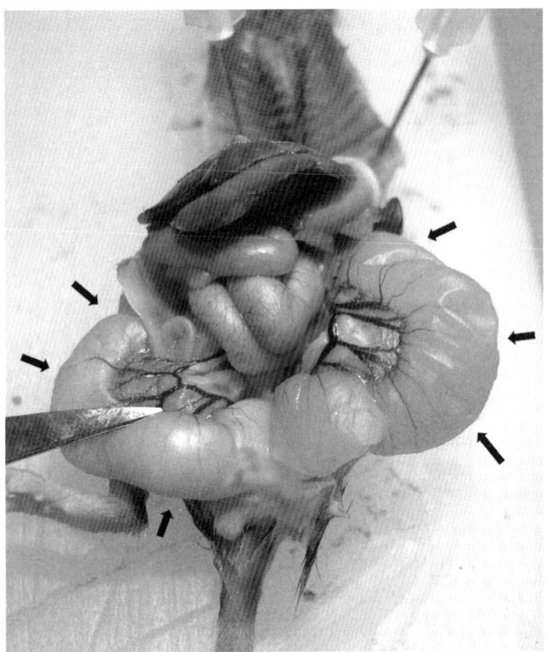

FIGURE 4.17. Necropsy photograph of marked hydrometra (arrows) in a female mouse. This animal had marked abdominal distension ante mortem. Courtesy of David Hobson.

Sudden Death

Mice die unexpectedly from dehydration, lack of access to feed, sudden environmental stressors or shock resulting in massive thymic involution or gastrointestinal hemorrhage, heat stress, trauma, urolithiasis in males, organophosphates, chronic renal disease, septicemia, and toxemia. Sendai virus and mouse hepatitis virus are particularly insidious killers of mice. Fighting and social incompatibility with resultant starvation may also result in death of subordinate animals.

References

Ackerman JI, Fox JG. Isolation of Pasteurella ureae from reproductive tracts of congenic mice. J Clin Microbiol. 1981, 13:1049–1053.

Anderson CK, Lozano EA. Pine needle toxicity in pregnant mice. Cornell Vet. 1977, 67:229–235.

Andrews AG, et al. Immune complex vasculitis with secondary ulcerative dermatitis in aged C57BL/6N Nia mice. Vet Pathol. 1994, 31:293–300.

Brownstein DG, Johnson E. Experimental nasal infection of normal and leukopenic mice with Pseudomonas aeruginosa. Vet Pathol. 1982, 19:169–178.

Davis JK, et al. The role of Klebsiella oxytoca in utero-ovarian infection of B6C3F1 mice. Lab Anim Sci. 1987, 37:159–166.

DeHeer DH, Edgington TS. Cellular events associated with the immunogenesis of antierythrocyte autoantibody responses of NZB mice. Transplant Rev. 1976, 31:116–155.

Duignan PJ, Percy DH. Diagnostic exercise: unexplained deaths in recently acquired C3H3 mice. Lab Anim Sci. 1992, 42:610–611.

Everitt JI, Ross PW, Davis TW. Urologic syndrome associated with wire caging in AKR mice. Lab Anim Sci. 1988, 38:609–611.

Fisk SK. Iatrogenic pneumothorax and pneumoderma in a mouse. Lab Anim Sci. 1976, 26:648.

Fredericks GR, et al. Ovulation rates and embryo degeneracy in female mice fed the phytoestrogen coumestrol. Proc Soc Exper Biol Med. 1981, 167:237–241.

Heatley JJ. Cardiovascular anatomy, physiology, and diseases of rodents and small exotic mammals. Vet Clin Exot Anim. 2009, 12:99–113.

Hoelter SM, et al. "Sighted C3H" mice—a tool for analyzing the influence of vision on mouse behavior? Front Biosci. 2008, 13:5810–5823.

Huerkamp MJ, Dillehay DL. Struvite uroliths in a male mouse. Lab Anim Sci. 1991, 41:642–643.

Kastenmayer RJ, Fain MA, Perdue KA. A retrospective study of idiopathic ulcerative dermatitis in mice with a C57BL/6 background. J Amer Assoc Lab Anim Sci. 2006, 45:8–12.

Ladd Beaumont S. Ocular disorders of pet mice and rats. Vet Clin Exot Anim. 2002, 5:311–324.

Lawson GW, Sato A, Fairbanks LA, Lawson PT. Vitamin E as a treatment for ulcerative dermatitis in C57BL/6 mice and strains with a C57BL/6 background. Contemp Top Lab Anim Sci. 2005, 44:18–21.

Maronpot RR, Chavannes J-M. Dacryoadenitis, conjunctivitis, and facial dermatitis of the mouse. Lab Anim Sci. 1977, 27:277–278.

Marsteller FA, Lynch CB. Reproductive responses to variation in temperature and food supply by house mice: I. Mating and pregnancy. Biol Reprod. 1987, 37:838–843.

———. Reproductive responses to variation in temperature and food supply by house mice: II. Lactation. Biol Reprod. 1987, 37:844–850.

Newton WM. Environmental impact on laboratory animals. Adv Vet Sci Comp Med. 1978, 22:1–28.

Randelia HP, Deo MG, Lalitha VS. Megaesophagus in mouse-histochemical studies. Gastroenterol. 1988, 94:1243–1244.

Randelia HP, Panicker KNS, Lalitha VS. Megaesophagus in the mouse; histochemical and ultrastructural studies. Lab Anim. 1990, 24:78–86.

Rao GN, et al. Utero-ovarian infection in aged B6C3F1 mice. Lab Anim Sci. 1987, 37:153–158.

Reeves WK, Cobb KD. Ectoparasites of house mice (Mus musculus) from pet stores in South Carolina, USA. Comp Parasitol. 2005, 72:193–195.

Schneemilch HS. A naturally acquired infection of laboratory mice with Klebsiella capsule type 6. Lab Anim. 1976, 10:305–310.

Seyfried TN. Audiogenic seizures in mice. Fed Proc. 1979, 38:2399–2404.

Simpson W, Simmons DJC. Two Actinobacillus species isolated from laboratory rodents. Lab Anim. 1980, 14:15–16.

Stewart DD, et al. An epizootic of necrotic dermatitis in laboratory mice caused by Lancefield group G streptococci. Lab Anim Sci. 1975, 25:296–302.

Taylor DM, Neal DL. An infected eczematous condition in mice: methods of treatment. Lab Anim. 1980, 14:325–328.

Van den Broek FA, Orutzigt CM, Beynen AC. Whisker trimming behaviour in A2G mice is not prevented by offering means of withdrawal from it. Lab Anim. 1993, 27:270–272.

Wullenweber M, Kaspareit-Rittinghausen J, Farouq M. Streptobacillus moniliformis epizootic in barrier-maintained C57BL/6J mice. Lab Anim Sci. 1990, 40:608–612.

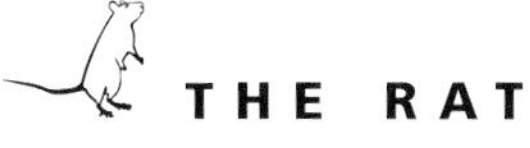

THE RAT

Skin Conditions

Alopecia

Hair loss or thinning without dermatitis is seen in some strains of rats, and hair loss may occur with accompanying dermatitis (Table 4.21). Dermatophytosis, abrasion on cages or bedding, and mutual grooming or barbering all produce hair loss with little or no grossly evident dermatitis.

Swelling and Masses

The most common subcutaneous masses in female rats are mammary tumors, a fibroadenoma in most cases, although adenocarcinomas do occur (Figure 4.18). These tumors may grow to become very large and can be removed surgically. Ovariohysterectomy is often curative, although tumors may still arise in neutered animals with prolactin-secreting pituitary adenomas. Other types of neoplasms do occur, such as fibrosarcoma, squamous cell carcinoma of the head, and rarely thyroid and salivary gland tumors. Auricular chrondromas and Zymbal's gland carcinomas occur commonly in some strains of rats (Figure 4.19). *Staphylococcus aureus, Pasteurella pneumotropica*, and *Klebsiella pneumoniae* abscesses occur uncommonly, as do arthropathies from *Streptobacillus* spp and *Erysipelothrix* spp infections. Cervical swelling may result from salivary gland inflammation, secondary to sialodacryoadenitis virus infection or multicentric lymphoma. *S. aureus* and *Pasteurella pneumotropica* may cause mastitis.

Dermatitis

Staphylococcus aureus, *Polyplax spinulosa*, and *Trichophyton mentagrophytes* are implicated occasionally as causative agents of rat dermatitis. *Ornithonyssus bacoti*, the tropical rat mite, is rare but has been reported in animals obtained from pet stores. Infection with this parasite is reportable, as it can transmit a variety of diseases to humans. Pruritis with secondary *Staphylococcus aureus* infection may result in ulcerative lesions on the neck and anterior trunk that are difficult to treat. Trimming the hind nails, topical treatment with zinc ointment, and administration of long-acting penicillin subcutaneously may help to resolve the condition. Infestation with the mite *Notoedres muris* may lead to a permanent and disfiguring auricular chondritis. *S. aureus* may also induce a gangrenous pododermatitis in colonies, which can be difficult to manage. Serotypes of the bacteria are often identical to those found on the skin of human handlers, suggesting that anthropozoonotic transmission of this bacterium may occur.

Fighting wounds are seen less commonly in group-housed rats of either sex but when present often occur on the side of the face or flank. Ringtail, as described for mice, also occurs in rat pups. Pododermatitis may be seen in rats housed on coarse or wet bedding, or when housed for prolonged periods of time on wire-bottom cages. Tail slip, as

Table 4.21. Common presenting skin conditions and differential diagnoses in rats.

Condition	Differential Diagnoses
Alopecia	Noninfectious Fighting/trauma Barbering Mechanical, e.g., feeder Nutritional deficiencies Infectious Dermatophytosis, e.g., *Trichophyton* spp Mite infestations, e.g., *Radfordia ensifera, Notoedres muris*
Swellings/Masses	Noninfectious Trauma/hemorrhage Neoplasia (mammary fibroadenoma, lymphoma, fibrosarcoma, Zymbal's gland carcinoma, squamous cell carcinoma) Infectious Abscesses, e.g., *Staphylococcus* spp, *Pasteurella pneumotropica* Granulomas Mastitis
Dermatitis	Noninfectious Fighting/bite wounds Nutritional deficiencies, e.g., low protein Rough bedding Infectious Bacterial, e.g., *Staphylococcus* spp Dermatophytosis, e.g., *Trichophyton* spp Parasitic, e.g., mites (*Notoedres* spp, *Demodex* spp), lice (*Polyplax spinulosa*)

described for gerbils, may occur in rats when they are picked up by the distal third of their tail. Treatment is as described for gerbils.

Gastrointestinal Conditions

Gastrointestinal disease is uncommon in rats. Malocclusion may occur from incisor overgrowth, leading to excess salivation and inability to prehend food.

Diarrhea associated with rotavirus infection has been reported in suckling rats but is generally mild and self-limiting. Tyzzer's disease with associated typhlitis is reported rarely in rats, although rats are common carriers of the bacterial spore. Pinworm (*S. muris, A. obvelata*) and cestode (*R. nana, Hymenolepis* spp) infections are generally subclinical, even in the face of high parasite burdens.

Cardiopulmonary Conditions

Rhinitis

Sniffling, sneezing, and serous nasal discharge are associated with respiratory mycoplasmosis commonly and less commonly with infection by

Corynebacterium kutscheri, Pasteurella pneumotropica, Streptococcus pneumoniae, S. zooepidemicus, and sialodacryoadenitis virus (coronavirus) infections (Table 4.22). A red ocular and nasal discharge, rich in lacrimal lipids and fluorescent porphyrins of Harderian gland origin, accompanies many debilitating diseases and stress conditions in rats (chromodacryorrhea).

Dyspnea

Myocardial fibrosis and degeneration may be seen commonly in older rats and may result in pulmonary edema and sudden collapse.

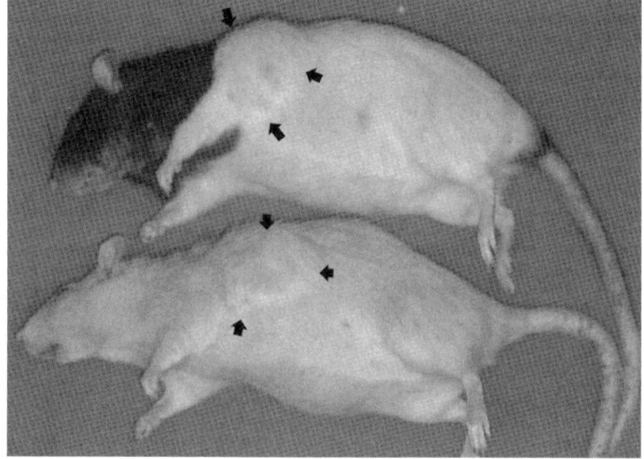

FIGURE 4.18. Mammary gland fibroadenomas (arrows) in aged sibling female rats.

Pneumonia in rats, often precipitated by ammonia-laden environments or under stressful or otherwise debilitating conditions, can be caused by *Mycoplasma pulmonis*, cilia-associated respiratory bacillus (CARB), *Streptococcus pneumoniae*, and *Pasteurella pneumotropica*. Less often *Corynebacterium kutscheri, Aspergillus* spp, *Streptococcus zooepidemicus*, and *Haemophilus* spp are involved.

Uncomplicated Sendai virus infection can cause death in pregnant or aged rats. These rats develop rough hair coats and dyspnea but not rhinitis. A putative new virus, termed rat respiratory virus, has been described in rats in North America and Europe. Affected animals may have no clinical signs but may die suddenly under anesthesia. Gross lesions consist of random, multifocal 1–4 mm flat to raised pale to plum-colored foci on the surface of the parenchyma. There is no evidence to date that the agent is zoonotic. Microscopically, lesions consist of perivascular infiltrates of neutrophils and macrophages (± lymphocytes) in 8- to 10-week-old rats. Lesions are most prominent in 10- to 12-week-old rats and consist of pyogranulomatous perivascular and peribronchiolar infiltrates with focal alveolitis, and hyperplasia of type II pneumocytes. The lesion resolves in older animals with just perivascular lymphoplasmacytic cuffing and multifocal alveolar

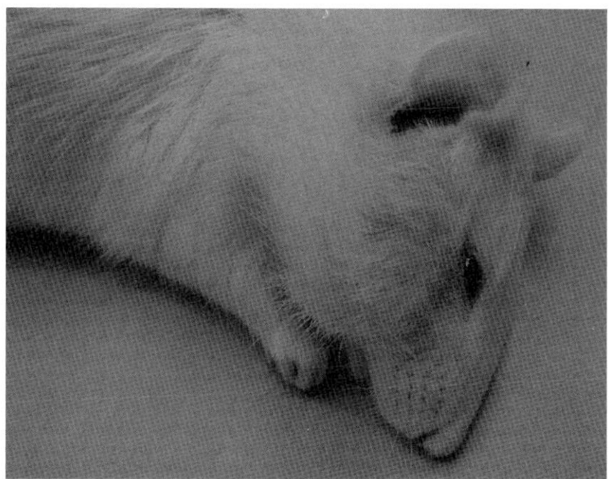

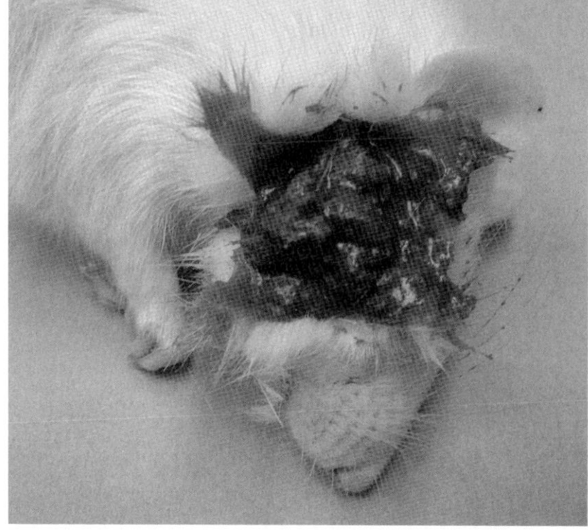

FIGURE 4.19. Facial swelling in a Fischer 344 rat at necropsy (left). Mass opened to demonstrate a Zymbal's gland carcinoma (right), a common neoplasm in aged F344 rats. Courtesy of Lisa B. Martin.

Table 4.22. Common presenting cardiopulmonary conditions and differential diagnoses in rats.

Condition	Differential Diagnoses
Nasal Discharge/ Rhinitis/Sneezing	Noninfectious
	Irritation (volatile oils from softwood bedding)
	Nasal foreign body
	Infectious
	Bacterial infection, e.g., *Mycoplasma pulmonis*, CARB, *Streptococcus pneumoniae, Corynebacterium kutscheri*
	Fungal, e.g., aspergillosis associated with corncob bedding
	Viral, e.g., SDAV
Dyspnea	Noninfectious
	Heat stress
	Primary cardiac disease (myocardial degeneration)
	Systemic disease
	Aspiration pneumonia
	Esophageal foreign body (choke)
	Neoplasia, e.g., lymphoma with chylothorax, pulmonary adenoma
	Infectious
	Larval migration through lungs
	Bacterial pneumonia, e.g., *Corynebacterium kutscheri, Streptococcus* spp, *Pasteurella pneumotropica, Staphylococcus aureus, Klebsiella pneumoniae*
	Viral infection, e.g., Sendai virus

macrophage aggregates. The virus has not been cultured and identified to date.

Chylothorax has been reported infrequently in rats and is associated with dyspnea. *Trichosomoides crassicauda*, a nematode that infects the urinary bladder of rats, may be associated with dyspnea and lung lesions during the time that larvae migrate through the lungs. Pulmonary adenoma is reported in aged rats.

Endocrine Conditions

Pituitary hyperplasia and adenoma are common conditions seen in aging rats of certain strains and are generally slow-growing, space-occupying masses that will eventually lead to neurologic signs such as seizures, head tilt, and paresis. Thyroid tumors (C cell origin) are common in older rats although they are rarely clinically important. Pancreatitis with destruction of pancreatic islets and resultant diabetes mellitus has been reported in rats. The condition is otherwise very rare in rats. Pancreatic islet cell tumor also occurs infrequently in older animals.

Nervous and Musculoskeletal Conditions

Head Tilt

Otitis media/interna, pituitary adenoma, and encephalitis may cause head tilt in rats. Otitis caused by *Mycoplasma pulmonis, Streptobacillus moniliformis, Streptococcus* spp, and *Pseudomonas aeruginosa* have all been reported (Table 4.23).

Incoordination and Seizures

Trauma, encephalitis, pituitary neoplasia, severe systemic disease, wasting, and otitis interna can lead to

Table 4.23. Common presenting nervous and musculoskeletal conditions and differential diagnoses in rats.

Condition	Differential Diagnoses
Head Tilt/Torticollis	Noninfectious Trauma Cerebrovascular accident Toxins, e.g., lead (paint) Neoplasia, e.g., pituitary adenoma Infectious Otitis media/interna secondary to bacterial infection, e.g., *Mycoplasma pulmonis, Staphylococcus aureus* Brain abscess
Seizures	Noninfectious Heat stroke Hypoxia Audiogenic seizure Severe systemic disease Neoplasia Infectious Bacterial encephalitis/meningitis/abscess, e.g., *Streptococcus* spp
Paresis/Paralysis	Noninfectious Trauma (leg/muscle) Fractures Osteoarthritis Degenerative disease, e.g., polyradiculoneuropathy Severe inanition Neoplasia, e.g., lymphoma, vertebral histiocytic sarcoma, pancreatic islet cell tumor (weakness, incoordination) Infectious Spinal abscess

incoordination in rats. Pancreatic islet cell tumor may lead to clinical signs of ataxia following pulsatile release of insulin with resulting hypoglycemia.

Paresis or Paralysis

Brain or spinal lesions (e.g., abscesses, phycomycosis, or neoplasia), trauma of the spinal cord, malnutrition, polyradiculoneuropathy, and ostearthritis can produce limb weakness or paralysis.

Abscesses at the head of the tail or in the perineum may extend into the spinal canal, resulting in myelitis.

Ocular Conditions

Chromodacryorrhea

Localized bacterial infections and sialodacryoadenitis virus produce blepharospasm, swelling, lacrimation, and sometimes a mucopurulent discharge. Red tears or chromodacryorrhea is a nonspecific sign of stress or underlying disease. The red pigments in tears are protoporphyrin IX and coproporphyrin III, synthesized de novo in the Harderian gland and expelled under parasympathetic discharge. The pigments are identified in dried tears by the orange-red fluorescence under ultraviolet light. The eyelids, nares, and forepaws may be smeared with the pigment. Unilateral involvement probably indicates atrophy of the secretory cells of one Harderian gland or blockage of a nasolacrimal duct.

Conjunctivitis

Conjunctivitis in rats with swelling and discharge may be caused by *Pasteurella pneumotropica, Streptococcus pneumoniae*, sialodacryoadenitis virus (SDAV), self-trauma, or dust or ammonia irritation. Conjunctivitis may be associated with other primary ocular diseases, including keratoconjunctivitis, uveitis, glaucoma, and corneal opacity. Hypovitaminosis A and SDAV are causes of keratoconjunctivitis.

Dacryoadenitis

Inflammation of the lacrimal glands is related to SDAV or rarely to bacterial infection of the glands.

Other Conditions

Corneal dystrophy is common in rats and is heritable. Corneal hypoxia, as occurs with certain injectable anesthetic agents, may lead to keratitis and ulceration. Supplemental oxygen, reversible anesthetic injectable agents, and sterile eye lubrication should always be used in rats to enhance postanesthetic recovery time and minimize the occurrence of this condition. Exophthalmos from Harderian gland enlargement (SDAV) can occur, as can microphthalmia.

Genitourinary Conditions

Renal Conditions

Chronic progressive nephrosis is a common life-threatening condition of older rats and is related to male sex, ad libitum feeding, age, and strain, for example, Sprague-Dawley rats (Table 4.24). Nephrocalcinosis is common in certain strains of rats and is more frequently seen in females as young as 7 weeks of age. Urolithiasis (commonly struvite) has been reported sporadically in rats fed normal diets (Figure 4.20). Hydronephrosis may be unilateral or bilateral and congenital or acquired in origin. Congenital hydronephrosis is often an incidental finding at necropsy, as are solitary renal cysts and renal polycystic disease. Acquired hydronephrosis may result from an ascending suppurative pyelonephritis and cystitis, commonly caused by *E. coli* or *Proteus* spp infection.

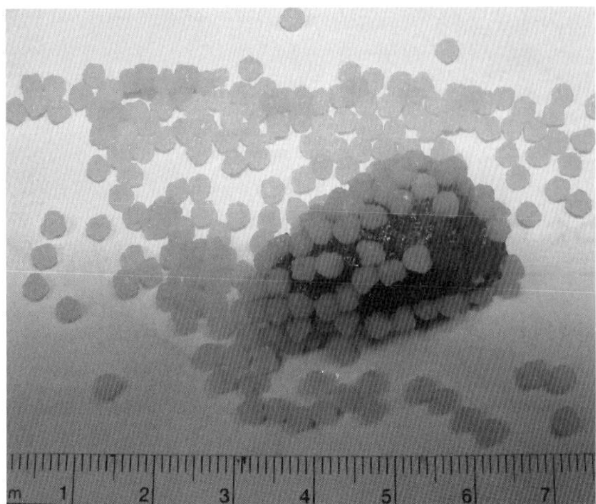

FIGURE 4.20. Uroliths from the urinary bladder of an 8-week-old female rat. Generally, animals have 1–10 stones; however, this case was somewhat unusual in that 266 stones were recovered. The urolith composition was largely calcium carbonate. Courtesy of Kresimir Pucaj.

Reproductive Conditions

Infertility

Rats younger than 70 days or older than 18 months of age may be sexually incompetent. Other causes of real or apparent infertility include vitamin E deficiency, protein deficiency, viral infection, for example, caused by Sendai virus, sialodacryoadenitis, rat virus, *Mycoplasma pulmonis*–related metritis, elevated temperature and humidity, constant light, and systemic disease. Vaginal prolapse may be seen rarely (Figure 4.21). Bacterial prostatitis may be seen in older males and cystic endometrial hyperplasia occurs in older female rats.

Litter Desertion or Death

Factors that may lead to destruction of neonates include excessive environmental noise, deformed or dead young, overcrowding, injured young, presence of the male parent, a small litter, dirty cage, lack of privacy, lack of nesting material, and agalactia.

Table 4.24. Common presenting genitourinary conditions and differential diagnoses in rats.

Condition	Differential Diagnoses
Renal Conditions	Noninfectious Chronic renal failure Polycystic kidney disease Urolithiasis Hydronephrosis Neoplasia, e.g., lymphoma Infectious Pyelonephritis/nephritis/cystitis secondary to bacterial infection, e.g., *Proteus* spp, *E. coli* Septicemia Renal abscess
Uterine Conditions	Noninfectious Cystic endometrial hyperplasia Infertility, e.g., inadequate protein or vitamin E content, inappropriate light cycle, senescence, immaturity, mate incompatibility, low ambient temperature Abortion, e.g., stress, hyperthermia, trauma Neoplasia, e.g., leiomyoma Hydrometra Infectious Pyometra/metritis following bacterial infection, e.g., *Pasteurella multocida, Staphylococcus aureus*
Mammary Gland Conditions	Noninfectious Neoplasia Infectious Mastitis, e.g., *S. aureus*
Male Reproductive Conditions	Noninfectious Trauma Neoplasia Infectious Bacterial infection, e.g., prostatitis

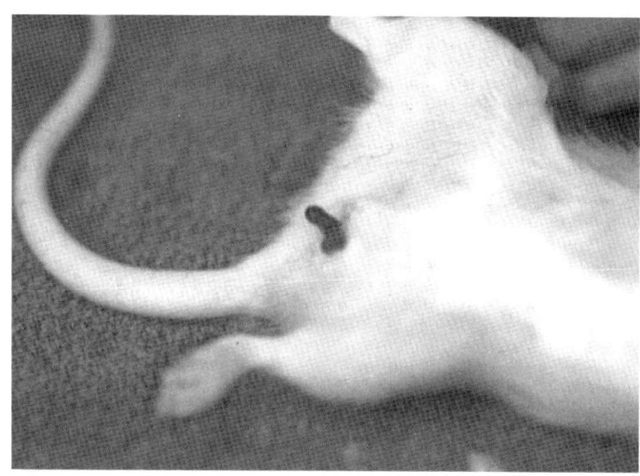

FIGURE 4.21. Vaginal prolapse in a female rat.

Sudden Death

Adult rats can die from inapparent pneumonia, chronic renal failure, overwhelming neoplasia, sudden shock or stress with massive thymic or gastrointestinal hemorrhage, lack of water, overheating or chilling, and ileus following administration of certain anesthetic agents (e.g., chloral hydrate).

References

Andrews EJ. Muzzle trauma in the rat associated with the use of feeding cups. Lab Anim Sci. 1977, 27:278.

Elwell MR, et al. Have you seen this? Inflammatory lesions in the lungs of rats. Toxicol Pathol. 1997, 25:529–531.

Gupta BN, Faith RE. Chylothorax in a rat. J Am Vet Med Assoc. 1977, 171:973–974.

Harkness JE, Ridgway MD. Chromodacryorrhea in laboratory rats (Rattus norvegicus): etiologic considerations. Lab Anim Sci. 1980, 30:841–844.

Heatley JJ. Cardiovascular anatomy, physiology, and diseases of rodents and small exotic mammals. Vet Clin Exot Anim. 2009, 12:99–113.

Herrenkohl LR. Prenatal stress reduced fertility and fecundity in female offspring. Science. 1979, 206:1097–1099.

Jackson NN, et al. Naturally acquired infections of Klebsiella pneumoniae in Wistar rats. Lab Anim. 1980, 14:356–361.

Ladd Beaumont S. Ocular disorders of pet mice and rats. Vet Clin Exot Anim. 2002, 5:311–324.

Livingston RS, et al. Serologic diagnosis of rat respiratory virus (RRV) infection. Contemp Top Lab Anim Sci. 2001, 40(4):58.

Lynch JJ, Katcher AH. Human handling and sudden death in laboratory rats. J Nerv Ment Dis. 1974, 159:362–365.

Marennikova SS, Shelukhina EM, Fimina VA. Pox infection in white rats. Lab Anim. 1978, 12:33–36.

Pucak GJ, Lee CS, Zaino AS. Effects of prolonged high temperature on testicular development and fertility in the male rat. Lab Anim Sci. 1977, 27:76–77.

Rapp JP, McGrath JT. Mycotic encephalitis in weaning rats. Lab Anim Sci. 1975, 25:477–480.

Reinhard GR, Harbison MH. Skin mass in rats. Lab Anim. 1988, 17:14–16.

Riley L. Idiopathic lung lesions in rats: search for an etiologic agent. Contemp Top Lab Anim Sci. 1997, 36(4):46–47.

Roberts SA, Gregory BJ. Facultative Pasteurella ophthalmitis in hooded lister rats. Lab Anim. 1980, 14:323–324.

Slaoui M, et al. Inflammatory lesions in the lungs of Wistar rats. Toxicol Pathol. 1998, 26:712–713.

Turner PV, Albassam MA. Susceptibility of rats to corneal lesions following anesthesia. Comp Med. 2005, 55:182–189.

Utsumi K, et al. Reproductive disorders in female SHR rats infected with sialodacryoadenitis virus. Adv Exp Med Biol. 1990, 276:525–532.

Williams DL. Ocular disease in rats: a review. Vet Ophth. 2002, 5:183–191.

Summary of Zoonotic Conditions of Rabbits and Rodents

Table 4.25. Summary of zoonotic conditions reported for rabbits and rodents.

Agent	Species Affected
Viral Disease	
Lymphocytic choriomeningitis virus	hamsters, guinea pigs, mice
Rabies virus	rabbits, guinea pigs
Hantavirus	rats, mice
Bacterial Disease	
Francisella tularensis	rabbits, hamsters
Salmonella spp	rabbits, guinea pigs, chinchillas, hamsters, mice, rats
Streptobacillis moniliformis	rats, mice
Spirillum minus	rats, mice
Pasteurella pneumotropica	mice, rats, hamsters, gerbils
Pasteurella multocida	rabbits, guinea pigs
Streptococcus pneumoniae	rats, guinea pigs
Campylobacter spp	hamsters
Yersinia spp	rabbits, wild rodents
Leptospira spp	rats, mice
Fungal Disease	
Trichophyton mentagrophytes	all
Parasitic Disease	
Trixacarus caviae	guinea pig
Hymenolepis spp/*Rodentolepis* spp	hamster, gerbil, rat, mouse

Chapter 5

Specific Diseases and Conditions

The diseases and conditions of rabbits and rodents described in this chapter were selected because of their substantial prevalence in pet and laboratory rabbits and rodents, public health significance, or potential importance to biomedical research. This listing is not complete. Tuberculosis, yersiniosis, mycotic infections other than dermatophytoses, many viral diseases, congenital abnormalities, and several nutritional conditions are referenced in chapter 4 but are not described further. References in this chapter are included at the end of each discussion of a disease or condition. Differences in normal flora, housing conditions, and diet result in significant differences in disease incidence in rabbits and rodents housed as pets, for food or fur production, or used in research. A major difference between research rabbits and rodents and pets of the same species is life span. The pet rabbit or rodent tends to live much longer than does the research animal, and the pet will show many more diseases and conditions that accompany aging. For example, most laboratory rabbits are younger than 3 years of age, whereas rabbits raised for other purposes may live 5–12 years. Pet rodents also tend to be more prone to husbandry-related conditions and nutritional diseases. Production animals are more likely to contract diseases associated with high-energy diets and high-prevalence infectious diseases. Laboratory animals typically live in conditions that exclude most of the more common diseases; congenital and heredity conditions are therefore more likely to be seen. Experimental conditions resulting in immunodeficiency may predispose animals to opportunistic diseases, and the experimental conditions themselves can result in iatrogenic disease.

ACARIASIS (MITE INFECTIONS)

General Discussion

Hosts

Most mite species affecting rabbits and rodents are host-specific; however, some, such as *Cheyletiella* spp, are freely contagious from one host species to another and can also transiently affect humans. Bites on nondefinitive hosts are generally not adaptive behavior for the mite, as other species usually represent accidental or dead-end hosts, which don't support species reproduction.

Etiology

Mites are small arachnids, similar to scorpions and spiders, and as adults, they have four pairs of legs and two body parts instead of three pairs of legs and three body parts, as seen on insects.

Transmission

Most mites of laboratory animals spend their entire life cycle on one host. Anatomic adaptations and feeding requirements confine mites to the host unless they are brushed onto the bedding or leave because of overpopulation or death of the host. Direct transfer from adult to suckling young is the most common route of spread. Mites are also spread by direct contact with infected hosts, pelage, debris, or bedding. Mites off the host usually die within 3 weeks. When laid, ova are attached either to hair shafts near the epidermis (surface-dwelling mites), or are laid in epidermal tunnels (burrowing mites), and hatch approximately 4 days after being deposited. Ova are resistant to environmental factors and may survive for long, indefinite periods off the host.

Predisposing Factors

Clinically apparent mite infections in debilitated or chronically diseased older hosts, in young hosts, or in animals housed in unsanitary or stressful environments are often more severe than infections in more vigorous individuals. This may be due to variations in self-grooming behavior or a suppressed immune response. Healthy infected animals in enzootically infected colonies become immune, and the mite population will begin to decline when the animals are 2–3 months of age. Introduction of new susceptible hosts into a colony at this time, that is, suckling young, weanlings, or new animals, will allow the cycle to continue. Through their pheromones, pet and laboratory rodents attract feral or wild rodents of like species. This contact provides an ideal opportunity for transfer of many diseases, including acariasis.

Diagnosis

Ectoparasites can be found on rodents and rabbits in many ways. Only a few methods are covered here. In the live animal, adult mites, such as the rabbit ear mite, can sometimes be seen moving on the host with the unaided eye. Loupes or a hand lens can be used to examine the fur, especially around the head, ears, neck, perianal region, and margins of lesions. A piece of filter paper placed within a vacuum hose will collect skin debris, including surface-dwelling mites, upon vacuuming the animal's body. The debris is transferred to a pool of mineral oil on a microscope slide and examined for eggs and parasites. The pelage can be brushed or combed over a dark background and the background examined for ectoparasites. The collected material is then examined carefully with a hand lens for live mites or picked up with clear cellophane tape and examined microscopically. Clear cellophane tape can also be applied directly to the skin to pick up debris, or a scalpel blade dipped in mineral oil can be used to take deep skin scrapings. Material is transferred to a microscope slide, a cover slip is placed on the slide, and it is examined microscopically for ova and mites. Skin biopsies of a mite-induced lesion may reveal hyperkeratosis, acanthosis, cutaneous ulcers, scabs, crusts, and secondary bacterial colonization. Sectioned profiles of mites and their eggs may also be seen.

When the host dies or is killed, the parasites migrate off the cool pelt and move toward the warmer tips of the hair. Cellophane tape can be applied to the fur and then placed on a glass slide and examined. If the pelt is placed on dark-colored paper surrounded by a frame of either double-gummed cellophane or packing tape or a bead of petroleum gel for several hours, the mites become trapped as they leave the pelt and try to cross the tape or gel. A more certain diagnosis may result if all or part of the pelt is cooled in a covered Petri dish or plastic bag in the refrigerator for at least 30 minutes, removed to a warmer atmosphere for 10 or more minutes, and then examined. If the diagnostic test relies on migration of live mites, it is important that the method of euthanasia does not kill the mites. If the host animal has been dead for some time, parasites may have completely migrated off the cold pelt, which may lead to an incorrect false negative result.

A portion of the pelt can be dissolved overnight in a 5% trypsin solution and then heated in 10% potassium hydroxide until cleared. The cloudy liquid is then passed through an 80-mesh brass filter. A xylene wash may be needed to remove body fat from the screen. The mites are retained on the filter and are identified and counted easily by microscopic examination.

Treatment

Treatments effective in one species of rodent are likely effective in others, with appropriate adjustments in dose based on body weight. Mites, once established in a colony, were more realistically controlled rather than eliminated before the advent of ivermectin and other drugs in the macrocyclic lactone family, a potent group of systemic parasiticides many of which were originally derived from *Streptomyces avermitilis* with a broad spectrum of action against many arachnids and nematodes. These chemicals have specific actions in invertebrate muscles and nerves and generally have a wide margin of safety in mammals because of a low affinity for similar receptor targets in mammals. These compounds do not readily cross the blood-brain barrier, though some breeds or strains with an incomplete blood-brain barrier develop neurological signs following application of recommended therapeutic doses. Treatment with pyrethrins or organophosphates can also be successfully employed.

Silicate dusts, alone or compounded with insecticides, abrade and desiccate ectoparasites and provide a mechanical alternative to potentially toxic chemicals. This material is mixed with contact bedding in the affected animals' cages.

With research animals, the consequences of treatment of ectoparasitism on subsequent use of the animals must be carefully evaluated to ensure the animals are not rendered unusable. Both reproduction and animal behavior may be altered by such treatments. People must be protected from excessive exposure to the products used in treatment. Appropriate drug withdrawal times must be observed for rabbits being shipped for food consumption.

Elimination of ectoparasites from the premises requires treatment and removal or containment of all possible host animals, thorough mechanical scrubbing, and, in severe cases, fumigation of the room with hydrogen peroxide or formaldehyde gas generated from paraformaldehyde. Fomites such as feed bags, carts, trash cans, and clothing and notebooks moved from room to room also must be cleaned to remove ectoparasites. Rooms should be repopulated with animals proven free of ectoparasites.

Prevention

In research facilities, mite infections are prevented by placing clean stock into clean premises and using dedicated equipment in animal rooms. Potentially infected animals should be separated, quarantined, and treated until determined to be free of infection, and the premises should be disinfected. Wild rodents must be excluded from the colony or housing room.

General References on Acariasis

Byford RL, Craig ME. Biology of Arthropods. In: Flynn's Parasites of Laboratory Animals, 2nd ed. Baker DG (ed.). Ames, IA: Wiley-Blackwell, 2007; 51–68.

Chitwood M, Lichtenfels JR. Identification of parasitic Metazoa in tissue sections. Exp Parasitol. 1972, 32:407–519.

Griffiths HJ. Some common parasites of small laboratory animals. Lab Anim. 1971, 5:123–135.

Levine JL, Lage AL. House mouse mites infesting laboratory rodents. Lab Anim Sci. 1984, 34:393–394.

Mullen GR, O'Connor BM. Mites (Acari). In: Medical and Veterinary Entomology. Mullen G, Durden L (eds.). Amsterdam: Academic Press, 2002, 449–516.

Owen DG. Parasites of Laboratory Animals. Lab Animal Handbook 12. London: Royal Society of Medical Services Ltd., 1992.

Pence DB. Diseases of Laboratory Animals. In: Mammalian Diseases and Arachnids, vol. II, Medico-Veterinary, Laboratory and Wildlife Diseases, and Control. Nutting WB (ed.). Boca Raton, FL: CRC Press, 1984; 129–187.

White SD, Bourdeau PJ, Meredith A. Dermatologic problems of rabbits. Sem Av Exot Pet Med. 2002, 11:141–150.

Acariasis in the Rabbit

Etiology

Mites commonly found on rabbits are members of the suborder Prostigmata, superfamily Cheyletidae. Commonly encountered rabbit mites include *Psoroptes cuniculi*, the rabbit ear mite (ear canker) (Figure 5.1), and *Cheyletiella parasitovorax* (walking dandruff) (Figure 5.2), a surface-dwelling fur mite that lives on the keratin layer of the skin and that has a broad host range, including guinea pigs, chinchillas, dogs, cats, and humans. *Leporacarus gibbus*, another fur mite, is less common but seen occasionally in both pet and research rabbits. Ear mite infections have the potential to cause great economic loss in meat-producing animals if not treated and controlled, and severe infestations may interfere with normal behaviors such as eating, drinking, and ambulating.

Demodex cuniculi mites reside in hair follicles. There have been only a few reports of *Demodex* spp in rabbits. Their presence is usually not associated with clinical signs. *Notoedres cati* and *Sarcoptes scabiei* are nonspecies-specific burrowing mites that rarely affect pet or research rabbits. *Sarcoptes scabiei*, a burrowing mange mite, can cause intense pruritus and dermal lesions of the head and neck.

Transmission

The egg-to-egg life cycle of *P. cuniculi* requires approximately 21 days. The entire life cycle of *C. parasitovorax* takes place on the animal and requires approximately 35 days.

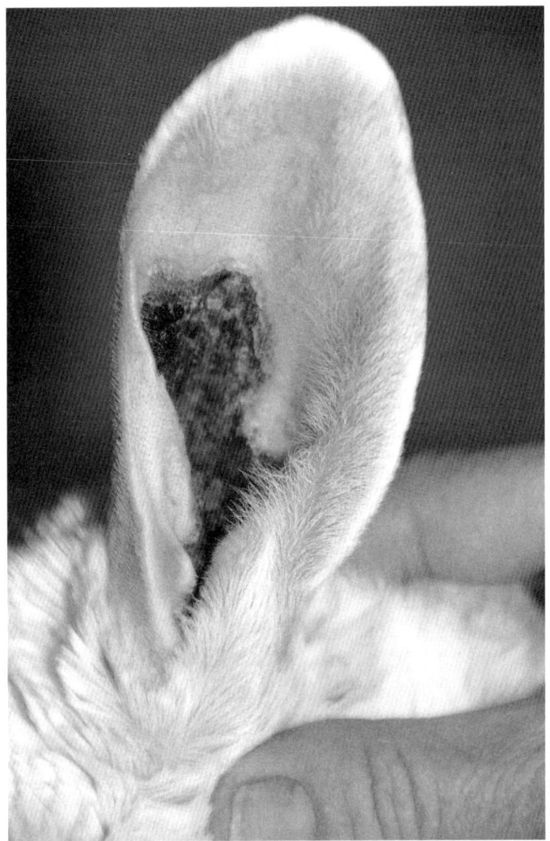

FIGURE 5.1. *Psoroptes cuniculi* infestation in a rabbit.

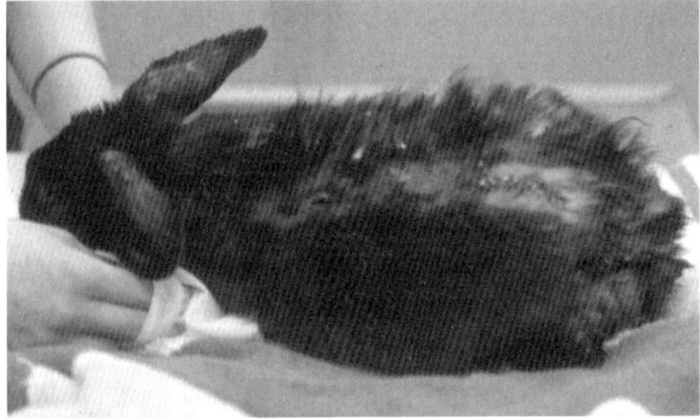

FIGURE 5.2. *Cheyletiella parasitovorax* infestation in a rabbit.

Clinical Signs

In rabbits, the nonburrowing *P. cuniculi* mites chew and pierce epidermal layers of the pinnae of the ear, inducing an inflammatory response and resulting in characteristic accumulations of multiple layers of thin, tan, flaky crust in the external ear canal. The mites are seen rarely on the skin of the adjacent head and throat or almost any other part of the body. Beneath the crusts the skin is hairless, moist, and raw. Secondary bacterial infections, though uncommon, may cause scratching, head shaking, and head tilt, if there is an accompanying unilateral bacterial otitis media. Extension of an uncomplicated mite infection to the middle and inner ears is not reported.

Cheyletiella parasitovorax may not cause clinical signs in rabbits or infestation may result in loose hair that can be pulled out in clumps. Affected skin may be slightly reddened, oily, hairless, and scaly in patches over the back, shoulders, and head. Rabbits with *Cheyletiella* mite infestations appear to have increased "dandruff" on the skin and deep in the fur.

The small *Leporacarus gibbus*, also a surface-dwelling fur mite of rabbits, is nonpathogenic even though it can be present in large numbers. *Leporacarus gibbus* is found predominantly on the abdomen and back of rabbits.

Diagnosis

In early or light infections, *Psoroptes* mites and lesions are deep in the concha or external ear canal and are easily overlooked. *Psoroptes cuniculi* mites are visualized readily with a pediatric otoscope. The mites move rapidly in the external ear canal, and they are large enough to be seen with the unaided eye, although they are covered frequently with debris. Examination of debris scrapings (in mineral oil) from the ear canal reveals round to oval mites with well-developed legs and bell-shaped suckers on the ends of the first and second pairs of legs of the female mite. Refractory cases should include a complete work-up with clear identification of the parasite. *Sarcoptes scabiei* mites may rarely be found infesting the ears of rabbits, inducing an intensely pruritic dermatitis with superficial canal and external ear crusting. This mite can only be identified with deep skin scrapings and the treatment is different, making definitive diagnosis all the more critical.

In the case of *C. parasitovorax* infections, examination of the fur may reveal pale yellow-to-white mites, approximately 0.3 mm long, with piercing chelicerae and large, curved papal hooks.

Treatment

In uncomplicated infestations of *Psoroptes cuniculi*, the mite can be eliminated (smothered) with mineral oil or oil-based insecticide preparations. One or 2 mL of the liquid preparations are massaged into each ear canal. The ear drum must be intact if using this technique. Acaricides are usually not ovicidal, and treatment is repeated approximately 7–14 days later to eliminate recently hatched immature mites before they can deposit ova. This should always be accompanied by an environmental clean-up at home for pets or in the viviarium.

Ivermectin (200–440 ug/kg, SC or IM) given every 7–18 days for three treatments has eliminated all *P. cuniculi* mites in several studies and appears to be safe for rabbits (note: ivermectin is not approved for meat rabbits). The 1% cattle formulation was used in a number of these studies. Ivermectin should not be used in rabbits intended for human consumption because of the potential for drug residues in major organs. Two 400 ug/kg doses given subcutaneously 7–14 days apart were also clinically effective and eradicated the infection. Ivermectin persisted in the skin of the body and ears long enough (9 and 13 days, respectively) to remove the new generation of mites as they hatched from ova. Also, at this dose, the maximum plasma concentration of 42 ng/mL was achieved approximately 2 days postinjection; however, the biological half-life in rabbits is not known, and ivermectin lacks ovicidal properties. Most current reports recommend treating at least twice at a 2- to 3-week interval.

Dermatitis has been described on the hind quarters above the tail due to *P. cuniculi* infection. After clipping and scrubbing with an iodine preparation, the area was treated twice per day with a topical application of Panalog®, an antimicrobial-steroid ointment.

More recent studies evaluating the activity of other macrocyclic lactones, such as selamectin and moxidectin, against *Psoroptes cuniculi* suggest that topical selamectin administered to the skin at the base of the neck of New Zealand white rabbits at a dose of 6–18 mg/kg either as a single dose or repeated at a 4-week interval is safe and efficacious in treating and removing all *P. cuniculi* mites. Moxidectin at 0.2 mg/kg given in two oral doses 10 days apart was very effective at eliminating *P. cuniculi* infestations in rabbits.

In severe cases, rabbits may need to be deeply sedated or anesthetized before attempting to clean the ears, and the use of a sebumolytic compound, antiseptic soap, and topical or systemic antibiotic given with a postprocedural antiinflammatory and analgesic drug, such as meloxicam, may be indicated.

Cheyletiella spp can be reduced by dusting adults, weanlings, and bedding with a permethrin powder at weekly intervals. Ivermectin given in multiple doses SC or SC and PO did not appear to effectively resolve *Cheyletiella* infestations in rabbits. Rabbits treated topically with a single dose of selamectin at 12 mg/kg had complete resolution of *Cheyletiella* infestation up to 5 weeks posttreatment.

Selamectin administered topically at the base of the neck at a dose of 10–12 mg/kg was only partially effective at killing sarcoptic mange mites in Angora rabbits. Doramectin 1% given at 0.2 mg/kg SC following two injections of moxidectin 1% at 0.2 mg/kg given 2 weeks apart was very effective at eliminating *Sarcoptes scabiei* from the ears of angora rabbits.

Prevention

Newly arriving rabbits, unless known to be free of ear mites, should be quarantined and treated twice with ivermectin at 400 ug/kg body weight SC at a 14-day interval before being placed in an established clean colony. New introductions, whether pet, breeder, or institutional, should always be quarantined away from other rabbits for up to 2 weeks postarrival, to ensure that they are free of opportunistic disease.

Public Health Significance

Psoroptes spp and *Leporacarus* spp mites of rabbits do not affect humans. *Cheyletiella parasitovorax*, in rare cases, can cause dermatitis in humans, especially children. *Notoedres cati* of rabbits also may cause transient dermatitis in humans. *Sarcoptes scabiei* is zoonotic and may induce intense pruritus in humans.

References

Curtis SK. Diagnostic exercise: moist dermatitis on the hind quarters of a rabbit. Lab Anim Sci. 1991, 41:623–624.

Curtis SK, Brooks DL. Eradication of ear mites from naturally infested conventional research rabbits using ivermectin. Lab Anim Sci. 1990, 40:406–408.

Curtis SK, Housley R, Brooks DL. Use of ivermectin for treatment of ear mite infection in rabbits. J Am Vet Med Assoc. 1990, 196:1139.

Flatt RE, Wiemers J. A survey of fur mites in domestic rabbits. Lab Anim Sci. 1976, 26:758–761.

Harvey RG. Demodex cuniculi in dwarf rabbits (Oryctolagus cuniculus): a case report. J Small Anim Prac. 1990, 31:204–207.

Hofin, L, Krau, L. Arthropod and Helminth Parasites. In: The Biology of the Laboratory Rabbit, 2nd ed. Manning PJ, Ringler DH, Newcomer CE (eds.). San Diego: Academic Press, 1994, 231–257.

Kim SH, Jun HK, Song KH, et al. Prevalence of fur mites in pet rabbits in South Korea. Vet Dermatol. 2008b, 19(3):189–190.

Kim SH, Lee JY, Jun HK, et al. Efficacy of selamectin in the treatment of cheyletiellosis in pet rabbits. Vet Dermatol. 2008a, 19(1):26–27.

Kurtdede A, Karaer Z, Acar A, et al. Use of selamectin for the treatment of psoroptic and sarcoptic mite infestation in rabbits. Vet Dermatol. 2007, 18:18–22.

McKellar QA, et al. Clinical and pharmacological properties of ivermectin in rabbits and guinea pigs. Vet Rec. 1992, 130:71–73.

McTier TL, Hair JA, Walstrom DJ, et al. Efficacy and safety of topical administration of selamectin for treatment of ear mite infestation in rabbits. J Am Vet Med Assoc. 2003, 223(3):322–324.

Mellgren M, Bergvall K. Treatment of rabbit cheyletiellosis with selamectin or ivermectin: a retrospective case study. Acta Vet Scand. 2008, 50:1–6.

Niekrasz MA, Curl JL, Curl JS. Rabbit fur mite (Listrophorus gibbus) infestation of New Zealand white rabbits. Contemp Top Lab Anim Sci. 1998, 37(4):73–75.

Pandey, VS. Effect of ivermectin on the ear mange mite, Psoroptes cuniculi, of rabbits. Br Vet J. 1989, 145:54–56.

Suckow MA, et al. Biology and Diseases of Rabbits. In: Laboratory Animal Medicine. Fox JG, Anderson LC, Loew FL, Quimby FW (eds.). Orlando: Academic Press, 2002; 329–364.

Uhlir J. Humoral and cellular immune response of rabbits to Psoroptes cuniculi, the rabbit scab mite. Vet Parasitol. 1991, 40:325–334.

Voyvoda H, Ulutas B, Eren H, et al. Use of doramectin for treatment of sarcoptic mange in five Angora rabbits. Vet Dermatol. 2005, 16(4):28–28.

Wagner R, Wendlberger U. Field efficacy of moxidectin in dogs and rabbits naturally infested with Sarcoptes spp., Demodex spp. and Psoroptes spp. mites. Vet Parasitol. 2000, 93(2):149–158.

Acariasis in the Guinea Pig

Etiology

The most common species of guinea pig mites is *Chirodiscoides caviae*, a small, generally harmless fur mite, and *Trixacarus caviae*, a burrowing sarcoptid mite. *Trixacarus* spp may be confused easily with *Sarcoptes* and *Notoedres* spp. Some early reports of the latter mite infections may have been caused by *Trixacarus* spp.

Clinical Signs

Trixacarus caviae of guinea pigs frequently produces a severe, dry, scaling, and crusting dermatitis and alopecia on the neck, shoulders, inner thighs, and abdomen, which often results in intense pruritus and self-mutilation, with frantic scratching culminating in seizure-like activity. Maximal parasite load is reached approximately 1 month after infection, then parasite numbers slowly regress if left untreated. Mortality of infected guinea pigs has been reported in rare cases. In contrast, few clinical signs or lesions may be seen with *C. caviae* infestation, even though the parasites may be numerous.

Diagnosis

The pelt can be examined effectively for *C. caviae* mites with a hand lens or a dissecting microscope. The mites concentrate in the lumbar region and lateral aspects of the rear legs. Adult *C. caviae* mites can be seen with the unaided eye moving in the fur. *C. caviae* mites are usually seen in pairs, which represent a noncopulatory union of juvenile males with more mature females, presumably to ensure the presence of a mate when both reach sexual maturity.

Lesions of *Trixacarus caviae* are typically severe. Burrows containing mites and ova may be seen histologically in the stratum corneum.

Treatment

Some have described the use of dichlorvos vapor to treat *C. caviae* infections. *Chirodiscoides* populations can be reduced by dusting adult and weanling guinea pigs and their bedding with a permethrin powder at weekly intervals. Eradication has also been reported in guinea pigs by spraying dilute (0.2 mg/mL) ivermectin on the coats of infested guinea pigs followed by applying undiluted drops of ivermectin (10 mg/mL) directly onto the coats.

Ivermectin has been used at 500 ug/kg via oral, SC, and topical routes to treat *T. caviae*. All routes resulted in an effective cure for *T. caviae* when a second dose was given 7 days after the first. Ivermectin has also been used SC at 200 ug/kg twice at a 10-day interval to treat guinea pig mange. By 21 days posttreatment, clinical signs had completely resolved. Side effects included subdermal necrosis at the injection site in younger animals and inflammation of the skin in the older animals, possibly due to the propylene glycol used as a diluent.

Public Health Significance

Chirodiscoides caviae do not affect humans. *Trixacarus caviae* may cause urticaria in humans but infestation is transient and self-limiting.

References

Bean-Knudsen DE, Wagner JE, Hall RD. Evaluation of the control of Myobia musculi infestations on laboratory mice with permethrin. Lab Anim Sci. 1986, 36:268–270.

Hirsjärvi P, Phyälä L. Ivermectin treatment of a colony of guinea pigs infested with fur mite (Chirodiscoides caviae). Lab Anim. 1995, 29(2):200–203.

Kummel BA, Estes SA, Arlian LG. Trixacarus caviae infestation of guinea pigs. J Am Vet Med Assoc. 1980, 177:903–908.

McKellar QA, et al. Clinical and pharmacological properties of ivermectin in rabbits and guinea pigs. Vet Rec. 1992, 130:71–73.

Rothwell TLW, et al. Haematological and pathological responses to experimental Trixacarus caviae infection in guinea pigs. J Comp Pathol. 1991, 104:179–185.

Thoday KL, Beresford-Jones WP. The diagnosis and treatment of mange in the guinea pig caused by Trixacarus (Caviacoptes) caviae. J Small Anim Pract. 1977, 18:591–595.

Wagner JE, Al-Rabiai S, Rings RW. Chirodiscoides caviae infestation in guinea pigs. Lab Anim Sci. 1972, 22:750–752.

Zajac A, Williams JF, Williams CSF. Mange caused by Trixacarus caviae in guinea pigs. J Am Vet Med Assoc. 1980, 177:900–903.

Zenoble RD, Greve JH. Sarcoptid mite infestation in a colony of guinea pigs. J Am Vet Med Assoc. 1980, 177:898–900.

Acariasis in the Hamster

Etiology

Several species of mites have been described in hamsters: *Demodex criceti* is found in epidermal pits and *D. aurati* is found in the pilosebaceous glands and hair follicles. *Notoedres* spp, a burrowing mite, can cause scabby lesions of the ears, feet, nose, and genital region. More recently, infestation with the tropical rat mite, *Ornithonyssus bacoti*, has been reported in pet hamsters and their owners. Presumably, these mites were transmitted to hamsters from the pet store of origin or from exposure to feral rodents in the home.

Clinical Signs

A *Demodex* spp infestation in hamsters is rarely associated with clinical signs, but it may cause alopecia, rough hair coat, and scaly, scabby dermatitis of the rump and back. Demodecosis is particularly common in male hamsters older than 1.5 years and is frequently secondary to chronic renal disease, intercurrent systemic disease, and malnutrition. Pruritus is not a prominent feature of demodecosis of hamsters.

Diagnosis

Demodex spp is difficult to detect. If *Demodex* infestation is suspected, a deep skin scraping with an oil- or glycerin-wetted scalpel blade will aid in the collection of mites. Scraped material is placed on a slide with a few drops of warmed 10% potassium hydroxide, coverslipped, allowed to sit 10 minutes, and then examined microscopically. Histologically, hair follicles are distorted, dilated, and filled with debris and mites.

Treatment

Amitraz (Mitaban®) is used for treating generalized demodecosis of dogs, localized infections in cats, and can be used with great caution to treat hamsters. Excessive exposure of hamsters to amitraz, as occurs with dipping, causes multisystem toxicity largely due to alpha2-adrenergic agonist effects. The hamster should be bathed first with a mild soap and water solution and towelled dry before being treated topically. A dilute amitraz-water mixture can be applied to affected areas with a cotton ball or toothbrush and allowed to air dry. Three to six topical treatments 14 days apart are recommended. Ivermectin has also been used with variable effect to treat demodecosis in hamsters and is much safer. Daily oral treatment with 0.3 mg/kg of ivermectin led to resolution of the infestation in 58% of animals in one study.

Public Health Significance

Demodex mites of hamsters do not affect humans. *Ornithonyssus bacoti*, the tropical rat mite, is zoonotic and can act as a vector to transmit other more serious diseases to humans.

References

Creel NB, Crowe MA, Mullen GR. Pet hamsters as a source of rat mite dermatitis. Cutis. 2003, 71(6):457–461.

Desch CE, Jr, Hurley RJ. Demodex sinocricetuli: new species of hair follicle mite (Acari:Demodecidae) from the Chinese form of the striped hamster, Cricetulus barabensis (Rodentia:Muridae). J Med Entomol. 1997, 34(3):317–320.

Estes PC, Richter CB, Franklin JA. Demodectic mange in the golden hamster. Lab Anim Sci. 1971, 21:825–828.

Flatt RE, Kerber WT. Demodectic mite infestation in golden hamsters. Lab Anim Digest. 1968, 4:6–7.

Hasegawa T. A case report of the management of demodicosis in the golden hamster. J Vet Med Sci. 1995, 57(2):337–338.

Nutting WB. Demodex aurati sp. nov. and D. criceti, ectoparasites of the golden hamster (Mesocricetus auratus). Parasitol. 1961, 51:515–522.

Nutting WB, Rauch H. Distribution of Demodex aurati in the host (Mesocricetus auratus) skin complex. J Parasitol. 1963, 49:323–329.

Owen D, Young C. The occurrence of Demodex aurati and Demodex criceti in the Syrian hamster (Mesocricetus auratus) in the United Kingdom. Vet Rec. 1973, 92:282–284.

Tani K, Iwanaga T, Sonoda K, et al. Ivermectin treatment of demodicosis in 56 hamsters. J Vet Med Sci. 2001, 63(11):1245–1247.

Acariasis in the Gerbil

Demodex mites occasionally infect gerbils, but demodecosis is not considered a significant clinical disease of healthy gerbils. *Demodex* mites have been seen in skin scrapings from a lesion on the tailhead of a gerbil. The mange described was similar to that seen in hamsters with *Demodex* infections. Treatment is uncertain. Avian mite (*Ornithonyssus silviarum* and *Dermanyssus gallinae*) infestation of pet gerbils has been reported with subsequent transmission of mites to their owners. The gerbils were interpreted to be accidental hosts.

References

Lucky AW, Sayers C, Argus JD, Lucky A. Avian mite bites acquired from a new source—pet gerbils: report of 2 cases and review of the literature. Arch Dermatol. 2001, 137(2):167–170.

Schwarzbrott SS, Wagner JE, Frisk CS. Demodecosis in the Mongolian gerbil (Meriones unguiculatus): a case report. Lab Anim Sci. 1974, 24:666–668.

Acariasis in the Mouse

Etiology

Mites found commonly on rodents are members of the suborder Prostigmata. Common species of mouse mites include *Myobia musculi, Myocoptes musculinus*, and *Radfordia affinis*, all of which are fur mites, and *Psorergates simplex*, a follicular mite that is rarely seen. *Ornithonyssus bacoti* has also been infrequently reported in pet and laboratory mice. Morphologically, *Myobia* and *Radfordia* are similar. *Myobia* has one terminal claw on each of the second pair of legs, whereas *Radfordia* has two. *Myocoptes* is a more oval mite with heavily chitinized "boxing gloves" on the third and fourth sets of legs. Mixed populations of *Myobia* and *Myocoptes* are common.

Transmission

Life cycles of all three species are direct with all stages occurring on the host. Hairless (glabrous) mice are therefore not suitable hosts for fur mites. *Myobia* ova hatch in 7–8 days. The egg-to-egg life cycle requires approximately 12–16 days. Typical infections are mixed, although *Myocoptes musculinus* is more common in North America.

Predisposing Factors

Black strains of mice are particularly susceptible to chronic hypersensitivity dermatitis that is frequently severe and associated with self-mutilation. In some cases, the pruritic effects of mite infections in these strains are interpreted to initiate self-mutilation. Fur mite infestation has been demonstrated to induce marked IgE production and mast cell degranulation in the skin of various mouse strains, particularly those of a C57BL/6 background. It should also be noted that chronic skin lesions are common in aged mite-free mice of the black strains so the condition must be worked up carefully in these strains.

Clinical Signs

Typically, even in very heavy infestations, *M. musculi* may cause signs no more dramatic than host scratching. In susceptible mice, hyperactive behavior, excessive scratching, and a roughened hair coat are seen, often with low parasite populations. Alopecia, epidermal scaling, and scant to extensive ulceration may occur; however, these signs are likely caused by a scratching response to the allergic or pruritic stimulus induced by the mites. The actual number of mites per mouse appears to have little bearing on the severity of the reaction and the extent of the lesions. *Myocoptes musculinus* and *R. affinis* may cause similar signs in mice, although they tend to induce less of an allergic response.

Psorergates simplex inhabits hair follicles. As mites and debris accumulate in the skin, follicular invaginations or cysts are visible as small (2 mm) white nodules in the skin of the head, neck, shoulder, and lumbar areas. These nodules are seen best at necropsy on the subcutaneous or underside of the reflected skin.

Diagnosis

Ectoparasites of mice and rats can be seen incidentally at the time of microscopic examination of perianal cellophane tape impressions for pinworm ova (*Syphacia* spp). Strips of heavy cellophane or clear packing tape can be pressed firmly against the fur of the live animal and examined microscopically for ectoparasites. The dorsal fur tape test is the most effective diagnostic procedure to assess the degree of fur mite infection, although a diagnosis can often be made by evaluating hair shafts plucked from the edge of the lesion. Mites are readily visualized from skin biopsies and skin sections taken at necropsy. Many systemic effects occur with chronic dermatitis, such as markedly enlarged lymph nodes and spleens, especially in black mice.

Treatment

Rederivation of mouse colonies by Caesarian section with cross-fostering onto mite-free dams is an effective means of treating mite infestations.

A "micro-dot" dermal delivery technique with undiluted ivermectin has been demonstrated to be efficacious for treating mite-infected mice. Two treatments of 2 mg/kg of 1% ivermectin on the skin between the scapulae are recommended at a 10-day interval (a volume of 5 μl for a 25-g mouse) eliminated pinworms and fur mites. Cross-fostering pups from infested dams between 0 and 36 hours after birth and treating weanlings topically with 0.2 mg/kg ivermectin at 9-day intervals was a successful means of eliminating fur mites from a colony of genetically engineered mice that could not be rederived by Caesarian section. Ivermectin has been reported to induce behavioral changes and neurotoxicity in some strains of mice. If this is relevant to a colony or an ongoing experiment, the effects should be evaluated on a small number of animals before routinely administering it to different strains of mice.

Moxidectin given to mice orally at 2 mg/kg and repeated at a 15-day interval was effective in eliminating *R. affinis* from a mouse colony with no adverse effects noted. A single dose of 0.5 mg/kg of moxidectin pour-on (0.5%) has also been used topically to eliminate *Myocoptes* spp from mouse colonies. Selamectin may not be as efficacious for long-term elimination of *Myocoptes* spp infection, when compared with moxidectin in mice.

The effectiveness of different methods of external application of trichlorphon (Neguvon®) and ivermectin was evaluated for treating *M. musculi* and *Myocoptes* spp infections in conventional laboratory mice as well as feeder colonies of mice. Ivermectin was found to be effective over a longer time period than was trichlorphon. There was no difference in the results obtained with different methods of application. Topical misting over the cages of a 0.1% solution of injectable ivermectin once weekly for 3 consecutive weeks was more practical than individual dipping for large colonies of mice. For mice being bred as feeder rodents for reptiles and raptors, the length of time that ivermectin and trichlorphon persist in the carcass is unknown.

Myobia spp, *Radfordia* spp, and *Myocoptes* spp infections can be reduced markedly by dusting adult and weanling mice and their bedding with permethrin powder at weekly intervals. Control of *Myobia* spp in mice was achieved by mixing 4.0g of 0.25% permethrin dust (Ectiban®) weekly into the bedding. Cotton balls containing 5–7.4% (w/w) active permethrin (Permanone 40®) have also been used as bedding and nesting material to treat mice with mites. After 4 weeks, mice were essentially mite-free and showed no adverse reactions.

Chlorpyrifos, an organophosphate, is reported to be nontoxic and efficacious in the control of *M. musculi*. The granules are applied in animal bedding at 6g per 27cm by 48cm (11 × 9in) shoebox cage twice weekly for 3 weeks.

Dichlorvos treatment may not completely eliminate mites from colonies. An infestation of *Radfordia affinis* in mice that had been previously unsuccessfully managed with dichlorvos in the bedding was eradicated using two applications of topical selamectin administered in conjunction with amitraz- and fipronil-treated nesting matenals changed weekly.

Ornithonyssus bacoti was successfully eliminated from a colony of infested mice by placing permethrin-impregnated cotton balls in the mouse cages for 8 weeks and treating the premises by spraying floors and walls of all rooms housing mice and adjacent hallways in the colony with pyrethrin spray.

SPECIFIC DISEASES AND CONDITIONS

Public Health Significance

Psorergates spp, *Myobia* spp, *Radfordia* spp, and *Myocoptes* spp mites of mice are not known to affect humans. *Ornithonyssus bacoti* can infect humans and transmit several arthropod-borne diseases.

References

Baumans V, et al. The effectiveness of Ivomec and Neguvon in the control of murine mites. Lab Anim. 1988, 22:243–245.

Baumans V, Havenaar R, Van Herck H. The use of repeated treatment with Ivomec and Neguvon spray in the control of murine fur mites and oxyurid worms. Lab Anim. 1988, 22:246–249.

Bean-Knudsen DE, Wagner JE, Hall RD. Evaluation of the control of Myobia musculi infestations on laboratory mice with permethrin. Lab Anim Sci. 1986, 36:268–270.

Bornstein DA, Scola J, Rath A, et al. Multimodal approach to treatment for control of fur mites. J Amer Assoc Lab Anim Sci. 2006, 45(4):29–32.

Cole JS, Sabol-Jones M, Karolewski B, et al. Ornithonyssus bacoti infestation and elimination from a mouse colony. Contemp Top Lab Anim Sci. 2005, 44(5):27–30.

Constantin ML. Effects of insecticides on acariasis in mice. Lab Anim. 1972, 6:279–286.

Csiza CK, McMartin DN. Apparent acaridal dermatitis in a C57BL/6 Nia mouse colony. Lab Anim Sci. 1976, 26:781–787.

Davis JA, et al. Behavioural effects of ivermectin in mice. Lab Anim Sci. 1999, 49(3):288–296.

Friedman S, Weisbroth SH. The parasitic ecology of the rodent mite, Myobia musculi. II. Genetic factors. Lab Anim Sci. 1975, 25:440–445.

———. The parasitic ecology of the rodent mite, Myobia musculi. IV. Life cycle. Lab Anim Sci. 1977, 27:34–37.

Green CJ, Needham JR. Control of mange mites in a large mouse colony. Lab Anim. 1974, 8:245–251.

Huerkamp MJ, Zitzow LA, Webb S, et al. Cross-fostering in combination with ivermectin therapy: a method to eradicate murine fur mites. Contemp Top Lab Anim Sci. 2005, 44(4):12–16.

Mather TN, Lausen NCG. A new insecticide delivery method for control of fur mite infestations in laboratory mice. Lab Anim. 1990, 19:25–29.

Mook DM, Benjamin KA. Use of selamectin and moxidectin in the treatment of mouse fur mites. J Amer Assoc Lab Anim Sci. 2008, 47(3):20–24.

Morita E, Kaneko S, Hiragun T, et al. Fur mites induce dermatitis associated with IgE hyperproduction in an inbred strain of mice, NC/Kuj. J Dermatol Sci. 1999, 19(1):37–43.

Pence BC, et al. The efficacy and safety of chlorpyrifos (Dursban®) for control of Myobia musculi infestation in mice. Lab Anim Sci. 1991, 41:139–142.

Pochanke V, Hatak S, Hengartner H, et al. Induction of IgE and allergic-type responses in fur mite–infested mice. Eur J Immunol. 2006, 36(9):2434–2445.

Pollicino P, Rossi L, Rambozzi L, et al. Oral administration of moxidectin for treatment of murine acariosis due to Radfordia affinis. Vet Parasitol. 2008, 151(2–4):355–357.

Pullium JK, Brooks WJ, Langley AD, et al. A single dose of topical moxidectin as an effective treatment for murine acariasis due to Myocoptes musculinus. Contemp Top Lab Anim Sci. 2005, 44(1):26–28. Erratum (dosage error in text) in: Contemp Top Lab Anim Sci. 2005, 44(3):56.
Sueta T, Miyoshi I, Okamura T, et al. Experimental eradication of pinworms (Syphacia obvelata and Aspiculuris tetraptera) from mice colonies using ivermectin. Exp Anim. 2002, 51(4):367–373.
Weisbroth SH, et al. The parasitic ecology of the rodent mite Myobia musculi. I. Grooming factors. Lab Anim Sci. 1974, 24:510–516.
Weisbroth SH, Friedman S, Scher S. The parasitic ecology of the rodent mite, Myobia musculi. III. Lesions in certain host strains. Lab Anim Sci. 1976, 26:725–735.
West WL, Schofield JC, Bennett BT. Efficacy of the "micro-dot" technique for administering topical 1% ivermectin for the control of pinworms and fur mites in mice. Contemp Top Lab Anim Sci. 1992, 31(6):7–10.

Acariasis in the Rat

Etiology

Most of the general information presented about clinical signs, diagnosis, and treatment of acariasis in other species of rodents, particularly mice, applies to the rat and is discussed in the earlier sections of this chapter regarding acariasis in other rodent species. Mites commonly found on rats, like those of mice, are members of the suborder Prostigmata. Representative species of rat mites include *Radfordia ensifera*, a surface-dwelling fur mite, and *Notoedres muris*, an infrequently seen burrowing ear mange mite. Rats rarely have *Demodex nanus* infections. *Ornithonyssus bacoti*, the tropical rat mite, also infests domesticated rats. It is not species-specific and is zoonotic. With the exception of *O. bacoti*, the mites described live on the skin surface and obtain nourishment from epithelial debris and tissue secretions. Life cycles are approximately 10–21 days, and ova hatch in approximately 8 days, although cycle lengths and intervals vary with host condition and environment.

Transmission

Ornithonyssus bacoti is a blood-sucking parasite that feeds on the host intermittently and most of the time lives off the host in the rodent's nests and bedding. Frequent bedding changes and nest removal preclude the possibility of the tropical rat mite completing its life cycle.

Clinical Signs

Alopecia, epidermal scaling, and superficial epidermal ulceration may occur in cases of mite infestations, but these signs are thought to be caused by a pruritic response to an allergic reaction induced by the mites. Secondary dermatitis caused by *Staphylococcus aureus* colonization may follow self-traumatization. *R. ensifera*, the rat fur mite, may cause clinical signs similar to those caused by mouse mites.

Notoedres muris infestation of the ears of rats may result in a severe proliferative and disfiguring aural dermatitis with intense pruritus most commonly involving the tips of the ears, and also the nose and forelegs.

Nymphal and adult forms of *O. bacoti* intermittently suck blood from the host; the loss of blood may cause anemia, decreased fertility, weakness, and death. As with fur mites, mammalian hosts may develop an allergic dermatitis to burrowing and biting mites, and the pruritic response may be intense.

Diagnosis

Diagnostic techniques are similar to methods described for other rodents. Engorged *Ornithonyssus* spp mites moving in the fur can be seen with the unaided eye. Ectoparasites of rats are sometimes seen at the time of microscopic examination of perianal cellophane tape impressions for pinworm ova. Additionally, wide strips of heavy cellophane or clear packing tape can be pressed firmly against the fur of the live animal and examined microscopically for ectoparasites.

Treatment

Treatment is similar to that for acariasis of mice and hamsters. *Radfordia* spp and *Ornithonyssus* spp can be reduced by dusting the adults, weanlings, and bedding with a permethrin powder at weekly intervals. *Ornithonyssus bacoti* can be controlled without pesticides by use of water moats and pans with liquid disinfectants placed strategically so the mites drown after leaving the host. Feral or wild rodents or infected bedding are likely sources of blood-sucking mites in a conventional facility.

Public Health Significance

Radfordia spp mites of rats do not affect humans. However, *Ornithonyssus bacoti* bites humans and can serve as a vector for murine typhus, tularemia, Q fever, plague, and other diseases.

References

Baker DG. Parasitic Diseases. In: The Laboratory Rat, 2nd ed. Suckow MA, Weisbroth SH, Franklin CL (eds.). Orlando: Academic Press, 2006, 453–478.

Baumstark J, Beck W, Hofmann H. Outbreak of tropical rat mite (Ornithonyssus bacoti) dermatitis in a home for disabled persons. Dermatol. 2007, 215(1):66–68.

Beck W. Occurrence of a house-infesting tropical rat mite (Ornithonyssus bacoti) on murides and human beings. Travel Med Infect Dis. 2008, 6(4):245–249.

Chung SL, Hwang SJ, Kwon SB, et al. Outbreak of rat mite dermatitis in medical students. Int J Dermatol. 1998, 37(8):591–594.

Desch CE, Jr. Redescription of Demodex nanus (Acari:Demodicidae) from Rattus norvegicus and R. rattus (Rodentia). J Med Entomol. 1987, 24:19–23.

Engel PM, Welzel J, Maass M, et al. Tropical rat mite dermatitis: case report and review. Clin Infect Dis. 1998, 27(6):1465–1469.

Kelaher J, Jogi R, Katta R. An outbreak of rat mite dermatitis in an animal research facility. Cutis. 2005, 75(5):282–286.

Kondo S, Taylor A, Chun S. Elimination of an infestation of rat fur mites (Radfordia ensifera) from a colony of Long Evans rats, using the micro-dot technique for topical administration of 1% ivermectin. Contemp Top Lab Anim Sci. 1998, 37(1):58–61.

Watson J. New building, old parasite: mesostigmatid mites—an ever-present threat to barrier rodent facilities. ILAR J. 2008, 49(3):303–309.

ANOREXIA AND REDUCED FOOD INTAKE

Etiology

Anorexia, a reduction of more than 25% of the daily food intake for 3 or more days or complete cessation of eating for more than 1 day, is a common and nonspecific sign in rabbits and rodents. It may arise from a number of underlying conditions including neophobia, lack of access to water, temperature extremes, food changes, an unpalatable or improperly compounded diet, toxin ingestion, gastric stasis, dental malocclusion or oral lacerations, pain, loss of olfaction, obesity, metabolic disorders such as renal failure or vitamin C deficiency in guinea pigs, infectious diseases, neoplasia, loss of cagemates, mechanical factors that prevent access to water and feed, and territorial and behavioral traits, for example, a dominant guinea pig hoarding and guarding feed and water supplies. Guinea pigs are especially susceptible to the detrimental effects of short-term anorexia because of their need for exogenous vitamin C, their tendency to develop ketosis, and their basic behavioral traits. Specifically, sick guinea pigs often appear to lack the will to live, readily go off feed, and sometimes must be gently coaxed into surviving. Guinea pigs are particularly neophobic in their food habits. A change from one food or flavor to another should be done gradually by using transitional mixtures. Young animals should be introduced to new foods that may be used as treats at a later time. This can help to overcome food neophobias seen in all species. It is also important to note that rodents that cannot access water will not eat and can rapidly become compromised. Excessively hard food pellets and elevated or nonfunctional sipper tubes or automatic watering devices may result in death, especially in weanlings.

Clinical Signs

Anorexia is a common presenting problem of pet guinea pigs, chinchillas, and rabbits. Clinical manifestations of anorexia are weight loss or failure to gain, absence of feces, increased susceptibility to disease, enteropathies, dehydration, loss of pups, and death. Irreversible ketosis may develop rapidly in guinea pigs and obese rabbits, even after these animals have resumed eating. It is important to determine if the animal seems hungry and would like to eat, which may be indicative of underlying dental disease, or if it is truly anorexic. The treatment should be adjusted accordingly. Anorexia should be considered a medical emergency in these species because of their small size, stoic natures, and rapid metabolism, and particularly if animals appear distressed or ill, are dehydrated, or in poor body condition. These animals may be in very fragile condition at the time of presentation and may die suddenly if handled roughly. At a minimum, animals should be provided with warmed fluids parenterally and a comfortable warm place to rest while the assessment of their condition is ongoing.

Diagnosis

Determination of the cause or causes of anorexia is based on history (caging, recent changes, diet, environment, and character of urine and feces); results of a physical examination (oral exam, body temperature, evaluation of the eyes and nostrils, respiratory, and digestive tracts); and on results of fecal, blood, and microbial examinations. Small mammal pets that refuse all food for 1 or more days are anorectic and because of their high metabolic rate should be treated as a clinical emergency—a "wait and see" approach is rarely successful in anorexia cases.

Treatment

Animals with mildly reduced food consumption that are not displaying other signs of illness are often treated successfully by providing free-choice grass hay, rehydrating with a balanced electrolyte solution (per os, subcutaneously, IP, or IV), and providing a quiet, low-stress environment.

Environmental or behavioral problems that result in anorexia may be overcome in the short term by offering small amounts of sweetened or preferred feeds (corn, oats, sunflower seeds, fresh greens and vegetables, alfalfa hay, apples), by changing feeds or feeders and waterers, by giving B vitamins (vitamin B complex at 0.20 mL/kg), or by reducing crowding or separating incompatible or dominant individuals.

Medical causes of anorexia in rabbits and rodents should be treated aggressively. Subcutaneous, intraperitoneal, or intraosseous administration of warmed isotonic fluids several times daily will improve hydration and help stabilize the animal. In dehydrated, depressed animals, fluids can be delivered via a sterile 20- to 22-gauge needle into the medullary cavity of the femur. Syringe-feeding nutritious, high-fiber slurry will help maintain nutritional status, prevent ileus from developing, and rehydrate the stomach contents. Commercial products are available, for example, Critical Care™, Oxbow® Pet Products (www.oxbowanimalhealth.com), and many homemade formulations, such as yogurt mixed with puréed vegetables, ground feed and glucose solution, or baby pablum with a small amount of psyllium fiber and probiotic powder, have also been used successfully.

Anorectic rabbits are often too weak or too ill to eat voluntarily but may tolerate placement of a nasogastric tube made of soft rubber (e.g., 5F pediatric feeding tube). The slurry fed to the rabbit must pass through the diameter of the tube. Because rabbits are herbivores, supplemental diets must be high in fiber, low in fat, and low in carbohydrates, to stimulate the gastrointestinal tract. Most human and carnivore replacement diets are too high in carbohydrates and fat, and too low in fiber to be suitable for replacement feeding of rabbits. Commercial formulations specifically for nasogastric feeding are available from Oxbow®. Rabbits with delayed gastric emptying may benefit from metoclopramide 0.2–0.5 mg/kg every 6–8 hours PO or SC, provided no obstruction is present. Critically ill guinea pigs should be supplemented with injectable vitamin C at 50–100 mg/pig/day. The use of analgesics should be considered, because pain may result in anorexia.

Once the animals begin eating again, they must be gradually weaned back onto a nutritionally balanced diet. Good-quality grass hay should be available free-choice for rabbits, guinea pigs, and chinchillas. Equine alfalfa cubes and small amounts of fresh fruits and vegetables, such as parsley, celery, carrots, and apples, can also be offered, along with the usual pelleted diet. Human oral caloric replacement products, for example, vanilla-flavored Ensure®, are often readily consumed by rats without prior training, and hamsters willingly accept rice baby cereal from a syringe. Introducing pet and laboratory rodents to these supplements before a potentially painful procedure will improve acceptance postoperatively and will facilitate provision of nutritional support.

Esophagostomy and gastrostomy tube placement is described for rabbits; however, these procedures are not commonly used because of the high potential for abscess formation at the site of implantation and poor tolerance of these devices by rabbits. Animals weakened by prolonged anorexia are usually poor surgical candidates.

A thorough dental examination is necessary in all cases of anorexia. Oral ulcers, excess saliva or food in the mouth, and wetting of the ventral cervical area are suggestive of a dental problem. Sharp points due to malocclusion are common on the lateral (buccal) edges of the upper cheek teeth (premolar and molar) and the medial (lingual) edges of the lower cheek teeth. It may be necessary to sedate the animal to conduct a thorough oral examination. In addition to malocclusion, the mouth should also be checked for foreign bodies and tooth root abscesses. Skull radiographs may be a useful adjunct procedure.

A commonly noted relationship exists between obesity in sedentary rabbits, anorexia, and eventual death. Rarely do rabbits live 3 full weeks after feces no longer appear in the pan. Limited feeding (85–142 g or 3–5 oz per day) of a consistent amount of feed to prevent obesity and overeating or feeding a high-fiber diet to nonpregnant adult rabbits prevents many anorexia problems.

References

Cheeke PR. Nutrition and Nutritional Diseases. In: The Biology of the Laboratory Rabbit, 2nd ed. Manning PJ, Ringler DH, Newcomer CE (eds.). San Diego: Academic Press, 1994, 321–333.

Harkness JE, et al. Weight loss and impaired reproduction in the hamster attributable to an unsuitable feeding apparatus. Lab Anim Sci. 1977, 27:117–118.

Hawkins MG, Graham JE. Emergency and critical care of rodents. 2007. Vet Clin Exot Anim. 2007, 10:501–531.

Hillyer EV. Approach to the anorexic rabbit. J Small Exot Anim Med. 1992, 1:106–108.

Paul-Murphy J. Critical care of the rabbit. Vet Clin Exot Anim. 2007, 10:437–461.

Suckow MA, Brammer DW, Rush HG, Chrisp CE. Biology and Diseases of Rabbits. In: Fox, JG, Anderson LC, Loew FL, Quimby FW (eds.). Laboratory Animal Medicine. Orlando: Academic Press, 2002; 329–364.

BORDETELLA BRONCHISEPTICA INFECTIONS

Hosts

Clinical infection with *Bordetella bronchiseptica* is common in guinea pigs, especially after stress. Epizootic respiratory disease caused by *B. bronchiseptica* can result in high mortality in guinea pigs. The bacterium may also be cultured from conventional laboratory guinea pigs as well as from pet animals, with no clinical signs. Outbreaks of *B. bronchiseptica* infection also have been reported in farmed chinchillas in Brazil. Dogs, rabbits, cats, swine, birds, humans, and primates may also develop clinical infections, but usually *B. bronchiseptica* is an opportunistic pathogen in these species. The hamster seems to be uniquely resistant to intranasal inoculation with *B. bronchiseptica*. Mice and rats, likewise, are not very susceptible to natural clinical disease but can be infected experimentally with the bacterium and may act as carriers in some situations. *Bordetella hinzii* is noted occasionally as a spontaneous infection-inducing upper respiratory disease in conventionally housed laboratory mice.

In experimental trials, *B. bronchiseptica* caused pneumonia and was more pathogenic for the respiratory system of weanling rats than was *Pasturella pneumotropica*. Young (8- to 10-week-old) specific pathogen free (SPF) rabbits, given hydrocortisone to simulate stress, developed similar degrees of pneumonia when inoculated with either *B. bronchiseptica* or *Pasteurella multocida*. A high percentage of commercial and laboratory-reared rabbits have antibodies to *B. bronchiseptica* and rarely have clinical signs associated with colonization.

Etiology

Bordetella bronchiseptica is a small, motile, Gram-negative bacillus or coccobacillus. After incubation for 48 hours at 37 °C on blood agar, *Bordetella* colonies are approximately 1 mm in diameter, yellowish-brown, and variably hemolytic. The bacterium does not ferment carbohydrates but does split urea.

Transmission

Transmission of *B. bronchiseptica* is by direct contact with clinically affected animals, carrier hosts, contaminated fomites, and respiratory aerosols. Interspecies transmission is likely. Although many surviving animals eventually develop immunity and eliminate the infection, subclinical infections and carrier animals are common, and *B. bronchiseptica* can be cultured from the upper respiratory tract and trachea of clinically normal animals. Uterine infections (metritis) have been reported.

Predisposing Factors

Many outbreaks of *B. bronchiseptica* infection are precipitated by stressors such as nutritional imbal-

SPECIFIC DISEASES AND CONDITIONS

ances, climatic and temperature changes, drafts, season (winter), crowding, feed changes, experimental procedures, intercurrent diseases, and marginal diets, especially those deficient in vitamin C, in the case of guinea pigs. Guinea pigs, particularly the young, pregnant, anorectic, ketotic, and aged, are susceptible. Contact with potential carrier species, such as rabbits, dogs, cats, and nonhuman primates, and mixing of guinea pigs from multiple sources should be minimized.

Clinical Signs

Clinical signs of *B. bronchiseptica* infection in guinea pigs are usually associated with pneumonia and vary from no signs to anorexia, inappetence, nasal and ocular discharge, dyspnea, and death. The incubation period is 5–7 days. The acute or epizootic form of the infection has a sudden onset and lasts 2–3 days. High mortality, abortions, and stillbirths are noted in guinea pigs during epizootics, which occur when the agent is introduced into uninfected susceptible colonies. Enzootic infections often follow epizootics. A decrease in immunity of individual animals from enzootically infected colonies may result in isolated cases or waves of clinical disease.

Rabbits frequently harbor *B. bronchiseptica* in their upper respiratory passages, including the paranasal sinuses. The usual consequence, through ciliary and epithelial damage, is a predisposition to other infections, particularly pasteurellosis, although primary *B. bronchiseptica* rhinitis is occasionally noted.

Necropsy Signs

The most common necropsy finding is discrete anteroventral consolidation of one or more lung lobes. The affected lung is firmer than normal and dark red or reddish-tan to gray. Mucopurulent exudate with otitis media, rhinitis, and tracheitis may be seen independently or may accompany bronchopneumonia. The histologic features of epizootic bronchopneumonia that characterize *B. bronchiseptica* infection in guinea pigs are suppuration, exudation, and hemorrhage. Additionally, there may be marked purulent bronchitis. The lumena of the air passageways contain substantial amounts of heterophils, mucus, and desquamated bronchiolar epithelium, which may extend to terminal bronchioles. Alveoli are packed characteristically with degenerating, protein-rich masses composed largely of cellular debris, primarily heterophils, and fibrin. Although rabbits are much less likely to develop overt disease than are guinea pigs, they may have similar lesions when affected.

Diagnosis

A definitive diagnosis is based on clinical signs and culture of *B. bronchiseptica* from exudate of the nasopharynx, trachea, bronchial lumen, or middle ear on 5–10% blood agar, MacConkey agar, or nutrient broth. Slow growth is characteristic and results in small 0.5 mm colonies at 24 hours. The pearl-like, variably hemolytic colonies reach a maximal size of 2–3 mm by 72 hours. When nasal swabs are used to screen animal colonies for carriers, MacConkey agar is the preferred culture medium because it retards growth of contaminants. Frequently, pure cultures of *B. bronchiseptica* can be recovered from the tympanic bullae of animals with suppurative otitis media. Other common causes of bacterial pneumonia in guinea pigs to be considered in the differential diagnosis are *Streptococcus zooepidemicus* and *S. pneumoniae*. Fresh isolates can be used in serodiagnosis with an agglutination test using known immune serum. Otitis media can be detected in living guinea pigs as tympanic membrane cloudiness visible through a pediatric otoscope, and by radiographic examination of the tympanic bullae. An ELISA serologic test has been reported to be more effective than culture in detecting guinea pigs infected with *B. bronchiseptica*. Other diagnostic tests include tube agglutination, microagglutination, and indirect immunofluorescence.

Treatment

Treatment of clinical *Bordetella* bronchopneumonia in rabbits and rodents is usually not practical except in individual pets, and even then treatment of chronic infections is palliative. Affected guinea pigs should be force-fed, as needed, and given fluids and ascorbic acid orally or by injection.

A variety of injectable and oral trimethoprim-sulfa products are available. Oral chloramphenicol palmitate or injectable chloramphenicol succinate (SC or IM) may be used at a dose of 30–50 mg/kg twice daily, and clients should be cautioned about potential hazards associated with handling this drug. Sulfamethazine in the drinking water at 4.0 mL of a 12.5% stock solution per 500 mL (166–517 mg/L) for 1–2 weeks may suppress, but rarely cures, an active infection. Experimentally, gentamicin, oxytetracycline, doxycycline, enrofloxacin, and marbofloxacin have all demonstrated good in vitro activity against this agent.

A fatal enterocolitis caused by clostridial toxin release after antibiotic therapy may develop in guinea pigs. Narrow-spectrum drugs with activity against anaerobic bacteria that may allow overgrowth of *C. difficile* include penicillin, cephalosporins, lincomycin, clindamycin, and erythromycin. Safer antibiotics for guinea pigs include chloramphenicol, enrofloxacin, trimethoprim-sulfa (sulfadiazine), or various aminoglycosides. Fluoroquinolone antibiotics should be used with caution in immature animals because of their toxic effects on developing cartilage. If diarrhea develops following administration of any antibiotic, antibiotics should be withdrawn.

Bordetella bronchiseptica was eliminated from a colony of guinea pigs without treatment through isolation and bacteriologic screening techniques. Embryo transfer has been successfully used to eliminate *B. bronchiseptica* infection in rabbits.

Prevention

Good husbandry, purchase of clean stock, and separation of possible carrier animals from healthy guinea pigs are essential. A *Bordetella*-free colony must be managed on the closed-colony principle (no entry of foreign animals allowed) or with entry restricted to guinea pigs from colonies that are known to be free of the organism. Guinea pigs with enzootic *B. bronchiseptica* infections are unsatisfactory for research because they may unexpectedly succumb to infection, particularly when stressed. Rabbits deserve special attention as a source of infection because *B. bronchiseptica* is a potential pathogen. Weanlings may be inapparent carriers of *B. bronchiseptica* and are housed frequently in the same facilities as guinea pigs.

A single IM injection of formalin-killed bacterin with incomplete Freund's adjuvant resulted in protective serologic titers in guinea pigs lasting 4–6 months. Prolonged use of an autogenous bacterin with intermittent sulfamethazine in the drinking water eliminated the carrier state in an affected colony. However, a colony may experience high morbidity and mortality before the bacterin can be developed.

Two IM injections of 0.2 mL of a nonadjuvanted bacterin developed for dogs (Bronchicine, Dellen Labs, Omaha, NE) at 3-week intervals followed by a booster injection every 6 months induced protective immunity against a lethal challenge of virulent *B. bronchiseptica* in strain 13/N guinea pigs. An attenuated bacterin prepared from the heat-sensitive (34 °C) porcine ts-S34 mutant of *B. bronchiseptica* was reported to grow in the guinea pigs' nasal passage but not in the lungs. Protective antibodies were produced after intranasal administration of the bacterin. Commercially available porcine *B. bronchiseptica* bacterins also protected guinea pigs against fatal pneumonias.

Public Health Significance

The importance of *B. bronchiseptica* infection in humans is likely minimal, although the organism is recovered occasionally from the human nasopharynx and could serve as a source of infection to guinea pigs. The organism can cause a whooping cough syndrome and bronchopneumonia in elderly persons. Classical whooping cough in children is caused by the related organism, *B. pertussis*.

References

Allen DG, Pringle JK, Smith DA. Handbook of Veterinary Drugs, 2nd ed. Philadelphia: Lippincott Williams & Wilkins, 1998.

Bemis DA, Shek WR, Clifford CB. Bordetella bronchiseptica infections of rats and mice. Comp Med. 2003, 53(1):11–20.

Boot R, et al. An enzyme-linked immunosorbent assay (ELISA) for monitoring guinea pigs and rabbits for Bordetella bronchiseptica antibodies. Lab Anim. 1993, 27:342–349.

Burek JD, et al. The pathology and pathogenesis of Bordetella bronchiseptica and Pasteurella pneumotropica infection in conventional and germ-free rats. Lab Anim Sci. 1972, 22:844–849.

Glass LS, Beasley JN. Infection with and antibody response to Pasteurella multocida and Bordetella bronchiseptica in immature rabbits. Lab Anim Sci. 1989, 39:406–410.

Harkness JE, Murray KA, Wagner JE. Biology and Diseases of Guinea Pigs. In: Laboratory Animal Medicine, 2nd ed. Fox JG, Anderson LC, Loew FM, Quimby FW (eds.). Orlando: Academic Press, 2002; 203–247.

Hayashimoto H, Yasuda M, Goto K, et al. Study of a Bordetella hinzii isolate from a laboratory mouse. Comp Med. 2008, 58(5):440–446.

Lazzari AM, et al. Infectious agents isolated from Chinchilla laniger. Ciencia Rural, Santa Maria. 2001, 31:337–340.

Matheme CM, Steffen EK, Wagner JE. Efficacy of commercially available vaccines in protecting guinea pigs against Bordetella bronchiseptica pneumonia. Lab Anim Sci. 1987, 37:191–194.

McKellar QA. Drug dosages for small mammals. In Pract. 1989, 11:57–61.

Park J-H, Seok S-H, Baek M-W, et al. Microbiological monitoring of guinea pigs raised conventionally at two breeding facilities in Korea. Exp Anim. 2006, 55(5):427–432.

Percy, DH, et al. Incidence of Pasteurella and Bordetella infections in fryer rabbits: an abattoir survey. J Appl Rabbit Res. 1988, 11:245–246.

Quesenberry KE. Guinea pigs. Vet Clin North Am Small Anim Pract. 1994, 24:67–87.

Rougier S, Galland D, Boucher S, et al. Epidemiology and susceptibility of pathogenic bacteria responsible for upper respiratory tract infections from pet rabbits. Vet Microbiol. 2006, 115:192–198.

Shimizu T. Prophylaxis of Bordetella bronchiseptica infection in guinea pigs by intranasal vaccination with live strain ts-534. Infect Immun. 1978, 22:318–321.

Simpson W, Simmons DJC. Problems associated with the identification of Bordetella bronchiseptica. Lab Anim. 1976, 10:47–48.

Stephenson EH, et al. Efficacy of a commercial bacterin in protecting Strain 13 guinea pigs against Bordetella bronchiseptica pneumonia. Lab Anim. 1989, 23:261–269.

Suzuki H, et al. An attempt at embryo transfer as a means of controlling Bordetella bronchiseptica infection in the rabbit. Exp Anim. 1990, 39(3):397–400.

Trahan CJ, et al. Airborne-induced experimental Bordetella bronchiseptica pneumonia in Strain 13 guinea pigs. Lab Anim. 1987, 21:226–232.

Tynes VV. Drug therapy in pet rodents. Vet Med. 1998, 93(11):988–991.

Wagner JE, et al. Otitis media of guinea pigs. Lab Anim Sci. 1976, 26:902–907.

Watson WT, et al. Experimental respiratory infection with Pasteurella multocida and Bordetella bronchiseptica in rabbits. Lab Anim Sci. 1975, 25:459–464.

Wullenweber M, Boot R. Interlaboratory comparison of enzyme-linked immunosorbent assay (ELISA) and indirect immunofluorescence (IIF) for detection of Bordetella bronchiseptica antibodies in guinea pigs. Lab Anim. 1994, 28(4):335–339.

BUPHTHALMIA IN RABBITS

Hosts

Buphthalmia occurs commonly in rabbits. In some aspects, the condition is similar to congenital glaucoma of humans.

Etiology

Primary buphthalmia in rabbits may also be known as hydrophthalmia, moon eye, or ox eye. The condition is caused by an autosomal recessive genetic defect with incomplete penetrance and has a variable age of onset in young rabbits.

Predisposing Factors

Age and strain are predisposing factors. Rabbits from a variety of strains, especially some stocks with New Zealand white backgrounds, are more likely than others to have the mutant gene for this congenital disease. Defects in the anterior chamber angle of the eye may be seen in nursing kits as young as 2–3 weeks of age. More commonly, signs of increasing intraocular pressure are evident at 3–7 months of age. The sclera is not mature and well developed in younger rabbits. This permits enlargement of the eye due to the increased intraocular pressure.

Clinical Signs

Clinical signs are usually seen postweaning and may include unilateral or bilateral progressive enlargement and flattening of the protruded globe, corneal clouding, scarring, vascularization, and conjunctivitis, which is frequently complicated by a *Pasteurella multocida* infection. The condition may be painful, but animals generally continue to eat and drink. Blindness occurs when the increased intraocular pressure becomes severe. In chronic cases, in which the ciliary body has become atrophied, the intraocular pressure regresses to almost normal, but the increased corneal diameter remains unchanged.

Necropsy Signs

Gross lesions involving one or both eyes include enlargement and protrusion of the eye, variable corneal changes manifested by alterations in color (bluish-gray), texture, and vascularity. The cornea may be opaque, edematous, and scarified, and the surrounding soft tissues, such as the conjunctiva and the sclera, may be reddened and swollen.

Histopathologic changes of a severely buphthalmic eye include abnormalities in the filtration apparatus, atrophy of the ciliary processes, and cupping of the optic nerve head. These microscopic lesions are evidence of chronic and severe intraocular pressure.

Diagnosis

Characteristic gross and microscopic lesions, increased intraocular pressure, and increased corneal diameter in New Zealand white rabbits provide a tentative diagnosis of congenital juvenile glaucoma or buphthalmia. Ophthalmic evaluations using an indirect ophthalmoscope with 30-D or 40-D lenses, biomicroscope (slit lamp), and applanation tonometer are essential in the examination of the eye and early diagnosis of the condition. Digital tonometry can be used for diagnosis in advanced cases. Normal intraocular pressure for rabbits ranges from 15 to 23 mm Hg. To facilitate visualization of the fundus and chambers of the eye, topical tropicamide solution may be used to dilate the pupils. Cupping of the optic nerve head without other concurrent clinical signs is considered a normal physiologic change in the rabbit.

Treatment

Laboratory rabbits with buphthalmia usually are not treated because of the poor prognosis and because animals do not generally appear to be in pain. Medical treatment is generally ineffective and surgical correction should be considered for pet rabbits with advanced disease and glaucoma (e.g., enucleation with silicon prosthesis implantation, laser cyclophotocoagulation, cyclocryotherapy).

Prevention

Because the condition is heritable, may be painful, and a blind eye is easily injured, breeding colonies should be monitored routinely for this defect, and affected animals should be culled along with their offspring, dams, and sires.

References

Bauck L. Ophthalmic conditions in pet rabbits and rodents. Comp Cont Educ Pract Vet. 1989, 11:258–266.

Boyt J, Love JA. Protruding eyes in New Zealand white rabbits. Lab Anim. 1989, 18:19–20.

Burrows AM, Smith TD, Atkinson CS, et al. Development of ocular hypertension in congenitally buphthalmic rabbits. Lab Anim Sci. 1995, 45(4):443–444.

Hanna BL, Sawin PB, Sheppard LB. Recessive buphthalmos in the rabbit. Genet. 1962, 47:519–529.

Lindsey JR, Fox RR. Inherited Diseases and Variations. In: The Biology of the Laboratory Rabbit, 2nd ed. Manning PJ, Ringler DH, Newcomer CE (eds.). San Diego: Academic Press, 1994, 293–319.

Wegner F, Fehr M. Common ophthalmic problems in pet rabbits. J Exot Vet Med. 2007, 16(3):158–167.

Williams DL. Laboratory animal ophthalmology. In: Gelatt KN (ed.). Veterinary Ophthalmology, 3rd ed. Baltimore: Lippincott Williams & Wilkins, 1999; 1209–1236.

CESTODIASIS (TAPEWORM INFESTATIONS)

Hosts

Cestodes or adult tapeworms and their intermediate forms infect a wide range of species worldwide. These include rabbits, hamsters, rats, mice, and gerbils. Guinea pigs rarely are infected with tapeworms.

Etiology

Rodentolepis nana, the dwarf tapeworm, is found in rodents, especially hamsters, and may infest primates. *Hymenolepis diminuta*, the rat tapeworm, may be found in rats and other rodents. Adults of *Taenia pisiformis* are found in the intestine of carnivores, and the larvae (*Cysticercus pisiformis*) in rabbits. The larval stage of *Taenia taeniaeformis*,

Cysticercus fasciolaris, occurs in mice and rats. Adult forms inhabit the intestines of cats and other carnivores. The larval stage of *Taenia (Multiceps) serialis, Coenurus serialis*, is found in intermuscular connective tissue of rabbits. The adult stage occurs in the small intestines of dogs and foxes.

Transmission

Rodentolepis nana has three life cycle variations. In the direct cycle, ova in proglottids are passed in the feces from one definitive host and are ingested by another. The prepatent period is 15–30 days. Tissue migration by the parasites occurs in this cycle, as it does in the second or autoinfection cycle variation in which ova mature in the intestinal lumen of the definitive host without leaving the intestine. In the third or indirect cycle, there is minimal host reaction because tissue migration does not occur; the ova are passed in the feces from a definitive host through an intermediate host, such as beetles, cockroaches, or fleas, to another definitive host following ingestion of the insects.

Hymenolepis diminuta ova appear in the feces of the definitive host and are ingested by insects. When the insects are eaten, the ova are passed to another definitive host. Because of the requirement for an intermediate insect host, *H. diminuta* infections are rarely noted in contemporary laboratory rodents, although they have been seen in imported genetically engineered mice.

Taenia ova are passed in proglottids in carnivore feces and are ingested by the rabbit or rodent usually during ingestion of feces-contaminated food. Embryos pass from the intestines via hepatic portal veins to the liver and, less often, lungs and mesenteric lymph nodes. Maturation in the liver requires 2–4 weeks, when the larvae leave the liver as cysticerci. The cycle is completed when the carnivore eats the rabbit or rodent.

Predisposing Factors

General debility and absence of previous exposure to cestodes predispose the host to the more serious effects of infection. Contamination of feed and bedding with carnivore and rodent feces contributes to the spread of cestodes to rabbits and rodents. Susceptibility and reaction to cestode infections vary with the host's sex, age, strain of animal, and virulence of the parasite. For example, DBA/2 mice are more susceptible to *Hymenolepis* spp infections than are C3H mice.

Clinical Signs

Infections with *Rodentolepis* and *Hymenolepis* species are typically subclinical in rodents. Prevalence of infection is common in pet rodents purchased from large distributors in which many rodent species from different breeders are mixed with little separation between species. When present in large numbers, cestode infections may cause catarrhal diarrhea, weight loss, and death.

Taenia infections are, with rare exception, subclinical in rabbits and rodents, but in heavy infections, nonspecific clinical signs including abdominal distention, lethargy, and weight loss may occur. A rabbit with *T. serialis* infection will develop a coenurus (bladder worm and cyst) in subcutaneous connective tissues, fascial and muscular planes, the brain, and within the abdomen. The coenurus forms daughter cysts with scolices that compromise the host further. Clinical signs depend on the extent to which tissues are affected or displaced. Exophthalmos due to intraocular *Taenia serialis* cyst formation has been reported in a pet dwarf rabbit and exophthalmos caused by an orbital *Taenia* coenurus has been reported in a chinchilla. *Taenia taeniaeformis*–induced metastatic hepatic sarcoma has also been reported in a pet rat.

Necropsy Signs

Adult worms are found in the small intestine and occasionally in the pancreatic and biliary ducts of rodents. Worm masses migrate into the anterior two-thirds of the small intestine after ingestion of a meal by the host. When the stomach is empty, the worms retreat to the posterior two-thirds of the small intestine.

Taenia pisiformis cysticerci, containing a single scolex and measuring up to 2 cm in diameter, are found attached to the mesentery and viscera of rabbits. Hepatic lesions resulting from migration of the larvae appear as pale streaks with sharp boundaries beneath the capsule of the liver. They grossly resemble the hepatic lesions of *Eimeria stiedae* infection, but *Eimeria* lesions are usually more concentric with less distinct edges.

There are usually between 1 and 10 *T. taeniaeformis* cysticerci, which appear as white to clear, thick-walled cysts in the rodent liver. The cysts, which grossly resemble abscesses, are several millimeters in diameter, contain a coiled strobila, and are nonreactive if undisturbed.

Taenia serialis cysts contain multiple scolices and are up to 5 cm in diameter. Most often they are found in the subcutis and in connective tissue of skeletal muscle in rabbits, but they may occur in other tissues.

Diagnosis

Rodentolepis nana is identified by its oval ova (44–62 × 30–55 um), which contain an embryo with three pairs of small hooks. The adult tapeworms (20–30 mm × 1 mm) occur in the small intestine or pancreatic and biliary ducts and are found at necropsy. Oncospheres (16–25 × 24–30 um) occur in the lamina propria of intestinal villi. *Rodentolepis* adult forms are approximately the size of a rodent villus in length and may be found interdigitating between villi, whereas *Hymenolepis* adults are considerably larger and are found in the intestinal lumen.

Hymenolepis diminuta adults are 20–60 um × 4 mm and the ova are 52–81 × 62–88 um. Because *Hymenolepis* ova are not shed individually but reach the environment in proglottids shed in the feces, flotation techniques to find ova in the feces are not reliable diagnostic tests.

Taenia pisiformis larvae in rabbits are recognized at necropsy in the liver as scattered white foci on the capsular surface or within the abdominal cavity as cysts with a single scolex. The larval cysts are usually between 0.5 and 2.0 cm in diameter. Histologically, the *Taenia* migration lesion in the hepatic parenchyma consists of focal granulomas that contain scattered heterophils. In contrast, *Eimeria stiedae* lesions seen with hepatic coccidiosis in rabbits involve the bile duct epithelium (destruction, hyperplasia, oocyst development) and adjacent portal tissue (fibrosis with chronic inflammatory cell infiltration).

Taenia serialis larvae may be detected by observation and palpation of cysts, aspiration of cyst fluid, or by demonstration of cysts at necropsy. *Taenia taeniaeformis* larvae in rodents are detected in the liver at necropsy.

SPECIFIC DISEASES AND CONDITIONS

Treatment

Thiabendazole (0.3% in the feed for 7–14 days) or uredofos (25 mg/kg in the drinking water or 125 ppm in the feed for 6 days) has been used successfully to treat cestode infections in mice. Praziquantel (Droncit®) in the feed at 140 ppm for 1 week eliminated *Rodentolepis* in mice. Mebendazole at 1 gm/kg of feed for 14 days killed cysticerci of *T. pisiformis*. This was approximately equivalent to a dose of 50 mg/kg BW per day. *Taenia* infections in rabbits are not treated. *Taenia serialis* cysts can be removed surgically unless they are too numerous or inaccessible. Treatment should be accompanied by husbandry changes to prevent reinfection.

Prevention

Cestode infections are prevented by excluding carnivores, wild rodents, arthropod vectors, and insects from rabbit and rodent colonies. Food and bedding should be clean, and dogs and cats in the immediate area of rabbits and rodents should be treated for tapeworms. High humidity favors the survival of cestode ova in the environment.

Public Health Significance

Some *Rodentolepis* spp are zoonotic for humans and may cause enteric disease; however, recent evidence suggests that the subspecies of *R. nana* that infects humans may be different from that infective for rodents. *Taenia pisiformis* does not affect humans, but *T. taeniaeformis* may, if the rodent is eaten and is not sufficiently cooked. *Taenia serialis* larvae can affect humans as they affect other intermediate hosts.

References

Ambu S, Kwa BH. Susceptibility of rats to Taenia taeniaeformis infection. J Helminthol. 1980, 54:43–44.

Arther RG, Cox DD, Schmidl JA. Praziquantel for control of Hymenolepis nana in mice. Lab Anim Sci. 1981, 31:301–302.

Ayuya JM, Williams JF. The immunological response of the rat to infection with Taenia taeniaeformis. VII. Immunizations by oral and parenteral administration of antigens. Immunol. 1979, 36:825–834.

Balk MW, Jones SR. Hepatic cysticercosis in a mouse colony. J Am Vet Med Assoc. 1970, 157:678–679.

Baskerville M, Wood M, Newton CM. Mebendazole for worming mice: effectiveness and side effects. Lab Anim. 1988, 22:263–268.

Craig PS. Circulating antigens, antibodies and immune complexes in experimental Taenia pisiformis infections of rabbits. Parasitol. 1984, 89:121–131.

Craig P, Akira I. Intestinal cestodes. Curr Opin Infect Dis. 2007, 20(5):524–532.

Duwel D, Brech K. Control of oxyuriasis in rabbits by fenbendazole. Lab Anim. 1981, 15:101–105.

Flatt RE, Campbell WW. Cysticercosis in rabbits: incidence and lesions of the naturally occurring disease in young domestic rabbits. Lab Anim Sci. 1974, 24:914–918.

Flatt RE, Moses RW. Lesions of experimental cysticercosis in domestic rabbits. Lab Anim Sci. 1975, 25:162–167.

Ghazal AM, Avery RA. Observations on coprophagy and the transmission of Hymenolepis nana infections in mice. Parasitol. 1976, 73:39–45.

Hasegawa H, Sato H, Iwakiri E, et al. Helminths collected from imported pet murids, with special reference to concomitant infection of the golden hamsters with three pinworm species of the genus Syphacia (Nematoda: Oxyuridae). J Parasitol. 2008, 94(3):752–754.

Heath DD, Christie MJ, Chevis RA. The lethal effect of mebendazole on secondary Echinococcus granulosus, cysticerci of Taenia pisiformis and tetrathyridia of Mesocestoides corti. Parasitol. 1975, 70:273–285.

Holmberg BJ, Hollingsworth SR, Osofsky A, et al. Taenia coenurus in the orbit of a chincilla. Vet Ophth. 2007, 10:53–59.

Hopkins CA. Diurnal movement of Hymenolepis diminuta in the rat. Parasitol. 1970, 60:255–271.

Insler GD, Roberts LS. Hymenolepis diminuta: lack of pathogenicity in the healthy rat host. Exp Parasitol. 1976, 39:351–357.

Irizarry-Rovira IR, Wolf A, Bolek M. Taenia taeniaeformis-induced metastatic hepatic sarcoma in a pet rat (Rattus norvegicus). J Exot Pet Med. 2007, 16(1):45–48.

Ito A. A simple method for collecting infective cysticercoids of Hymenolepis nana from the mouse intestine. J Parasitol. 1977, 63:167–168.

Ito A, Baker DG. Biology of the Cestodes. In: Flynn's Parasites of Laboratory Animals. Baker DG (ed.). Ames, IA: Blackwell, 2007; 37–42.

Kwa BH, Liew FY. Studies on the mechanism of long term survival of Taenia taeniaeformis in rats. J Helminthol. 1978, 52:1–6.

Lussier G, Loew FM. Natural Hymenolepis nana infection in Mongolian gerbils (Meriones unguiculatus). Can Vet J. 1970, 11:105–107.

Macnish MG, Morgan UM, Behnke JM, et al. Failure to infect laboratory rodent hosts with human isolates of Rodentolepis (= Hymenolepis) nana. J Helminthol. 2002, 76(1):37–43.

Macnish MG, Ryan UM, Behnke JM, et al. Detection of the rodent tapeworm Rodentolepis (= Hymenolepis) microstoma in humans. A new zoonosis? Int J Parasitol. 2003, 33(10):1079–1085.

Mitchell GF, Rajasekariah GR, Rickard MD. A mechanism to account for mouse strain variation in resistance to the larval cestode Taenia taeniaeformis. Immunol. 1980, 39:481–489.

O'Reilly A, McCowan C, Hardman C, et al. Taenia serialis causing exophthalmos in a pet rabbit. Vet Ophth. 2002, 5:227–230.

Rajasekariah GR, Rickard MD, O'Donnell IJ. Taenia pisiformis: protective immunization of rabbits with solubilized oncospheral antigens. Exp Parasitol. 1985, 59:321–327.

Read CP. Hymenolepis diminuta in the Syrian hamster. J Parasitol. 1951, 37:324.

Ronald NC, Wagner JE. Treatment of Hymenolepis nana in hamsters with Yomesan (niclosamide). Lab Anim Sci. 1975, 25:219–220.

Simmons DJC, Walkey M. Capillaria and Hymenolepis in a wild rat: hazards to barrier maintained laboratory animals. Lab Anim. 1971, 5:49–55.

Taffs LF. Further studies on the efficacy of thiabendazole given in the diet of mice infected with H. nana, S. obvelata and A. tetraptera. Vet Rec. 1976, 99:143–144.

Tena D, Simón MP, Gimeno C, et al. Human Infection with Hymenolepis diminuta: case report from Spain. J Clin Microbiol. 1998, 36(8):2375–2376.

Tucek PC, Woodard JC, Moreland AF. Fibrosarcoma associated with Cysticercus fasciolaris. Lab Anim Sci. 1973, 23:401–407.

Worley DE. Quantitative studies on the migration and development of Taenia pisiformis larvae in laboratory rabbits. Lab Anim Sci. 1974, 24:517–522.

CILIA-ASSOCIATED RESPIRATORY BACILLUS INFECTIONS

Hosts

Naturally occurring infections by the cilia-associated respiratory bacillus (CARB) have been reported in rats, mice, rabbits, guinea pigs, hamsters, cattle, goats, swine, cats, dogs, and wild rats.

Etiology

CARB has evolved a unique mode of orientation and colonization between and parallel to the cilia of the respiratory epithelium. The organism, because of its motility, is classified tentatively among the gliding bacteria. Despite this classification, the bacterium lacks structures analogous to flagellae, pili, and axial filaments. Sequencing of the 16S rRNA gene suggests that the bacterium is most closely related to others in the *Flavobacter/Flexibacter* group. The strains affecting rabbits and rats are species-specific and share less than 50% sequence homology. A comparison of the rabbit CARB 16S rRNA sequence suggests that it is most closely related to other members within the *Helicobacter* genus. Isolates of rat origin were more pathogenic for mice than were those of rabbit origin.

The bacterium is filamentous, 0.2 um wide and 6–8 um long, with a trilaminar cell wall. The bacterium is capable of colonizing the respiratory tract (upper nasal respiratory passages, trachea, lungs, and middle ear) and acting as a primary pathogen as well as exacerbating infections caused by other agents. Pathogenicity is highly correlated with bacterial strain, and in experimental CARB infections in rats, there was little difference in susceptibility to infection between F344, Lewis, and Sprague-Dawley rats.

Predisposing Factors

Host species, CARB strains (e.g., rat or rabbit origin), and the presence of other respiratory pathogens such as Sendai virus, *Pasteurella multocida*, and *Mycoplasma pulmonis*, acting as co-pathogens, are factors that predispose to clinical disease. Results of pathogenesis studies, using an isolate of mouse origin, suggested that mice are highly susceptible, followed by hamsters, rabbits, and guinea pigs (rats were not evaluated). Sex and age of the animal did not seem to influence susceptibility to the bacterium. Use of a homologous strain of CARB (mouse origin) likely skewed the study results.

Transmission

Transmission is primarily by direct contact with infected animals, that is, dam to suckling offspring. Interspecies transmission does occur, but pathogenicity of the organism may be more variable and is generally less virulent in a nonhomologous host. Experimental inoculation of rabbits with rat-origin CARB resulted in seroconversion without histopathologic lesions. Experimental infection was accomplished by using lung homogenate of infected animals, CARB cultured in embryonated ova, or organisms grown on artificial media. Airborne transmission is an unlikely route for spread of infection.

Clinical Signs

Most early reports of CARB infection involved coinfection with common respiratory pathogens such as Sendai virus and *Mycoplasma pulmonis*. It is difficult to identify the exact role of CARB in the pathogenesis of the observed respiratory disease in such cases. CARB infection has been observed as an uncomplicated, naturally occurring disease, and the clinical signs are very similar to those seen with *Mycoplasma pulmonis*.

Experimentally transmitted and naturally occurring uncomplicated CARB infections have similar clinicopathologic characteristics. Although infected rodents are often asymptomatic, signs such as increased respiratory noises, for example, wheezing and crackling, decreased activity, weight loss, and rough hair coat may be observed.

Necropsy Signs

Necropsy signs are variable and will depend upon the pathogenicity of the bacterial strain involved and the chronicity of the infection. In some cases in rabbits, no gross lesions were associated with natural infection by CARB nor in rabbits and guinea pigs experimentally inoculated with rat-origin CARB. Nonspecific gross lesions in the lungs, including failure to deflate (emphysema), areas of consolidation and atelectasis, scattered pale foci on the pleural surface, and clear to mucoid exudate in the trachea have been reported in infected rabbits.

A multifocal to coalescing pyogranulomatous bronchopneumonia with bronchiectasis, enlarged mediastinal and bronchial lymph nodes, and dilated bronchi are seen in naturally infected rats and mice and in experimentally infected hamsters.

Histopathologic lesions attributed to CARB infection vary between and within species. The bacilli are argyrophilic and readily detected with a Warthin-Starry stain. Consistent findings include observation of CARB interdigitating between cilia in ciliated respiratory epithelial cells with a moderate to marked mixed inflammatory infiltrate in the lamina propria around bronchi and bronchioles. The location of the organisms leads to interference with the mucociliary apparatus, and there may be secondary infection with other opportunitistic agents in chronic cases. More severe and advanced lesions in rats include thickening of the bronchiolar epithelium with goblet cell proliferation, sloughing of epithelial cells, and bronchiectasis. Pyogranulomatous bronchopneumonia and tympanitis are reported in rats.

In rabbits, CARB infection causes mild hypertrophy and hyperplasia of the laryngeal, tracheal, and bronchial epithelium with few, if any, damaged cilia. There is a concurrent mild inflammatory infiltrate composed of heterophils, lymphocytes, and plasma cells in the lamina propria.

Diagnosis

In laboratory animal facilities, a soiled bedding transfer sentinel system may not detect the presence of the bacterium. Direct contact is required between the sentinels and the affected animals for efficient transfer of the bacilli. A PCR assay is available and is rapid, specific, and sensitive for diagnosis of CARB strains of rats and mice. Serological tests, such as ELISA and immunofluorescent antibody (IFA), are sensitive in detecting serum antibodies to CARB, but they lack specificity. Histopathologic examinations of formalin-fixed, decalcified, silver-stained sections of the respiratory tract are useful to confirm presence of the argyrophilic bacilli between cilia in the epithelium of the trachea, lungs, and nasal turbinates. CARB can be cultured in artificial media and examined using electron microscopy for ultrastructural morphology. Other characteristics such as PAS-positive, Gram-negative, nonacid-fast, and nonsporeforming habits offer methods for additional diagnostic confirmation.

Treatment

Culture and antibiotic sensitivity testing have demonstrated that the CARB organism is sensitive to sulfonamides (sulfamethamazine), procaine penicillin G, ampicillin, chloramphenicol, neomycin, gentamicin, and streptomycin. Many of these agents can be given in the water. No data exist to show the efficacy of antimicrobial therapy in eliminating CARB from enzootically infected colonies or in chronically infected pets. In such cases, antibiotic treatment may be intermittent and palliative. Other complicating factors and diseases should not be overlooked when attempting to treat CARB infections.

Prevention

Routine serologic screening, using animals from CARB-free colonies for replacement breeders or as pets, and excellent husbandry practices are suitable control measures. Other measures are quarantine and isolation of infected animals and Caesarean rederivation of valuable replacements.

Public Health Significance

Cilia-associated respiratory bacillus infection or disease has not been reported in humans, to date.

References

Brogden KA, Cutup RC, Lehmkuhl HD. Cilia-associated respiratory bacillus in wild rats in central Iowa. J Wildl Dis. 1993, 29:123–126.

Cundiff DD, Besch-Williford C. Respiratory disease in a colony of rats. Lab Anim. 1992, 21(6):16–19.

Cundiff DD, Besch-Williford CL, Hook RR, Jr, et al. Characterization of cilia-associated respiratory bacillus in rabbits and analysis of the 16S rRNA gene sequence. Lab Anim Sci. 1995, 45(1):22–26.

Cundiff DD, et al. Characterization of cilia-associated respiratory bacillus isolates from rats and rabbits. Lab Anim Sci. 1994, 44:305–312.

Cundiff DD, et al. Detection of cilia-associated respiratory bacillus by PCR. J Clin Microbiol. 1994, 32:1930–1934.

Cundiff DD, Riley LK, Franklin CL, et al. Failure of a soiled bedding sentinel system to detect cilia-associated respiratory bacillus infection in rats. Lab Anim Sci. 1995, 45:219–221.

Franklin CL, Pletz JD, Riley LK, et al. Detection of cilia-associated respiratory (CAR) bacillus in nasal-swab specimens from infected rats by use of polymerase chain reaction. Lab Anim Sci. 1999, 49(1):114–117.

Hastie AT, Evans LP, Allen AM. Two types of bacteria adherent to bovine respiratory tract ciliated epithelium. Vet Pathol. 1993, 30:12–19.

Itoh T, et al. Naturally occurring CAR bacillus infection in a laboratory rat colony and epizootiological observations. Exp Anim. 1986, 36:387–393.

Kawano A, Nenoi M, Matsushita S, et al. Sequence of 16S rRNA gene of rat-origin cilia-associated respiratory (CAR) bacillus SMR strain. J Vet Med Sci. 2000, 62(7):797–800.

Kurisu K, et al. Cilia-associated respiratory bacillus infection in rabbits. Lab Anim Sci. 1990, 40:413–415.
Matsushita S. Spontaneous respiratory disease associated with cilia-associated respiratory (CAR) bacillus in a rat. Jpn J Vet Sci. 1986, 48:437–440.
Matsushita S, et al. Transmission experiments of cilia-associated respiratory bacillus in mice, rabbits, and guinea pigs. Lab Anim. 1989, 23:96–102.
Matsushita S, Joshima H. Pathology of rats intranasally inoculated with the cilia-associated respiratory bacillus. Lab Anim. 1989, 23:89–95.
Matsushita S, Kashima M, Joshima H. Serodiagnosis of cilia-associated respiratory bacillus infection by the indirect immunofluorescence assay technique. Lab Anim. 1987, 21:356–359.
Matsushita S, Suzuki E. Prevention and treatment of cilia-associated respiratory bacillus in mice by use of antibiotics. Lab Anim Sci. 1995, 45(5):503–507.
Medina LV, et al. Respiratory disease in a rat colony: identification of CAR bacillus without other respiratory pathogens by standard diagnostic screening methods. Lab Anim Sci. 1994, 44:521–525.
Ramos-Vara JA, Franklin C, Miller MA. Bronchitis and bronchiolitis in a cat with cilia-associated respiratory bacillus-like organisms. Vet Pathol. 2002, 39:501–504.
Schoeb TR, Davidson MK, Davis JK. Pathogenicity of cilia-associated respiratory (CAR) bacillus isolates for F344, LEW, and SD rats. Vet Pathol. 1997, 34(4):263–270.
Schoeb TR, et al. Cultivation of cilia-associated respiratory bacillus in artificial medium and determination of 165 rRNA gene sequence. J Clin Microbiol. 1993, 31:2751–2757.
Shoji Y, Itoh T, Kagiyama N. Enzyme-linked immunosorbent assay for detection of serum antibody to CAR bacillus. Exp Anim. 1988, 37:67–72.
———. Pathogenesis of CAR bacillus in rabbits, guinea pigs, Syrian hamsters, and mice. Lab Anim Sci. 1991, 41:567–571.
———. Propagation of CAR bacillus in artificial media. Exp Anim. 1992, 41:231–234.
Van Zwieten MJ, et al. Respiratory disease in rats associated with a filamentous bacterium: a preliminary report. Lab Anim Sci. 1980, 30:215–221.
Waggie KS, Spencer TH, Allen AM. Cilia-associated respiratory (CAR) bacillus infection in New Zealand white rabbits. Lab Anim Sci. 1987, 37:533.
Yokos IT, Kagiyama N. Pathogenesis of CAR bacillus in rabbits, guinea pigs, Syrian hamsters, and mice. Lab Anim Sci. 1991, 41:567–571.

COCCIDIOSIS (HEPATIC) IN RABBITS

Hosts

Coccidia strains are highly host-specific, and within the host, reside in specific anatomic locations. Hepatic coccidiosis is a protozoal disease of rabbits and wild lagomorphs and was the first protozoal disease and protozoan identified by Van Leeuwenhoek in 1678.

Etiology

Eimeria stiedae is potentially a highly pathogenic protozoan commonly found in domestic rabbits. Sporulated oocysts excyst in the duodenum and pass via blood and lymph to the liver and other organs. Schizogony and gametogony occur in the biliary epithelium, and unsporulated oocysts pass via bile ducts to the intestine. The prepatent period is 15–18 days.

Transmission

Transmission of *E. stiedae* is by ingestion of sporulated oocysts passed in the feces. Sporulation requires 2 or more days outside the host, and reinfection is unlikely to occur with coprophagy. Long-lasting immunity develops after initial exposure. Coccidial oocysts are extremely resistant, and viable oocysts may be found in soil, feed, and on personnel, vegetables, caging, and utensils. Oocysts remain infectious in the environment for several months.

Predisposing Factors

Factors predisposing to clinical coccidiosis include lack of immunity to a specific coccidium, number of oocysts ingested, and general disease resistance of the host. Although 3- to 4-week-old rabbits may have oocysts in their feces, the disease is usually more severe clinically in 5- to 8-week-old weanling rabbits, especially those in unsanitary, contaminated environments.

Clinical Signs

Infection with *Eimeria stiedae* is usually subclinical, but consequences in an animal without previous exposure are dependent on the number of oocysts ingested. Anorexia, failure to gain weight, weight loss, a pot-bellied abdomen, icterus, diarrhea, debilitation, and death can occur. In young, susceptible animals exposed to many oocysts, mortality can reach 50% or higher. Hepatic coccidiosis can be expected to alter many liver and serum components and other physiologic functions so that infected rabbits are generally unsuitable for research. Infected rabbits should not be purchased when uninfected rabbits from other sources are available.

Necropsy

The most common sign of hepatic coccidiosis at necropsy is few to numerous, focal to coalescing, yellow-white linear tracts or nodules on the liver surface (Figure 5.3). These foci are irregularly shaped, raised, and, when cut, may ooze a yellow-green fluid. The cords are several millimeters in diameter and course into the body of the liver following the path of affected bile ducts. The gallbladder and major extrahepatic ducts may be thickened, distended, and contain yellow-green fluid. The number of foci and the degree of hepatomegaly are directly related to the number of infective oocysts ingested. The liver is usually enlarged, up to several times normal size, in severe infections. Hepatic fibrosis with inspissated bile in affected ducts may be evident on cutting the liver. Grossly, bile duct hyperplasia may be so extreme as to resemble neoplasia.

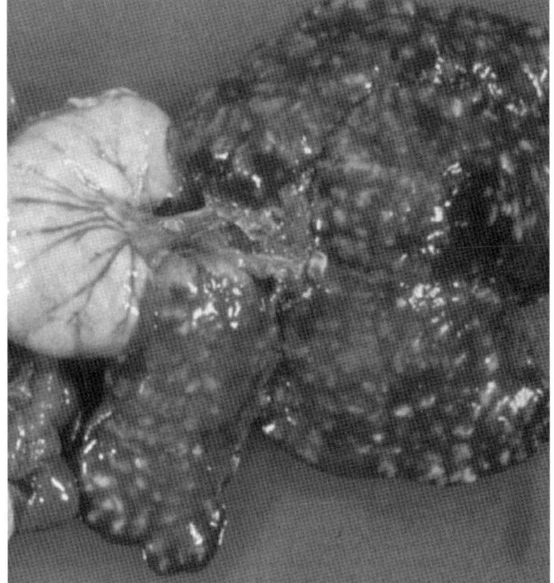

FIGURE 5.3. Liver and gallbladder from a rabbit with severe hepatic coccidiosis due to *Eimeria stiedae* infection.

The microscopic lesion consists primarily of papillary hyperplasia of the biliary epithelium, which usually contains coccidia intracellularly in various stages of development. Occasionally, infection and compression of hepatocytes adjacent to portal areas result in mixed inflammatory cell infiltration and fibrosis. Sometimes enlarged bile ducts will rupture, releasing contents into surrounding tissue, initiating a severe granulomatous response. Histopathologic examination of livers from rabbits recovered from active hepatic coccidiosis demonstrate periportal fibrosis and varying amounts of lymphoplasmacytic infiltration. Remnants of lesions may remain for the life of the rabbit and may confound subsequent pathology interpretation.

Diagnosis

Diagnosis is by recognition of characteristic lesions at necropsy. Flotation and concentration-flotation methods are used to detect oocysts in the feces or bile. *E. stiedae* fecal oocysts are elongated ellipsoidal bodies, about 20 × 37 um and distinguishable from other oocysts of the rabbit based on size, shape, and structure. Oocytes may also be found in the bile. The oocysts are smooth and light yellow, with a wide thin micropyle and residual body, and the sporocyst has a terminal knob (Stiedae body). Histologically, developmental coccidial stages can be demonstrated in the bile duct epithelium. In heavy primary infections, especially in young rabbits, death may occur before oocysts appear in the feces. Examination of direct smears prepared from cut surfaces of liver lesions at necropsy is an excellent diagnostic technique.

Treatment

Hepatic coccidiosis is best prevented or controlled through rigid sanitation practices. Effective treatment is possible only during a short, inapparent stage early in the asexual part of the protozoan life cycle. For all practical purposes, hepatic coccidiosis, ordinarily a subclinical disease, is untreatable. Treatments used for intestinal coccidiosis may be of value in controlling hepatic coccidiosis; however, robenidine, a commonly used coccidiostat for intestinal coccidiosis in meat rabbits, is not effective against *Eimeria stiedae*. In commercial meat rabbit production facilities, sulphonamides are typically used as a preventative. Note that ionophores that are commonly used to treat coccidiosis in poultry are toxic to rabbits.

Prevention

Prevention of coccidiosis rests primarily with the use of good husbandry and sanitation, that is, clean stock, proper equipment, regular environmental sanitation, and vector control. The use of coccidiostats often results in frustration because of confusion about dosages and regimens and the reappearance of the disease when the drug is removed.

Adult rabbits may be asymptomatic carriers of *Eimeria* spp. This state, combined with the difficulty of eliminating oocysts from caging, bedding, and soil, makes coccidiosis difficult to eliminate from a rabbit colony. Control of coccidiosis requires screening resident and incoming animals for oocysts in the feces, culling infected animals, and strict cleaning and disinfecting procedures. Oocysts are commonly found in the feces of clinically healthy rabbits, and a "clean" pet, breeding doe, or conventionally housed rabbit is rare.

Detergents, disinfectants, and a scrub brush vigorously applied to cages will remove the organic material in which viable oocysts reside, but no commonly used disinfectant, used as directed, kills coccidial oocysts. Hot 2% lye solution, flaming, heat sterilization (e.g., 120°C for 20 minutes), and small hazardous molecules as 10% ammonia solution, methylbromide, and carbon disulfide may be used to kill oocysts. Cleaning with and exposure to pressurized hot water and steam are perhaps the most practical methods for eliminating oocysts from an environment. Soil removal, where appropriate, may also be used. The use of sipper tube waterers and hopper feeders is extremely important in preventing coccidiosis, as is elimination of vermin and education of handlers.

Drugs, especially sulphonamides, are used to prevent coccidiosis; however, the only drug product approved for use in rabbits by the U.S. Food and Drug Administration is a specific preparation of sulfaquinoxaline (Sulfaquinoxaline Premix 40%®), which is no longer marketed. Other sulfaquinoxaline products, though unapproved for rabbits, are available. Rabbits so treated should not be slaughtered for food until the required 10-day withdrawal period has passed. The responsibilities for residues remaining at slaughter lie with the owner or prescribing veterinarian. Sulfonamides also have a variety of side effects that can adversely affect medical research. These effects range from inhibition of phagocytosis to nephrotoxicity to blood clotting disorders.

Rabbit feeds supplemented with 0.025–0.03% sulfaquinoxaline and fed continuously during the critical weaning period (3–8 weeks) are reported to reduce coccidiosis and acute pasteurellosis in young rabbits. Sulfaquinoxaline may also be added to the drinking water at 0.025–0.1%. This drug is given continuously for 4–8 weeks or for alternating "on-off-on" 2-week periods, the intent being to have the drug present at adequate levels when oocysts excyst.

Other prophylactic regimens include daily ingestion of succinyl sulfathiazole (0.625 g), sulfamethazine 0.05–1.0% in the feed, and sulfadimethoxine at 75 mg/kg for 7 days. Sulfamethazine (0.2%) and sulfamethoxine (0.5–0.7 g/L) may be administered in the drinking water on a 5-day on-off schedule. Toltrazuril (50 ppm in the drinking water) has been used with ivermectin (1 mg/kg SC) to good effect in treating experimental infections of *E. stiedae* in rabbits. These drugs may control the protozoan until the body's defenses overcome the infection.

The most important consideration in controlling coccidiosis is to prevent rabbits from contacting infective feces or contaminated food and water containers by frequent cleaning, use of self-cleaning cages (wire or barred floors), and using external feeders and waterers. Coccidiostats may provide a short-term palliative treatment until husbandry and management practices can be revised to control infection of susceptible stock.

Public Health Significance

Eimeria species of rabbits do not affect humans.

References

Barriga OO, Arnoni JV. Eimeria stiedae: weight, oocyst output, and hepatic function of rabbits with graded infections. Exp Parasitol. 1979, 48:407–414.

Cama Y, Atasever A, Eraslan G, et al. Eimeria stiedae: experimental infection in rabbits and the effect of treatment with toltrazuril and ivermectin. Exp Parasitol. 2008, 119:164–172.

Chapman MP. The use of sulfaquinoxaline in the control of liver coccidiosis in domestic rabbits. Vet Med. 1948, 43:375–379.

Gracey JF, Collins DS, Huey RJ. Meat Hygiene, 10th ed. San Diego: Elsevier Health Sciences, 1999; 289.

Horton-Smith C, Taylor EL, Turtle EE. Ammonia fumigation for coccidial disinfection. Vet Rec. 1940, 52:829–832.

Levine, ND. Parasites of Rabbits. In: Parasites of Laboratory Animals, 2nd ed. Baker DG (ed.). Ames, IA: Wiley-Blackwell, 2007; 451–500.

Long PL, Bums Brown W, Goodship G. The effect of methyl bromide on coccidial oocysts determined under controlled conditions. Vet Rec. 1972, 90:562–566.

Norton CC, Catchpole J, Rose ME. Eimeria stiedae in rabbits: the presence of an oocyst residuum. Parasitol. 1977, 75:1–7.

Pakes SP, Gerrity LW. Protozoal Diseases. In: The Biology of the Laboratory Rabbit, 2nd ed. Manning PJ, Ringler DH, Newcomer CE (eds.). San Diego: Academic Press, 1994, 205–229.

Peeters JE, Geeroms R. Efficacy of Toltrazuril against intestinal and hepatic coccidiosis in rabbits. Vet Parasitol. 1986, 22:21–35.

Schmidt RE. Protozoal diseases of rabbits and rodents. Sem Av Exot Pet Med. 1995, 4(3):126–130.

Smetana H. Coccidiosis of the liver in rabbits. I. Experimental study on the excystation of oocysts of Eimeria stiedae. Arch Pathol. 1933, 15:176–192.

Suckow MA, Brammer DW, Rush HG, et al. Biology and Diseases of Rabbits. In: Laboratory Animal Medicine, 2nd ed. Anderson LC, Quimby FW, Fox JG, Lowe FM (eds.). San Diego: Academic Press, 2002; 329–364.

Tsunoda K, et al. Clinical effectiveness of sulfamethoxine and sulfadimethoxine in spontaneous coccidial infections in rabbits. Jpn J Vet Sci. 1968, 30:109–117.

COCCIDIOSIS (INTESTINAL)

Hosts

Intestinal coccidiosis occurs frequently in rabbits, and the protozoa (caused by different species) may occasionally be transmitted from wild rodents, in which they are common, to laboratory or pet rats and mice. Laboratory or pet guinea pigs occasionally have intestinal coccidia.

Etiology

Coccidiosis is the only major enteric protozoal parasitic disease of domestic rabbits. The disease can be caused by concurrent infection with several different *Eimeria* species of varying pathogenicity. Different *Eimeria* species have distinct and sometimes overlapping ecological niches within the intestinal tract, with the result that mixed-species infections are common, particularly in rabbits. Many diarrhea outbreaks attributed to coccidia are in fact caused primarily by other agents, and it is important to ascertain that coccidia are present prior to initiating treatment. Although coccidiosis is generally a sign of poor environmental hygiene, it can occasionally be seen in well-managed rabbits.

In North America, the primary species inducing intestinal coccidiosis in rabbits are *Eimeria magna*, *E. perforans*, *E. media*, and *E. irresidua*. *Eimeria magna* and *E. irresidua* tend to be more pathogenic species. Differentiation of oocysts to definitively speciate coccidia is not useful in planning therapy or prevention, except that necropsy will determine if affected rabbits also have hepatic coccidia, *E. stiedae*, which will also result in coccidial oocysts in the feces. Prepatent periods among *Eimeria* species range from 2 to 10 days. Sporulation at 20 °C requires 22 hours for *E. perforans* to 70 hours for *E. piriformis*.

Eimeria falciformis is the most common coccidial agent infecting the large intestine of the mouse, while *E. caviae* infects guinea pigs, *E. nieschulzi* affects the rat, and *E. chinchilla* is found in chinchillas. Prepatent periods range from 7 to 10 days for each of these species. Host immunity develops against each species; however, immunity against one species will not prevent infection by another species later in life.

The transmission, predisposing factors, treatment, prevention, and public health significance of intestinal coccidiosis are similar to those of hepatic coccidiosis, discussed in the previous section of this chapter. Diarrhea associated with intestinal coccidiosis can be treated symptomatically but is often unsuccessful. In addition to being a direct cause of disease in rabbits, coccidia may predispose animals to bacterial enteritis, particularly clostridial enterotoxemias and colibacillosis.

Clinical Signs

Coccidia frequently reside in the intestine more as innocuous flora than as pathogenic organisms. This characteristic is common in immunocompetent adult animals; however, the introduction of new *Eimeria* species into immunologically naive young or old animals can produce a range of clinical signs depending on susceptibility of host, extent of infection, and strain of the causative organism. New additions to the household or colony should always be quarantined and ascertained to be free of disease before mixing with established animals.

Intestinal coccidiosis in commercial or pet rabbits is most often a subclinical disease associated with growth retardation and reduced feed conversion. In clinically evident diarrheal outbreaks, the course from first signs to death may vary from several hours to months. Most deaths occur after ingestion of large quantities of oocysts of pathogenic species and may be seen in weanlings from 1 to 3 months of age with a peak at 6–8 weeks, although younger and older rabbits may be affected. In an acute infection, deaths may occur without diarrhea, with rapid onset of intermittent or continuous diarrhea, or a few rabbits may be initially affected with prevalence increasing over several days until most are affected or dead. Inappetence, depression, weight loss, watery to mucoid feces, sometimes containing blood, subnormal temperature, and polydipsia are common clinical signs. Chronic infections occur as well, in which case pasty brown to black diarrhea may continue for weeks or months. Rabbits that survive may be cachectic, grow slowly, have intermittent pasty feces, or develop intussusception.

In rodents, coccidia are generally considered nonpathogenic; however, *E. caviae* infections in guinea pigs may occasionally result in diarrhea and death.

Diagnosis

Diagnosis involves finding characteristic forms of the protozoa on microscopic examination of intestinal scrapings (wet mounts or impression smears) together with histologic lesions or by detecting oocysts in the feces. It may be difficult to determine if oocysts found in feces are associated with primary clinical disease or if they are the product of an incidental, low-grade infection in a resistant host. Oocysts of various *Eimeria* species have distinct morphologic traits. For example, *E. flavescens* has oocysts that are smaller and more ovoid in shape than the yellow, broadly ellipsoidal or ovoidal *E. irresidua* oocysts. Serologic tests for antibody to *Eimeria* spp are performed uncommonly for all species.

Necropsy

In rabbits, no gross lesions may be evident, or there may be segmental dilatation of the small intestine with watery or hemorrhagic content, and serosal hyperemia and edema. Mucosal ulceration may proceed from focal desquamation to coalescing ulcers and Peyer's patch enlargement. Petechiation may be evident on the cecal and colonic serosa.

Both asexual and sexual forms of coccidia infect the mucosal epithelium, leading to swelling and eventual rupture of parasitized cells. Loss of mucosal integrity may lead to ulceration, mixed inflammatory cell infiltration, and increased susceptibility to other pathogenic agents.

Treatment

Treatments recommended for hepatic coccidiosis of rabbits can be applied to intestinal coccidiosis. Some of the various coccidiostats that have been used in rabbits are listed in Table 5.1. Treatments should continue for at least 5 consecutive days and be repeated after 5 days. Resistance to common commercial coccidiostats is common. As for hepatic coccidiosis, improved hygiene and environmental

Table 5.1. Coccidiostats commonly used in rabbits.

Drug	Dosage
Sulfaquinoxaline	1 g/L in water; 125–250 ppm in feed
Sulfamethazine	0.77 g/L in water; 0.5–1% in feed
Sulfadimethoxine	75–100 mg/kg; 0.5–0.7 g/L in water
Sulfadimerazine	2 g/L in water

decontamination (10% ammonia) of caging, food hoppers, sipper tubes, toys, and so forth are critical for successful elimination of the organism. Separation of weanlings from infected and shedding older rabbits may help to break the cycle of infection. Coccidiosis is common in wild rabbits and pet rabbits should not be allowed to contact feces from feral animals.

Guinea pigs and other rodents affected with coccidiosis have been safely and successfully treated with 2% sulfamethazine in water for 7–10 days.

References

Chowdury AA, Fraser GC. Coccidia (Eimeria spp) of domestic rabbits in New South Wales. Austr Vet J. 2008, 86:365–366.

Gregory MW, Catchpole J. Coccidiosis in rabbits: the pathology of Eimeria flavescens infection. Int J Parasitol. 1986, 16:131–145.

Owen DG. Parasites of Laboratory Animals. Laboratory Animal Handbook 12. London: Royal Society of Medicine Services Limited, 1992; 50–53, 63–68, 117–119.

Pakes SP, Gerrity LW. Protozoal Diseases. In: The Biology of the Laboratory Rabbit, 2nd ed. Manning PJ, Ringler DH, Newcomer CE (eds.). San Diego: Academic Press, 1994; 205–229.

Patterson LT. Rabbit coccidiosis. Vet Hum Toxicol. 1987, 29(Suppl 1):73–79.

Peeters JE, et al. Coccidiosis in rabbits: a field study. Res Vet Sci. 1981, 30:328–334.

Peeters JE, Geeroms R. Efficacy of Toltrazuril against intestinal and hepatic coccidiosis in rabbits. Vet Parasitol. 1986, 22:21–35.

Percy DH, Barthold SW. Rabbit. In: Pathology of Laboratory Rodents and Rabbits, 3rd ed. Ames, IA: Wiley-Blackwell, 2007; 287–290.

Schmidt RE. Protozoal diseases of rabbits and rodents. Sem Av Exot Pet Med. 1995, 4(3):126–130.

Weisbroth SH, Scher S. Fatal intussusceptions associated with intestinal coccidiosis (Eimeria perforans) in a rabbit. Lab Anim Sci. 1975, 25:7–81.

CORONAVIRUS INFECTIONS

These enveloped RNA viruses are species-specific and affect a variety of hosts including mice, guinea pigs, ferrets, cats, dogs, pigs, calves, and humans. In general, young animals are selectively affected, and older immunocompetent animals are relatively refractory to infection and clinical disease. Coronavirus strains may be nonspecific in terms of the organ system affected and induce generalized disease, or they may target the gastrointestinal tract, resulting in diarrhea. Increased susceptibility of very young animals to intestinal coronavirus infection is due, in large part, to decreased turnover of intestinal epithelial cells. For example, as mice mature, the rate of enterocyte turnover increases, allowing an enhanced production of new enterocytes to compensate for loss of cells infected by the virus.

Rabbit

Coronavirus infections occur naturally in rabbits and may play a role in some enzootics of diarrheal disease in this species. Carrier animals have been identified. It has been suggested that carriers may be responsible for the persistence of the infection in some rabbitries where there is a high incidence of mortality due to enteritis. Studies evaluating the prevalence of this virus in rabbitries suggest a rate of 3–40%, although the overall prevalence of infection among pet and laboratory rabbits is unknown, because testing for the agent is not routinely conducted. There is no specific treatment for this condition in rabbits beyond supportive nursing care. Secondary bacterial or protozoal infections are common, and the virus may induce myocarditis that progresses to dilated cardiomyopathy in survivors. Affected animals should be kept warm, clean, stress-free, and dry and be provided with good nutrition and fluids, as needed. Attention should be paid to overall hygiene, and animals with diarrhea should be handled after unaffected animals to minimize viral spread between animals. There is no commercial serologic test available for this virus. Circumstantial confirmation of infection may be obtained by isolation of viral particles from the feces of young animals with diarrhea.

References

Alexander LK, Keene BW, Yount BL, et al. ECG changes after rabbit coronavirus infection. J Electrocardiol. 1999, 32(1):21–32.

Deeb BJ, et al. Prevalence of coronavirus antibodies in rabbits. Lab Anim Sci. 1993, 43:431–433.

Descoteaux JP, Lussier G, Berthiaume L, et al. An enteric coronavirus of the rabbit: detection by immunoelectron microscopy and identification of structural polypeptides. Arch Virol. 1985, 84:241–250.

Eaton P. Preliminary observations on enteritis associated with a coronavirus-like agent in rabbits. Lab Anim. 1984, 18:71–74.

Small JD, Aurelian L, Squire RA, et al. Rabbit cardiomyopathy associated with a virus antigenically related to human coronavirus strain 229E. Am J Pathol. 1979, 95(3):709–729.

Small JD, Woods RD. Relatedness of rabbit coronavirus to other coronaviruses. Adv Exp Med Biol. 1987, 218:521–527.

Guinea Pig

A coronavirus has been reported in guinea pigs that is antigenically related to other coronaviruses, including rat and human coronaviruses. Viral infection has been associated with diarrhea and wasting in young guinea pigs. Chronic fecal excretion of coronavirus-like particles has been observed in asymptomatic adult guinea pigs. The significance of these findings requires further study, but it is likely that coronavirus infections play a role in some cases of enteritis in guinea pigs, particularly in young animals. The virus is transmitted by fecal-oral contact, reinforcing the need for good environmental hygiene. The prevalence of viral infection among guinea pig populations is unknown, and there is no commercial diagnostic test for this agent. Definitive diagnosis would require isolation of virus particles from the feces of affected guinea pigs.

References

Jaax GP, Jaax NK, Petrali JP, et al. Coronavirus-like virions associated with a wasting syndrome in guinea pigs. Lab Anim Sci. 1990, 40:375–378.

Marshall JA, Doultree JC. Chronic excretion of coronavirus-like particles in laboratory guinea pigs. Lab Anim Sci. 1996, 46:104–106.

Mice

Mice are the hosts for the coronavirus mouse hepatitis virus (MHV). Mouse hepatitis virus infection is widespread, often difficult to detect, highly contagious, and has manifold effects on the host's immune system. It continues to be one of the most prevalent viral infections in rodent colonies in North America and Europe.

Etiology

There are many genetically related strains of MHV, and because it is an RNA virus, it is capable of high mutation rates resulting in antigenic drift. Because of varied tissue affinities, antigenic variation, and differential host susceptibilities, the viral strains induce a wide spectrum of disease in mice. Immmunity to the virus is strain-specific and short-lived, and colonies in which the virus has been eliminated can readily become reinfected following another exposure. In addition, many genetically modified strains of mice are not fully immunocompetent, and these animals may not be readily able to clear the viral infection. This has given rise to the common misconception that the virus has a latent phase.

Transmission

Mouse hepatitis virus infection is highly contagious. The virus is disseminated by respiratory aerosol, in the feces, and possibly through the placenta. Because of the ubiquitous and highly contagious nature of MHV in wild rodents and resident mouse populations, the infection can be difficult to exclude from contemporary research animal facilities. The virus may survive for a few to several days outside the host in feces and on fomites. Incoming animals and mouse biologic materials should be determined to be free of infection before mixing with the general mouse population. Shared animal equipment should also be thoroughly cleaned between users.

Predisposing Factors

Depending on the virus strain, MHV has tissue tropism for the gastrointestinal tract (enterotropic) or has systemic effects (polytropic), and clinical signs are related to the system of primary infection. Polytropic strains often replicate in the nasal epithelium and disseminate to other tissues from this site of primary infection. A number of stressors may induce overt clinical disease in infected animals, including but not limited to debilitation, neoplasia, immune system suppression or alteration, X-irradiation, splenectomy, neonatal thymectomy, or infection with other pathogens.

Genotype and other host factors substantially influence the outcome of MHV infections. For

SPECIFIC DISEASES AND CONDITIONS

example, immunocompetent adults are generally more resistant to clinical disease than are weanlings, and BALB/c mice are more susceptible than SJL mice.

Clinical Signs

Most MHV infections are enzootic and subclinical. Despite this, animals with active infections typically have immune and physiologic perturbations that can alter the outcome of experimental manipulations performed during the acute phase of viral infection. These changes, coupled with the high prevalence of the disease and highly contagious nature of the virus, contribute to the fact that MHV continues to be one of the most commonly encountered and devastating infections of large research colonies.

Susceptible suckling mice, usually between 7 and 13 days of age, can develop a severe, epizootic, diarrheal disease with high mortality or encephalitis with tremors and spasticity. The diarrheic fluid is yellow and sticky and resembles diarrheal disease of rotavirus and reovirus infections of suckling mice. Pups infected with MHV are often acutely sick, dehydrated, and refuse to nurse, resulting in the loss of the characteristic milk spot (milk-containing stomach visible through the skin). In older mice, loss of weight, breeding inefficiency, jaundice, and death may result.

Mouse hepatitis virus alters lymphocyte differentiation, immunoglobulin responses to sheep red blood cells, phagocytosis, tumor growth, antibody response, interferon production, infection with other agents, and hepatic enzyme activity. Athymic nude and SCID mice typically cannot clear the infection, and these mice develop chronic progressive emaciation or wasting syndrome with an associated persistent infection of the intestinal tract or nasal mucosa.

Necropsy Signs

A prominent lesion with some strains of MHV in immunodeficient adult mice is a multifocal necrotizing hepatitis, characterized by gray or red foci on the liver surface. These foci may contain multinucleated giant cells as well as other components of an acute inflammatory response.

Depending on the strain of enterotropic mouse coronavirus involved, replication may occur at various sites in the small and large intestine, but manifestations and lesions are usually confined to changes in the small intestine. In the small intestine, coronaviruses replicate selectively in the relatively well-differentiated enterocytes lining villi. The loss of these enterocytes results in collapse of villi and subsequent villous fusion and atrophy. Enteritis in suckling mice is typically seen as a flaccid gut distended with gas and yellow fluid. Histopathologic changes consist of villous atrophy, fusion, vacuolation, desquamation, and syncytial cell formation in the absorptive epithelium at the tip of the villi. Secondary bacterial or protozoal overgrowth is common.

Neurotropic strains of the virus disseminate by viremia and the lymphatics and replicate in the endothelium and parenchyma of the brain, where they cause vascular-oriented encephalitis with neuronal chromatolysis and neurodegeneration.

Diagnosis

Clinical history, necropsy, and histopathologic features are helpful in establishing a diagnosis of MHV infection. Multinucleated giant cells in the nasal epithelium, liver, or absorptive epithelium of the small or large intestine are highly indicative, if not pathognomonic, of MHV infection. Use of a "Swiss roll" technique greatly facilitates histopathologic examination of the entire gastrointestinal tract. In this technique, the intestine is opened along its length, the feces are removed, the intestine is rerolled along its length usually around a short stick or toothpick, frozen or fixed, and then embedded in paraffin and sectioned.

An ELISA or IFA test is used commonly to detect serum antibody to MHV infection. PCR may also be used to detect antigen in fecal pellets and mesenteric lymph nodes during the acute phase of infection. Female mice usually have higher titers than do males because they ingest the infected feces of sucklings. Strains of mice vary in their serologic responsiveness to various strains of mouse hepatitis viruses. C57BL/6 mice produce a high antibody titer and are a good sentinel strain for MHV infection. DBA/2 mice, on the other hand, are poor responders for antibody production and should not be used to test for MHV if other strains are available. Positive serology should be confirmed by repeat testing, testing of additional animals, or use of a second diagnostic assay. False positive results may occur due to nonspecific color reactions or subclinical infections of mice with rat coronaviruses.

Treatment

A satisfactory treatment for MHV infection does not exist. Maternally derived, passive immunity prevented MHV infection in 1-week-old pups that were challenged with a homologous strain of MHV. Pups that were challenged with a heterologous strain were only partially protected.

Because MHV is an RNA virus, it may be possible to eliminate the virus from an enzootically infected breeding colony of immunocompetent mice by complete cessation of breeding of seropositive animals, without new colony introductions, for an 8-week period, coupled with rigorous environmental decontamination. This is often not practical with large breeding operations, which may more reliably eliminate the virus from colonies by embryo transfer of pups from infected to clean foster dams.

Prevention

Because the source of MHV and other infections is usually other mice, feral or domestic, exclusion of infected animals is paramount to maintaining disease-free populations. The use of embryo transfer or Caesarean-derived mice in a barrier-sustained colony, repeated serologic testing of breeding females, histopathologic examination of dead weanlings, and the use of exclusion filter top cages, gloves, disinfected forceps for handling mice, and laminar flow units are proven preventive measures for minimizing opportunities for MHV spread within a facility. Soiled bedding transfer for sentinel detection of MHV in a colony is not necessarily foolproof, and false negatives may occur, depending on the viral load of infected animals and time of peak viral shedding versus bedding sampling.

Appropriately used, a microisolator caging system provides an effective barrier against MHV infection at the cage level and also protects mice against other infectious agents. C57BL/6 mice housed on soiled bedding have been used as sentinels for detection of MHV from infected mice that were housed in microisolators. Along with use of the microisolator caging system, rigorous sanitary procedures must be practiced.

Public Health Significance

Mouse hepatitis virus does not affect humans.

References

Barthold SW. Host age and genotypic effects on enterotropic mouse hepatitis virus infection. Lab Anim Sci. 1987, 37:36–40.

———. Research Complications and State of Knowledge of Rodent Coronaviruses. In: Complications of Viral and Mycoplasma Infections in Rodents to Toxicology Research and Testing. Hamm TE, Jr (ed.). Washington, DC: Hemisphere Press, 1986; 53–90.

Barthold SW, Beck DS, Smith AL. Enterotopic coronavirus (mouse hepatitis virus) in mice: influence of host age and strain on infection and disease. Lab Anim Sci. 1993, 43:276–284.

Barthold SW, Smith AL. Duration of mouse hepatitis virus infection: studies in immunocompetent and chemically immunosuppressed mice. Lab Anim Sci. 1990, 40:133–137.

Boorman GA, et al. Peritoneal macrophage alterations caused by naturally occurring mouse hepatitis virus. Am J Pathol. 1982, 106:110–117.

Casebolt DB, Qian B, Stephensen CB. Detection of enterotropic mouse hepatitis virus fecal excretion by polymerase chain reaction. Lab Anim Sci. 1997, 47(1):6–10.

Dillehay DL, Lehner DM, Huerkamp MJ. The effectiveness of a microisolator cage system and sentinel mice for controlling and detecting MHV and Sendai virus infections. Lab Anim Sci. 1990, 40:367–370.

Garlinghouse LE, Jr, Smith AL. Responses of mice susceptible or resistant to lethal infection with mouse hepatitis virus, strain JHM, after exposure by a natural route. Lab Anim Sci. 1985, 35:469–472.

Homberger FR. Enterotropic mouse hepatitis virus. Lab Anim. 1997, 31(2):97–115.

Homberger FR, Barthold SW, Smith AL. Duration and strain-specificity of immunity to enterotropic mouse hepatitis virus. Lab Anim Sci. 1992, 42:347–351.

Katami K, et al. Vertical transmission of mouse hepatitis virus infection in mice. Jpn J Exp Med. 1978, 48:481–490.

Kunita S, et al. Sequence analysis and molecular detection of mouse hepatitis virus using the polymerase chain reaction. Lab Anim Sci. 1992, 42:593–598.

Lavi E, et al. Limbic encephalitis after inhalation of a murine coronavirus. Lab Invest. 1988, 58:31–36.

Li LH, et al. Effect of mouse hepatitis virus infection on combination therapy of P388 leukemia with

cyclophosphamide and pyrimidinones. Lab Anim Sci. 1987, 37:41–44.
Navas-Martin S, Weiss SR. SARS: lessons learned from other coronaviruses. Viral Immunol. 2003, 16(4):461–474.
Peters RL, et al. Enzyme-linked immunosorbent assay for detection of antibodies to murine hepatitis virus. J Clin Microbiol. 1979, 10:595–597.
Rodriguez-Cuesta J, et al. Effect of asymptomatic natural infections due to common mouse pathogens on the metastatic progression of B16 murine melanoma in C57BL/6 mice. Clin Exper Metast. 2005, 22:549–558.
Shek WR. Role of housing modalities on management and surveillance strategies for adventitious agents of rodents. ILAR J. 2008, 49(3):316–325.
Smith PC, Nucifora M, Reuter JD, et al. Reliability of soiled bedding transfer for detection of mouse parvovirus and mouse hepatitis virus. Comp Med. 2007, 57(1):90–96.
Ward JM, Collins MJ, Jr, Parker JC. Naturally occurring mouse hepatitis virus infection in the nude mouse. Lab Anim Sci. 1977, 27:372–376.
Weir EC, et al. Elimination of mouse hepatitis virus from a mouse breeding colony by temporary cessation of breeding. Lab Anim Sci. 1985, 35:524.

Rats

Rats are the natural hosts for the highly contagious coronavirus sialodacryoadenitis virus (SDAV). The self-limiting clinical disease, sialodacryoadenitis (SDA), caused by this agent is seen worldwide, primarily in young rats. Mice may develop a transient interstitial pneumonia with seroconversion.

Etiology

SDAV is a coronavirus (RNA) antigenically related to the mouse hepatitis viruses (MHVs), rat coronavirus (RCV), and human coronaviruses. SDAV is highly infectious and epitheliotropic and replicates in the cytoplasm, most notably in cells of the respiratory epithelium, and in salivary, lacrimal, and Harderian glands. In contrast, other forms of RCV infection do not generally infect the salivary glands.

Transmission

Passage among exposed rats is exceptionally rapid by respiratory aerosol or direct contact with respiratory secretions. The respiratory tract is the primary portal of entry. Infected animals secrete the virus for approximately 7 days. The disease can be endemic, but like MHV, SDAV does not exist in a latent carrier state in immunocompetent animals. Mortality is usually low but morbidity and subclinical infection commonly reach 100%. Extension of the infection from the respiratory epithelium is via ducts of the salivary, lacrimal, and Harderian glands. The virus has not been detected in feces.

Athymic rats carry and can transmit the infection for 6 months or longer after inoculation. Prior infection of immunocompetent rats with SDAV protect them against development of typical salivary gland lesions after reinoculation with SDAV for up to 15 months after infection. Immunocompetent rats reinfected with homologous RCV will transmit virus to naive contacts as early as 6 months after initial infection.

Predisposing Factors

Healthy, naive rats of both sexes and all ages are susceptible to SDAV infection, although the severity and site of the lesions vary among hosts of different ages and strains. Susceptible, young animals, 2–4 weeks of age and with no maternal antibody, develop more serious forms of the disease with the highest mortality.

Clinical Signs

Sialodacryoadenitis is a highly infectious enzootic or epizootic disease of rats. Whereas clinical signs are seen in a colony for several weeks during an epizootic, individual animals show signs for up to a week. Signs include squinting, photophobia, blinking, and eye rubbing followed by sneezing and cervical swelling within 5–7 days postinfection. Sneezing is associated with acute rhinitis. Swelling under the neck is caused by cervical edema, enlarged cervical lymph nodes, and necrotic and inflamed salivary glands. Bilateral or unilateral suborbital or periorbital swelling, prominent or bulging eyes, and often chromodacryorrhea ("red tears") and ophthalmic lesions develop secondary to decreased lacrimation; self-mutilation may occur as a result of scratching the eyes and other affected areas. Very young animals may enucleate the eyeball.

During the infection rats usually remain active and continue to eat, although certain behavioral activities may be suppressed, for example, pain may reduce food intake and complicate feeding studies.

Pneumotropic strains of rat coronaviruses may cause an interstitial pneumonia in young rats, particularly of the Fischer 344 strain. This infection may be exacerbated fatally by concomitant Sendai virus infection or mycoplasmosis. There may be high mortality associated with general anesthesia during the pneumonic phase of the disease.

Necropsy Signs

The infection progresses rapidly from the respiratory epithelium to the lacrimal and serous or serous-mucous mixed salivary glands, associated lymph nodes, and contiguous tissues. Affected glands are enlarged, edematous, pale, and often reddened. The thymus becomes atrophic; however, this sign and the chromodacryorrhea may be stress responses. The salivary, Harderian, and exorbital lacrimal glands may all be affected as a group or individually. Lesions are frequently unilateral, and paired salivary and lacrimal glands should be harvested for histopathologic examination.

The glands will return to normal or become permanently scarred, depending upon the severity of the infection and the degree of tissue damage, within 2–4 weeks of infection. Ophthalmic lesions are frequently associated with loss of tears, self-trauma, and inflammation, and range from keratitis sicca to multiple inflammatory sites on and around the eye to corneal ulceration to enucleation.

Immunofluorescent studies demonstrate viral antigen in the respiratory epithelium, lacrimal and salivary glands, and lymph nodes. Epithelial cells of the respiratory tract and ducts and acini of the salivary, lacrimal, and Harderian glands undergo severe necrosis and inflammation. As the virus is eliminated from the lesion in about a week, the restoration process ensues. Provided the basement membranes are intact, tissues will regenerate with minimal permanent scarring. The ductal epithelium undergoes transient squamous metaplasia, and acinar repair is characterized by regenerative hyperplasia. Harderian glands may also have prominent squamous metaplasia. Accompanying changes include persistent mixed inflammatory cell infiltration of the interstitium, tubular blockage, secondary cystic and metaplastic changes, and hyperplasia of local lymph nodes. Athymic rats develop chronic, active lesions that persist in target organs for months.

Diagnosis

Mouse hepatitis virus antigens cross-react with SDAV antibody in the serum and are often used in ELISA tests. Diagnosis of SDAV is based on clinical signs, histologic lesions, and the detection of serum antibodies. Harderian gland lesions caused by damage associated with blood collection from the retroorbital sinus can be confused with lesions of SDAV infection. Conjunctivitis from other causes may mimic secondary signs of an SDAV infection. Rats without antibody titers to mouse hepatitis virus or rat coronavirus antigens can be assumed to be free of SDAV antibodies. Virus neutralization, IFA, and immunohistochemical tests may also be useful. Acute infections may be detected by PCR of salivary or Harderian gland tissue.

Treatment

Nursing support by providing the animal with a warm, comfortable environment, tasty food treats, sterile ophthalmic lubricant, and fluids will help to make the pet rat more comfortable during the course of disease, which will last approximately 1–3 weeks. Treatment with antibiotics during the rapid course of the disease can alleviate the effects of secondary ophthalmic trauma and bacterial infections from agents such as *Pasteurella pneumotropica*, *Actinobacillus* spp, and *Staphylococcus aureus*. Laboratory rats are rarely treated because of the potential risk associated with keeping infected animals in a facility and are humanely culled.

Prevention

Susceptible colonies can be isolated and quarantined, but the virus is highly infectious and strict isolation and microisolator caging are usually required to prevent an outbreak from infecting an entire facility. Except in cases of severe keratitis or when eye enucleation is required, the disease usually produces no long-term disability. Immunocompetent rats will clear the infection after exposure to SDAV but may become reinfected with new strains subsequently, as there is little interstrain cross-protectivity.

Public Health Significance

There are no reports of human susceptibility to SDAV.

References

Barthold SW, de Souza MS, Smith AL. Susceptibility of laboratory mice to intranasal and contact infection with coronaviruses of other species. Lab Anim Sci. 1990, 40:481–485.

Brammer D, et al. Elimination of sialodacryoadenitis virus from a rat production colony by using seropositive breeding animals. Lab Anim Sci. 1993, 43:633–634.

Hajjar AM, et al. Chronic sialodacryoadenitis virus (SDAV) infection in athymic rats. Lab Anim Sci. 1991, 41:22–25.

Hanna PE, et al. Sialodacryoadenitis in the rat: effects of immunosuppression on the course of the disease. Amer J Vet Res. 1984, 45:2077–2083.

Jacoby RO, Gaertner DJ. Viral Diseases. In: The Laboratory Rat. Suckow MA, Weisbroth SH, Franklin CL (eds.). Orlando: Academic Press, 2006, 423–452.

La Regina M, et al. Transmission of sialodacryoadenitis virus (SDVA) from infected rats to rats and mice through handling, close contact, and soiled bedding. Lab Anim Sci. 1992, 42:344–346.

Percy DH, et al. Duration of protection from reinfection following exposure to sialodacryoadenitis virus in Wistar rats. Lab Anim Sci. 1990, 40:144–149.

Percy DH, Williams KL, Paturzo FX. A comparison of the sensitivity and specificity of sialodacryoadenitis virus, Parker's rat coronavirus, and mouse hepatitis virus-infected cells as a source of antigen for the detection of antibody to rat coronaviruses. Arch Virol. 1991, 119:175–180.

Peters RL, Collins MJ. Use of mouse hepatitis virus antigen in an enzyme-linked immunosorbent assay for rat coronaviruses. Lab Anim Sci. 1981, 31:472–475.

Schoeb TR, Lindsey JR. Exacerbation of murine respiratory mycoplasmosis by sialodacryoadenitis virus infection in gnotobiotic F344 rats. Vet Pathol. 1987, 24:392–399.

Utsumi K, et al. Reproductive disorders in female rats infected with sialodacryoadenitis virus. Exp Anim. 1991, 40:361–365.

Weir EC, et al. Infection of SDAV-immune rats with SDAV and rat coronavirus. Lab Anim Sci. 1990, 40:363–366.

———. Persistence of sialodacryoadenitis virus in athymic rats. Lab Anim Sci. 1990, 40:138–143.

Weisbroth SH, Peress N. Ophthalmic lesions and dacryoadenitis: a naturally occurring aspect of sialodacryoadenitis virus infection of the laboratory rat. Lab Anim Sci. 1977, 27:466–473.

CORYNEBACTERIUM KUTSCHERI INFECTIONS

Hosts

Mice and rats are the primary laboratory species affected by *Corynebacterium kutscheri*. Isolation has been reported in the hamster and guinea pig.

Etiology

Corynebacterium kutscheri is a Gram-positive, nonmotile, diphtheroid bacillus that causes corynebacteriosis or pseudotuberculosis. After 48 hours of aerobic incubation on 5% blood agar, colonies are circular, 1–4 mm in diameter, translucent, gray to yellow, smooth, and nonhemolytic.

Transmission

Corynebacterium kutscheri is carried in the oral cavity, colon, rectum, and submaxillary lymph nodes, and transmission is by the oral-fecal route. Prenatal transmission has been demonstrated experimentally. Infected animals may shed the bacterium into the environment for extended periods of time. For example, the organism has been detected in the feces of mice up to 5 months postinfection. *Corynebacterium* spp have also been isolated from the conjunctiva of normal, apparently healthy rabbits and guinea pigs. Pet rodents, and rats in particular, may transmit the bacterium to their human handlers.

Predisposing Factors

Corynebacterium kutscheri is considered an opportunistic pathogen in immunocompetent animals. Infections in mice and rats are typically inapparent and become overt after immunosuppression or other stressful manipulations. Nutritional deficiencies, concomitant infections (e.g., salmonellosis or mousepox), corticosterone administration to induce immunsuppression, pregnancy, irradiation, inadequate hygiene, and possibly anemia are predisposing stressors. Rats infected with SDAV, Sendai virus, or parvovirus do not convert preexisting subclinical *C. kutscheri* infections into clinically apparent diseases. Susceptibility to the bacterium varies among inbred strains of mice. Strain A mice, for example, are highly susceptible. Strains of mice sensitive to *C.*

kutscheri infection tend to be resistant to *Salmonella* spp infections and vice versa. Rats are more resistant to acute spontaneous pseudotuberculosis than are mice.

Clinical Signs

The infection is usually latent and subclinical. The acute clinical disease, with high morbidity and low variable mortality (2–10%), is characterized by a rough hair coat, emaciation, rapid respiration, hunched posture, abnormal gait, nasal and ocular discharge, septic swollen joints, and lethargy. In cutaneous infections, the skin is abscessed, ulcerated, and underlaid by fistulous tracts. Loss of necrotic extremities mimics clinical signs associated with mousepox in mice. Death usually occurs within a week. A chronic infection, with low morbidity and mortality, may be inapparent or produce nonspecific signs.

Necropsy Signs

Hematogenous extension of the organism from the oral cavity via small abrasions or from regional lymph nodes results in focal embolic abscessation in a variety of organs, most notably the kidneys, lungs, heart, mesentery, and liver. The brain, middle ear, lymphatic system, joints, and skin may also be affected. The lesions are scattered, gray to light yellow, and raised with caseopurulent foci up to 15 mm in diameter. There are usually no splenic lesions as in salmonellosis and mousepox. Rats may develop a severe pneumonia with a striking target-like pattern caused by multifocal abscesses against the dark red parenchyma of the lung. The central necrotic portion of each lesion often has an umbilicated appearance.

Histologically, the lesions are chronic and consist of a pyogranulomatous infiltrate around the central necrotic core, surrounded by a mantle of infiltrating lymphocytes, plasma cells, and fibroblasts. Abundant clumps of the Gram-positive bacteria are evident on smear preparations and in tissue sections. Lung lesions eventually become granulomatous, hence the reason for calling the disease pseudotuberculosis.

Diagnosis

Examination of Giemsa-, Gram-, and silver-stained impression smears from affected tissues or tissue sections often reveals bacteria surrounding the areas of necrotic debris typically arranged in characteristic "Chinese character" patterns and consisting of Gram-positive short, plump rods. Definitive diagnosis requires characterization of bacteria cultured on blood agar or serologic testing. The isolation rate of *C. kutscheri* is highest in specimens collected from the oral cavities and the submaxillary lymph nodes. The organism can also be recovered from the cecum and conjunctiva. Cortisone acetate or cyclophosphamide can be used to trigger latent infections with subsequent culture in diagnostic screening of rat and mouse colonies. The agent is difficult to recover from animals latently infected in enzootically affected colonies, although oral swabs of the gingiva may be helpful. ELISA and DNA hybridization assays can also be used to detect evidence of infection.

Treatment

The bacterium is sensitive to a variety of antibiotics, including ampicillin, chloramphenicol, and tetracycline. Antibiotic therapy does not eliminate infection but may suppress clinical disease. When treatments are withdrawn, overt disease may resume.

Prevention

Prevention of a *C. kutscheri* outbreak involves selection of clean stock and use of good husbandry practices that take into consideration the fact that *C. kutscheri* survives in the environment. Latently infected carrier animals may be difficult to detect and may be culture-negative. Immunologically compromised mice and rats should be isolated and carefully observed for signs of the disease.

Public Health Significance

Corynebacterium kutscheri is primarily a rodent pathogen, but a case of chorioamnionitis has been reported in humans and abscessation has been reported in human handlers following a bite from a subclinically infected rat.

References

Amao H, Akimoto T, Komukai T, et al. Detection of Corynebacterium kutscheri from the oral cavity of rats. Exp Anim. 2002, 5:99–102.

SPECIFIC DISEASES AND CONDITIONS

Amao H, Kanamoto T, Komukai Y, et al. Isolation of Corynebacterium kutscheri from aged Syrian hamsters (Mesocricetus auratus). Lab Anim Sci. 1991, 41:265–268.

Amao H, Moriguchi N, Komukai Y, et al. Detection of Corynebacterium kutscheri in the faeces of subclinically infected mice. Lab Anim. 2008, 42(3):376–382.

Baker DG. Natural pathogens of laboratory mice, rats, and rabbits and their effects on research. Clin Microbiol Rev. 1998, 11(2):231–266.

Barthold SW, Brownstein DG. The effect of selected viruses on Corynebacterium kutscheri infection in rats. Lab Anim Sci. 1988, 38:580–583.

Brownstein DG, et al. Experimental Corynebacterium kutscheri infection in rats: bacteriology and serology. Lab Anim Sci. 1985, 35:135–138.

Cooper SC, McLellan GJ, Rycroft AN. Conjunctival flora observed in 70 healthy domestic rabbits (Oryctolagus cuniculus). Vet Rec. 2001, 149(8):232–235.

Coster ME, Stiles J, Krohne SG, et al. Results of diagnostic ophthalmic testing in healthy guinea pigs. J Am Vet Med Assoc. 2008, 232(12):1825–1833.

Fitter WF, DeSa DJ, Richardson H. Chorioamnionitis and funisitis due to Corynebacterium kutscheri. Arch Dis Child. 1979, 55:710–712.

Fox JG, et al. Comparison of methods to diagnose an epizootic of Corynebacterium kutscheri pneumonia in rats. Lab Anim Sci. 1987, 37:72–75.

Hirst RG, Wallace ME. Inherited resistance to Corynebacterium kutscheri in mice. Infect Immun. 1976, 14:475–482.

Holmes NE, Korman TM. Corynebacterium kutscheri infection of skin and soft tissue following rat bite. J Clin Microbiol. 2007, 45(10):3468–3469.

Pierce-Chase CH, Fauve RM, Dubos R. Corynebacterial pseudotuberculosis in mice. I. Comparative susceptibility of mouse strains to experimental infection with Corynebacterium kutscheri. Vet Pathol. 1964, 5:227–237.

Suzuki E, Mochida K, Nakagawa M. Naturally occurring subclinical Corynebacterium kutscheri infection in laboratory rats: strain and age related antibody response. Lab Anim Sci. 1988, 38:42–45.

CRYPTOSPORIDIOSIS

Hosts

Cryptosporidiosis may be an important cause of enterocolitis and diarrhea in guinea pigs, chinchillas, rats, nonhuman primates, young ruminants (calves and lambs), foals, snakes, birds, and humans. Asymptomatic infections have been reported in mice, hamsters, and rabbits.

Etiology

Cryptosporidium spp was identified first by Tyzzer in 1907 in the pyloric glands of laboratory mice. Protozoans of the genus *Cryptosporidium* are small (3–6 um), intracellular, coccidian parasites that typically infect the absorptive surface of epithelial cells covering intestinal villi. Less often, epithelial cells of the respiratory and biliary mucosa may be infected. During infection, cryptosporidia fuse with host membranes, invaginate between microvilli, and ultimately lie within the apex of absorptive epithelial cells or, on occasion, within the cytoplasm of M cells in Peyer's patches. Cryptosporidia produce sporulated infective oocysts. Like other enteric coccidia, only one host is required to complete the life cycle (monoxenous).

Originally, cryptosporidia were considered highly host-specific, as are most coccidia, and each new species was named or speciated based on the host species from which it was recovered. More recent experimental and naturally occurring cross-species transmissions among mammals indicate that *Cryptosporidium* spp is not a host-specific parasite. The parasite has received increasing attention in recent years because of the potential public health significance.

Transmission

Transmission of cryptosporidia occurs with ingestion of mature and infective sporulated oocysts. Oocysts in the feces of animals with cryptosporidiosis are infective immediately for other animals. Indirect transmission may occur through contact with oocyst-contaminated food, water, or fomites. Excystation is believed to occur by digestion of the oocyst wall in the gastrointestinal tract of the host. The organism can exist in a latent form for months outside the host.

Predisposing Factors

In immunocompetent hosts, cryptosporidiosis usually occurs as a transient bout of diarrhea with low mortality, but chronic infections may occur in young animals. In immunocompromised individuals, persistent and recurrent infections frequently occur. Recently weaned animals, particularly guinea pigs, are most likely to show clinical signs. Stress caused by shipping and overcrowding may contribute to the severity of disease. Heavily contaminated environments may increase intestinal microbial load and exacerbate clinical signs.

Clinical Signs

Cryptosporidial infections are frequently subclinical and asymptomatic. Lethargy, rough hair coat, failure to gain or maintain weight, and weight loss have all been reported in natural and experimental infections in mice, rats, and rabbits. In guinea pigs, failure to gain weight, watery diarrhea, and occasionally death have been associated with cryptosporidiosis.

Necropsy Signs

There are typically no gross lesions associated with subclinical cryptosporidiosis in rabbits and rodents. Guinea pigs with clinical signs may show emaciation, hyperemia of the small intestine, serosal edema of the cecal wall, and watery content throughout the intestines.

Microscopic examination of affected areas of the intestine in acute cases may demonstrate sloughing of enterocytes at the tips of villi, edema of the lamina propria, and hyperplasia of the crypt epithelium. Villous atrophy, fusion, and hyperplasia may be seen, depending upon the stage of infection, and lymphocytic infiltration in the lamina propria is observed in chronic cases. In Giemsa-stained sections, the organisms may be visualized along the microvillous border of enterocytes. In immunodeficient mice, the ability of the organism to colonize the intestinal tract depends on the makeup of the resident intestinal microflora. In a comparison of susceptibility to *C. parvum*, infections were delayed in mice with intestinal flora compared with germ-free mice. Colonization of the biliary system with cryptosporidia has been observed in immunodeficient mice.

Diagnosis

Diagnosis is made by recognition of clinical signs, characteristic lesions such as parasites in microscopic sections, or by identification of oocysts in the feces. Cryptosporidial oocysts are overlooked frequently in fecal sample analysis because of their small size ($7 \times 5\,um$) and their morphologic similarity to yeast. Diagnosis of cryptosporidiosis may be facilitated by concentration techniques, such as oocyst flotation from fecal specimens and subsequent examination of meniscal fluid by light or phase-contrast microscopy. Examination of fresh or formalin-fixed fecal smears stained with acid-fast or Giemsa stains may aid in the detection of oocysts. Phase-contrast examination of impressions or scrapings of the ileal mucosa made at necropsy will also reveal the small, mature, birefringent oocysts.

Treatment

Treatments effective for other coccidial species appear to be ineffective for *Cryptosporidium* spp. Supportive care, such as provision of warmth and fluids, should be provided.

Prevention

Prevention of transmission of cryptosporidia is based on the use of husbandry and sanitation procedures that preclude exposure to carrier animals and contaminated objects. Many animal species, especially lambs and calves, may be carriers and sources of infection. Contact between these species or their feces and rabbit or rodent species can result in infection. Oocysts in the environment may be destroyed by treatment with 5% ammonia solution followed by thorough drying or exposure to temperatures below 0 °C or above 65 °C.

Public Health Significance

Because of their infectious nature and tendency to cross species lines, *Cryptosporidium* spp is a potential public health hazard. Infant mice and guinea pigs may be infected with *C. parvum*, the human cryptosporidial species, and feral rats may be carriers of this agent. Caution is warranted in the handling of potentially infected animals, specimens, and material from the suspected carrier's environment and as always, thorough hand-washing procedures should be used after handling any pet or laboratory animals. Cryptosporidial infections have been documented in veterinary students and animal handlers who care for calves with cryptosporidiosis. Lack of host specificity suggests that rabbits and rodents shedding the organism could result in human infection.

The course of cryptosporidiosis in humans is determined largely by the host's immune status. Infection may be asymptomatic or cause profuse, watery diarrhea, abdominal pain, and anorexia. Diarrhea is self-limiting in immunocompetent people, whereas immunocompromised individuals develop chronic, severe diarrhea, which may contribute to the death of the patient. Cryptosporidia cause severe, irreversible diarrhea in human patients with immunologic disorders, especially acquired immune deficiency syndrome (AIDS).

References

Campbell I, et al. Effect of disinfectants on survival of cryptosporidium oocysts. Vet Rec. 1982, 111:414–415.

Chrisp CE, Mason P, Perryman LE. Comparison of Cryptosporidium parvum and Cryptosporidium wrairi by reactivity with monoclonal antibodies and ability to infect severe combined immunodeficient mice. Infect Immun. 1995, 63(1):360–362.

Davis AJ, Jenkins SJ. Cryptosporidiosis and proliferative ileitis in a hamster. Vet Pathol. 1986, 23:632–633.

Gibson SV, Wagner JE. Cryptosporidiosis in guinea pigs: a retrospective study. J Am Vet Med Assoc. 1986, 189:1033–1034.

Harp JA, et al. Resistance of severe combined immundeficient mice to infection with Cryptosporidium parvum: the importance of intestinal microflora. Infect Immun. 1992, 60:3509–3512.

Kimura A, Edagawa A, Okada K, et al. Detection and genotyping of Cryptosporidium from brown rats (Rattus norvegicus) captured in an urban area of Japan. Parasitol Res. 2007, 100(6):1417–1420.

Kuhls TL, et al. Cryptosporidiosis in adult and neonatal mice with severe combined immunodeficiency. J Comp Pathol. 1992, 106:399–410.

Marcial MA, Madara JL. Cryptosporidium: cellular localization, structural analysis of absorptive cell-parasite membrane-membrane interactions in guinea pigs, and suggestion of protozoan transport by M cells. Gastroenterol. 1986, 90:583–594.

Moody KD, Brownstein DG, Johnson EA. Cryptosporidiosis in suckling laboratory rats. Lab Anim Sci. 1991, 41:625–627.

Ramirez NE, Ward LA, Sreevatsan S. A review of the biology and epidemiology of cryptosporidiosis in humans and animals. Microbes Infect. 2004, 6(8):773–785.

Soave R, Ma P. Cryptosporidiosis: traveler's diarrhea in two families. Arch Intern Med. 1985, 145:70–72.

Sunnotel O, Lowery CJ, Moore JE, et al. Cryptosporidiosis. Lett Appl Microbiol. 2006, 43:7–16.

DERMATOPHYTOSIS (RINGWORM)

Hosts

Dermatophytes are fungal pathogens that use keratin as a nutrient source and affect a range of animals. Most reports of ringworm or dermatophytosis in small mammals refer to rabbits and guinea pigs, although chinchillas, hamsters, and other small rodent species may be subclinically infected, with reported prevalence rates of 5–30%.

Etiology

Trichophyton mentagrophytes is the organism typically encountered in rabbit and rodent dermatophytoses. Several cultural variants of *T. mentagrophytes* exist, a circumstance that leads to confusion in the literature and in the diagnostic laboratory. *Microsporum canis* is infrequently isolated from rabbits and rodents and is thought to be acquired from other domestic animals, such as dogs and cats.

Transmission

Although clinical infections are uncommon, asymptomatic carriers of the dermatophyte are common, and they pose a continuing threat to other animals and caregivers. Dermatophytes are readily transmitted by direct contact with spores on hair coats, in bedding, on grooming equipment, and elsewhere within the environment.

Predisposing Factors

Husbandry and nutritional, environmental, and experimental stress are all potential factors that increase exposure or reduce resistance, predisposing animals to dermatophytoses. Genetic background, overcrowding, inappropriate heat and humidity, ectoparasitism, age, and pregnancy have also been implicated as predisposing factors.

Clinical Signs

Most animals that carry *T. mentagrophytes* have few or no clinical signs of infection. Lesions in guinea pigs usually arise on the face and spread over the back and limbs. Lesions are oval to patchy, hairless and scaling, with crusts or scabs over raised areas. Hamsters present with similar signs. Pruritus, if present, is usually mild. In chinchillas, lesions appear on the nose, behind the ears, or on the front feet, and may spread to any part of the body (Figure 5.4). Lesions on the rat tend to occur over the back, whereas tail lesions may be seen in mice. Scant to complete focal hair loss, erythema, scaling skin, and scabs are signs of ringworm infection in mice.

Characteristically, in young rabbits, lesions are more generalized than focal, but there may be 2–3 cm hairless areas with reddening and slight to heavy crust formations over the snout, face, forelimbs, or ears. Fur loss on the footpads and toes of rabbits may be due to a progressive mycotic pododermatitis condition wherein treatment is most effective during the early stages. Rabbits may chew their feet and exacerbate the clinical condition.

Diagnosis

The diagnosis may be established by microscopic examination of skin scrapings or plucked hairs taken from the periphery of the lesion and mounted in 10% KOH under a petrolatum-ringed coverslip. Scrapings should be inoculated onto a suitable agar culture medium and cultivated aerobically at room temperature for at least 10 days. Dermatophyte test medium (DTM) with color indicators is commonly used for culture (growth of saphrophytic fungi does not result in colorimetric change of the medium). Specimens for routine culture screenings can be collected by using a sterile toothbrush or surgical scrub brush to dislodge hair and cellular debris directly onto the agar surface, or the brush with scrapings can be inoculated onto the agar. Histologic sections stained with periodic acid Schiff (PAS) or methenamine silver will aid in confirming a diagnosis. Ultraviolet fluorescence (i.e., use of a Wood's lamp) is only diagnostic for some forms of *Microsporum canis*.

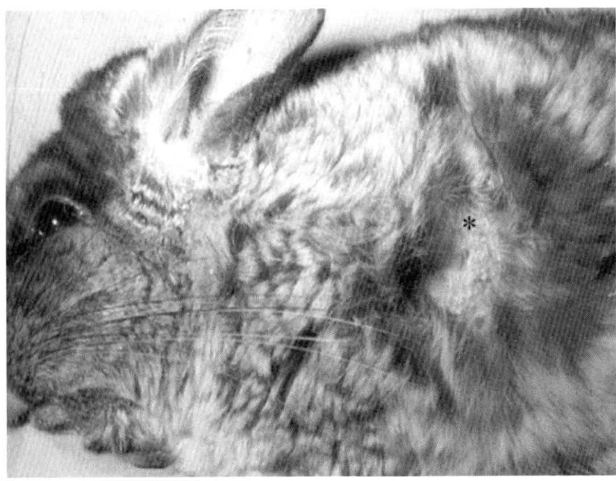

FIGURE 5.4. Dermatophytosis (circular patch of alopecia marked by *) in a chinchilla, caused by infection with *Trichophyton mentagrophytes*.

Treatment

Successful treatment of ringworm involves elimination of the organism, not just the lesions. Treatment should be undertaken only after consideration of the public health significance of the fungus.

Topical and systemic antifungal agents are available. Topical antifungal creams or lotions, such as those containing clotrimazole or miconazole, can be applied twice daily to affected areas for 2–4 weeks. Griseofulvin can be administered at 25 mg/kg body weight daily in the water for 14 days or as an oral solution of 15–25 mg/kg/day. Griseofulvin is teratogenic and should not be given to pregnant animals. Fluconazole at 16 mg/kg/day has been used with great success in guinea pigs. Dipping the affected toes in an iodine solution several times daily for weeks may be necessary to destroy infective fungus in nail beds. Topical antifungal shampoos that are approved for cats are safe for guinea pigs and chinchillas as well.

A 1% solution of copper sulfate and a metastabilized chlorous acid/chloride dioxide compound (LD disinfectant®) was reported to be effective in treating *T. mentagrophytes* infections in rabbits. The latter compound is nontoxic, nonmutagenic, and nonirritating. LD disinfectant® is used commonly as an environmental disinfectant, and cages and other materials can be soaked in this fungicide for decontamination. Together, LD disinfectant® and copper sulfate may serve as economically feasible alternatives to conventional dermatophyte treatments when large numbers of animals are involved.

Lime sulfur dips (1:40 with water) can be used once weekly for chinchillas. Animals should not be rinsed after bathing but instead toweled dry. Care should be taken not to get the solution in the eyes or ears, as the solution is irritating. Owners should be warned that this treatment, though relatively effective and nontoxic, has an unpleasant odor and can stain fabrics. This can be combined with griseofulvin at 25 mg/kg PO daily for greater effectiveness over a 4- to 6-week treatment period. Captan, an antifungal powder, has been used in the past as a fungicide added to chinchilla sandbaths; however, it is categorized as a probable human carcinogen and should be avoided in favor of safer alternative treatments.

It is important that the environment be effectively sanitized to eliminate fungal spores. Hair and skin dust should be vacuumed and surfaces wiped with dilute bleach. Any towels or bedding used for animal grooming should be washed in hot water with bleach.

Prevention

Maintenance of high husbandry standards is a protective measure particularly with young, aged, pregnant, or recently arrived animals. Culture screening for dermatophytes, optimal adjustment of temperature and humidity, removal of ectoparasites, culling carriers, and sterilization of contaminated equipment are other preventive measures. Hypochlorite (bleach), benzalkonium chloride, and glutaraldehyde are all effective in the environmental control of ringworm in small animals.

Public Health Significance

Trichophyton mentagrophytes may infect animal caregivers before it is observed on the animals. The fungus is infectious for humans, particularly very young or infirm persons. Animal caregivers should always wash their hands carefully before handling animals in other rooms, and grooming equipment should never be shared between rooms or species without disinfection in between.

References

Canny CJ, Gamble CS. Fungal diseases of rabbits. Vet Clin Exot Anim. 2003, 6:429–433.

Cheeke PR, Patton MM, Templeton GS. Rabbit Production, 6th ed. Danville, IL: Interstate Printers and Publishers, Inc., 1987.

Chermette R, Ferreiro L, Guillot J. Dermatophytoses in animals. Mycopathologia. 2008, 166:385–405.

Donnelly TM, Rush EM, Lackner PA. Ringworm in small exotic pets. J Exot Pet Med. 2000, 9(2):82–93.

Marshall KL. Fungal diseases in small mammals: therapeutic trends and zoonotic considerations. Vet Clin Exot Anim. 2003, 6:415–427.

Pollock C. Fungal diseases of laboratory rodents. Vet Clin Exot Anim. 2003, 6:401–403.

Reuber MD. Carcinogenicity of captan. J Environ Pathol Toxicol Oncol. 1989, 9(2):127–143.

ENCEPHALITOZOONOSIS

Hosts

Among small mammals, rabbits are the principal animal infected by encephalitozoonosis, although rodents may be subclinically infected. The disease is common in rabbits, and the infection frequently complicates research and may present as sudden death in pet rabbits.

Etiology

The disease is caused by infection with *Encephalitozoon cuniculi*, an obligate, intracellular, microsporidian, protozoal parasite.

Transmission

Urine-oral contact is the usual route of transmission between rabbits and within rodent colonies. The major exchange of spores occurs between the doe and her young between the fourth and sixth weeks of life. The young seroconvert during the seventh to ninth week of life. The organism enters the intestine, passes via phagocytes to the bloodstream, and is distributed to other organs. Spores appear in the kidneys approximately 35 days postinfection. Transplacental and respiratory transmission has also been described for guinea pigs and rabbits.

Predisposing Factors

As with other host-parasite interactions, the severity of infection depends on host resistance and infective dose. Young rabbits and other susceptible species, in which maternal antibodies subside at approximately 4 weeks, are at an increased risk to develop clinical disease if they are housed in unsanitary conditions and eat or drink from crocks that are contaminated with spore-containing urine from infected dams. Prevalence within guinea pig colonies depends on husbandry conditions. Guinea pigs housed with infected rabbits are at greater risk of becoming infected than if rabbits are housed separately.

Clinical Signs

Most cases of encephalitozoonosis are chronic and subclinical and are usually diagnosed on postmortem examination. Less commonly, poor growth, tremors, torticollis, paresis, convulsions, and death may occur weeks after ingestion of infective spores. In a recent study examining seroprevalence of *Encephalitozoon* in pet rabbits, of animals showing clinical signs, 75% showed neurological symptoms, 14.6% demonstrated phacoclastic uveitis, and 3.5% suffered from renal failure, while 6.9% of the animals had combined symptoms. Vestibular disease dominated within the rabbits that showed neurological symptoms. *Encephalitozoon cuniculi* infections in mice depress host immunity early in the course of infection.

Necropsy Signs

Encephalitozoon has a predilection for the kidney and later the eye and brain, although the lungs, heart, and liver may be transiently affected during the first few weeks after ingestion. The infection is terminated after between 40 and 70 days in the kidney, by which time lesions may be forming in the brain.

In the more acute stages of the disease, the kidneys may be enlarged with grossly apparent small white foci within the cortex. Chronic renal infection is evidenced by numerous, randomly scattered, small (1–3 mm) pits on the cortical surface. The granulomatous brain lesions and renal pitting, caused by tissue destruction and scarring, remain for the life of the animal. Cerebral lesions are not evident grossly, although uveitis may sometimes be seen in dwarf rabbits infected with *E. cuniculi*.

Diagnosis

In rabbits with neurologic signs, serology can help to confirm the diagnosis, although seropositivity does not necessarily indicate that *E. cuniculi* is causative, as many seropositive individuals exist with no symptoms. CT scans or MRI may assist with diagnosis of multifocal cerebral lesions characteristic of the disease. There is no correlation between serum antibody titer and severity of clinical disease, and antibodies may persist for greater than 1 year postinfection.

Within the kidney, microscopic lesions include interstitial granulomatous nephritis. Frequently, organisms are seen to be encysted and quiescent in the brains of infected rabbits with no other signs of host reactivity. More active lesions are evidenced by pyogranulomatous inflammation and necrosis within the cerebral parenchyma with lymphoplasmacytic perivascular cuffing. In paraffin-embedded sections, organisms may be identified with Gram (positive), Giemsa, or carbol fuschin stains, in which they appear as oval or crescent-shaped trophozoites approximately 1 µm in length or as pseudocysts 8–12 µm in diameter.

In most cases, histopathologic findings, coupled with serologic testing, remain the preferred method of diagnostic monitoring for *Encephalitozoon* infections. Pathologists should be aware of the potential for residual lesions of encephalitozoonosis, which can contribute to background effects in the brain and kidney of rabbits and guinea pigs.

Treatment

No effective treatment exists for encephalitozoonosis and some clinical signs may be irreversible. Infected laboratory rabbits are generally culled. Animals with acute episodes of vestibular disease may recover well without treatment. In one study, almost 50% of seropositive rabbits demonstrating neurologic signs, such as head tilt and circling, spontaneously resolved between 2 and 4 weeks later.

Treatment is three-pronged and aimed at elimination of the parasite, reduction of inflammation, and treatment of other associated signs. No currently marketed drugs have label efficacy for *E. cuniculi*. Albendazole (20–25 mg/kg for up to 30 days), fenbendazole (20 mg/kg for at least 28 days), and oxytetracycline have been reported to be efficacious, with claims of fenbendazole eliminating infection, while human HIV patients infected with *E. cuniculi* take fenbendazole for life. Reducing inflammation is accomplished via corticosteroids such as dexamethasone. Acute neurological signs in rabbits can be treated with a single injection of dexamethasone of 1–2 mg/kg, while ongoing inflammation can be treated with 0.2 mg/kg of dexamethasone, a dose less likely to induce immunosuppression. Diazepam (1–2 mg/kg SC or IV) and prochlorperazine (0.2–0.5 mg/kg PO up to three times daily) can be used to treat acute seizures and vertigo, respectively. Nonspecific supportive care should be given to animals with general signs of renal failure, such as providing warmth, fluids, and a comfortable, quiet area to rest. Lens removal is curative for rabbits demonstrating *Encephalitozoon*-induced phacoclastic uveitis.

Elimination of an infection from an existing colony is difficult, and *E. cuniculi*–positive rabbits will sometimes be found in rabbits from reputable commercial vendors. Extensive serologic testing and culling of seropositive animals should be used along with good sanitary procedures using disinfectants and hot water to reduce or eliminate infective spores from the environment. Spores may remain viable for 4 weeks or more in dry conditions.

Prevention

Selection of rabbits free of *E. cuniculi* is the best means of preventing colony infection. Urine and fecal transmission are reduced if cages are kept clean and if sipper tubes or automatic waterers and hopper feeders are used instead of bowls, pans, or other feeding or watering devices that are easily contaminated with urine.

Public Health Significance

Several cases of suspected *Encephalitozoon* encephalitis have been reported in immunocompromised patients, and human-adapted strains of *E. cuniculi* exist. Owners, veterinarians, and caregivers should always wash their hands after handling or examining rabbits.

References

Bywater JEC, Kellett BS. The eradication of Encephalitozoon cuniculi from a specific pathogen free rabbit colony. Lab Anim Sci. 1978, 28:402–404.

Cox JC. Altered immune responsiveness associated with Encephalitozoon cuniculi infection in rabbits. Infect Immun. 1977, 15:392–395.

Didier ES, Didier PJ, Snowden KF, et al. Microsporidiosis in mammals. Microbes Infect. 2000, 2:709–720.

Didier ES, Shadduck JA. Modulated immune responsiveness associated with experimental Encephalitozoon cuniculi infection in BALB/c mice. Lab Anim Sci. 1988, 38:680–684.

Felche LM, Sigler RL. Phacoemulsification for the management of Encephalitozoon cuniculi–induced phacoclastic uveitis in a rabbit. Vet Ophth. 2002, 5:211–215.

Gannon J. The course of infection of Encephalitozoon cuniculi in immunodeficient and immunocompetent mice. Lab Anim. 1980, 14:189–192.

Greenstein G, et al. The incidence of Encephalitozoon cuniculi in a commercial barrier-maintained rabbit breeding colony. Lab Anim. 1991, 25:287–290.

Harcourt-Brown FM. Encephalitozoon cuniculi infection in rabbits. Sem Av Exot Pet Med. 2004, 13(2):86–93.

Hunt RD, King NW, Foster HL. Encephalitozoonosis: Evidence for vertical transmission. J Infect Dis. 1972, 126:212–214.

Illanes OG, et al. Spontaneous encephalitozoonosis in an experimental group of guinea pigs. J Vet Diagn Invest. 1993, 5:649–651.

Keeble EJ, Shaw DJ. Seroprevalence of antibodies to Encephalitozoon cuniculi in domestic rabbits in the United Kingdom. Vet Rec. 2006, 158:539–544.

Kunzel F, Gruber A, Tichy A, et al. Clinical symptoms and diagnosis of encephalitozoonosis in pet rabbits. Vet Parasitol. 2008, 151:115–124.

Liu JJ, Greeley EH, Shadduck JA. Murine encephalitozoonosis: the effect of age and mode of transmission on occurrence of infection. Lab Anim Sci. 1988, 38:675–679.

Owen DG, Gannon J. Investigation into the transplacental transmission of Encephalitozoon cuniculi in rabbits. Lab Anim. 1980, 14:35–38.

Suter C, Müller-Doblies UU, Hatt JM, et al. Prevention and treatment of Encephalitozoon cuniculi infection in rabbits with fenbendazole. Vet Rec. 2001, 148(15):478–480.

Valencakova A, Balent P, Petrovova E, et al. Encephalitozoonosis in household pet Nederland Dwarf rabbits (Oryctolagus cuniculus). Vet Parasitol. 2008, 153:265–269.

Waller T. Sensitivity of Encephalitozoon cuniculi to various temperatures, disinfectants and drugs. Lab Anim. 1979, 13:227–230.

ENTEROPATHIES

General Discussion

Introduction

The gastrointestinal tract of rabbits and rodents is normally colonized by a complex array of symbionts and commensals that have important effects on immune function and nutrient uptake. Detailed studies have been conducted to characterize these populations in different animal species. Innate defenses, such as epithelial production of defensins, mucins, and various lectins, minimize bacterial overgrowth and maintain the mucosal barrier. Commensal populations of bacteria are important for tolerizing the gut to various antigens. The intestinal ecosystem is dynamic and also has spatial diversity.

The balance or imbalance of intestinal microorganisms may play a critical role in the development of disease. In a study of experimental ulcer formation associated with nonsteroidal antiinflammatory drugs (NSAIDs) in rats, factors released by Gram-positive bacteria (i.e., *Lactobacillus* spp) in the small intestine appeared to play a protective role in impairing ulcer development. Conversely, NSAID-associated ileal ulcers were seen following overgrowth by Gram-negative enteric bacteria, and they were interpreted to play an important role in promoting ulcer development.

Gastroenteropathies in rabbits and other hindgut fermenting rodents such as guinea pigs, chinchillas, and hamsters result in nonspecific clinical signs and high mortality rates. The enduring challenge of determining the causes and pathogenesis of gastroenteropathies has resulted in confusion regarding potential treatments and prognosis. This causes considerable frustration for pet owners and for veterinary practitioners alike, because beyond the identification of an ongoing enteritis and offering of a guarded prognosis, the next step is generally to admit ignorance or to prescribe treatments that may be ineffective. Appropriate husbandry and diet are the most important measures to prevent enteropathies, and prevention is far more successful than treatment.

Etiology

There are a variety of events that may disrupt the microbial balance within the gut and lead to clinical disease. These include exposure to pathogenic organisms (viral, bacterial, and/or parasitic), therapy with narrow-spectrum antibiotics, and dietary or drug-induced alterations. Weanlings are most susceptible to enteric disruption because of the convergence of waning of passive maternal immunity, change in diet from high-protein/-fat (milk-based) to one that is high in fiber and fermentation-based, movement and separation of animals to new locations, and other species-specific factors discussed below.

Frequently two or more organisms may act in concert to produce disease. An additive effect in the intensity of the disease occurs in mice or rabbits co-infected with rotavirus and a pathogenic strain of *E. coli*. Intestinal tract disease in rabbits is frequently attributable to dual infections with pathogenic bacteria (e.g., proliferative enterocolitis associated with an enteropathogenic strain of *E. coli* and *Lawsonia intracellularis*). A similar pattern has been observed in certain parasitic infections. For example, in outbreaks of intestinal coccidiosis in domestic rabbits, there may be a striking increase in the number of coliform bacteria in the intestine compared with those present in healthy animals. Similarly, when comparing the intensity of intestinal disease in germ-free and conventional immunodeficient mice inoculated with *Cryptosporidium parvum*, impaired colonization and reduced intensity of disease were seen in mice with defined intestinal flora. These findings were attributed to nonspecific mechanisms provided by the commensal bacterial organisms.

Predisposition

The low pH (~1–2) of the rabbit stomach inhibits bacterial growth, such that the stomach and small intestine are essentially sterile. Weanling rabbits (3–14 weeks old) are very susceptible to diarrhea, in part because their stomach pH of 5–6.5 is not low enough to kill ingested bacteria; however, the higher pH permits them to acquire their gut flora. During lactation, milk components (8 and 10 carbon fatty acids) restrict intestinal microbial growth, but during the susceptible period, the naive gut and low gastric acidity favor passage and colonization by microbes, including potential pathogens. Adult rabbits may carry small populations of the same pathogens but are able to compensate for them because other commensal bacteria keep bacterial growth in check.

Predisposing factors for enteritis in all species include genetic background, concurrent infection, loss of maternal or acquired antibody, exposure to animals shedding pathogens, environmental stress, and dietary factors. Also, rabbit kits weighing less than 60 g at birth are weaker and more susceptible to disease. In many cases of enteritis, particularly in the rabbit, the primary predisposing factors may be dietary. Excessive food consumption for any reason, including eating more in cold weather or return to full feed after kindling, may lead to premature and abrupt exposure to high carbohydrate levels in the hindgut and predispose to enteritis, as may prolonged feeding of a diet low in fiber.

The pathogenesis of bacterial overgrowth is similar regardless of the species affected. Abnormal microbial action or other transitory chemical effects may lead to a fermentation-induced transient acidosis that reduces normal bacterial flora numbers and variety. This event is followed by a rising pH in the presence of high carbohydrates and proliferation or toxin production by certain bacteria. These events may cause gut hypomotility, which results in digesta retention and changes in substrate, bacterial populations, and osmolarity. Increased intestinal pH causes dissociation of volatile fatty acids, removing the inhibiting effect of undissociated fatty acids on bacterial proliferation. Additionally, a low-protein diet leads to a decrease in the number and size of Peyer's patches. This may result in decreased resistance to enteritis, while adverse stress leads to intestinal hypomotility and variable feed intake. Green feed, season of the year, water deprivation, changes in water salinity, and fiber particle size have uncertain roles in predisposing animals to enteritis.

Enteritis also may result from dysbiosis, leading to coliform or, more likely, clostridial proliferation after antibiotic administration. Antibiotics most often involved include orally administered procaine penicillin, ampicillin, lincomycin, amoxicillin, erythromycin and other macrolide antibiotics, cephalosporins, clindamycin, and other drugs that reduce certain Gram-positive flora. Diarrhea and other signs of enterotoxemia usually appear within 1–3 days of antibiotic administration and most cases result in death.

Clinical Signs

General signs of enteritis include sudden death with few clinical signs or, in animals living hours to days, anorexia, listlessness, rough hair coat, dehydration, polydipsia, bloat, borborygmus, weight loss, tooth grinding, diarrhea (Figure 5.5), and death. Feces are unformed, may be watery, soft, or tarry, have a foul odor, and may contain blood or mucus, and coprophagy often ceases. Rabbits may die within hours or days, or they may have abnormal stool and anal impaction over several months. Rabbits recovering from a bout of enteritis will often have profound production of mucoid stools.

Diarrhea can result from increased mucosal permeability (enterotoxemia, coccidiosis), hypersecretion (enterotoxemia), and malabsorption (viruses). Death occurs from loss of electrolytes and water, acidosis, and from the manifold effects of toxins.

Clinicopathologic changes include acidosis; decreased serum glucose, protein, albumin, calcium, and alkaline phosphatase; and increased serum aspartate transferase, blood urea nitrogen, phosphorus, cholesterol, and uric acid. Enterotoxic effects may lead to impaired metabolic pathways and renal and hepatic dysfunction.

Necropsy Findings

It is imperative during large-scale epizootics of enteropathy in breeding colonies or at production

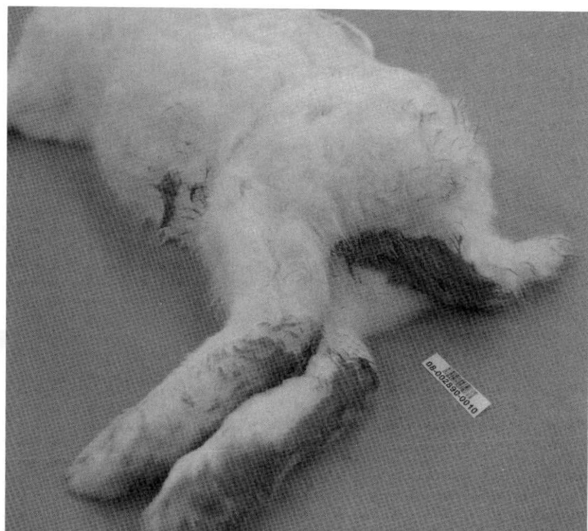

FIGURE 5.5. Soiled hocks and perineum are a common presentation in rabbits with enteropathies. Courtesy of Marina Brash.

facilities that moribund animals be submitted alive to the pathology service for necropsy. Tissue decomposition in cases of enteritis is rapid, and optimal sampling of gut tissues for diagnostic purposes must be done as soon as possible after death if any hope of making a definitive diagnosis is entertained.

Gross signs of enteritis at necropsy include a discolored large intestine (gray-green is normal), fluid intestinal content with or without hemorrhage, and dehydration. A thickened corrugated appearance to the serosa may be indicative of *Lawnsonia intracellularis* infection (discussed elsewhere in this chapter). The additional findings of focal hepatic and myocardial necrosis may occur with Tyzzer's disease (discussed separately in this chapter), and cecal impaction may occur in rabbits with mucoid enteropathy.

Diagnosis

Except for a few enteric conditions linked to specific pathogens or signs (e.g., severe coccidiosis, salmonellosis, Tyzzer's disease), diagnoses are frequently challenging in cases or outbreaks of enteritis. Fecal flotation, smears, wet mounts of cecal smears, culture, histopathology, serology, and electron microscopy may all be useful techniques. Certain bacteria, such as *Clostridium difficile*, are ubiquitous and toxin elaboration must be demonstrated to correlate bacterial presence with a pathogenic effect.

Prevention

Prevention of enteritis is critically important. Primary preventive considerations include selection of healthy stock (from health records and initial and thorough diagnostic screening); proper husbandry practices; strict sanitation; use of hopper feeders and sipper tube waterers; and, above all, appropriate management of feeding practices. Cages and equipment must be designed to prevent fecal contamination of feed and water and promote ease of sanitation by brush, water, heat, and chemicals. Nesting materials and boxes for young animals should be sanitizable, or preferably, disposable. Only if these practices fail should feed or water additives be considered as short-term measures. Vaccines for rotavirus and enterotoxemia (*Clostridium* spp) have been evaluated experimentally for rabbits but are not available commercially.

The current literature emphasizes the critical balance of fiber (lignocellulose) and carbohydrate (starch) in the feed and the ability to digest dietary carbohydrate to absorbable glucose before the starch reaches the cecum and colon, where it may be fermented. General measures to be observed are (1) dietary changes, especially changes in total carbohydrate consumed, should be gradual and made over 4–5 days; (2) dietary fiber should be kept between 17% and 23% to promote gut motility and dilute carbohydrate content; (3) feed should be restricted when a weaned litter is moved to a new cage; (4) feed to a recently delivered doe should be increased gradually to full feed; and (5) a higher fiber diet should be fed to young for the first 2 weeks postweaning and then gradually increased to higher energy growth diets. All these critically important steps are intended to prevent undigested carbohydrate from passing into the large intestine.

Use of 250 ppm copper sulfate ($CuSO_4$) in the feed reduces mortality caused by enteritis based on the hypothesis that copper may interfere with clostridial growth and enterotoxin production. Higher fiber diets augment the copper effect. With $CuSO_4$ use, liver and fecal copper levels increase 20–30 times, but muscle copper level is unchanged.

Various commercial preparations of live or dead lactobacilli, other bacteria (e.g., *Streptococcus* spp, *Bacillus* spp), yeasts, molds, acidifiers, and salts are available for use in rabbits and mixtures are added to either food or water. These products are purported to reduce weanling mortality, although the beneficial effect is more pronounced in colonies with higher incidences of enteritis. The postulated effects of these products in 3- to 10-week-old rabbits are to decrease intestinal pH, provide buffers, compete with pathogenic organisms, and provide amylase activity. Most lactobacilli added to the diet are killed in the highly acid environment of the rabbit's stomach, and if they do survive that passage, they are killed by bile, do not adhere to the intestinal wall, and do not colonize. Any beneficial mechanism, therefore, is unknown or unproven.

Off-label antibiotic mixtures (e.g., bacitracin-methylene disalicylate [BMD]), similar to those used for necrotic enteritis in chickens, are frequently added to commercial rabbit feed to manage or prevent ongoing enteritis issues. The responsibility for ensuring that no drug residues are present in meat produced for human consumption lies with the prescribing veterinarian and the producer.

Treatment

Because the disease process is usually advanced when clinical signs are first noted, treatment of enteropathies is often unrewarding. Elimination of the sickest animals and thorough equipment sanitization must accompany treatment of an infected herd. A fundamental step in treatment is to change the diet by increasing fiber and decreasing the protein-energy to some effective ratio of the two components (e.g., 14% crude protein and 20% crude fiber), which varies among colonies.

Symptomatic treatment may be indicated for acute diarrheas in individual or colony animals. This consists primarily of maintaining hydration with appropriate warmed fluids given orally or parenterally, providing analgesics, maintaining core body temperature (38.5–40 °C), providing some form of enteral nutrition such as herbivore-specific critical care formula, and softening and removal of feces impacted around the anus. B vitamin supplements are often given because these animals are not practicing coprophagia. Because a specific etiologic diagnosis is difficult to determine, a balanced electrolyte solution such as lactated Ringer's solution is preferred, with or without added saline or glucose. The quantity given (IV, IO, PO, SC, or IP) is based on the usual calculation of degree of dehydration plus additional maintenance requirements. For example, a weanling rabbit (1–2 kg) with 10% weight loss would require 100–200 mL fluid above maintenance. Fluids given PO, SC, or IP can be divided and given as boluses three or four times a day. Fluids given by the intravenous or intraosseous route at the appropriate rate may be used to provide more rapid rehydration.

Body temperature can be maintained by placing the animal on a thermostatically controlled heating pad, by careful use of a heatlamp, by placing oatbags or bags of warmed (25–30 °C) liquid around the convalescing animal, or using other small animal rewarming devices. Animals with enteritis are depressed and may grind their teeth, in part from visceral pain. If analgesics are used, nonopioids should be selected, because of the inhibitory effect of opioids on gut motility.

Beyond fluids, warmth, and possibly an analgesic to make the animal more comfortable, other treatments are unproven. Bismuth subsalicylate in a flavored medium may be given at 0.3–0.6 mL/kg every 4–6 hours (rabbits and rats will lick the suspension from a syringe tip), as may a 1:1 mixture of yogurt and a high-caloric supplement. Further down the list of useful treatments are antimicrobials, such as trimethoprim-sulfa (15 mg/kg every 12 hours), chloramphenicol (20–50 mg/kg every 6 hours), metronidazole (10–15 mg/kg every 12 hours), or any one of several sulfonamides. There is little evidence from controlled studies that these drugs, or any combination among them, are efficacious in resolving enteritis.

References

Bing SR, Kinouchi T, Kataoka K, et al. Protective effects of a culture supernatant of Lactobacillus acidophilus and antioxidants on ileal ulcer formation in rats treated with a nonsteroidal antiinflammatory drug. Microbiol Immunol. 1998, 42(11):745–753.

Blankenship-Paris TL, et al. Clostridium difficile infection in hamsters fed an atherogenic diet. Vet Pathol. 1995, 32:269–273.

Butzner JD, Gall DG. Refeeding enhances intestinal repair during an acute enteritis in infant rabbits subjected to protein-energy malnutrition. Pediatr Res. 1991, 29:594–600.

Cheeke PR. Rabbit Feeding and Nutrition. Cunha TJ (ed.). Orlando: Academic Press, 1987.

Cheeke PR, Grobner MA, Patton NM. Fiber digestion and utilization in rabbits. J Appl Rabbit Res. 1986, 9:25–30.

Elliott SN, Buret A, McKnight W, et al. Bacteria rapidly colonize and modulate healing of gastric ulcers in rats. Am J Physiol. 1998, 275(3 Pt 1):G425–432.

Erlandsen SL, Chase DG. Morphological alterations in the microvillus border of villus epithelial cells produced by intestinal microorganisms. J Clin Nutr. 1974, 27:1277–1286.

Foster TL, Winans L, Jr, Carski TR. Evaluation of Lactobacillus preparation in enterotoxigenic E. coli–induced rabbit ileal loop reaction. Am J Gastroenterol. 1980, 73:238–243.

Gascon M, Verde M. Study of biochemical profiles in diarrheal rabbits. J Appl Rabbit Res. 1985, 8:141–143.

Harp JA, et al. Resistance of severe combined immunodeficient mice to infection with Cryptosporidium

parvum: the importance of intestinal microflora. Infect Immun. 1992, 60:3509–3512.
Hollister AG, et al. Effects of dietary probiotics and acidifiers on performance of weanling rabbits. J Appl Rabbit Res. 2001, 13:6–9.
Hooper LV, et al. 2001. Commensal host-bacterial relationships in the gut. Science. 2001, 292:1115–1118.
Katz L, et al. Experimental clindamycin associated colitis in rabbits. Gastroenterol. 1978, 74(2 Pt 1):246–252.
Lelkes L, Chang C-L. Microbial dysbiosis in rabbit mucoid enteropathy. Lab Anim Sci. 1987, 37:757–764.
Loliger HC. Prophylactic measures in control of rabbit diseases and disorders. J Appl Rabbit Res. 1987, 10:175–180.
Lowe BR, et al. Clostridium difficile–associated cecitis in guinea pigs exposed to penicillin. Amer J Vet Res. 1980, 41:1277–1279.
Moon HW. Mechanisms in the pathogenesis of diarrhea: a review. J Am Vet Med Assoc. 1978, 172:443–448.
Newsome PM, Coney KA. Synergistic rotavirus and Escherichia coli diarrheal infection of mice. Infect Immun. 1985, 47:573–574.
Olfert ED. Ampicillin toxicity in rabbits. Can Vet J. 1981, 22:217.
Patton NM, et al. The effect of dietary copper sulfate on enteritis in fryer rabbits. J Appl Rabbit Res. 1982, 5:78–82.
Peeters JE, Geeroms R, Dussart P. Efficacy of antimicrobials against enteropathogenic Escherichia coli in rabbit. J Appl Rabbit Res. 1986, 9:12–13.
Pote LM, Cheeke PR, Patton NM. Use of greens as a supplement to a pelleted diet for growing rabbits. J Appl Rabbit Res. 1980, 3:15–20.
Sarma-Rupavtarm RB, et al. Spatial distribution and stability of eight microbial species of the altered Schaedler flora in the mouse gastrointestinal tract. Appl Env Microbiol. 2004, 70:2791–2800.
Schauer DB, et al. Proliferative enterocolitis associated with a dual infection with enteropathogenic Escherichia coli and Lawsonia intracellularis in rabbits. J Clin Microbiol. 1998, 36:1700–1703.
Smith HW. The antimicrobial activity of the stomach contents of suckling rabbits. J Pathol Bacteriol. 1966, 91:1–9.
———. Observations on the flora of the alimentary tract of animals and factors affecting its composition. J Pathol Bacteriol. 1965, 89:95–122.
Thilstead JP, et al. Fatal diarrhea in rabbits resulting from the feeding of antibiotic contaminated feed. J Am Vet Med Assoc. 1981, 179:360–362.
Uejima M, et al. Role of intestinal bacteria in ileal ulcer formation in rats treated with a nonsteroidal antiinflammatory drug. Microbiol Immunol. 1996, 40:553–560.
Whitney JC. Treatment of enteric disease in rabbit. Vet Rec. 1974, 95:553.
Yu B, Tsen HY. Lactobacillus cells in the rabbit digestive tract and the factors affecting their distribution. J Appl Bacteriol. 1993, 75:269–275.

Clostridial Enterotoxemia

Hosts

Fatal enterotoxemia due to *Clostridium* spp proliferation and toxin production can occur in rabbits, hamsters, chinchillas, and guinea pigs either as a sporadic, spontaneous outbreak or after administration of one of several antibiotics.

Etiology

Clostridial infections play an important role in intestinal disorders of laboratory and domestic animals. There are several predisposing factors recognized to contribute to the development of clinical disease due to these Gram-positive, anaerobic, spore-forming pathogens, particularly events that disrupt the normal microbial population. These include inappropriate antibiotic administration and rapid dietary and environmental changes. Oral treatment with antibiotics directed primarily against Gram-positive bacteria (e.g., penicillins, cephalosporins, and macrolides) has been associated with an overgrowth of *C. difficile* in guinea pigs, chinchillas, hamsters, gerbils, and rabbits.

The essential virulence factors of *C. difficile* are toxin A (a potent enterotoxin) and toxin B (a potent cytotoxin). The disease has a neural component as well, leading to release of substance P and subsequent mast cell degranulation. *C. difficile*–induced enterotoxemia is also reported in dogs (e.g., following metronidazole therapy for *Giardia* spp), nonhuman primates (e.g., following clindamycin therapy), and swine. Humans and animals commonly carry *C. difficile* asymptomatically. The bacterial spores usually proliferate only after the disruption of the normal gut flora, for example, following antibiotic treatment, because the normal flora competitively limits growth of *C. difficile* in healthy individuals. Because guinea pigs, chinchillas, and rabbits are hindgut fermenters, the antibiotic-associated disruption in gut flora occurs primarily in the cecum and colon, resulting in profuse diarrhea associated with acute typhlocolitis. Colonization of the jejunum also occurs in rabbits, and death may be peracute. In hamsters, necrotizing typhlitis has been reported in animals fed an atherogenic diet. Hamsters are exquisitely sensitive to *C. difficile*, and clostridial enteropathies may occur in the absence of identifiable predisposing factors.

In rabbits fed a high-carbohydrate diet, clostridial enteropathy has been attributed to infections with either *C. perfringens* or *C. spiroforme*. *Clostridium spiroforme* is an anaerobic, Gram-positive, spore-forming, nonmotile, C-shaped bacillus. The bacilli may have a terminal spore body and may link end-to-end to produce helical forms. *C. spiroforme* may be the more important clostridial pathogen in rabbits. *C. perfringens* is classified into five types, A–E, based on production of one or more of the four major toxins (alpha, beta, epsilon, and iota). The syndrome following infection typically involves enterotoxemia and enteritis, usually involving the proximal gastrointestinal tract. Detection of enterotoxin in the feces of affected animals is the most sensitive means of confirming infection.

C. spiroforme causes iota enterotoxemia in rabbits, usually in the cecum. The toxin has two polypeptide components that act synergistically; one component may be an ADP-ribosylating enzyme and the other involved in cell surface binding. The toxin is produced within a pH range of 6.0–7.5 and depends on certain cations as cofactors for production or activation. It produces increased vascular permeability and is neutralized by specific antiserum. Outbreaks of clostridial enteropathy with mortality are common in commercial rabbitries and occasionally occur in the research environment. Increasing the fiber content of the feed may help to reduce the incidence of the disease.

Outbreaks of fatal diarrhea within 3–6 days or more after antibiotic administration to guinea pigs and hamsters have been attributed to *C. difficile* and *C. sordellii*; these organisms also infect humans, hares, and other rodents. The cecal and colonic lesions are primarily necrotizing and hemorrhagic with or without mucosal hyperplasia. Spontaneous typhlitis resembling that induced by antibiotic administration has also been observed in an SPF guinea pig colony.

Administration of lincomycin may be associated with development of enterotoxemia in hamsters. Administration of lincomycin or clindamycin has also been associated with development of enterotoxemia in rabbits.

Transmission

Clostridium spp are likely present in low numbers in the large intestine of rabbits and rodents. Transmission is primarily by the fecal-oral route, although clinical cases likely arise from proliferation of organisms already resident within the patient's cecum.

Predisposing Factors

Enterotoxemia in rabbits usually occurs in weanling fryers 4–8 weeks old when passively acquired maternal immunity has decreased, body growth is rapid, and intestinal microbes are populating the intestine. The disease, however, may also affect adults on high-caloric diets or does returned to full feed immediately after kindling. Factors described in the "General Discussion" section on "Enteropathies" are applicable.

Clinical Signs

The course of the disease is rapid in weanling rabbits. Affected animals may die with no other clinical signs, may develop and survive a mild diarrhea, or, more likely, over 6–48 hours may exhibit anorexia, polydipsia, immobility, profuse watery to hemorrhagic diarrhea, cyanosis, tooth grinding, hypothermia, recumbency, paralysis, or convulsions, and death. Mortality can be from a few to most colony animals, but a range of 25–60% is common. In older rabbits, such as does returning to full feed postkindling, deaths may be sporadic. Antibiotic-induced disease is primarily seen in adults treated for reasons other than for enteritis.

A "young doe syndrome" occurs in primiparous and early multiparous does and may be a form of clostridial enterotoxemia. Affected rabbits die suddenly when their litters are 1–4 weeks of age. A few days preceding death, the does go off feed, some salivate profusely, and diarrhea may or may not be seen.

The cause of neonatal or milk enterotoxemia is uncertain, but it may be caused by a toxin passed in low amounts through the milk or by *Clostridium* spp passed into the neonatal gut. Young die suddenly during the first 3 days postpartum. This problem, which can produce great economic loss in a rabbitry, is more common during the winter months and may be linked with overfeeding of kits.

Hamsters with adult-onset *C. difficile* enteritis have diarrhea, dehydration, roughened hair coat, and a hunched posture. The most commonly encountered sign is profuse diarrhea. Animals with acute watery or hemorrhagic diarrhea have high mortality.

Necropsy Signs

Clostridium spiroforme infection results in acute exudation, edema, and inflammatory cell infiltration followed by various degrees of mucosal necrosis and pseudomembrane formation. Portions of the small intestine, cecum, and colon are dilated and contain gas and watery brown, occasionally hemorrhagic, malodorous content. Petechiae and ecchymoses often are seen subserosally on the cecum, with hemorrhage and ulceration on the mucosal surface. Mucous exudation is rare. Proliferative changes of cryptal epithelium may occur, with clumps of desquamated cells in the lumen.

Clostridium spiroforme is rarely isolated from healthy rabbits, and when the organism is identified its source presumably is the environment or spore-containing feed. Asymptomatic carriers exist.

Outbreaks of epizootic rabbit enteropathy have been described in commercial rabbitries by several groups across Europe in recent years. Mortality was described to be highest in weanlings (6- to 8-week-old animals). Grossly, there was marked diffuse dilatation of the gastrointestinal tract with liquid contents in affected animals. *E. coli* (nonenteropathogenic) and *C. perfringens* (alpha toxin positive) were the most common isolates from cecal samples. Coccidial oocysts were noted in feces of many animals, but no *Cryptosporidium* spp.

Histopathologically, in hamsters with *C. difficile* typhlitis, there is cecal necrosis, epithelial denudation, vascular congestion, and hemorrhage. More chronically affected hamsters have cecal mucosal hyperplasia.

Diagnosis

Diagnosis of clostridial enteropathy requires strict anaerobic culture conditions or demonstration of the enterotoxin from the feces. Identification of the typical Gram-positive coiled and curved organisms (*C. spiroforme*) on direct smear of the terminal ileum or cecum is a useful and rapid procedure assisting with confirming the diagnosis.

The primary methods for diagnosis include Gram staining of cecal smears (most practical but may be negative despite positive identification of cecal iota toxin), isolation of the toxigenic organisms on special media, cytotoxicity assays, and neutralization of toxic cecal filtrate with specific antiserum. The toxemia itself has been rarely, if ever, demonstrated, and a septicemia is not part of the disease.

A diagnosis is established by (1) correlating clinical signs and necropsy findings with age, medication, and treatment history; (2) performing diagnostic tests and ancillary procedures such as bacterial culture of cecal contents, especially for *E. coli*, *Salmonella* spp, and other enteric pathogens; (3) demonstrating organisms in histologic sections; or (4) demonstrating presence of toxin in intestinal contents.

Treatment

Treatment of clostridial diarrhea is discussed in this chapter under the "General Discussion" section for "Enteropathies." There is little to no evidence that antibiotics are effective or helpful in treating individual cases or outbreaks of enterotoxemia.

Supportive treatment should be started and antibiotics withdrawn immediately in animals that develop diarrhea during antibiotic treatment. Cholestyramine (Questran®) at 2 g/20 mL water, PO, every 24 hours has been demonstrated to bind to clostridial and other bacterial toxins in humans and may be useful in rabbits.

Prevention

Prevention of *C. spiroforme* enteritis follows the general recommendations discussed previously. As mentioned, when reviewed over a range of different trials, antimicrobial administration is not efficacious in preventing the disease and may exacerbate an existing problem.

An experimental bacterin prepared from a formalinized, alum-precipitated antigen (antitoxin) has been used to protect against an intraperitoneal challenge of *C. spiroforme* toxin. The vaccine was given to rabbits at weaning and boosted 14 days later. No protection was passed to the young. Antibody levels detected by ELISA plateaued at 17 days and remained at that level throughout the 42-day trial.

"Young doe syndrome" can be prevented by increasing the amount of feed provided after kindling by 10–25 g per day, rather than all at once, until ad libitum levels are reached.

Public Health Significance

Whereas *C. perfringens* affects a variety of species, *C. spiroforme* is primarily a rabbit pathogen, although this clostridium has been associated with diarrhea in one human case report. *Clostridium difficile* is a spore-forming, Gram-variable bacterium that has been identified as part of the gut flora in neonatal humans, and it is considered normal indigenous gut flora of young mammals of several species, including the hamster, rabbit, and guinea pig. Generally, the bacterium causes no clinical signs unless there is bacterial overgrowth. *C. difficile* has also been associated with a range of serious gastrointestinal illnesses in humans and is considered to be an emerging zoonotic disease. Recent studies involving PCR ribotyping of *C. difficile* from a range of species, including pigs, dogs, and horses, have demonstrated identical types in these species and in humans. It is unknown whether rabbits may be a reservoir for *C. difficile* ribotypes relevant for humans.

References

Babudieri S, et al. Diarrhea associated with toxigenic Clostridium spiroforme. J Infect Dis. 1986, 12:278–279.

Bartlett JG, et al. Antibiotic-induced lethal enterocolitis in hamsters: studies with eleven agents and evidence to support the pathogenic role of toxin producing clostridia. Amer J Vet Res. 1978, 39:1525–1530.

Baskerville M, Wood M, SeAm JH. Clostridium perfringens type E. enterotoxaemia in rabbits. Vet Rec. 1980, 107:18–19.

Boot R, Angulo AF, Walvoort HC. Clostridium difficile–associated typhlitis in specific pathogen free guinea pigs in the absence of antimicrobial treatment. Lab Anim. 1989, 23:203–207.

Borriello SP, Carman RJ. Association of iotalike toxin and Clostridium spiroforme with both spontaneous and antibiotic-associated diarrhea and colitis in rabbits. J Clin Microbiol. 1983, 17:414–418.

Borriello SP, Davies HA, Carman RJ. Cellular morphology of Clostridium spiroforme. Vet Microbiol. 1986, 11:191–195.

Boss SM, et al. Use of vancomycin hydrochloride for treatment of Clostridium difficile enteritis in Syrian hamsters. Lab Anim Sci. 1994, 44:31–37.

Butt MT, et al. A cytotoxicity assay for Clostridium spiroforme enterotoxin in cecal fluid of rabbits. Lab Anim Sci. 1994, 44:52–54.

Carman RJ, Borriello SP. Laboratory diagnosis of Clostridium spiroforme mediated diarrhea (iota enterotoxaemia) of rabbits. Vet Rec. 1983, 113:184–185.

Carman RJ, Evans RH. Experimental and spontaneous clostridial enteropathies of laboratory and free living lagomorphs. Lab Anim Sci. 1984, 34:443–452.

Chang J, Rohwer RG. Clostridium difficile infection in adult hamsters. Lab Anim Sci. 1991, 41:548–552.

Cheeke PR, Patton NM. Carbohydrate-overload of the hindgut—a probable cause of enteritis. J Appl Rabbit Res. 1980, 3:20–23.

Eaton P, Femie DS. Enterotoxaemia involving Clostridium perfringens iota toxin in a hysterectomy-derived rabbit colony. Lab Anim. 1980, 14:347–351.

Ellis TM, Gregory AR, Logue GD. Evaluation of a toxoid for protection of rabbits against enterotoxaemia experimentally induced by trypsin-activated supernatant of Clostridium spiroforme. Vet Microbiol. 1991, 28:93–102.

Fekety R, et al. Antibiotic-associated colitis: effects of antibiotics on Clostridium difficile and the disease in hamsters. Rev Infect Dis. 1979, 1:386–396.

Holmes HT, Sonn RJ, Patton NM. Isolation of Clostridium spiroforme from rabbits. Lab Anim Sci. 1988, 38:167–168.

Kaur T, Ganguly NK. Modulation of gut physiology through enteric toxins. Molec Cell Biochem. 2003, 253:15–19.

Keel MK, Songer JG. The comparative pathology of Clostridium difficile–associated disease. Vet Pathol. 2006, 43:225–240.

Knoop FC. Clindamycin-associated enterocolitis in guinea pigs: evidence for a bacterial toxin. Infect Immun. 1979, 23:31–33.

Lipman NS, et al. Utilization of cholestyramine resin as a preventive treatment for antibiotic (clindamycin) induced enterotoxaemia in the rabbit. Lab Anim. 1992, 26:1–8.

Lowe BR, Fox JG, Bartlett JG. Clostridium difficile–associated cecitis in guinea pigs exposed to penicillin. Amer J Vet Res. 1980, 41:1277–1279.

Matsushita S, Matsusumoto T. Spontaneous necrotic enteritis in young RFM/Ms mice. Lab Anim. 1986, 20:114–117.

Patton NM, Cheeke PR. Etiology and treatment of young doe syndrome. J Appl Rabbit Res. 1980, 3:23–24.
Patton NM, et al. The effect of dietary copper sulfate on enteritis in fryer rabbits. J Appl Rabbit Res. 1982, 5:78–82.
Peeters JE, et al. Significance of Clostridium spiroforme in the enteritis-complex of commercial rabbits. Vet Microbiol. 1986, 12:25–31.
Perkins SE, et al. Detection of Clostridium difficile toxins from the small intestine and cecum of rabbits with naturally acquired enterotoxemia. Lab Anim Sci. 1995, 45(4):379–384.
Rehg JE, Lu Y-S. Clostridium difficile colitis in a rabbit following antibiotic therapy for pasteurellosis. J Am Vet Med Assoc. 1981, 179:1296–1297.
Rehg JE, Yarbrough BA, Pakes SP. Toxicity of cecal filtrates from guinea pigs with penicillin-associated colitis. Lab Anim Sci. 1980, 30:524–531.
Ryden EB, et al. Clostridium difficile typhlitis associated with cecal mucosal hyperplasia in Syrian hamsters. Lab Anim Sci. 1991, 41:553–558.
Ryden EB, et al. Non-antibiotic-associated Clostridium difficile enterotoxemia in Syrian hamsters. Lab Anim Sci. 1990, 40:544.
Thilsted JP, et al. Fatal diarrhea in rabbits resulting from the feeding of antibiotic-contaminated feed. J Am Vet Med Assoc. 1981, 179:360–361.
Yonushonis WP, et al. Diagnosis of spontaneous Clostridium spiroforme iota enterotoxemia in a barrier rabbit breeding colony. Lab Anim Sci. 1987, 37:69–71.

Colibacillosis

Hosts

Escherichia coli is the most common etiological agent for diarrhea in animals. Rabbits and rodent species of all ages may be affected by enteritis induced by the bacterium.

Etiology

There are seven classes of pathogenic *E. coli*, including enteropathogenic *E. coli* (EPEC), enterohemorrhagic *E. coli* (EHEC), enteroinvasive *E. coli* (EIEC), enterotoxigenic *E. coli* (ETEC), enteroaggregative *E. coli* (EAEC), diarrhea-associated hemolytic *E. coli* (DHEC), and cytolethal descending toxin (CDT)-producing *E. coli*. Many pathogenic *E. coli* are capable of producing heat stabile or labile toxins. The heat labile toxin closely resembles cholera toxin. The toxins are elaborated directly into the cytoplasm of the cell, where they induce increased cell permeability leading to cell death. Additional virulence factors including EPEC strains secrete a collection of proteins that interfere with the host cell metabolism; ETEC strains adhere to intestinal epithelial cells and produce enterotoxins that cause cell death and a secretory diarrhea; EIEC strains invade and multiply in enterocytes, causing exudative enteritis and endotoxemia; and EHEC (attaching and effacing) embed in enterocyte cytoplasmic membranes, efface microvilli, and produce a Shiga-like toxin, with resulting damage to the mucosa, inducing hemorrhage and diarrhea.

Younger animals are particularly susceptible to coliform infections. The clinical signs associated with a pathogenic coliform infection (severe watery to hemorrhagic diarrhea with anorexia and wasting) may be attributable solely to the organism, but frequently other microorganisms are involved in the disease process. For example, in domestic rabbits, an outbreak of diarrhea in suckling or weanling animals may be attributable only to infection with EHEC. In other cases, there may be two or more pathogens acting in concert to produce clinical disease. Concurrent infections with a pathogenic strain of *E. coli* have been shown to have an additive effect in animals infected with rotavirus or intestinal coccidiosis. It is likely that strains of *E. coli* play a similar additive role in mixed microbial infections in other species. Immunodeficient animals may be particularly at risk. In laboratory rodents, enteritis due to EIEC has been reported in immunocompromised mice.

The causative agents in rabbits are among the hundreds of biotypes or serotypes of the Gram-negative, facultatively anaerobic bacteria. Pathogenic serotypes of *E. coli* cultured from rabbits with acute diarrhea include 015, 0153, 0157, 0128, and an unclassified serogroup OX1; however, other types, some thought to be nonpathogenic, also have been cultured during diarrheal outbreaks. The gastrointestinal tracts of rabbits, guinea pigs, and gerbils normally have few or no *E. coli*, whereas other rodents carry the organism in low numbers.

Other probable coliform diseases in small rodents include diarrhea in gerbils and enteritis in hamsters, which may occur alone or in combination with a proliferative or hyperplastic lesion of the ileum. After antibiotic injections, guinea pigs and hamsters may die within 2–6 days; coliform or clostridial overgrowth has been implicated as the cause.

Transmission

Transmission of *E. coli* is by the fecal-oral route. The clinical disease, however, probably develops from activation of a preexisting component of the intestinal flora.

Predisposing Factors

Predisposing factors for colibacillosis include change of diet, entrance of pathogenic organisms into the uncolonized gut of weanlings, high-carbohydrate–low-fiber diets, adverse stress such as chilling of neonates, cecal pH greater than 6.8, other disease, or alteration of the microflora with antibiotics active against Gram-positive or anaerobic bacteria. Factors that predispose to diarrhea or other enteropathies in rabbits and rodents are discussed in more detail in the "General Discussion" section for "Enteropathies" in this chapter.

Clinical Signs

Signs attributed to *E. coli* infection may be similar to those of other enteric infections, and the signs and lesions of experimental *E. coli* infections in healthy rabbits and rodents range from mild to severe (Figure 5.6). Morbidity and mortality can range from mild transient diarrhea in a few young animals to death of entire litters from profuse, watery, and bloody diarrhea. Early nonspecific signs of colibacillosis include acute onset, fever, depression, reduced water and food intake, weight loss, and peracute death within 6–72 hours of infection. Within hours or a few days, perineal staining occurs with watery, foul-smelling brown to yellow diarrhea, sometimes with blood and mucus. Because of the effects of various *E. coli* serotypes and of receptor maturation, outbreaks may be seen in sucklings, weanlings, or adults. Signs in all groups vary from mild to severe, and death may occur within hours of appearance of signs to several weeks later.

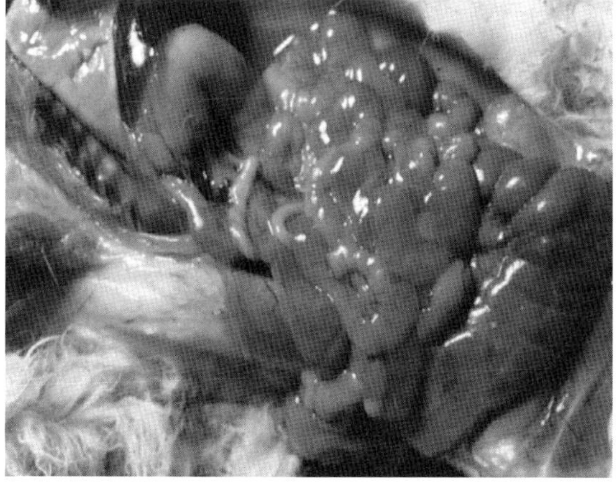

FIGURE 5.6. Coliform enteritis in a weanling rabbit. Note the flaccid, fluid-filled loops of small intestine.

Necropsy Signs

Depending on the strain of *E. coli* involved, lesions may be confined primarily to the small or large intestine. Microscopically, identifiable bacilli may be evident lining the mucosal surface in close apposition to the microvilli, and there is swelling and sloughing of enterocytes in affected regions. Effacement of the mucosa and villous atrophy are typical changes seen during the acute stages of the disease. Diarrhea is usually accompanied by dehydration and electrolyte imbalance in affected hosts, with variable mortality. Persistent infections may occur, particularly in immunocompromised animals. Gross signs of colibacillosis include cecal hemorrhage and edema and a watery brown, fetid, luminal content. Other nonspecific changes include enlarged mesenteric nodes and congested kidneys. Microscopically, there are hemorrhages and edema within the gut wall, loss of epithelium, and inflammatory infiltrates within the submucosa and mucosa.

Diagnosis

Specific diagnosis is through clinical signs and isolation of pathogenic strains of *E. coli* classified by culture, microscopy, serotype, and biotype. Demonstration of bacterial attachment and effacement of intestinal epithelium further confirm the diagnosis. The most practical method is culture of feces on MacConkey's medium and recovery of nonhemolytic, facultatively anaerobic *E. coli*. Samples must be fresh for optimal results.

Treatment

Infection with EPEC strains of low pathogenicity can be treated symptomatically and with strict hygienic measures, including vigorous culling of dehydrated and obviously sick young and thorough washing and disinfection of the environment. Chloramphenicol may be useful in some circumstances, and supportive care for dehydration and general debility can be helpful in management of individual cases.

Prevention

Prevention of colibacillosis follows the recommendations in the "General Discussion" section on "Enteropathies" in this chapter. Highly pathogenic coliforms, either in sucklings or in weanlings, are difficult to eliminate, and destruction of the affected colony may be necessary.

An orally administered enteric-coated protease preparation to prevent ETEC attachment and a formalin-killed bacterin given per os over 10 days to stimulate local and systemic responses have been tested to reduce the coliform component of the enteritis complex, but neither product is available commercially. Trials using large populations of live *Lactobacillus acidophilus* or *L. bulgaricus* have inhibited ETEC effects, but their preventive effects on EPEC infection are unreported.

Public Health Significance

It is important to note that EHEC is considered to be an emerging human pathogen. Rabbits, both from pet and commercial sources, are reported to be reservoirs of this bacterium and may carry EHEC subclinically. Experimental infection of rabbits with EHEC has led to renal hypoxia and damage, similar to what is seen in humans with hemolytic uremic syndrome (HUS). Appropriate hand washing is required after handling or examining sick animals to minimize the risk of disease transmission.

References

Camguilhem R, Muon A. Protection of weaned rabbits against experimental Escherichia coli 0103 intestinal infection by oral formalin-killed vaccine. Vet Microbiol. 1990, 21:353–362.

Cantey JR, Blake RK. Diarrhea due to Escherichia coli in the rabbit: a novel mechanism. J Infect Dis. 1977, 135:454–462.

Cantey JR, O'Hanley PD, Blake RK. A rabbit model of diarrhea due to invasive Escherichia coli. J Infect Dis. 1977, 136:640–648.

Caprioli A, et al. Enterohemorrhagic E coli: emerging issues on virulence and modes of transmission. Vet Res. 2005, 36:289–311.

Dean P, et al. EPEC's weapons of mass subversion. Curr Opin Microbiol. 2005, 8:28–34.

Farrar WE, Jr, Kent TH. Enteritis and coliform bacteremia in guinea pigs given penicillin. Am J Pathol. 1965, 47:629–642.

Foster TL, Winans L, Jr, Carski TR. Evaluation of Lactobacillus preparation in enterotoxigenic E. coli–induced rabbit ileal loop reactions. Am J Gastroenterol. 1980, 73:238–243.

Frisk CS, Wagner JE, Owens DR. Hamster (Mesocricetus auratus) enteritis caused by epithelial cell-invasive Escherichia coli. Infect Immun. 1981, 31:1232–1238.

Garcia A, et al. Renal injury is a consistent finding in Dutch belted rabbits experimentally infected with enterohemorrhagic E coli. J Infect Dis. 2006, 193:1125–1134.

Garcia A, Fox JG. The rabbit as a new reservoir host of enterohemorrhagic E coli. Emerg Infect Dis. 2003, 9:1592–1597.

Garmendia J, et al. Enteropathogenic and enterohemorrhagic E coli infections: translocation, translocation, translocation. Infect Immun. 2005, 73:2573–2585.

Glantz PJ. Serotypes of Escherichia coli associated with colibacillosis in neonatal animals. Ann NY Acad Sci. 1971, 176:67–79.

———. Unclassified Escherichia coli serogroup OX1 isolated from fatal diarrhea of rabbits. Can J Comp Med. 1970, 34:47–49.

Moon HW, et al. Attaching and effacing activities of rabbit and human enteropathogenic Escherichia coli in pig and rabbit intestines. Infect Immun. 1983, 41:1340–1351.

Muon A, Esslinger J, Camguilhem R. Adhesion of Escherichia coli strains isolated from diarrheic weaned rabbits to intestinal villi and HeLa cells. Infect Immun. 1990, 158:2690–2695.

Mynott TL, Chandler DS, Luke RKJ. Efficacy of enteric coated protease in preventing attachment of enterotoxigenic Escherichia coli and diarrheal disease in the RITARD model. Infect Immun. 1991, 59:3708–3714.

Peeters JE, et al. Pathogenic properties of Escherichia coli strains isolated from diarrheic commercial rabbits. J Clin Microbiol. 1984, 20:34–39.

Peeters JE, Geeroms R, Dussart P. Efficacy of antimicrobials against enteropathogenic Escherichia coli in rabbit. J Appl Rabbit Res. 1986, 9:9–13.

Peeters JE, Geeroms R, Orskov F. Biotype, serotype, and pathogenicity of attaching and effacing enteropathogenic

Escherichia coli strains isolated from diarrheic commercial rabbits. Infect Immun. 1988, 56:1442–1448.
Robins-Brown RM, et al. Adherence characteristics of attaching and effacing strains of Escherichia coli from rabbits. Infect Immun. 1994, 62:1584–1592.
Shauer DB et al. Proliferative enterocolitis associated with a dual infection with enteropathogenic Escherichia coli and Lawsonia intracellularis in rabbits. J Clin Microbiol. 1998, 36:1700–1703.
Small JD. Fatal enterocolitis in hamsters given lincomycin hydrochloride. Lab Anim Care. 1968, 18:411–420.
Spears KJ, et al. A comparison of enteropathogenic and enterohemorrhagic E. coli pathogenesis. FEMS Microbiol Lett. 2006, 255:187–202.
Thouless ME et al. The effect of combined rotavirus and Escherichia coli infections in rabbits. Lab Anim Sci. 1996, 46:381–385.
Waggie KS, et al. Cecocolitis in immunodeficient mice associated with an enteroinvasive lactose negative E. coli. Lab Anim Sci. 1981, 38:389–393.

Mucoid Enteropathy

Hosts

Mucoid enteropathy (ME) of rabbits is a distinct disease with unusual characteristics and, in this description, is not a catarrhal diarrhea. The disease occurs in adults, but weanling rabbits 7–10 weeks of age are the most susceptible.

Etiology

Much has been written about ME. Research reports and reviews contain descriptions of numerous methods for diagnosis and prevention, but little is certain as to its etiology or treatment. The disease is characterized by minimal inflammation, hypersecretion, and accumulation of mucus in the small and large intestines. Mucoid enteropathy may occur concurrent with other enteric diseases such as coccidiosis, clostridial enterotoxemia, Tyzzer's disease, and colibacillosis, which obscure the classic signs of ME.

The etiology of mucoid enteropathy remains unknown. When serum (but not plasma) of rabbits with mucoid enteropathy is placed on the free-living, mucus-secreting coelomate, *Sipunculus nudus*, the urn cells of that invertebrate secrete copious mucus. Mucus-stimulating substance (MSS), a postulated blood-borne factor, adheres to certain cell receptors and elicits mucus release. In ME, the lectin-binding activity of colon goblet cell mucin is changed from normal mucin.

Transmission

If an infectious organism or its enterotoxin is involved, transmission is most likely by the fecal-oral route. Sterile cecal filtrates stimulate excessive mucus production in colonic mucosal explants, suggesting transmission of a physical factor.

Predisposing Factors

Dietary changes, dietary fiber less than 6% or greater than 22%, antibiotic influences, environmental stress, and encounters with bacteria are all considered factors predisposing to ME. The disease is more common in the spring, in certain rabbit families, in young does with their first litter, in does with large litters, and in young fryers with high food intake.

Clinical Signs

Disease outbreaks diagnosed as ME have occurred in both weanling (4–12 weeks old) and adult animals. Abdominal distention, slushing of intestinal contents, lethargy, hunched posture, polydipsia, rough hair coat, tooth grinding, rapid weight loss from anorexia and diarrhea, dehydration, clear or yellow-brown mucus diarrhea, staining of the perineum, subnormal temperature (37.2–38.3 °C; normal is 38.9–40 °C), cold extremities, and death may be seen in cases of ME, although many of these signs are common to other enteropathies. Distinguishing signs of the condition are the subnormal temperature, copious quantities of clear mucus diarrhea sometimes preceded by constipation, occurrence in adults, and necropsy signs.

Clinical signs precede death by 1–3 days in an acute form, which is nearly indistinguishable from other enteropathies, or by 7–9 days in the longer-term condition. As the disease progresses, mucoid diarrhea becomes profuse or constipation occurs, and in either case animals die. Weight loss may reach 20–25% of original body weight. Mortality may reach 70% or more, with no sex differences. Does with litters in the nest box may succumb. Abdominal palpation may reveal a firm, impacted cecum or ballotable fluid-filled intestines.

Clinical laboratory findings are those associated typically with dehydration, for example, increased hematocrit. Depending on the stage of the disease, total leukocyte counts, serum lipase, glucose, albumin, globulins, phosphorus, and blood urea nitrogen may be elevated. Calcium, potassium, sodium, and chloride may be decreased.

Necropsy Signs

Lesions of subacute, uncomplicated mucoid enteropathy are derived from the hypersecretion of electrolytes, water, and mucus from ostensibly normal epithelium, or at most from an epithelium with mild edema and slight to moderate mixed inflammatory cell infiltration. The esophagus and stomach are usually free of lesions. The small intestine is either empty or contains fluid and mucus with a progressive increase in goblet cell size and number from the duodenum to ileum.

In acute (1–3 days) stages, the digestive tract contains a watery fluid with pockets of gas. In these stages, the cecum, lymphoid appendix, sacculus rotundus, colon, gallbladder, bile ducts, pancreatic ducts, and even the tracheal mucosa exhibit characteristic goblet cell hyperplasia and increased mucus-secreting activity.

The excessive discharge of mucus (mixture of neutral and acidic mucins, proteins, cells, bacteria, ions, and water), especially into the colon and distal ileum, results in formation of a clear to yellow, semifluid to gel plug that can be removed in large masses from an opened colon at necropsy. The jelly mass in some rabbits may be mixed with chyme or secreted fluid, resulting in a colored discharge from the rectum.

A critical gross lesion of uncomplicated mucoid enteropathy in the longer-term stages is an inspissated, firm, dry or clay-like mass of ingesta filling the cecum, adhering to the cecal wall, and possibly obstructing the ileo-cecal junction. The static cecal mass and the gelatinous colonic plug underlie constipation. Goblet cell ducts are depleted of acidic mucus and are plugged and dilated. Death follows ileus and impaction.

Histologically, the primary change is goblet cell hyperplasia of the ileum, cecum, appendix, sacculated colon, and colon.

Diagnosis

Diagnosis of ME is based on clinical and necropsy signs. Culture of the gut or a fecal examination may be indicated to detect or rule out clostridial infections, colibacillosis, salmonellosis, coccidiosis, and other parasitic diseases.

Treatment

Intense fluid therapy given by stomach tube or subcutaneously, coupled with an enema or laxative to remove the mucus mass, may help in some cases, as may antibiotic administration to control bacterial overgrowth. The prognosis is generally poor in most cases, but antibiotics, fluids, electrolyte solutions, vitamins, and analgesics can be tried.

Prevention

The usual recommendations to prevent enteritis in rabbits apply to the prevention of mucoid enteropathy as well; fiber should be added to the diet, but not more than 22% crude fiber because in one case, higher fiber seemed to predispose to the disease.

Public Health Significance

There is no known public health hazard with ME.

References

Bang GG, Bang FB. Mucus-stimulating substances in human body fluids assayed in an invertebrate mucous cell system. Johns Hopkins Med J. 1979, 145:209–216.

Cheeke P, Patton NM. Effect of alfalfa and dietary fiber on the growth performance of weanling rabbits. Lab Anim Sci. 1978, 28:167–172.

Hotchkiss CE, Merritt AM. Mucus secretagogue activity in cecal contents of rabbits with mucoid enteropathy. Lab Anim Sci. 1996, 46(2):179–186.

Itagaki S-I, et al. Lectin histochemical changes of colon goblet cell mucin in rabbit mucoid enteropathy. Lab Anim Sci. 1994, 44:82–84.

Lelkes L, Chang C-L. Microbial dysbiosis in rabbit mucoid enteropathy. Lab Anim Sci. 1987, 37:757–764.

Patton NM, Cheeke P. A precautionary note on high fiber levels and mucoid enteritis. J Appl Rabbit Res. 1981, 4:56.

Sinkovics G. Intestinal flora studies in rabbit mucoid enteritis. Vet Rec. 1976, 98:151–152.

Toofanian F, Hamar DW. Cecal short-chain fatty acids in experimental rabbit mucoid enteropathy. Lab Anim Sci. 1986, 87:2423–2425.

Toofanian F, Targowski S. Stimulation of colonic goblet cells by cecal filtrates from rabbits with experimental mucoid enteropathy. Lab Anim Sci. 1986, 36:157–160.

Van Kruiningen HJ, Williams CB. Mucoid enteritis of rabbits. Comparison to cholera and cystic fibrosis. Vet Pathol. 1972, 9:53–77.

EPILEPSY IN GERBILS

Etiology

Pet owners, animal technicians, and others not familiar with gerbils may become alarmed on witnessing, for the first time, the spontaneous tonic-clonic seizures or convulsions seen commonly in gerbils. These reflex epileptiform seizures are precipitated by novel or excitement-producing experiences such as handling and unfamiliar environments.

Predisposing Factors

Seizure-resistant and seizure-sensitive strains of gerbils exist. Incidence of seizure susceptibility in normal populations is approximately 20% but approaches 100% in some lines. Seizure traits may be influenced as well by cage, diet, age, and environmental determinants. Adverse stress decreases the threshold to trigger seizures in adults.

Clinical Signs

Seizures vary from a mild hypnotic state characterized by cessation of motor activity and spasms or twitching of vibrissae and pinnae to severe myoclonic convulsions followed by tonic extensor rigidity and body flattening. Violent kicking of the hind legs occurs after the seizure motor manifestation has faded. Seizures last from approximately 30 seconds to 2 minutes. Gerbils begin having seizures at approximately 45 days of age, although the onset is extremely variable. Usually the refractory period following a severe seizure is several days and may be due to an adaptation or habituation effect. Although the characteristic clinical signs appear severe, there are no apparent lasting or long-term adverse effects and normal activity is resumed within a few minutes.

Diagnosis

Characteristic clinical signs and ease of inducing such signs consistently are adequate information for a presumptive diagnosis of epilepsy. Differential diagnoses should include encephalitis, poisoning, toxemia, and trauma in all cases of convulsions.

Prevention and Treatment

Frequent handling from an early age may suppress development of seizures. Phenobarbital has been evaluated experimentally for seizure control in gerbils; however, efficacious doses of anticonvulsant drugs for pets have not been reported and these drugs are generally not recommended because of the short duration of most seizures.

References

Cox B, Lomax P. Brain amines and spontaneous epileptic seizures in the Mongolian gerbil. Pharmacol Biochem Behav. 1976, 4:203–267.

Cutler MG, Mackintosh, JH. Epilepsy and behavior of the Mongolian gerbil: an ethological study. Physiol Behav. 1989, 46:561–566.

Goldblatt D. Seizure disorder in gerbils. Neurol. 1968, 18:303–304.

Goldblatt D, et al. The effect of anticonvulsants on seizures in gerbils. Neurol. 1971, 21:433–434.

Kaplan H. What triggers seizures in the gerbil, Meriones unguiculatus? Life Sci. 1975, 17:693–698.

Kaplan H, Silverman WP. Early experience affects seizure latency and post seizure recovery time in the Mongolian gerbil. Neuropsychol. 1978, 16:649–652.

Loskota WJ, Lomax P, Rich ST. The gerbil as a model for the study of the epilepsies. Seizure patterns and ontogenesis. Epilepsy. 1974, 15:109–119.

Paul LA, Schain RJ, Bailey BG. Structural correlates of seizure behavior in the Mongolian gerbil. Science. 1981, 213:924–926.

Schonfeld AR, Glick SD. Effect of handling-induced seizures and passive avoidance learning in the Mongolian gerbil (Meriones unguiculatus). Behav Biol. 1978, 24:101–106.

Simmet T, Seregi A, Hertting G. Characterization of seizure-induced cysteinylleukotriene formation in brain tissue of convulsion-prone gerbils. J Neurochem. 1988, 50:1738–1742.

Watanabe KS, et al. Effects of phenobarbital on seizure activity in the gerbil. Pediatr Res. 1978, 12:918–922.

GASTRIC STASIS IN RABBITS

Hosts

Previously, gastric stasis in rabbits and other small mammal pets was thought to be due to accumulation of masses of hair in the stomach (trichobezoar or "wool block" in Angora rabbits). This was confusing for the practitioner, in terms of etiology, because rabbits may have large gastric hair balls and never show clinical signs, they may have a small, obstructing hair mass in the pylorus and die, or they may show all or most clinical signs ordinarily associated with an obstructive gastric mass yet have no gastric or duodenal blockage. More recent evidence suggests that hair accumulates in the stomach because of an underlying motility disorder known as gastric stasis. Prognosis is often guarded in cases of prolonged gastric or intestinal hypomotility.

Etiology and Predisposing Factors

Gastric stasis generally arises because of defects in propulsion (hypomotility) or because of obstructions. Hypomotility can be caused by low-fiber–high-carbohydrate diets, obesity, lack of exercise, pain, or a variety of management or psychological stressors. Obstructions may result from impaction of ingested hair or foreign bodies combined with chronic dehydration.

Gastric stasis leads to anorexia, lethargy, ileus, constipation, and, occasionally, rupture of the intestine with subsequent peritonitis and death. Rough handling, molting, and ingestion of large amounts of fur are other predisposing factors.

Clinical Signs

The pattern of signs suggesting gastric or duodenal stasis or obstruction is a lack of interest in food, anorexia, progressive emaciation, increased water consumption, and scant feces. These signs may also occur with incisor overgrowth, oral or esophageal abscesses, pain, loss of sense of smell, foul-smelling feed, heat stress, lack of access to drinking water, and various systemic diseases. The stomach is usually readily palpated and may feel distended and doughy. Emaciation can be determined by comparing hypaxial muscle mass among rabbits.

Necropsy

Hair found normally in a rabbit's stomach is loose and mixed with food or cecotrophs. When collections of entangled, matted, and compacted hair are retained in the stomach, they become trichobezoars (Figure 5.7). There may be several trichobezoars, most weighing 6 grams or less, or a large mass may fill the fundus and extend into the pylorus. Most hair balls reported weigh between 1 and 24 grams, but they can weigh over 100 grams. The mass or masses may be loose or firm, but most are soft yet cohesive.

Associated lesions include focal gastric hyperemia, inflammation, and ulceration; hepatic lipidosis due to obesity; and, rarely, ante mortem gastric rupture and peritonitis.

Diagnosis

Ante mortem determination of a gastric or duodenal obstruction can be difficult. Clinical signs of pro-

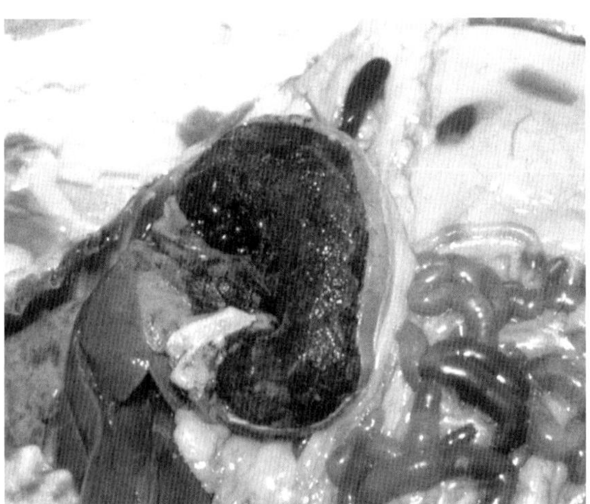

FIGURE 5.7. Postmortem specimen from an anorectic rabbit with gastric stasis. There is accumulation of hair within the stomach.

gressive emaciation and absence of fecal pellets are important indications. Whether or not trichobezoars are palpable is debatable, but a large, firm mass in the epigastric region of the abdomen should receive attention. Soft or smaller nodules cannot be distinguished from other stomach contents, especially masses of mucus-linked cecotrophs. Palpation may rupture an inflamed stomach.

Contrast radiography would seem to be useful, but results are often inconclusive, especially if the material is in the pylorus or if cecotrophs are present. Radiologic procedures that have been described are per os administration of (1) 30 mL liquid barium sulfate followed by radiographs taken at 300 MA, 84 KY, 0.05 sec, at 36 inches, or (2) 15 mL of liquid barium sulfate, rolling the rabbit to disperse the medium, and then delivery of 60 mL air. A 5–8 Fr pediatric feeding tube can be readily passed through the ventral meatus of the nose into the stomach to facilitate delivery of contrast material.

Treatment

Following diagnosis, medical treatment for suspected gastric stasis should be considered urgent. Animals are often fragile at this point and must be handled gently. Aggressive fluid therapy is indicated to rehydrate obstructive gastric masses. In addition, animals may require analgesics such as meloxicam (0.5 mg/kg PO 1–2 times daily) as well as promotility agents (e.g., metaclopromide, 0.5 mg/kg PO or SC 1–3 times daily), provided that a complete obstruction is not suspected. Nasogastric or syringe feeding of liquid herbivore critical care supplements is necessary to provide nutritional support. Percutaneous pharyngostomy tubes have been used for force-feeding rabbits and are generally well tolerated, although they may require an Elizabethan collar for protection.

Gastrotomy to remove stomach masses carries a poor prognosis and should be a last resort. Pre- and postsurgical supportive therapy should be intense and should include parenteral fluids (e.g., lactated Ringer's), pain medication, and an antibiotic (e.g., trimethoprim-sulfa, 15–30 mg/kg twice daily, IM or PO). The stomach is elevated with stay sutures through a 4-cm cranial celiotomy incision, and an incision made on the greater curvature. The hair masses are removed and the incisions closed. Rabbits usually continue to be anorectic for 1 to several days postoperatively, and the rabbit may have to be force-fed. A mixture of a high-caloric supplement, yogurt or *Lactobacillus* product, and 50% dextrose has been used to stimulate eating (30 mL per feeding). Various vegetables, shredded wheat, raspberry jam, canned pumpkin and moistened rabbit feed slurry have also been recommended. Commercial herbivore critical care nutritional supplements are also available. To prevent recurrence, the rabbit should be fed a high-fiber feed or given supplemental hay, as well as opportunities for exercise.

Prevention

Avoiding stress and obesity, provision of a high-fiber feed and ad lib palatable water, careful restraint, routine grooming (brushing or clipping) to remove excess hair, and environmental enrichment are reasonable recommendations for prevention.

References

Gillett NA, Brooks DL, Tillman PL. Medical and surgical management of gastric obstruction from a hair ball in the rabbit. J Am Vet Med Assoc. 1983, 183:1176–1178.

Jackson G. Intestinal stasis and rupture in rabbits. Vet Rec. 1991, 129:287–289.

Jenkins JR, Brown SA. A Practitioner's Guide to Rabbits and Ferrets. Lakewood, CA: American Animal Hospital Association, 1993.

Lee KJ, Johnson WD, Lang CM. Acute peritonitis in the rabbit (Oryctolagus cuniculus) resulting from a gastric trichobezoar. Lab Anim Sci. 1978, 28:202–204.

Paul-Murphy J. Critical care of the rabbit. Vet Clin Exot Anim. 2007, 10:437–461.

Reusch B. Rabbit gastroenterology. Vet Clin Exot Pract. 2005, 8:351–375.

Sebesteny A. Acute obstruction of the duodenum of a rabbit following the apparently successful treatment of a hair ball. Lab Anim. 1977, 11:135.

Turner PV, Chen HC, Taylor WM. Pharmacokinetics of meloxicam in rabbits after single and repeat oral dosing. Comp Med. 2006, 56(1):63–67.

Wagner JL, Hackel DB, Samsell, AG. Spontaneous deaths in rabbits resulting from gastric trichobezoars. Lab Anim Sci. 1974, 24:826–830.

HANTAVIRUS INFECTIONS

Hosts

Rodents are the primary reservoir hosts worldwide of the Hantaan and related viruses that cause hantavirus pulmonary syndrome (HPS) and hemorrhagic fever with renal syndrome (HFRS). Susceptible reservoir rodents include *Rattus norvegicus* and *R. rattus* (rats), *Peromyscus* spp (white-footed mouse), and *Microtus* spp (voles) in the United States, and *Clethrionomys* spp (voles) and *Apodemus* spp (field mice) in other parts of the world. In the laboratory, the rat is the primary animal associated with spread of hantaviruses. Rabbits, guinea pigs, cats, and dogs have been found to be seropositive occasionally when kept in the same room as infected rats.

Mice may become infected with hantaviruses, and wild mice such as *Peromyscus maniculatus* have been identified as the primary hantavirus reservoir and cause of HFRS outbreaks in humans in the U.S. Southwest. Humans are considered to be accidental hosts.

Etiology

Both HFRS and HPS are caused by infection with one of the hantaviruses of the arthropod-borne family, Bunyaviridae. Hemorrhagic fever with renal syndrome (HFRS) refers to a group of clinically similar diseases that occur throughout Europe and Asia. Hantaviruses that can cause HFRS include Hantaan virus, Puumala virus, Dobrava virus, and Seoul virus. Hemorrhagic fever with renal syndrome is a febrile disease with renal involvement that has occurred primarily among researchers and animal technicians working with infected rats or cell cultures. Between 1975 and 1981, 102 cases of HFRS were detected in 15 Japanese institutions.

Hantavirus pulmonary syndrome (HPS) refers to a clinical syndrome caused by a number of hantaviruses in North and South America. In the United States, the Sin Nombre virus causes most cases of this condition, and increases in seroprevalence in mice occur in certain years when forage is plentiful. HPS can also be due to infection by at least 11 other named and unnamed hantaviruses.

Transmission

Hantaviruses infect most major wild mouse and rat populations in the United States. Seroepidemiologic studies suggest an antibody prevalence rate of up to 8% in wild murids. Infected rodents shed virus in saliva, urine, and feces for many weeks, and possibly the infection persists for a lifetime, but the duration of shedding and infectivity is unknown. The average incubation period is 12–16 days. The virus is probably not transmitted directly between humans.

Biting may be an important mode of transmission among free-living rodents because of infectious virus in saliva. Transmission may also occur by contact with fomites contaminated with rodent excreta or urine, by direct introduction into broken skin or the conjunctiva, by ingestion of contaminated food or water, or by aerosols.

Predisposing Factors

Predisposing factors among rodents include fighting, biting, and possibly grooming. There is no significant difference in survival, growth rate, body size, and fertility between seronegative and seropositive wild-caught brown Norway rats, and the virus appears to have little or no impact on demographics in Norway rat populations.

Clinical Signs

Clinical signs and lesions have not been reported in laboratory rats or mice, although they develop high antibody titers.

Diagnosis

Hantaviral infection can be diagnosed by detection of specific serum antibodies with enzyme-linked immunosorbent assay techniques (ELISA).

Prevention

The best approach to disease control and prevention is risk reduction through environmental hygiene practices that deter wild rodents from colonizing homes, laboratory buildings, and work environments. Control of wild rodents without concurrent control of fleas may increase risk of human plague as rodent fleas seek an alternative food source. Routes by which wild rodents might contaminate laboratory stocks must be eliminated. Laboratory work with these viruses must be done under appropriate conditions for controlling hazardous Biosafety Level 3 agents. Testing for hantaviruses should be conducted when potentially infected laboratory rats and possibly other rodent species are to be shipped from Asia, the United Kingdom, France, and Belgium or other areas of the world where the viruses may exist to other uninfected countries and areas. Testing should be done in advance of shipment or during quarantine of the animals after arrival. Wild-caught mice of the genera mentioned previously should also be tested, particularly if they originate from locations where the virus is known to be endemic.

Areas in which hantaviruses are being studied must be sanitized appropriately. Hantaviruses are susceptible to 1% sodium hypochlorite, 2% glutaraldehyde, and 70% ethanol. A 10% sodium hypochlorite solution has been recommended for heavily soiled areas. Hantaviruses are also susceptible to acid (pH 5) conditions and can be inactivated by heating at 60°C (140°F) for 1 hour.

Public Health Significance

Although not likely to cause clinical disease in rodents, hantaviruses may cause serious disease and death in humans. Clinical features of HFRS in people include acute high fever, severe malaise, myalgia, headaches, diarrhea, nausea and vomiting, proteinuria, oliguria, hemorrhagic manifestations, and possibly death. Pet animals should not be allowed to contact wild rodents or their droppings because of the risk for disease transmission.

Laboratory personnel have contracted disease from infected laboratory rats in Japan, France, Belgium, Korea, and Singapore. Most infections in humans result from aerosols generated by infected rodents or when dried rodent droppings have been disturbed in rural residences, garages, and sheds during spring cleaning. Wearing respiratory protection is advised for these procedures to reduce risk. Worldwide, lymphocytic choriomeningitis and hantavirus infections are potentially the most important zoonotic pathogens of laboratory rodents that do not originate from known negative sources. Specific pathogen free rats and mice are of little risk for transmission of these pathogens. Feral rodents are not recommended as pets for this reason.

References

Baek LJ, et al. Leaky virus: a new hantavirus isolated from Mus musculus in the United States. J Gen Virol. 1988, 69:3129–3132.

Chan YC, Wong TW, Yap EH. Haemorrhagic fever with renal syndrome: clinical, virological and epidemiological perspective. Ann Acad Med. 1987, 16:696–701.

Childs JE, et al. Effect of hantaviral infection on survival, growth and fertility in wild rat (Rattus norvegicus) populations of Baltimore, Maryland. J Wildl Dis. 1989, 25:469–476.

———. Epizootiology of hantavirus infections of Baltimore: isolation of a virus from Norway rats and characteristics of infected rat populations. Am J Epidemiol. 1987, 126:55–68.

Jay M, Ascher MS, Chomel BB, et al. Seroepidemiologic studies of hantavirus infection among wild rodents in California. Emerg Infect Dis. 1997, 3(2):183–190.

Kawamata J, et al. Control of laboratory acquired hemorrhagic fever with renal syndrome (HFRS) in Japan. Lab Anim Sci. 1987, 37:431–436.

LeDuc JW. Epidemiology of Hantaan and related viruses. Lab Anim Sci. 1987, 37:413–418.

LeDuc JW., et al. Hantaan-like viruses from domestic rats captured in the United States. Am J Trop Med Hyg. 1984, 33:992–998.

Lee HW, Johnson KM. Laboratory-acquired infections with Hantaan virus, the etiologic agent of Korean hemorrhagic fever. J Infect Dis. 1982, 146:645–651.

Lee PW, et al. Pathogenesis of experimental Hantaan virus infection in laboratory rats. Arch Virol. 1986, 88:57–66.

Morita C, et al. Age-dependent transmission of hemorrhagic fever with renal syndrome (HERS) virus in rats. Arch Virol. 1985, 85:145–149.

Quimby FW. Zoonotic implications of Hantaanlike viruses: an introduction. Lab Anim Sci. 1987, 37:411–412.

Rand MS. Hantavirus: an overview and update. Lab Anim Sci. 1994, 44:301–304.

Takahashi Y, et al. Comparison of immunofluorescence and hemagglutination inhibition tests and enzyme-linked immunosorbent assay for detection of serum antibody in rats infected with hemorrhagic fever with renal syndrome virus. J Clin Microbiol. 1986, 24:712–715.

Tsai TF. Serologic and virological evidence of a Hantaan virus-related enzootic in the United States. J Infect Dis. 1985, 152:126–136.

Zeier M, Handermann M, Bahr U, et al. New ecological aspects of hantavirus infection: a change of a paradigm and a challenge of prevention—a review. Virus Genes. 2005, 30(2):157–180.

HEAT PROSTRATION

Hosts

All animals are susceptible to heat prostration or heat stroke, but adult rabbits, chinchillas, and guinea pigs are cold-adapted species and are particularly susceptible to increased ambient temperatures.

Etiology

High ambient temperatures alone or in combination with any of the predisposing factors listed below may lead to failure of thermoregulatory mechanisms and an increased body temperature beyond a level compatible with life.

Predisposing Factors

Predisposing factors to heat stroke include an ambient temperature greater than 28 °C (85 °F), high humidity (more than 70%), a thick hair coat, obesity, older age, pregnancy, direct sunlight, poor ventilation, insufficient or warm water, crowding, history of recent transportation by common carrier, confinement in a vehicle, transportation delay, adverse stress, and anxiety. Heat stroke victims, like food deprivation cases, may present without a complete history. This makes a thorough clinical examination essential.

Clinical Signs

Signs of heat stress include hyperemia of peripheral vessels in the extremities, rapid respiration, hyperthermia (rectal temperature above 41 °C or 105 °F), cyanosis, prostration, death, or unexplained mortality in otherwise healthy animals, especially groups of animals. Mortality is greatest in the uppermost cages in tiered row breeder settings because heat rises. There may be blood-tinged fluid in the nares and coming from the mouth. Food intake drops and water intake is increased greatly. Rodents have large salivary glands and respond to overheating by profuse salivation. Excess saliva escaping from the corners of the mouth is groomed over the face and sides of the body with the forepaws, cooling the animal. Thus, the saliva wets the body and cools the animal through evaporation.

Chronically heat-stressed rabbits eat and grow less, consume more water, and at temperatures of 32 °C (90 °F) and above for several days or even weeks, males become sterile. This is reversible if the ambient temperature returns to normal. Younger bucks 5–7 months of age are less susceptible to heat-induced sterility.

Necropsy Signs

Signs of heat stroke include hyperemia of tissues, particularly of the lungs and intestinal wall, and often dehydration and copious salivation.

Diagnosis

The history of acute onset in hot weather and the absence of evidence of ketosis or infectious or toxic disease support a diagnosis of heat stroke. Rodents with acute heat stroke or suffocation will have evidence of excessive salivation from the corners of the mouth. Fur may be wet and matted, and extremities (ears, tail, scrotum, and feet) may be hyperemic and cyanotic.

Treatment

Heat-stressed animals can be sprayed with water, carefully dipped into a cool bath (not an ice water bath), or wrapped in a dampened cloth until the rectal temperature returns to normal. Supportive care and corticosteroids may be administered as well as IV or IO fluid therapy. The fluid bag can be put in ice water or the IV tubing can be run through ice water. Cool water enemas can be tried for animals that will tolerate this treatment. Efforts to lower body temperature should be discontinued around 103 °F to preclude rebound hypothermia and shivering. Monitoring for acute renal failure or metabolic acidosis should be considered in select cases. The prognosis is usually guarded to poor, particularly if the body temperature has exceeded 41.1 °C (106 °F).

Prevention

Obese and heavily furred animals are particularly susceptible and should be conditioned to higher ambient temperatures, culled, or potentially groomed and given a haircut. Prevention of heat stress includes provision of shade; adequate air circulation, feed, and water; water sprays; or a container of ice placed in the cage.

References

Besch EL, Woods JE. Heat dissipation biorhythms of laboratory animals. Lab Anim Sci. 1977, 27:54–59.
Oloufa MM, Bogart R, McKenzie FF. Effect of environmental temperature and the thyroid gland on fertility in the male rabbit. Fertil Steril. 1951, 2:223–229.
Paul-Murphy J. Critical care of the rabbit. Vet Clin Exot Anim. 2007, 10:437–461.
Pucak GJ, Lee CS, Zaino AS. Effects of prolonged high temperature on testicular development and fertility in the male rat. Lab Anim Sci. 1977, 27:76–77.
Rathore AK. High temperature exposure of male rabbits: fertility of does mated to bucks subjected to 1 and 2 days of heat treatment. Br Vet J. 1970, 126:168–172.

HELICOBACTER INFECTIONS

Hosts

Helicobacter spp are important pathogens of laboratory animals, particularly rodents. *Helicobacter* spp is the most common bacterial contaminant of research rodents in Europe and North America. Various *Helicobacter* spp infect mice, rats, guinea pigs, rabbits, hamsters, gerbils, ferrets, dogs, cats, humans, and other animal species. There are no reports of *Helicobacter* spp infections in chinchillas.

Etiology

Discovery of *Helicobacter hepaticus* occurred during an investigation into an unexpectedly high background incidence of hepatic tumors and hepatitis in control A/JCr mice in a carcinogenesis study. Subclinical infection may have profound systemic effects, confounding research. In one study, infection of mice with *Helicobacter* spp resulted in altered gene expression in cecal tissues, prior to the onset of clinical signs in the mice, leading to upregulation of 25 genes and downregulation of 3 others. Colonization of the intestine in mice is dependent upon production of a cytolethal distending toxin by the bacterium.

Helicobacter hepaticus and *Helicobacter bilus* are the two primary pathologic species in mice. Other species detected in mice include *H. muridarum, H. (Flexispira) rappini, H. rodentium*, and *H. typhlonicus*. These bacteria are microaerophilic, curved to spiral rods with variable numbers of flagella.

H. hepaticus and *H. bilis*, separately or in combination, are associated with a chronic typhlocolitis in immunodeficient mice. Confinement within the biliary system appears to afford protection against circulating antibody in chronically infected mice.

H. bilis has been reported to cause proliferative and ulcerative typhlocolitis and proctitis in nude rats. In addition to the hepatic lesions associated with *H. hepaticus* infections in immunocompetent and immunodeficient laboratory mice, wasting and chronic enterocolitis have been observed in immunocompromised mice and rats infected with *H. hepaticus, H. bilis, H. typhlonicus, H. rodentium*, or *H. muridarium*.

Spontaneous *Helicobacter* spp infections have been reported in hamsters and gerbils. In one report in gerbils, attempts to rid the colony of *Helicobacter* spp infection resulted in a *C. difficile* enterotoxemia. *Helicobacter* spp infection is a classic example of chronic inflammation resulting in neoplasia induction. This model is used to reliably reproduce various gastrointestinal and hepatic tumors. Infection in hamsters with naturally occurring species may result in gastric adenocarcinoma and intestinal metaplasia.

Predisposing Factors

There is a strain-related variation in susceptibility to the disease. A/J, BALB/c, Swiss-Webster, and ICR mice are susceptible to typhlocolitis, while C57BL/6 mice are relatively resistant. An autoimmune component has been recognized in chronically infected mice with active hepatitis. There is a gender pattern of disease susceptibility to *H. hepaticus*, with male mice being more susceptible to hepatitis and females to enterocolitis.

Clinical Signs

Infection in mice may result in diarrhea, rectal prolapse, chronic weight loss, and anemia. Signs of cholangiohepatitis may be nonspecific.

Necropsy Signs

At necropsy, lesions may be present in both the small and large intestine, but they are usually most extensive in the large intestine. Chronic proliferative typhlitis, colitis, and proctitis with hyperplasia of mucosal epithelial cells, patchy disruption of the normal mucosal architecture, and mild mononuclear cell infiltration in the lamina propria are typical histologic findings in mice. In silver-stained sections of intestine, numerous spiral-shaped bacilli are evident within crypts and on the surface of the affected mucosa.

Infections with *Helicobacter hepaticus* in many immunocompetent strains of mice may result in chronic cholangiohepatitis, and in the immunocompromised host, chronic proliferative enteritis involving the cecum, colon, and rectum are possible sequelae. The typical findings in cases of hepatitis are focal necrosis with hepatocytomegaly, ductular cell hyperplasia, and pericholangitis. *Helicobacter* spp infection may confound results of various experimental studies, particularly of those that use mice for inflammatory disease models. Hepatic tumors have been observed in A/J mice chronically infected with *H. hepaticus*. The bacteria are best demonstrated within bile canaliculi with the Steiner modification of the Warthin-Starry stain.

Transmission

Bacterial transmission is orofecal. Contaminated bedding is one possible source of infection. Chronic inapparent shedding is common. The organism may reside in the intestinal tract and in the bile canaliculi of the liver for months to years. Transplantable cell lines have been reported to be positive for *Helicobacter* spp contamination, and all biologics should be ascertained to be free of infectious organisms prior to injection into live animals.

Diagnosis

Infections are typically diagnosed based on serology or histologic lesions, with confirmation of bacterial presence using silver or Giemsa stains. Culture of the bacterium is difficult and requires specific media and microaerophilic conditions, whereas PCR of fecal pellets is a rapid and sensitive test for the bacteria. For *H. bilis*, the most sensitive test for diagnosis is by PCR or culture of feces, regardless of mouse strain. Colony monitoring by serology alone may be challenging, as seroconversion to bacterial presence may take several weeks, assuming that infected animals are shedding sufficient numbers of bacteria in the feces.

Because *Helicobacter* spp are able to rapidly hydrolyze urea to form urease, in human medicine, a presumptive diagnosis of *H. pylori* infection is made by inoculating a small piece of a gastric biopsy onto a direct urea slant and incubating it at 35 °C. The slant is examined at 1 and 4 hours postinoculation and a positive reaction (intense pink-red to red-violet color) is presumptive evidence of *H. pylori* infection. Anecdotally, this test has also been used in laboratory animal medicine; however, speciation of the bacteria is important to determine clinical significance of positive reactions.

Treatment

Helicobacter spp was reported to be eradicated successfully in experimentally inoculated mice using a combination therapy that included metronidazole, tetracycline, and bismuth subcitrate. Other antibiotics that were tried with variable effectiveness included erythromycin and amoxicillin. Tetracycline, when used alone, was ineffective.

Prevention

Helicobacter spp infections can largely be eliminated from colonies by cross-fostering pups within 48 hours of birth onto clean dams. Caesarean rederivation onto clean dams will also eliminate the bacteria. Traffic flow and personnel handling of animals should move from cleanest to dirtiest to minimize the possibility of colony contamination. Thought must be given to optimal husbandry practices on weekends, when reduced personnel are usually present. Shared equipment, for example, Morris water mazes, elevated plus mazes, and so forth, must be carefully cleaned between animals and between users with animals of differing health status.

Public Health Significance

Helicobacter hepaticus does not infect humans, although *H. pylori* (a human *Helicobacter* sp) readily infects mice, gerbils, and guinea pigs and causes a severe gastritis.

References

Bergin IL, et al. Eradication of enteric helicobacters in Mongolian gerbils is complicated by the occurrence of C. difficile enterotoxemia. Comp Med. 2005, 55:265–268.

SPECIFIC DISEASES AND CONDITIONS

Chichlowski M, Sharp JM, Vanderford DA, et al. Helicobacter typhlonicus and Helicobacter rodentium differentially affect the severity of colon inflammation and inflammation-associated neoplasia in IL10-deficient mice. Comp Med. 2008, 58(6):536–541.

DeBock M, et al. Helicobacter felis and Helicobacter bizzozeronii induce gastric parietal cell loss in Mongolian gerbils. Microbes Infect. 2006, 8:503–510.

Fox JG. Chronic inflammation is the culprit: rodent models of infectious gastrointestinal and liver cancer. Toxicol Pathol. 2005, 33(7):827–828.

Fox JG, et al. Helicobacter bilis, sp. nov., a novel Helicobacter species isolated from bile, livers, and intestines of inbred mice. J Clin Microbiol. 1995, 33:445–454.

Ge Z, et al. Cytolethal distending toxin is essential for Helicobacter hepaticus colonization in outbred Swiss Webster mice. Infect Immun. 2005, 73:3559–3567.

Goto K, Ishihar K-I, Kuzuoka A, et al. Contamination of transplantable human tumor-bearing lines by Helicobacter hepaticus and its elimination. J Clin Microbiol. 2001, 39:3703–3704.

Haines DC, et al. Inflammatory large bowel disease in immunodeficient rats naturally and experimentally infected with Helicobacter bilis. Vet Pathol. 1998, 35:202–208.

Hodzic E, et al. Evaluation of diagnostic methods for Helicobacter bilis infection in laboratory mice. Comp Med. 2001, 51(5):406–412.

Li X, et al. SCID/NCr mice naturally infected with Helicobacter hepaticus develop progressive hepatitis, proliferative typhlitis and colitis. Infect Immun. 1998, 66:5477–5484.

Livingston RS, et al. Sex influence on chronic intestinal inflammation in Helicobacter hepaticus-infected A/JCr mice. Comp Med. 2004, 54:301–308.

Mahler M, et al. Comparison of four diagnostic methods for detection of Helicobacter species in laboratory mice. Lab Anim Sci. 1998, 48(1):85–91.

Mahler M, Janke C, Wagner S, et al. Differential susceptibility of inbred mouse strains to Helicobacter pylori infection. Scand J Gastroenterol. 2002, 37:267–278.

Myles MH, et al. Pathogenicity of Helicobacter rodentium in A/JCr and SCID mice. Comp Med. 2004, 54:549–557.

Nambiar PR, et al. Gastritis-associated adenocarcinoma and intestinal metaplasia in a Syrian hamster naturally infected with Helicobacter species. Vet Pathol. 2005, 42:386–390.

Nambiar PR, et al. Progressive proliferative and dysplastic typhlocolitis in aging Syrian hamsters naturally infected with Helicobacter spp: a spontaneous model of inflammatory bowel disease. Vet Pathol. 2006, 43:2–14.

Simmons JH, et al. Helicobacter mesocricetorum sp. nov., a novel Helicobacter isolated from the feces of Syrian hamsters. J Clin Microbiol. 2000, 38:1811–1817.

Singletary KB, Kloster CA, Baker DG. Optimal age at cross fostering for derivation of Helicobacter hepaticus-free mice. Comp Med. 2003, 53:259–264.

Solvnick JV, Schauer DB. Emergence of diverse Helicobacter species in the pathogenesis of gastric and enterohepatic disease. Clin Microbiol Rev. 2001, 14:59–97.

Truett GE, Walker JA, Baker DG. Eradication of infection with Helicobacter spp by use of neonatal transfer. Comp Med. 2000, 50:444–451.

Van den Bulck K, et al. First report on the occurrence of "Helicobacter heilmannii" in the stomach of rabbits. Vet Res Commun. 2005, 29:271–279.

Ward JM, et al. Chronic active hepatitis and associated liver tumors in mice caused by a persistent bacterial infection with a novel Helicobacter species. J Nat Canc Instit. 1994, 86:1222–1227.

Ward JM, et al. Chronic active hepatitis in mice caused by Helicobacter hepaticus. Am J Pathol. 1994, 145:959–968.

Ward JM, et al. Inflammatory large bowel disease in immunodeficient mice naturally infected with Helicobacter hepaticus. Lab Anim Sci. 1996, 46:15–20.

Watson J, et al. Successful rederivation of contaminated immunocompetent mice using neonatal transfer with iodine immersion. Comp Med. 2005, 55(5):465–469.

Whary MT, Fox JG. Natural and experimental Helicobacter infections. Comp Med. 2004, 54:128–158.

HEMATURIA AND PIGMENTED URINE

Hosts

Bloody urine or hematuria and urine otherwise pigmented are seen more commonly in rabbits than in rodents. Urine of adult rabbits is normally turbid with a yellow-brown tint and has an alkaline pH of approximately 8.2. Urine of young rabbits, which is more acidic, is free of precipitate. The urine first appears turbid or cloudy when young rabbits begin to eat green feed and grains. The turbid appearance of the urine is due to the abundance of crystal precipitate (some ammonium magnesium phosphate but mostly calcium carbonate) seen in normal alkaline urine. Crystals dissolve if the urine becomes acidic (pH 6–7), as is the case in adult rabbits with fasting, food deprivation, or inappetence. Guinea pigs and chinchillas also may produce urine with a turbid appearance due to calcium crystal excretion.

Etiology

In rabbits, if the urine contains blood, then uterine adenocarcinoma, urolithiasis, and cystitis are likely causes. Other less frequent causes are bladder polyps, pyelonephritis, renal infarcts, disseminated intravascular coagulation (DIC), leptospirosis, ruptured endometrial venous aneurysms, hemangiomatosis, and abortion. An intermittent benign asymptomatic hematuria has been reported in Lewis × Brown Norway rats due to intermittent rupture of hemorrhagic, papillary, proliferative masses in the renal pelvis. Infections due to *E. coli, Klebsiella* spp, *Pasteurella multocida, Encephalitozoon cuniculi*, and other bacterial, parasitic, or viral agents are possible causes of pyelonephritis. Plant toxicosis or trauma also can cause hematuria, and renal failure has been reported in guinea pigs following ingestion of oxalate-containing houseplants.

Some cases of red urine in rabbits are due to porphyrin-pigmented basic urine and urobilin from heme degradation. The intensity of the color is heightened by dehydration (usually because of water restriction) and excess dietary calcium. Calcium and magnesium are excreted principally in the urine of rabbits; however, calcium is excreted primarily in the bile of other mammals.

Chronic renal disease, although common, is unlikely to result in hematuria. Metastatic mineralization is not an uncommon cause of renal disease in guinea pigs over 1 year of age. Unthriftiness and muscle stiffness may result if soft tissues are similarly affected. This may result from feeding rabbit pellets to guinea pigs or from giving animals multivitamin supplements. To achieve adequate levels of vitamin C with these supplements vitamin D toxicosis is often created. Rabbits are also sensitive to vitamin D intoxication and adults are more sensitive than younger animals. Clinical signs may be nonspecific and radiographic evidence of multiorgan mineralization may be diagnostic in some cases. Certain drugs may have nephrotoxic properties, particularly in dehydrated animals. Examples include gentamicin, tiletamine/zolazepam (Telazol®), and many nonsteroidal antiinflammatory drugs.

Similarly, most rodent species are susceptible to a chronic degenerative renal disease that may be strain- or sex-specific, linked to ad libitum feeding or related to high protein levels or inappropriate protein formulations in the diet. This does not produce hematuria.

Predisposing Factors

Normal cloudy, yellow-tan tinted urine may appear darker if an animal is dehydrated. The cloudy red urine, commonly seen in apparently healthy rabbits, is often mistaken by inexperienced rabbit owners and caretakers as blood in the urine. Rabbits that are fed carrots and other fresh foods high in carotene are likely to exhibit more red pigment in the urine than are animals on lower carotene foods.

Intact adult does have a high incidence of uterine adenocarcinoma. Discharge associated with this neoplasm may appear in the urine. The incidence of uterine adenocarcinoma is breed-specific and may be as high as 80% in the New Zealand white breed but is rarely reported in rex and Belgian breeds. The varieties of breeds seen in pet practice will include those likely to develop this tumor. Predisposing factors for urolithiasis and cystitis include systemic or local bacterial, viral, or parasitic infections and dietary imbalances.

Clinical Signs

Animals with true bleeding episodes and hematuria may be clinically pale or anemic and show other signs associated with their primary disease, especially if the condition is chronic. Regardless of the specific etiology, hematuria is frequently the most prominent feature in clinical disease, whereas reddish pigment in the urine is observed commonly in nonclinical (nondiseased) cases.

Reproductive disturbances such as decreased fertility, small litter size, increased incidence of stillborn and retained fetuses, desertion of a litter, dystocias, and fetal resorption are clinical signs highly correlated with uterine adenocarcinoma in older female breeder rabbits. Nonspecific signs such as anorexia, loss of condition, and depression may be associated with either systemic or localized conditions such as urolithiasis with or without cystitis, pyelonephritis, toxicosis, or trauma.

Necropsy Signs

Gross lesions associated with hematuria depend on the cause. The uterus may be unilaterally or bilaterally enlarged with variations in color and have a nodular appearance in some cases. If endometrial hyperplasia is implicated, cystic ovaries are seen. If metastasis of an adenocarcinoma has occurred, gross nodular lesions may be found in any major organ including lungs, liver, and bone marrow. In endometrial hemangiomatosis, the uterine horns are enlarged and turgid, and, on cross-section, contain red-tinged watery fluid and a variable number of red-purple, firm, ovoid, pedunculated masses. In cases of urolithiasis, concretions may be found anywhere in the bladder, urethra, ureter, or renal pelvis. Infection of rabbits with *E. cuniculi* may be apparent grossly in the kidneys as multiple, small, pale foci. Cystitis may be accompanied by gross changes in the bladder mucosa secondary to urine stasis.

Histologic lesions in uterine endometrial hyperplasia include proliferative changes of the endometrial glands and formation of papillary or polypoid cauliflower-like growths projecting from the luminal surface of the uterus. Uterine adenocarcinoma is characterized by anaplasia of the endometrial cells, proliferation of the endometrium with scattered mitotic figures, and a myxomatous appearance of the proliferating cells. The microscopic appearance of uterine hemangiomas includes congested and hemorrhagic polypoid nodules with laminated thrombi consisting of layers of fibrin and red cells in the vascular spaces. Microthrombi, hemorrhages, and cell necrosis may be seen in cases of disseminated intravascular coagulation, whereas microabscesses and infarcts may be seen in systemic or local infections.

Diagnosis

Red urine from clinically ill animals with obvious signs of dehydration, bacterial infections, and other concurrent diseases or conditions can be differentiated from the urine of healthy animals by urinalysis, including urine cytology. Thorough physical examination, abdominal palpation, ultrasonography, radiography, ancillary blood tests (hemograms and serum chemistry for azotemia), and biopsy results are helpful in making a diagnosis. Culture and isolation of bacteria from a cystocentesis sample are useful in ruling out an infectious process.

Histopathologic examination of uterine tissue is essential to differentiate between benign uterine hyperplasia and the early stages of uterine adenocarcinoma. This facilitates an accurate prognosis so that therapeutic management may be prescribed.

Treatment

The treatment will depend on the inciting cause. Aggressive and prudent use of antibiotics, such as trimethoprim-sulfa, may be necessary to eliminate infection, and surgery may be indicated in cases of urolithiasis, uterine hyperplasia, and adenocarcinoma that has not metastasized. Rabbits with malignant neoplasia (e.g., uterine adenocarcinoma) have a poor prognosis once metastasis has occurred, at which time symptomatic treatment is at best palliative.

Prevention

Abundant fresh clean water should be provided ad libitum to prevent dehydration, and parenteral fluid replacement should be used in emergencies and life-threatening conditions. Neutering of pubescent females will prevent uterine tumor development in later years. Feeding a balanced diet, reduction of stress, and good husbandry practices are measures that may prevent some cases of hematuria.

References

Baum I. What's your diagnosis? Hematuria in a rabbit. Lab Anim. 1992, 21:16–18.

Bray MV, et al. Endometrial venous aneurysms in three New Zealand white rabbits. Lab Anim Sci. 1992, 42:360–362.

Fisher PG. Exotic mammal renal disease: causes and clinical presentation. Vet Clin Exot Pract. 2006, 9:33–67.

Garibaldi BA, et al. Hematuria in rabbits. Lab Anim Sci. 1987, 37:762–772.

Holowaychuk MK. Renal failure in a guinea pig (Cavia porcellus) following ingestion of oxalate containing plants. Can Vet J. 2006, 47:787–789.

Paul-Murphy J. Critical care of the rabbit. Vet Clin Exot Anim. 2007, 10:437–461.

Toft JD. Commonly observed spontaneous neoplasms in rabbits, rats, guinea pigs, hamsters, and gerbils. Sem Av Exot Pet Med. 1992, 1:80.

Treloar AF, Armstrong A. Intermittent hematuria in a colony of Lewis X Brown Norway hybrid rats. Lab Anim Sci. 1993, 43:640–641.

HYPOVITAMINOSIS C (SCURVY) IN GUINEA PIGS

Hosts

Guinea pigs and primates, including humans, are among a small number of animal species with an absolute requirement for dietary or exogenous L-ascorbic acid or vitamin C, a vitamin active in certain biologic oxidation and reduction systems. Other animals that require vitamin C are a few species of fruit-eating bats, channel catfish, and certain birds, such as the red-vented bulbul. Although closely related to guinea pigs, chinchillas are able to synthesize enough vitamin C to meet their daily needs and are not susceptible to scurvy.

Etiology

The expression of the hepatic microsomal enzyme L-gulonolactone oxidase is genetically controlled. Guinea pigs, primates, and the other species that normally require ascorbic acid in their diet lack the gene necessary to produce the oxidase, which is one of several enzymes involved in the conversion of L-gulonolactone to L-ascorbic acid. Ascorbic acid is essential in the hydroxylase reactions necessary for formation and cross-linking of hydroxyproline and hydroxylysine in collagen and in the metabolism of cholesterol to bile acids, amino acids, and carbohydrates. A deficiency leads to fragmentation of collagen and intercellular ground substance. Because vitamin C is water-soluble, there is no internal storage depot and guinea pigs require vitamin C daily.

Predisposing Factors

Age, sex, amount of stored vitamin, diet, pregnancy, lactation, concomitant disease, and environmental conditions all affect the duration of onset and the magnitude of signs seen with ascorbic acid deficiency. Young guinea pigs show signs of deficiency within 2 weeks or less if vitamin C is withheld completely. Guinea pigs up to 6 weeks of age catabolize vitamin C much faster than those older than 4 months, and guinea pigs may show individual adaptations to dietary levels of vitamin C.

Ascorbic acid content of feed is reduced by dampness, light, heat, and prolonged storage. Up to 50% of vitamin C activity in stored feed is lost within 6 weeks. Similarly, up to 50% of vitamin C activity is lost within 24 hours when in water, such as in an open crock or bowl.

Clinical Signs

Pet or research guinea pigs with scurvy are lethargic, weak, anorexic, and often found hunched or lying in the cage. Many exhibit a characteristic "bunny-hopping" gait due to inability to extend their stifles. They may vocalize or bite from pain when restrained and often have enlarged limb joints and costochondral junctions, a rough hair coat, diarrhea, weight loss, bruising, and conjunctival and nasal discharge (Figure 5.8). Animals may grind their teeth and salivate excessively, and opportunistic infections are common. Young, growing animals are more susceptible to bone deformities than are older animals. A combined deficiency of vitamins E and C may produce signs of paralysis and death, related to spinal cord and brain degeneration.

Differential diagnoses for lameness, diarrhea, upper respiratory tract disease, or anorexia in guinea pigs should always include consideration of hypovitaminosis C among possible causes. Parenteral vitamin C supplementation should be part of the therapeutic regimen for any sick guinea pig.

Necropsy Signs

Gross lesions of scurvy are related to abnormalities of bones, cartilage and blood vessels. Signs, most prominent in growing animals, include hemorrhage into the subperiosteum, subcutaneous and periarticular tissues, skeletal muscle and intestine, and separation at the epidiaphyseal junction (Figures 5.9 and 5.10). Adrenal glands are usually markedly enlarged.

The consequences of aberrant synthesis of collagen cement substance and connective tissue are evident microscopically, most notably in young animals. Persistence of epiphyseal cartilage with

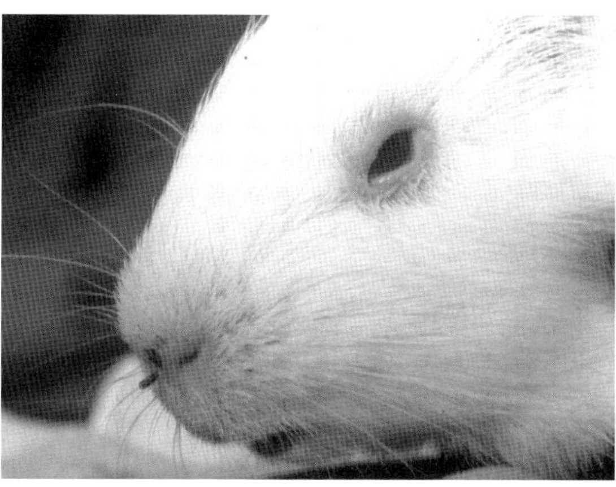

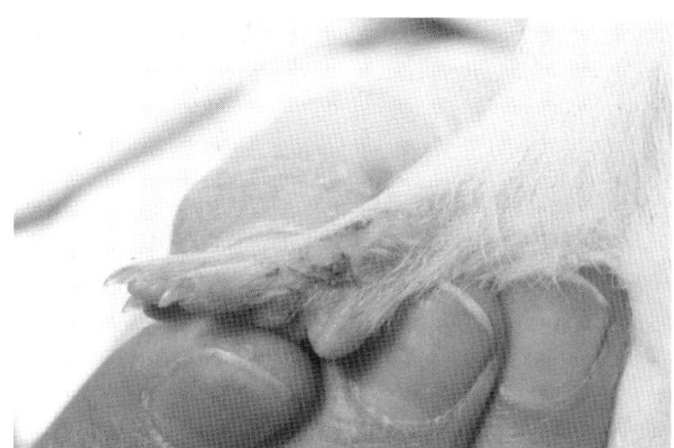

FIGURE 5.8. Conjunctivitis and nasal discharge (left) in a guinea pig with hypovitaminosis C. The nasal discharge has been transferred to the forepaws of this animal during grooming (right).

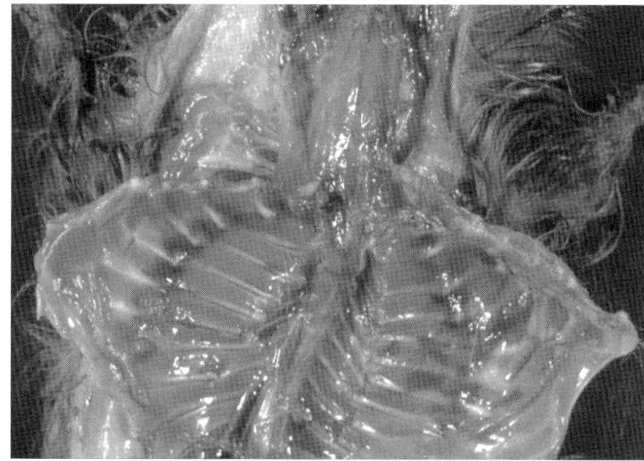

FIGURE 5.9. Hemorrhage and edema along the costochondral junctions of a guinea pig with hypovitaminosis C.

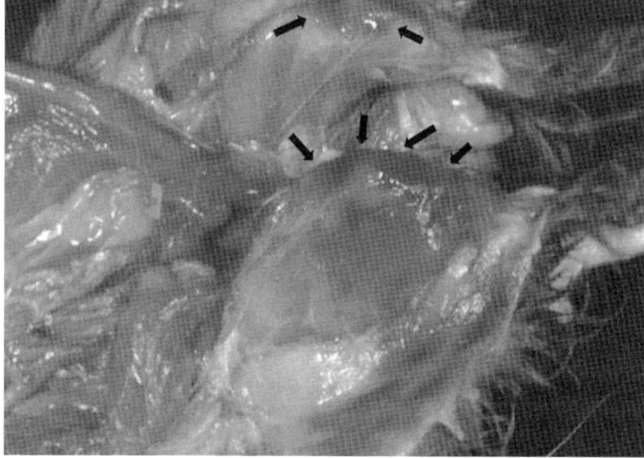

FIGURE 5.10. Stifle joints of a guinea pig with hypovitaminosis C, demonstrating periarticular edema and hemorrhage (arrows).

impaired ossification (scorbutic lattice), microfractures, and subperiosteal hemorrhage are common features. In the absence of new bone formation, the calcified cartilage lattice is thickened and relatively susceptible to mechanical forces, resulting in microfractures and hemorrhage. Proliferation of poorly differentiated fusiform mesenchymal cells is seen in affected areas (periosteal and periarticular tissues). Endothelial junctional defects in skeletal muscle lead to hemorrhage and fragmentation of myofilaments. Scurvy leads to decreased macrophage migration and decreased phagocytic activity of neutrophils. Gross and histologic lesions may be more subtle in an older guinea pig.

Diagnosis

A thorough dietary history and observation of clinical signs, particularly joint stiffness, provide a tentative diagnosis. Many pet guinea pig owners believe they are providing adequate vitamin C by feeding the appropriate pellets, supplementing with multivitamins in the water, and feeding fresh fruits and vegetables. They may not be aware that stored guinea pig pellets lose up to 50% of vitamin C activity within 6 weeks, small mammal multivitamin supplements do not contain sufficient vitamin C for guinea pigs, and the vitamin C content of fresh fruits and vegetables varies greatly; for example, one medium-size carrot contains only 4 mg, and the vitamin C content of iceberg lettuce is negligible (Table 5.2).

Necropsy findings, such as hemorrhage around joints and enlarged costochondral junctions, further support the diagnosis. Marginal deficiencies, especially in adults, and early cases often are difficult to diagnose from the nonspecific signs of weakness and anorexia. Secondary bacterial or metabolic diseases may obscure subtle signs of vitamin C deficiency. Subclinical vitamin C deficiency should be suspected with any ill guinea pig.

Treatment

Active ascorbic acid supplied daily, or at least every third day, via feed, water, or parenteral injection at 5–10 mg/kg body weight for maintenance or 30 mg/kg during pregnancy or 25–50 mg/kg during deficiency will frequently reverse the consequences of a deficiency. Clinical recovery usually requires around 1 week of therapy and may not be complete. Malocclusion due to microfractures of the mandible is a possible sequela. If the abrupt change in the taste of the feed or water causes the guinea pig to refuse the diet or to drink, then giving ascorbic acid per os may be necessary. Multivitamins should not be used because of the potential for toxic overdose of vitamins other than C.

Any sick guinea pig should be treated with daily vitamin C, preferably by the parenteral route. The benefits of empirically administering vitamin C vastly outweigh any risk associated with repeated injections.

Prevention

Provision of adequate, fresh, stabilized vitamin C in feed or water at recommended daily levels (200 mg/L in the drinking water) will prevent hypovitaminosis C. The instability of the vitamin-water solution, as well as the presence of chlorine in water, warrants daily vitamin-water changes. Metal, hard water, and heat also cause accelerated deterioration of ascorbic acid in solution. L-ascorbic acid phosphate is more stable against oxidation or hydrolysis in neutral or alkaline solutions. Commercial guinea pig feeds contain an approximately 800 mg/kg diet of vitamin C when milled. To ensure adequate vitamin C, feed should be stored at less than 22 °C and be used within 90 days of milling, although some newer irradiated

Table 5.2. Vitamin C content of some fruits and vegetables.

Fruit/Vegetable	Amount	Vitamin C Content (mg)
apple, w/skin	1 medium	8
apricots	3 medium	11
banana	1 medium	10
blackberries	1/2 cup	16
blueberries	1/2 cup	7
cantaloupe	1/2 cup	31
grapefruit	1/2 medium	38
guava	1 medium	165
honeydew melon	1/2 cup	16
kiwifruit	1 medium	70
mango	1/2 medium	29
nectarine	1 medium	7
orange	1 medium	70
papaya	1/2 cup	46
peach	1 medium	6
pear	1 medium	7
pineapple	1/2 cup	46
raspberries	1/2 cup	17
strawberries	7	49
Mandarin orange	1 medium	22
broccoli	1/2 cup	41
cabbage, green	1/2 cup	12
carrot	1 medium	4
cauliflower	1/2 cup	25
celery	1 stalk	1
cucumber	4 slices	1
lettuce, iceberg	1 cup	2
lettuce, romaine	1 cup	14
parsley	100 gram	133
peas, snowpeas	10	20
pepper, green	1/2 medium	66
pepper, red	1/2 medium	113
pepper, yellow	1/2 medium	171
tomato, red	1 small	16

References:
Nutrient Content of Some Common Foods, Health Canada, Ottawa, 2008.
http://fnic.nal.usda.gov/nal_display/index.php?info_center-4&tax_level-1

guinea pig diets contain a stabilized potentiated form of vitamin C and have a 6-month shelf life. Tablets containing 50 mg vitamin C are available for guinea pigs (Daily C, Oxbow®, www.oxbowanimalhealth.com) or human orange-flavored supplements (broken into halves or quarters) can be used to provide the daily requirement. Many guinea pigs regard these tablets as a tasty treat and eagerly take them from the hand, or the tablet can be pushed into the side of the mouth behind the fleshy cheek invaginations, where they are chewed and swallowed. Adequate daily ascorbic acid is contained in a quarter orange, a half-handful of parsley, or in a few pieces of sweet red or yellow pepper. The vitamin C content of other fruits and vegetables is listed in Table 5.2. Kale, broccoli, cabbage, brussels sprouts, and other members of the Brassica family are relatively high in vitamin C but also result in gas production, so should be fed only in very small amounts to avoid bloat. Cabbage also contains potentially goitrogenic and estrogenic substances.

The water-soluble nature of vitamin C makes overdose very unlikely if animals are well hydrated, so any combination of the above forms of supplementation may be used safely. Any excess ascorbic acid is eliminated in the urine.

References

Burk RF, Christensen JM, Maguire MJ, et al. A combined deficiency of vitamins E and C causes severe central nervous system damage in guinea pigs. J Nutr. 2006, 136(6):1576–1581.

Clarke GL, et al. Subclinical scurvy in the guinea pig. Vet Pathol. 1980, 17:40–44.

Deqkwitz E, Bodeker R-H. Indications for adaptation to differently high vitamin C supplies in guinea pigs. 1. Development of ascorbic acid levels after altered dosing. Z Emahrungswiss. 1989, 28:327–337.

Eva JK, Fifield R, Rickett M. Decomposition of supplementary vitamin C in diets compounded for laboratory animals. Lab Anim. 1976, 10:157–159.

Fulimer HM, Martin GR, Bums JJ. Role of ascorbic acid in the formation and maintenance of dental structures. Ann NY Acad Sci. 1961, 92:286–294.

Gangulay R, et al. Macrophage function in vitamin C-deficient guinea pigs. Am J Clin Nutr. 1976, 29:762–765.

Gore I, Fujinami T, Shirahama T. Endothelial changes produced by ascorbic acid deficiency in guinea pigs. Arch Pathol. 1965, 80:371–376.

Hickman DL, Wasson K, Ehrhart EJ. Morbidity and mortality in a group of young guinea pigs. Subclinical hypovitaminosis C. Lab Anim. 2003, 32(9):23–25.

Lykkesfeldt J, Trueba GP, Poulsen HE, et al. Vitamin C deficiency in weanling guinea pigs: differential expression of oxidative stress and DNA repair in liver and brain. B J Nutr. 2007, 98(6):1116–1119.

Ness R. Hypovitaminosis C in the guinea pig. J Small Exot Anim Med. 1991, 1:1.

Peterson FJ, Babish JG, Rivers JM. Excessive ascorbic acid consumption and drug metabolism in guinea pigs. Nutr Reports Int. 1982, 26:1037–1043.

Sato P, Udenfriend S. Scurvy-prone animals, including man, monkey, and guinea pig, do not express the gene for gulonolactone oxidase. Arch Biochem Biophys. 1978, 187:158–162.

Schwartz ER, Leveille C, Oh WH. Experimentally-induced osteoarthritis in guinea pigs: effect of surgical procedure and dietary intake of vitamin C. Lab Anim Sci. 1981, 31:683–687.

Smith DF, Balagura S. Taste and physiological need in vitamin C intake by guinea pigs. Physiol Behav. 1975, 14:545–549.

Zloch Z, Ginter E. Influence of age on the kinetics of vitamin C catabolism in guinea-pigs. Physiol Bohemoslov. 1988, 37:459–466.

LAWSONIA INFECTIONS (PROLIFERATIVE ILEITIS OF HAMSTERS)

Hosts

Young Syrian hamsters are highly susceptible to proliferative ileitis caused by infection with *Lawsonia intracellularis*. Infections may occur when they are either naturally or experimentally inoculated per os with intestinal or fecal material from affected animals. Rabbits, some strains of mice, ferrets, and pigs are also susceptible to infection and disease with this agent.

Etiology

Lawsonia intracellularis is an obligate, intracellular nonmotile, Gram-negative, and agyrophilic organism occurring as curved to straight short rods. Depending upon the circumstances and the species affected, the clinical presentation may vary from an acute onset of profuse diarrhea and dehydration with high mortality (regional ileitis in hamsters) to an asymptomatic carrier state, to animals with chronic diarrhea, weight loss, and variable mortality (e.g., proliferative enteropathy in rabbits). Proliferative ileitis is a convenient name for the disease because both hyperplastic and inflammatory components are included. Alternative names in hamsters are "wet tail" and "transmissible ileal hyperplasia."

Changes associated with this disease are likely to have a significant effect on intestinal absorption of water and nutrients. In a study of changes in intestinal absorption in infected rabbits, abnormalities noted included decreased basal intestinal water; sodium, chloride, and glucose absorption; and elevated basal adenylate cyclase activity.

In addition to intestinal disease associated with primary infections with this organism, cases of proliferative enteropathy associated with a dual infection of *L. intracellularis* and an enteropathogenic strain of *E. coli* have been documented in hamsters. Similar cases of dual infections are seen frequently in commercial rabbitries.

Transmission

The bacterium is passed from weanling to weanling or from adult to weanling by the fecal-oral route. There is no subspecies specificity, and the bacterium may readily be transmitted between pigs and rabbits, and rabbits and calves.

Predisposing Factors

Recently weaned hamsters (3–6 weeks of age) are most often affected clinically. Improper diet, intercurrent disease, exposure to infected animals, primiparous litters, crowding, dietary changes, and shipping predispose to development of the disease.

Clinical Signs

Proliferative ileitis has acute, subacute, and clinical consequences. The acute condition involves lethargy, matted hair coat, hunched posture, anorexia, irritability, watery diarrhea, emaciation, and death within 48 hours. In subacute cases, survivors do not gain weight and may die at any time from ileal obstruction, intussusception, peritonitis, or impaction. Hamsters with intussusceptions may have bloody diarrhea and a prolapsed rectum and colon.

Necropsy Signs

Lesions of *Lawsonia intracellularis* infection are usually most extensive in the terminal small intestine. Typical changes are those of proliferative ileitis, with increased mitotic activity of crypt epithelium, and lymphocytic and histiocytic cell infiltration into the lamina propria. Blunting and fusion of adjacent villi, dilatation of lacteals, and marked distortion of the normal architecture are seen in advanced cases.

Diagnosis

Diagnosis of proliferative ileitis is based on the clinical observation of diarrhea ("wet tail") and on the enlarged, thickened, and corrugated appearance of the distal small intestine in weanling hamsters and other animals. Young hamsters often have enteritis without ileal proliferation. In Steiner or Warthin-Starry silver-stained sections of affected ileum, usually large numbers of bacilli are aligned within the apical cytoplasm of enterocytes, with sparing of the microvillous border. The bacterium has stringent growth requirements and cannot be cultured in cell-free media because of a metabolic requirement for preformed mitochondrial triphosphate energy sources. A commercial tissue PCR test for bacterium identification in the ileum is available in some labs.

In rabbits, the disease is often mild and may be an incidental finding at necropsy. In mice, the bacterium predominantly affects the cecum, with similar proliferative and inflammatory changes, as described for hamsters.

Treatment

Treatment includes supportive fluids (oral or parenteral electrolytes or lactated Ringer's solution) for dehydration, an antidiarrheal, such as bismuth subsalicylate, up to 2 mL PO, and appropriate antibiotics such as chloramphenicol, tetracycline, enrofloxacin, metronidazole, or trimethoprim-sulfa, which can be administered orally or via the drinking water. Despite treatment, many hamsters will die of this disease.

Prevention

Affected animals should be isolated to prevent transmission of the disease, and cages and the environment should be thoroughly disinfected. Otherwise, high husbandry standards, frequent bedding changes, absence of environmental stressors, and use of cage filter lids may reduce the transmission of the bacterium within a colony or facility.

Public Health Significance

Proliferative ileitis is not known to be transmissible to humans.

References

Amend NK, et al. Transmission of enteritis in the Syrian hamster. Lab Anim Sci. 1976, 26:566–572.

Cooper DM, et al. Comparative aspects of proliferative enteritis. J Am Vet Med Assoc. 1998, 212:1446–1451.

Duhamel GE, et al. Subclinical proliferative enteropathy in sentinel rabbits associated with Lawsonia intracellularis. Vet Pathol. 1998, 35:300–303.

Frisk CS, Wagner JE. Experimental hamster enteritis: an electron microscopic study. Amer J Vet Res. 1977, 38:1861–1868.

———. Hamster enteritis: a review. Lab Anim. 1977, 11:79–85.

Go YY, Lee JK, Ye JY, et al. Experimental reproduction of proliferative enteropathy and the role of IFN-gamma in protective immunity against Lawsonia intracellularis in mice. J Vet Sci. 2005, 6(4):357–359.

Horiuchi N, Watarai M, Kobayashi Y, et al. Proliferative enteropathy involving Lawsonia intracellularis infection in rabbits (Oryctolagus cuniculus). J Vet Med Sci. 2008, 70(4):389–392.

Jacoby RO. Transmissible ileal hyperplasia of hamsters. 1. Histogenesis and immunocytochemistry. Am J Pathol. 1978, 91:433–450.

La Regina M, Fales WH, Wagner JE. Effects of antibiotic treatment on the occurrence of experimentally induced proliferative ileitis of hamsters. Lab Anim Sci. 1980, 30:38–41.

McNeil PE, et al. Control of an outbreak of wettail in a closed colony of hamsters (Mesocricetus auratus). Vet Rec. 1986, 119:272–273.

Murakata K, Sato A, Yoshiya M, et al. Infection of different strains of mice with Lawsonia intracellularis derived from rabbit or porcine proliferative enteropathy. J Comp Pathol. 2008, 139(1):8–15.

Shauer DB, et al. Proliferative enterocolitis associated with a dual infection with enteropathogenic Escherichia coli and Lawsonia intracellularis in rabbits. J Clin Microbiol. 1998, 36:1700–1703.

LISTERIOSIS

Hosts

Listeriosis is most commonly detected in rabbits and chinchillas, where it generally causes sporadic deaths or limited epizootics, particularly in pregnant animals.

Etiology

Listeria monocytogenes is a Gram-positive, motile nonsporeforming rod that is capable of growing at cold temperatures.

Predisposing Factors

Animals in advanced pregnancy are most frequently clinically affected, probably because the pregnant uterus and placenta present the most favorable environment for growth of the organism. Listeriosis in nonpregnant animals is often associated with predisposing factors (e.g., experimental manipulations, etc.) that may impair the normal immune response.

Transmission

The bacterium may be introduced into a herd via infected animals, by contact with a contaminated environment, or by contaminated feed. Feed may become contaminated because of inappropriate storage or processing methods, or hay may be contaminated in the field by wild rodents prior to processing. The method of transmission is fecal-oral. Equipment, cages, feed, and water contaminated with infected feces are the most important factors involved in the spread of the disease to other animals within the herd.

Clinical Signs

Affected animals may show signs of anorexia, lethargy, bruxism, and slow wasting. Animals more commonly present with constipation because of dehydration and reduced food intake, and rectal prolapse may occur. Central nervous signs such as blindness, head tilt, or convulsions may occur rarely in advanced cases. In pregnant animals, late-term abortions are seen. A high mortality rate is common in affected animals.

Necropsy Signs

In affected animals, there is often focal hepatic and splenic necrosis, lymphadenopathy, ecchymoses, acute metritis, hydrothorax, ascites, and anasarca. Histologically, there are foci of coagulation necrosis in the liver, with neutrophilic infiltrates. In animals that succumb during the perinatal period, acute suppurative metritis and placentitis may be observed.

Diagnosis

A presumptive diagnosis may be made from the history and gross findings. The organism is readily cultured using cold enrichment techniques from affected tissues.

Treatment

In other species, including humans, oral penicillins are the drugs of choice for treating listeriosis. These should not be used in rabbits and chinchillas because of the concern for antibiotic toxicity. Tetracycline and chloramphenicol have been used to effectively treat animals; however, treatment must be initiated early in the course of the disease to be curative. Chloramphenicol may induce infertility.

Prevention

Purchase of animals from clean breeding colonies is important for preventing this condition. In addition, high sanitation standards for equipment, water bottles, and pens will minimize transmission. Dust baths should be changed frequently and shouldn't be shared between cages of chinchillas. Any sick animals should be isolated from healthy ones and appropriate hand-washing regimes should be followed before and after handling sick animals. All food shoud be stored properly to minimize contamination by vermin. Hay can be autoclaved before feeding to kill any bacteria present.

Public Health Significance

The public health aspect is an important consideration when determining whether to treat or euthanize an animal, because treatment may not preclude a long-term carrier state. The organism may be harbored as an inapparent infection in various species.

References

Ayroud M, Chirino-Trejo M, Kumor L. Listeriosis in rabbits. Can Vet J. 1991, 32:44.

Finley GG, Long JR. An epizootic of listeriosis in chinchillas. Can Vet J. 1971, 18:164–167.

Iida T, Kanzaki M, Nakama A, et al. Detection of Listeria monocytogenes in humans, animals and foods. J Vet Med Sci. 1998, 60(12):1341–1343.

Kimpe A, Decostere A, Hermans K, et al. Isolation of Listeria ivanovii from a septicaemic chinchilla (Chinchilla lanigera). Vet Rec. 2004, 154(25):791–792.

Vetesi F, Kemenes F. Studies on listeriosis in pregnant rabbits. Acta Vet Acad Scient Hungaricae. 1967, 17:27–38.

Watson GL, Evans MG. Listeriosis in the rabbit. Vet Path. 1985, 22:191–193.

Wilkerson MJ, Melendy A, Stauber E. An outbreak of listeriosis in a breeding colony of chinchillas. J Vet Diagn Invest. 1997, 9(3):320–323.

LYMPHOCYTIC CHORIOMENINGITIS VIRUS INFECTION

Hosts

The natural reservoir host for the lymphocytic choriomeningitis virus (LCMV) is the wild mouse, in which the prevalence of infection varies and may approach 100% in some regions. Natural infections occur in mice, guinea pigs, man, monkeys, and wild mice (*Apodemus sylvaticus*). A variety of other species can be infected experimentally. Infection can be transmitted readily to hamsters, which were the source of several hundred cases of lymphocytic choriomeningitis in humans in the United States in the 1970s, and more recently, resulted in the deaths of four people in the United States who received organ transplants from an infected individual. Since the 2005 outbreak, significant measures have been taken to eliminate the infection from small mammal pets distributed and sold in pet stores across the United States. Transplantable tumors of mice, hamsters, and guinea pigs; tissue culture cell lines; and virus and protozoan stocks may become persistently contaminated with LCMV and act as a source of virus to inoculated animals.

Etiology

LCMV is an enveloped arenavirus (RNA). On the basis of clinical signs, viscerotropic and neurotropic strains exist. The virus is widespread in Europe and the Americas and is rare in laboratory mice, but common in wild mice, which are presumed to be the natural host for the virus. Hamsters pose a serious risk because they develop persistent infections following natural exposure as adults, unlike mice. Rats are not naturally susceptible.

Transmission

In utero transmission is common in an infected mouse population, but bite wounds may be a more common route of transmission in hamsters. The virus is passed in the urine, saliva, milk, and feces and enters susceptible individuals via traumatized skin, the conjunctiva, or respiratory passages. Blood-sucking arthropod vectors, such as ticks, lice, and mosquitoes, as well as dust or other fomites, may be transmission vehicles. Animals infected prenatally shed the virus for approximately 9 months, whereas animals infected postnatally shed the virus for 2–3 months. Mice have been accidentally infected by the inoculation of LCMV-contaminated transplantable murine tumors.

Predisposing Factors

Factors that predispose to the entry or persistence of LCMV infection in a colony include wild rodent invasion; introduction of carrier animals; use of infected tumors, cell lines, and other biologic products; decreased host resistance; and cutaneous traumatization.

Clinical Signs

The clinical signs of lymphocytic choriomeningitis are almost always subclinical but depend on the host's resistance and age when infected, although the various categories of the disease are not always delineated. If mice are exposed in utero or as neonates, they develop immunologic tolerance, allowing persistence and chronic shedding. Tolerance eventually breaks down later in life with lymphocytic infiltration of multiple organs and antigen-antibody complex glomerulonephritis. Adoptive transfer of T cells from immune mice to subclinically infected mice leads to clinical disease (lymphocytic choriomeningitis) and death. Virus strains are classified as "docile" or "aggressive" and "viscerotropic" and "neurotropic" for experimental purposes. Neonates survive when inoculated intracerebrally because their immune system is immature and no inflammatory reaction results. Adult mice inoculated intracerebrally die. These two experiments are used as bioassays for the virus.

Signs of the acute infection in mice continue for 1 or 2 weeks and include decreased growth, rough hair coat, hunched posture, blepharitis, weakness, photophobia, tremors, and convulsions. The terminal stage of the persistent tolerant infection, which occurs over several weeks in 5- to 12-month-old mice, is characterized by weight loss, blepharitis, impaired reproductive performance, and runted litters.

Necropsy Signs

The important necropsy signs are microscopic. Visceral organs, including the liver, kidneys, lungs, pancreas, blood vessels, and meninges, are infiltrated by lymphocytes and there may be moderate to marked necrosis of lymphoid follicles in multiple organs. A glomerulonephritis of probable immune complex origin is a characteristic feature of terminal persistent tolerant infection. Pituitary dwarfism has been produced in newborn mice inoculated with LCMV.

Diagnosis

Except for cases of persistent tolerant infection, infected animals either die or develop circulating antibodies, which can be detected serologically by neutralizing antibody, IFA, or ELISA techniques.

Mouse antibody production (MAP) tests or PCR-based screening tests may be useful in screening suspect tumors and other biologic materials for LCMV.

Because infections are asymptomatic with nonspecific clinical signs, virus isolation and serology are preferred diagnostic procedures.

Prevention

Screening diagnostic tests are methods for monitoring and maintaining an LCMV-free colony. Filter cage covers reduce aerosol transmission, and the exclusion of insect and wild rodent vectors from the colony prevents introduction of the virus. The potential for vertical or transuterine passage of the LCMV complicates eradication.

Public Health Significance

Lymphocytic choriomeningitis may be transmitted from infected animals to humans through direct or indirect contact with feces or urine or with infected murine tissues. LCMV is also transmitted by biting. Humans are typically exposed to the virus when bitten by pets or by contact with contaminated urine (ingestion, inhalation, dermal contact). In immunocompetent individuals, the disease may be asymptomatic or associated with mild flu-like disease; however, fatalities have been reported in immunocompromised individuals following exposure. The bacterium has been transmitted by subclinically infected donors to human organ recipients with fatal consequences. Care must be taken in handling, bleeding, or processing tissues from suspect infected animals.

References

Armstrong D, et al. Meningitis due to lymphocytic choriomeningitis virus endemic in a hamster colony. J Am Med Assoc. 1969, 209:265–267.

Baum SC, et al. Epidemic nonmeningitic lymphocytic choriomeningitis virus infection: an outbreak in a population of laboratory personnel. N Eng J Med. 1966, 274:934–936.

Bhatt PN, et al. Contamination of transplantable murine tumors with LCMV. Lab Anim Sci. 1986, 36:136–139.

Biggar RJ, et al. Lymphocytic choriomeningitis outbreak associated with pet hamsters: fifty-seven cases from New York state. J Am Med Assoc. 1975, 232:494–500.

Bowen GS, et al. Laboratory studies of a lymphocytic choriomeningitis virus outbreak in man and laboratory animals. Am J Epidemiol. 1975, 102:233–240.

Deibel R, et al. Lymphocytic choriomeningitis virus in man. Serologic evidence of association with pet hamsters. J Am Med Assoc. 1975, 232:501–504.

De Souza M, Smith AL. Comparison of isolation in cell culture with conventional and modified mouse antibody production tests for detection of murine viruses. J Clin Microbiol. 1989, 27:185–187.

Hirsch MS, et al. Lymphocytic choriomeningitis virus infection traced to a pet hamster. N Engl J Med. 1974, 291:610–612.

Hotchin, J. The contamination of laboratory animals with lymphocytic choriomeningitis virus. Am J Pathol. 1971, 64:747–769.

Hotchin J, et al. Lymphocytic choriomeningitis in a hamster colony causes infection of hospital personnel. Science. 1974, 135:1173–1174.

Ike F, et al. Lymphocytic choriomeningitis infection undetected by dirty-bedding sentinel monitoring and revealed after embryo transfer of an inbred strain derived from wild mice. Comp Med. 2007, 57:272–281.

Ivanov AP, Bashkirtsev VN, Tkachenko EA. Enzyme-linked immunosorbent assay for detection of arenaviruses. Arch Virol. 1981, 67:71–74.

Lymphocytic Choriomeningitis Virus Infection in Organ Transplant Recipients—Massachusetts, Rhode Island, 2005. MMWR. May 26, 2005/54(Dispatch); 1–2.

Parker JC, et al. Lymphocytic choriomeningitis virus infection in fetal, newborn, and young adult Syrian hamsters (Mesocricetus auratus). Infect Immun. 1976, 13:967–981.

Rodriguez M, et al. Pituitary dwarfism in mice persistently infected with LCMV. Lab Invest. 1983, 49:48–53.

Saron MF, et al. Lymphocytic choriomeningitis virus-induced immunodepression; inherent defect of B and T lymphocytes. J Virol. 1990, 65:4076–4083.

Skinner HH, Knight EH. The potential role of Syrian hamsters and other small animals as reservoirs of lymphocytic choriomeningitis virus. J Small Anim Pract. 1979, 20:145–161.

MALOCCLUSION AND DENTAL DISEASE

Hosts

Dental disease is very common in small mammal pets. Malocclusion is seen commonly in the incisors of rabbits (mandibular prognathism) and the premolar and molar teeth (cheek teeth) of guinea pigs, while crown elongation is seen frequently in chinchillas. Overgrowth of incisors is occasionally seen in rats, mice, hamsters, and gerbils.

Etiology and Predisposing Factors

Both rabbits and rodents are monophyodont, with one set of dentition throughout life. The incisors of rabbits and rodents grow throughout life, as well as the cheek teeth of chinchillas, guinea pigs, and rabbits. For both rabbits and rodents, the incisors grow at a rapid rate of approximately 55–100 mm per year. Malocclusion and tooth overgrowth result when, for genetic, dietary, infectious (abscesses), or traumatic reasons, open-rooted teeth do not occlude properly and therefore do not wear normally. Loss or malalignment of all or part of a tooth usually leads to overgrowth of the opposing tooth. Teeth that are dead because of infected roots are usually discolored.

In the rabbit, incisor overgrowth can create a condition known as "buck teeth." The underlying cause of this malocclusion in the rabbit is an autosomal recessive trait that results in an abnormally short skull, in the region of the maxillary diastema, relative to the length of the normal longer mandible. Incisor overgrowth is more common in the dwarf breeds.

Overgrowth of the open-rooted cheek teeth is the most common dental problem of pet rabbits and is likely indicative of dietary mismanagement in pet settings. Commercial diets, although convenient to feed, do not promote normal chewing patterns seen with less energy-dense grasses consumed by wild rabbits.

Malocclusion in guinea pigs is most pronounced in the most rostral cheek teeth (Figure 5.11). The condition is difficult to detect because of the abundance of loose skin in the edentulous diastema. The condition may be linked to a history of intermittent periods of poor nutrition, for example, vitamin C deficiency, or it may have a genetic basis, which can result in narrowing of the gap between mandibles. In guinea pigs, the lower cheek teeth overgrow in a lingual direction, which in part pins the tongue to the floor of the mouth and results in difficulty in prehension and deglutition. The upper cheek teeth overgrow laterally and sharp points that develop on these teeth will lacerate the buccal mucosa.

Parvovirus infections may cause epidemic incisor loss with high mortality in suckling and weanling hamsters.

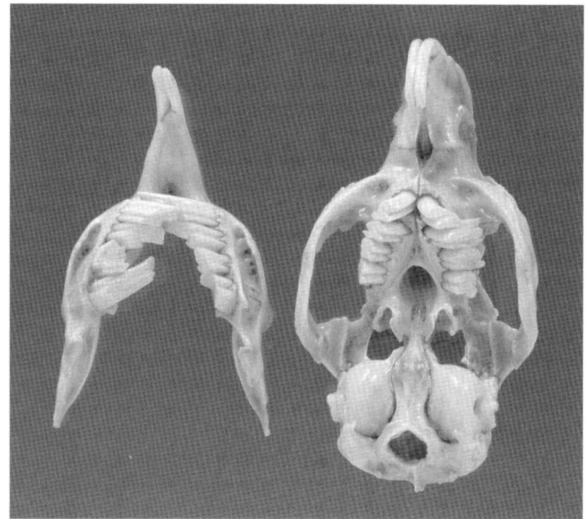

FIGURE 5.11. Skull from a guinea pig that had presented with anorexia. There is overgrowth of the upper and lower incisors as well as the cheek teeth. Overgrowth of the lower cheek teeth had resulted in tongue entrapment.

Clinical Signs

Overgrown teeth result in trauma to the inner cheeks, tongue, and mouth, which may cause dysphagia, ptyalism (slobbering), blood in the cage, anorexia, weight loss, starvation, and eventually death. The drooling around the mouth and onto the forequarters predisposes to moist dermatitis. Malocclusion is a common cause of chronic weight loss in rabbits and rodents, especially guinea pigs and chinchillas. For this reason, inspection of the mouth is an essential component of the physical examination.

The small gape makes it difficult to perform a thorough evaluation of the teeth, and insertion of a speculum can be stressful, especially in guinea pigs. The most rostral cheek teeth in guinea pigs can be assessed for overgrowth by inserting the pinky finger into the diastema, pressing it firmly onto the teeth, withdrawing the finger, and examining the width between the depressions made in the skin. Anesthesia is usually required for a complete evaluation, and sharp points and lingual and buccal lacerations must be actively sought. The close apposition of the cheeks to the upper arcades precludes visual inspection in all but the largest rabbits; however, a wooden applicator stick can be used to check for laterally growing points by inserting it horizontally between the teeth and the cheek and sliding it ventrally. If the stick moves freely, points are unlikely; however, if the stick gets caught, points may be present.

Treatment

Dental equipment designed specifically for rabbits and rodents, such as molar cutters, rasps, speculums, and cheek dilators, is readily available from veterinary suppliers. Use of nail trimmers, side-cutters, or other types of clippers is not appropriate as they may crack or split the teeth longitudinally, leading to pulp exposure, pain, and abscessation.

Recognition of the normal length and appearance of rabbit and rodent incisors is critical to avoid unnecessary trimming, which could harm the animal. In particular, the lower incisors of guinea pigs and hamsters often appear overgrown to the uninitiated. In addition, the intermandibular joint of hamsters, rats, and mice is somewhat flexible and allows the lower incisors to mildly splay apart, which should not be misinterpreted as a fracture. Treatment of incisor overgrowth involves repeated filing or use of a dental burr in a low-speed dental handpiece. In very severe cases, extraction of all the incisors may be necessary to preclude retrimming visits every 4–6 weeks.

Access to the cheek teeth is more difficult and animals must be anesthetized and care taken to guard against trauma to the cheeks, gums, and tongue while performing dental work. Use of an appropriately sized speculum and cheek dilators can greatly assist in the examination. An adjustable table-top dental positioner for rabbits has recently become available, which greatly facilitates examination and access. An otoscope or nasal speculum with light source and a narrow tongue depressor may also be helpful. Cheek tooth elongation can be corrected by using molar cutters, rasps, or a flat fissure burr in conjunction with visualizing the amount of tooth that can be removed with a lateral radiograph. This procedure may need to be repeated at 4- to 8-week intervals. The animals should be gradually switched over to a more natural diet that includes more grass hay and less pelleted feed in the intervening time. In chronically affected animals, revisits at 6- to 8-week intervals may be required for cheek tooth reductions for the rest of the animal's life.

Cheek tooth extraction may be necessary in cases of tooth root abscesses. It is important to protect the empty sockets to prevent impaction of food debris with subsequent abscessation. Commercially available gel preparations are available for this purpose. Maxillary tooth extraction is often very traumatic for the rabbit and carries a guarded prognosis. It is critical to remember that removal of a cheek tooth creates a malocclusion in the opposing tooth that will require regular attention throughout the animal's life.

Prevention

Animals with malocclusion should not be used for breeding. Because of the long narrow mouth and fleshy tongue of these species, adequate visualization of the teeth is difficult, even with cheek dilators in a heavily sedated animal. Radiographs should be considered a necessary and routine diagnostic procedure whenever dental problems are suspected, to ensure adequate visualization of all bony structures.

References

Capello V. Diagnosis and treatment of dental disease in pet rodents. J Exot Pet Med. 2008, 17(2):114–123.

Crossley DA. Dental disease in chinchillas in the UK. J Small Anim Pract. 2001, 42(1):12–19.

———. Oral biology and disorders of lagomorphs. Vet Clin Exot Anim. 2003, 6:629–659.

Crossley DA, Miguélez MM. Skull size and cheek-tooth length in wild-caught and captive-bred chinchillas. Arch Oral Biol. 2001, 46(10):919–928.

Fox RR, Gary DD. Mandibular prognathism in the rabbit: genetic studies. J Hered. 1971, 62:23–27.

Gibson SV, Rottinghaus AA, Wagner JE. Mortality in weanling hamsters associated with tooth loss. Lab Anim Sci. 1983, 33:497.

Gracis M. Clinical technique: normal dental radiography of rabbits, guinea pigs and chinchillas. J Exot Pet Med. 2008, 17:78–86.

Harcourt-Brown FM. The progressive syndrome of acquired dental disease in rabbits. J Exot Pet Med. 2007, 16(3):146–157.

Huang CM, Mi MP, Vogt DW. Mandibular prognathism in the rabbit: discrimination between single-focus and multifactorial models of inheritance. J Hered. 1981, 72:296–298.

Jekl V, Hauptman K, Knotek Z. Quantitative and qualitative assessments of intraoral lesions in 180 small herbivorous mammals. Vet Rec. 2008, 162(14):442–449.

Legendre LFJ. Oral disorders of exotic rodents. Vet Clin Exot Anim. 2003, 6:601–628.

Lennox AM. Diagnosis and treatment of dental disease in pet rabbits. J Exot Pet Med. 2008, 17(2):107–113.

Reiter AM. Pathophysiology of dental disease in the rabbit, guinea pig, and chinchilla. J Exot Pet Med. 2008, 17(2):70–77.

Rest JR, Richards T, Ball SE. Malocclusion in inbred strain-2 weanling guinea pigs. Lab Anim. 1982, 16:84–87.

MASTITIS

Hosts

Guinea pigs, rabbits, rats, and hamsters are affected most commonly.

Etiology

Acute inflammation of the mammary gland is most often encountered during lactation, when milk provides an excellent medium for bacterial growth, the glands are pendulous and easily injured, and the young traumatize the teats. Mastitis is established when one or several genera of microorganisms (*Pasteurella* spp, *Klebsiella* spp, coliform bacilli, *Streptococcus* spp, *Staphylococcus* spp, or *Pseudomonas* spp) enter the gland via the bloodstream, through a cutaneous lesion, or via the teat canal.

Predisposing Factors and Clinical Signs

An unsanitary environment, abrasive bedding, inappropriate caging, biting young, and mammary impaction after early weaning or death of neonates predisposes the dam to mastitis. The affected glands become diffusely or focally enlarged, firm, hyperemic, warm, and cyanotic. One or more glands may be affected and glands may dribble purulent material. Depression and death from septicemia or toxemia often follow.

Among pet and laboratory rabbits and rodents, guinea pigs are most often affected with mastitis. Causative agents are usually an alpha-hemolytic *Streptococcus* spp or *Escherichia coli*, although *Klebsiella* spp and *Staphylococcus* spp may also be involved. In acute cases, the affected gland is red-purple, and the milk may appear bloody. Maternal neglect of sucklings and death of the sow usually occur within hours to days. A chronic, suppurative mastitis may occur also.

Rabbit mastitis may be diffuse or focal and suppurative. When it is diffuse, the lesion is known as "blue breasts" or "caked udder." Affected rabbits are usually lactating and *Staphylococcus* spp, *Pasteurella* spp, or *Streptococcus* spp are generally the causative agents. Clinical signs include fever that exceeds 40 °C (104 °F), anorexia, depression, death of neonates, and death of the doe from septicemia.

In rats, small isolated mammary gland abscesses are more common than acute diffuse mastitis. *Pasteurella pneumotropica* and *S. aureus* are often cultured.

A case of mastitis was reported in an 11-month-old hamster due to a galactogenic *E. coli* infection. Incisors from suckling pups were believed to be the source of trauma. Clinical signs included firm discrete subcutaneous nodules.

Treatment and Prevention

Treatment of an acute infection in rabbits includes lancing and flushing the abscesses, if present, and administration of antibiotics. All glands should be examined carefully for signs of infection. Trimethoprim-sulfa, chloramphenicol, or enrofloxacin may be useful antibiotics for treating mastitis in small rodents. The infected animal's environment should be disinfected.

References

Frisk CS, Wagner JE, Owens DR. Streptococcal mastitis in golden hamsters. Lab Anim Sci. 1976, 26:97.

Gupta BN, Langham RF, Conner GH. Endotoxin-induced mastitis in the guinea pig. Amer J Vet Res. 1971, 32:1785–1793.

———. Mastitis in guinea pigs. Amer J Vet Res. 1970, 31:1703–1707.

Hong CC, Ediger RD. Chronic necrotizing mastitis in rats caused by Pasteurella pneumotropica. Lab Anim Sci. 1978, 28:317–320.

Huerkamp MJ, Dillehay DL. Coliform mastitis in a golden Syrian hamster. Lab Anim Sci. 1990, 40:325–327.

Kinder RJ, Jr, et al. Bacterial mastitis in guinea pigs. Lab Anim Sci. 1976, 26:214–217.

MOUSEPOX (ECTROMELIA VIRUS)

Hosts

The mouse is the only natural host of ectromelia virus, which causes mousepox in many countries worldwide. The term ectromelia refers to an absence or shortening of a limb. Experimental infection of other laboratory rodent species with this virus results in a brief, noncontagious infection with antibody production. Epizootic mousepox has occurred in many areas of the world for decades. This highly infectious and potentially devastating disease occurs as sporadic outbreaks in North America, generally associated with using contaminated biologics in susceptible mouse strains. Clinically, the disease is most severe among certain inbred strains, especially BALB/c, DBA, CBA, C3H, and A. C57BL/6 strains are resistant, and infections are frequently inapparent.

Etiology

Ectromelia virus is a large (175 × 290 nm), oval to brick-shaped, cytoplasmic, double-stranded DNA orthopoxvirus, with a characteristic dumbbell-shaped nucleus. It is classified in the family Poxviridae, Vaccinia subgroup, and is similar to vaccinia and variola in many ways.

Transmission

The virus is stable in dry environments. The probable transmission routes are respiratory aerosol, biting and skin abrasions, contact with skin debris, excretions from the oropharynx and genital tracts, cannibalism, and ingestion of contaminated feces. The virus is excreted from the intestinal tract for long periods after infection.

Urine, ectoparasites, other animals, humans, fomites, and infected tissues or biologics may disseminate the virus. Approximately 10 days after infection, characteristic skin lesions develop, and virus is shed into the environment. The virus is spread from cage to cage by animal handlers and among institutions by investigators who exchange infected mice or mouse tissues, for example, tumors, cell lines, hybridoma lines, and sera. The virus in these products may remain viable in ultracold freezers for decades.

Predisposing Factors

Different mouse strains vary in susceptibility to ectromelia virus, although such differences have been determined on the basis of a few outbreaks. In recent outbreaks high mortality was observed among BALB/c, DBA, A, and CBA mice. Mice of these strains tended to die suddenly with few or no skin lesions. C3H mice were susceptible, but death was delayed, and skin lesions developed frequently. C57BL/6 and black congenic strains of mice were resistant.

Clinical Signs

Mousepox infections may be asymptomatic, latent, acute, subacute, or chronic. Clinical signs vary widely, and the nature of clinical disease expressed is dependent largely on mouse genotype.

The acute, systemic form of infectious mousepox with high morbidity and mortality occurs in epizootic outbreaks in susceptible strains. Clinical signs of acute mousepox include hunched posture, rough hair coat, conjunctivitis, swelling of the face or extremities, diarrhea, and high mortality. The cutaneous rash, an important source of virus dissemination, is seen seldomly in acute outbreaks.

The subacute to chronic, enzootic, or cutaneous forms involve a generalized papular rash with eventual swelling, ulceration, and amputation of appendages and variable mortality. The cutaneous lesions of mousepox may resemble those associated with mite allergies, *Corynebacterium* spp arthritis infections, and bite wounds.

Necropsy Signs

The gross lesions associated with acute mousepox are hyperemia and edema of the viscera, enlarged Peyer's patches, lymphoid hyperplasia, splenomegaly, a peritoneal exudate, and, as the disease progresses, hemorrhage into the intestinal lumen and focal necrosis of the spleen, liver, pancreas, lymph nodes, thymus, and other organs.

In the subacute to chronic forms, focal necrosis becomes more extensive; the vesicular, cutaneous pox lesions become crusted; and swelling and necrosis of the extremities occur. Scars in the spleen are pathognomonic for prior ectromelia virus infection.

Histopathologic changes are characterized by massive splenic necrosis that originates in the lymphoid follicles and spreads throughout the organ. Hepatic necrosis often involves a large portion of the liver. Necrosis of Peyer's patches, lymph nodes, and thymus resembles microscopic changes seen in the spleen. Characteristic eosinophilic, type A, cytoplasmic inclusions can be found in infected epithelial cells early in the rash at sites of focal epidermal hyperplasia and erosion. Infected hepatocytes adjacent to areas of hepatic necrosis contain basophilic, type B, intracytoplasmic inclusion bodies.

Diagnosis

Mousepox is diagnosed by clinical and gross necropsy signs and by the demonstration of intracytoplasmic, eosinophilic inclusion bodies (Marechal bodies) in the epithelial cells of the skin, small intestine, and pancreas. When inapparent infections are suspected, susceptible, disease-free mice can be introduced into the colony as sentinel animals.

Finding splenic and hepatic necrosis and other typical lesions allows a diagnosis of acute mousepox. Confirmation is achieved through electron microscopy of affected organs, which reveals characteristic poxviruses. Caution is necessary because vaccination with live vaccinia virus may introduce viruses with the same morphologic characteristics as the natural infection. The virus can be isolated from the spleen and liver during early stages of disease by culture on mouse fibroblasts (L929), Vero, or HeLa cells, and it grows well on the chorioallantoic membrane of hen's eggs. Virus can be demonstrated in tissues by immunocytochemical methods, for example, fluorescent antibody.

Serologic testing is useful for screening suspect colonies and for detecting latent infections. Possible prior vaccination is a consideration in interpretation of serologic results. The IHD-T strain of vaccinia virus is used commonly in vaccination outside of North America; however, no hemagglutination-inhibiting antibody is produced, and the HAI test can be used for screening vaccinated colonies. Vaccination interferes with the more sensitive ELISA and IFA tests. The ELISA test or PCR is more sensitive and is used commonly as the primary serologic test. The IFA test is highly sensitive and specific and is used as a secondary or confirmatory procedure.

Treatment

A satisfactory treatment does not exist for infectious mousepox. Vaccination using a live IHD-T strain of vaccinia virus cultured in egg embryos may be used to limit outbreaks in small closed colonies; however, elimination of affected colonies is preferred to preclude the possibility of establishing an enzootic disease.

Prevention

Selection of ectromelia-free stock, careful husbandry and quarantine measures, serologic screening tests, and the use of disease-free, susceptible, sentinel mice are measures used to prevent latent carriers from entering the colony. Particular care should be taken with inbred and congenic strains from sources where mousepox has been enzootic. Imported mice or mouse tissues, mice from unknown sources, or suspect mice should be strictly quarantined. Mouse tissue destined for transmission to susceptible mice should be checked for ectromelia virus by passage through susceptible hosts or tested via MAP or PCR assays. Infected colonies must be eliminated, and rooms and equipment sanitized and disinfected thoroughly because the virus remains viable in dry environments. Several disinfectants are effective: vapor phase formaldehyde, iodophores (150–300 ppm), and sodium hypochlorite (1,000 ppm available chlorine). Dead animals, animal wastes, and contaminated bedding should be isolated and incinerated. Movement into and out of suspect colonies should be limited strictly. Intrauterine infections with ectromelia virus limit the effectiveness of hysterectomy derivation to eliminate the infection.

Susceptible mice may be vaccinated with the IHD-T strain, which does not produce HAI antibodies and does not interfere with subsequent HAI serologic testing. The vaccine is given by scarification at the tail base. If a vaccination "take" (lesion at scarification site) is not obvious, a latent carrier or immune state should be suspected. Successive passage of tumor lines through at least two vaccinated mice results in loss of ectromelia virus from that tumor line.

Public Health Significance

Humans are not susceptible to infection by the ectromelia virus.

References

Allen AM, et al. Pathology and diagnosis of mousepox. Lab Anim Sci. 1981, 31:599–608.

Bhatt PN, et al. Transmission of mousepox in genetically resistant or susceptible mice. Lab Anim Sci. 1985, 35:523–524.

Bhatt PN, Jacoby RO. Effect of vaccination on the clinical response, pathogenesis and transmission of mousepox. Lab Anim Sci. 1987, 37:610–614.
———. Mousepox in inbred mice innately resistant or susceptible to lethal infection with ectromelia virus. I. Clinical responses. Lab Anim Sci. 1987, 37:11–15.
———. Mousepox in inbred mice innately resistant or susceptible to lethal infection with ectromelia virus. III. Experimental transmission of infection and derivation of virus-free progeny from previously infected dams. Lab Anim Sci. 1987, 37:23–27.
Buller RML, Wallace GD. Reexamination of the efficacy of vaccination against mousepox. Lab Anim Sci. 1985, 35:473–476.
Dick EJ, Jr, Kittell CL, Meyer H, et al. Mousepox outbreak in a laboratory mouse colony. Lab Anim Sci. 1996, 46(6):602–611.
Esteban DJ, Buller RM. Ectromelia virus: the causative agent of mousepox. J Gen Virol. 2005, 86(Pt 10): 2645–2659.
Fenner F. Mousepox (infectious ectromelia): past, present, and future. Lab Anim Sci. 1981, 31:553–559.
———. Wallace P. Rowe lecture. Poxviruses of laboratory animals. Lab Anim Sci. 1990, 40(5):469–480.
Jacoby RO, Bhatt PN. Mousepox in inbred mice innately resistant or susceptible to lethal infection with ectromelia virus. II. Pathogenesis. Lab Anim Sci. 1987, 37:16–22.
Lipman NS, Nguyen H, Perkins S. Mousepox: a threat to U.S. mouse colonies. Lab Anim Sci. 1999, 49(3):229.
Lipman NS, Perkins S, Nguyen H, Pfeffer M, Meyer H. Mousepox resulting from use of ectromelia virus-contaminated, imported mouse serum. Comp Med. 2000, 50(4):426–435.
Wallace GD, Buller RML. Kinetics of ectromelia virus (mousepox) transmission and clinical response in C57BL/6J, BALB/cByJ and AKR/J inbred mice. Lab Anim Sci. 1985, 35:41–46.
Wallace GD, Buller RML, Morse HC. Genetic determinants of resistance to ectromelia (mousepox) virus-induced mortality. J Virol. 1985, 55:890–891.

MURINE ENCEPHALOMYELITIS

Hosts

Laboratory mice and rats are the natural hosts of generally asymptomatic infections with Theiler's murine encephalomyelitis viruses (TMEVs). The disease is sometimes referred to as mouse polio. Wild mice may be a source of infection. Laboratory rats, Syrian hamsters, and infant cotton rats can be infected experimentally with the mouse strains. Rats also have their own distinct strains of theilovirus (RTV) and commonly demonstrate weak cross-reactive titers to mouse GDVII virus in routine ELISA serodiagnostic testing. No lesions have been reported in rats.

Etiology

Strains of the TMEV picornaviruses (RNA) vary in their virulence for mice. GDVII and FA, both highly neurovirulent strains, and Theiler's original (TO) are among the more widely studied and reported strains. There may be differential strain susceptibility to viral infection in mice and rats, and sentinels should be selected carefully if this agent is to be detected. For example, a recent study suggested that SD rats are more susceptible to RTV infection with longer periods of viral shedding than CD rats. Similar strain-related differences in susceptibility are noted in mice. BALB/c and C57BL/6 mice tend to be resistant, whereas DBA/2, SJL, SWR, and CD-1 outbred mice are more susceptible.

The TMEV viruses should not be confused with the encephalomyocarditis viruses, which are picornaviruses with a predilection to cause heart damage.

Transmission

Spread of the infection is exclusively by the fecal-oral route because most strains of the virus that infect mice naturally replicate in the intestine. In colonies that are infected enzootically, mice become infected around the time of weaning, at approximately 3 weeks of age. In infected colonies, mice normally develop immunity and only a small percentage (e.g., <1%) may develop clinical disease. In the typical disease, affected mice develop flaccid posterior paralysis with or without convulsions. Severity of CNS signs is viral strain, host age, and genotype dependent. Unlike the transient intestinal infection, the virus in the CNS form of the disease may persist in the brain and spinal cord for the life of the mouse.

Clinical Signs

Infections with wild-type strains of TMEV and RTV are usually subclinical; however, small numbers of mice may develop an extended viremia with dissemination of the virus to the spinal cord and brain, causing paralysis of the rear legs (rarely), circling, rolling, and other signs of CNS disease. There is little or no mortality. Signs of CNS disease in mice are by no means pathognomonic of mouse polio, and CNS signs in mice may be associated with disease processes other than mouse polio.

Necropsy Signs

In mice with CNS signs, there is nonsuppurative meningoencephalitis and myelitis with selective involvement of the gray matter. In SCID mice, marked vacuolation of neurons and glial cells in the cerebrospinal axis is a feature of the disease.

Diagnosis

Clinical signs are of limited value due to their low prevalence. Diagnosis is based usually on serologic testing using either ELISA or IFA tests. Viral isolation, microscopic immune-related lesions of poliomyelitis, and demyelination in the CNS are useful also in establishing a diagnosis. Infection may resemble polio of humans.

Infected mice are an important model of polio in humans; therefore, this disease of mice has been studied extensively. Much of the credit for the current success in controlling human polio worldwide can be attributed to continuing research using laboratory mice in polio research.

Control and Prevention

Use of barrier conditions and mice proven free of mouse polio by serologic testing are the methods used most commonly to prevent introduction of the disease into viral-free mouse colonies. Hysterectomy and rederivation are effective means of eliminating the infection.

Public Health Significance

A number of TMEVs have recently been isolated from human clinical cases, one of which was a child with severe respiratory disease. The relationship to rodent exposure is unknown.

References

Brownstein D, et al. Duration, patterns of transmission of Theiler's mouse encephalomyelitis virus infection. Lab Anim Sci. 1989, 39:299–301.

Chiu CY, Greninger AL, Kanada K, et al. Identification of cardioviruses related to Theiler's murine encephalomyelitis virus in human infections. Proc Natl Acad Sci USA. 2008, 105(37):14124–14129.

Drake MT, Riley LK, Livingston RS. Differential susceptibility of SD and CD rats to a novel rat theilovirus. Comp Med. 2008, 58(5):458–464.

Easterbrook JD, Kaplan JB, Glass GE, et al. A survey of rodent-borne pathogens carried by wild-caught Norway rats: a potential threat to laboratory rodent colonies. Lab Anim. 2008, 42(1):92–98.

Gomez RM, et al. Theiler's mouse encephalomyelitis virus-induced cardiac and skeletal muscle disease. J Virol. 1996, 70:8926–8933.

Lindsey MD, Rodriguez M. Characterization of the inflammatory response in the central nervous system of mice susceptible or resistant to demyelination by Theiler's virus. J Immunol. 1989, 142:2677–2682.

Lipman NS, Newcomer CE, Fox JD. Rederivation of MHV and MEV antibody positive mice by cross-fostering and use of a microisolator caging system. Lab Anim Sci. 1987, 37:195–199.

Melvold RW, et al. Variations in genetic control of susceptibility to Theiler's murine encephalomyelitis virus (TMEV)-induced demyelinating disease. I. Differences between susceptible SJL/J and resistant BALB/c strains map near the T cell beta chain constant gene on chromosome 6. J Immunol. 1987, 138:1429–1433.

Ohsawa K, Watanabe Y, Miyata H, Sato H. Genetic analysis of a Theiler-like virus isolated from rats. Comp Med. 2003, 53(2):191–196.

Pritchett-Corning KR, Cosentino J, Clifford CB. Contemporary prevalence of infectious agents in laboratory mice and rats. Lab Anim. 2008, 165–173.

Rodrigues DM, Martins SS, Gilioli R, et al. Theiler's murine encephalomyelitis virus in nonbarrier rat colonies. Comp Med. 2005, 55(5):459–464.

Rozengurt N, Sanchez S. A spontaneous outbreak of Theiler's encephalomyelitis in a colony of severe combined immunodeficient mice in the UK. Lab Anim. 1993, 27:229–234.

MURINE MYCOPLASMOSIS

Hosts

Rats and mice are the principal natural hosts of respiratory and genital infections caused by *Mycoplasma pulmonis*. Infection and disease are common in pets, nonbarrier-housed rats and mice, and wild rodents.

Rabbits, guinea pigs, and other rodents may on occasion carry the organism, but they are generally not affected clinically.

Etiology

Mycoplasmas are very small pleomorphic organisms with no distinctive cell wall. They are bounded by a triple-layered membrane. They vary from ovoid to filamentous forms. *Mycoplasma pulmonis*, which may accompany viral or bacterial infections, is an extracellular pathogen that colonizes mucosal surfaces and is responsible for the clinical signs and lesions of murine mycoplasmosis. Bacteria that may accompany *M. pulmonis* in respiratory disease include *Pasteurella pneumotropica*, *Actinobacillus* spp, *Streptococcus pneumoniae*, *Bordetella bronchiseptica*, CARB, and *Corynebacterium kutscheri*.

Mycoplasma arthritidis, though usually causing inapparent infections of rats and mice, may cause polyarthritis in rats with swelling of joints and toes.

Transmission

Mycoplasma pulmonis is carried in the upper respiratory tract. Transmission of contagious mycoplasmal infections is by direct contact between mother and young, respiratory aerosol over short distances, sexual transfer, exposure to animal carriers, and in utero passage.

Predisposing Factors

Agents that damage the protective capacity of the respiratory epithelium predispose to *M. pulmonis* infection. Such agents include ammonia, sulfur dioxide, Sendai virus, and other bacterial infections. Ammonia gas in an animal colony is generated from urine and feces by urease-positive bacteria. Factors that are involved in ammonia accumulation include poor ventilation and sanitation, cage crowding, bacterial growth, and room overheating. The metaplastic and ciliary inhibiting effects of ammonia can extend an innocuous upper respiratory infection into a bronchopneumonia.

Clinical Signs

Although *M. pulmonis* infections are usually subclinical, at least to the casual observer, clinical signs occur and represent three major foci of infection: upper respiratory tract, lower respiratory tract, and urogenital tract. In all areas, the clinical onset is usually slow and progressive, but acute episodes may occur in young and susceptible animals.

The upper respiratory disease, involving the nasal passages and middle ears, is signaled by sniffling, occasional squinting, rough hair coat, and sneezing. If the inner ear becomes involved, torticollis or head tilt may occur.

Lower respiratory disease is initiated or exacerbated by ammonia gas, bacterial infections, or Sendai virus infection, and is characterized by lethargy, rough hair coat, hunched posture, chattering, weight loss, labored breathing, and eventually death. Porphyrin may accumulate around the eyes and external nares. Unless the respiratory infections are complicated by a bacterial infection, the terminal clinical stages of mycoplasmosis may last weeks or months. Geriatric pet rats commonly develop this form of the disease.

In the ascending genital infection, which is common, infertility, embryonic resorptions, and small litters occur.

Necropsy Signs

Upper respiratory infection is characterized by serous to purulent inflammation in affected tissues. In murine mycoplasmosis, unilateral or bilateral otitis media is a common finding, often the only gross abnormality. The pulmonary lesions in the early stages of the disease are well-demarcated foci of firm red or gray atelectasis and consolidation. As the disease progresses, inflammatory debris accumulates in the air passages, resulting in bulging, mucopurulent areas of bronchiectasis that give the lung a "cobblestone" appearance. The content of these lumps is pyogranulomatous and yellow-gray.

Microscopic lesions may be acute or chronic and begin with neutrophils in airways, hyperplasia of mucosal epithelium, and lymphoid proliferation in the submucosa of the bronchi and progress to bronchiolar invasion, consolidation, bronchiectasis, and pulmonary abscesses.

The genital infection, which may exist independently of the respiratory infection, is an ascending process that may involve the entire reproductive tract. Older females are more often affected. Metritis, pyometra, and purulent oophoritis and salpingitis characterize the serious genital infection.

Diagnosis

Diagnosis of murine mycoplasmosis is based on clinical signs and can be made presumptively based upon serologic tests (ELISA, MFI). Definitive diagnosis is based upon gross and microscopic lesions and on the cultural isolation of *M. pulmonis* from the nasal pharynx, tympanic bullae, trachea, uterus, or lungs. The organism may be carried in the upper respiratory passages in the absence of clinical disease. Culture of *M. pulmonis* requires special media enriched with yeast extract and 10% swine or horse serum. The plates are incubated at 37 °C in an atmosphere of normal or reduced oxygen and increased humidity.

CARB may produce lesions that resemble those associated with respiratory mycoplasmosis. A distinguishing feature is that large numbers of CARB can be found among cilia in the ciliated respiratory epithelium of the nasal passages, trachea, and other airways in silver-stained sections. An ELISA test can be used to detect serum antibody to CARB.

Treatment

Elimination of mycoplasmal infections in large populations of rats and mice is, for all practical purposes, impossible without rederivation. Antimicrobials placed in the drinking water may have a palliative effect, suppressing clinical signs. Tetracycline hydrochloride at 5 mg/mL given fresh daily for 5 days or longer in deionized drinking water may suppress clinical signs if rats drink the concentrated solution. Others have suggested that adding tetracycline to the drinking water is ineffective in controlling infectious disease and may, in fact, be detrimental in other ways. Some tetracycline solutions at this concentration in tap water form a scale that blocks the sipper tube. Use of distilled water reduces this effect. Lower levels of tetracycline may have an effect to reduce secondary bacterial complications. In vitro, tetracycline and tylosin have been more effective against *M. pulmonis* than are tiamulin, spectinomycin, lincomycin, and gentamicin. Enrofloxacin at 5–10 mg/kg every 12 hr IM, SC, or PO combined with doxycycline hyclate, 5 mg/kg PO every 12 hours, for 5–10 days may suppress clinical signs.

Sulfamethamazine at 0.02% in the drinking water or 1 mg/4 g feed, tylosin at 66 mg/L (2.5 g/10 gal) for 21 days, and chloramphenicol at 30 mg/kg body weight for 5 days are other treatment suggestions, but the prognosis for recovery remains poor, and treatment should not be advocated as a method to eliminate *Mycoplasma* spp from a colony.

Prevention

Prevention of murine mycoplasmosis involves placing rodents free of *M. pulmonis* into a barrier facility. Strict husbandry standards, exclusion of wild rodents, serologic and postmortem monitoring, good ventilation, and low population densities in the cage and room help to maintain a colony free of *M. pulmonis*.

Public Health Significance

Mycoplasma pulmonis has recently been detected, isolated, and sequenced in animal facility workers exposed to infected rats. The mode of transmission is unknown.

References

Aguila HN, et al. Experimental Mycoplasma pulmonis infection of rats suppresses humoral but not cellular immune response. Lab Anim Sci. 1988, 38:138–142.

Banerjee AK, et al. Naturally occurring genital mycoplasmosis in mice. Lab Anim. 1985, 19:275–276.

Broderson JR, Lindsey JR, Crawford JE. The role of environmental ammonia in respiratory mycoplasmosis of rats. Am J Pathol. 1976, 35:115–130.

Carter KK, et al. Tylosin concentrations in rat serum and lung tissue after administration in drinking water. Lab Anim Sci. 1987, 37:468–470.

Donnelly TM. Disease Problems of Small Rodents. In: Ferrets, Rabbits, and Rodents: Clinical Medicine and Surgery, 2nd ed. Quesenberry KE, Carpenter JE (eds.). St. Louis: Saunders, 2004; 299–315.

Easterbrook JD, Kaplan JB, Glass GE, et al. A survey of rodent-borne pathogens carried by wild-caught Norway rats: a potential threat to laboratory rodent colonies. Lab Anim. 2008, 42(1):92–98.

Ferreira JB, Yamaguti M, Marques LM, et al. Detection of Mycoplasma pulmonis in laboratory rats and technicians. Zoonoses Public Health. 2008, 55(5):229–234.

Ganaway JR, et al. Isolation, propagation, and characterization of a newly recognized pathogen, cilia-associated respiratory bacillus of rats: an etiological agent of chronic respiratory disease. Infect Immun. 1983, 47:472–479.

Harwick HJ, et al. Arthritis in mice due to infection with Mycoplasma pulmonis. I. Clinical and microbiologic features. J Infect Dis. 1973, 128:533–540.
Lai WC, et al. Mycoplasma pulmonis depresses humoral and cell-mediated responses in mice. Lab Anim Sci. 1989, 39:11–15.
Nichols PW, et al. Pulmonary clearance of Mycoplasma pulmonis in rats with respiratory viral infections or of susceptible genotype. Lab Anim Sci. 1992, 42:454–457.
Pinson DM, et al. Promotion of Mycoplasma pulmonis growth in rat tracheal organ cultures by ammonium chloride. Lab Anim Sci. 1988, 38:143–147.
Porter WP, et al. Absence of therapeutic blood concentrations of tetracycline in rats after administration in drinking water. Lab Anim Sci. 1985, 35:71–75.
Schoeb TR, Davidson MK, Lindsey JR. Intracage ammonia promotes growth of Mycoplasma pulmonis in respiratory tracts of rats. Infect Immun. 1982, 38:212–217.
Seok S, Park J, Cho S, et al. Health surveillance of specific pathogen-free and conventionally-housed mice and rats in Korea. Exp Anim. 2005, 54(1):85–92.
Stunkard JA, Schmidt JP, Cordano JT. Consumption of oxytetracycline in drinking water by healthy mice. Lab Anim Sci. 1971, 21:121–122.
Van Zwieten MJ, et al. Respiratory disease in rats associated with a filamentous bacterium. Lab Anim Sci. 1980, 30:215–221.

MURINE NOROVIRUS INFECTIONS

Host

To date, the only known host for this virus is the mouse.

Etiology

Mouse norovirus is a single-stranded RNA virus within the Caliciviridae family. The virus was first reported in mice in 2003, from a colony of immunodeficient mice (RAG/STAT–/–) experiencing increased mortality. Subsequently, the virus was isolated and characterized as a norovirus, named murine norovirus 1 (MNV-1), and it was thought that a requirement of STAT1-dependent innate immunity had to be present for resistance to the murine norovirus. Mice lacking both interferon α/β and interferon γ receptors are also very susceptible to lethal infection, demonstrating that interferons are needed for resistance to MNV-1. At least six distinct strains have been identified to date. In any regions where viral monitoring has been initiated in recent years, the prevalence of MNV has been high and reported at 30% or greater.

Transmission

The virus is thought to be transmitted by the fecal-oral route. Although autoclaving of materials is also effective, a 1:10 dilution of bleach is the only disinfectant that is currently known to kill the virus. Quaternary ammonium compounds and mild detergents are ineffective. Rederivation is an effective means for exclusion of MNV-1 from susceptible populations. Cross-fostering pups from MNV-positive dams to MNV-negative dams within 3 days of birth is also highly effective at eliminating the virus from infected colonies. The infection is chronic.

Predisposing Conditions

Defects in innate immunity were initially thought to be necessary for viral infection. Mild histologic lesions have been noted in subclinically infected immunocompetent outbred mouse stocks, suggesting that there may be a significant interstrain variability in infection and disease susceptibility.

Clinical and Necropsy Signs

MNV inoculation of RAG/STAT–/– mice, which have defects in both innate and acquired immunity, leads to lesions of encephalitis, cerebral vasculitis, pneumonia, meningitis, and hepatitis. Immunocompetent mice (129 wild-type) seroconvert to MNV-1 capsid protein after oral or intracerebral inoculation but have no clinical signs or tissue pathology. These mice have only a transient infection as evidenced by a lack of viral RNA from tissues by 3 days postinoculation. In mice deficient in T and B lymphocytes, MNV-1 causes persistent infection but no clinical signs.

Histologic lesions (mild, multifocal hepatic necrosis) have been reported in outbred sentinel female mice (Swiss-Webster). In this naturally occurring outbreak, there were no clinical or gross signs in affected mice; however, animals were serologically positive and had histologic lesions consistent with the infection in the liver (cross-reacted with MNV antibodies by IHC).

Diagnosis

The virus can be detected by serology, but this requires careful selection of sentinel animals. CD-1 mice showed poor to no seroconversion at 3 weeks postinfection. Animals maintained on dirty bedding also showed a poor antibody response at 4 weeks postexposure, but this was improved after 5–6 weeks of exposure. These findings point with the need for a longer period of time before detectable antibodies are present in the serum compared with other viruses. PCR can be used to detect MNV-2, -3 and -4 from the spleen, jejunum, and mesenteric lymph nodes at up to 8 weeks postinfection. Jejunum and mesenteric lymph nodes are the best tissues to select. In one study, fecal shedding was still reported for MNV-2, -3 and -4 at week 8 postinfection.

Public Health Signficance

Currently there is no evidence for zoonotic transmission of MNV.

References

Compton SR. Prevention of murine norovirus infection in neonatal mice by fostering. J Amer Assoc Lab Anim Sci. 2008, 47(3):25–30.

Hsu CC, et al. Development of a microsphere-based serologic multiplexed fluorescent immunoassay and a reverse transcriptase PCR assay to detect murine norovirus 1 infection in mice. Clin Diag Lab Immunol. 2005, 12(10):1145–1151.

Hsu CC, Riley LK, Wills HM, et al. Persistent infection with and serologic cross-reactivity of three novel murine noroviruses. Comp Med. 2006, 56(4):247–251.

Karst SM, et al. STAT1-dependent innate immunity to a Norwalk-like virus. Science. 2003, 299:1575–1578.

Kastenmayer RJ, Perdue KA, Elkins WR. Eradication of murine norovirus from a mouse barrier facility. J Amer Assoc Lab Anim Sci. 2008, 47(1):26–30.

Lencioni KC, Seamons A, Treuting PM, et al. Murine norovirus: an intercurrent variable in a mouse model of bacteria-induced inflammatory bowel disease. Comp Med. 2008, 58:522–533.

Manuel CA, Hsu CC, Riley LK, et al. Soiled-bedding sentinel detection of murine norovirus 4. J Amer Assoc Lab Anim Sci. 2008, 47(3):31–36.

Mumphrey SM, Changotra H, Moore TN, et al. Murine norovirus 1 infection is associated with histopathological changes in immunocompetent hosts, but clinical disease is prevented by STAT1-dependent interferon responses. J Virol. 2007, 81(7):3251–3263.

Perdue KA, Green KY, Copeland M, et al. Naturally occurring murine norovirus infection in a large research institution. J Amer Assoc Lab Anim Sci. 2007, 46(4):39–45.

Scipioni A, Mauroy A, Vinjé J, et al. Animal noroviruses. Vet J. 2008, 178(1):32–45.

Ward JM, Wobus CE, Thackray LB, et al. Pathology of immunodeficient mice with naturally occurring murine norovirus infection. Toxicol Pathol. 2006, 34(6):708–715.

Wobus CE, et al. Replication of norovirus in cell culture reveals a tropism for dendritic cells and macrophages. PLoS Biol. 2004, 2(12) e432:2076–2084.

MYIASIS (FLY STRIKE) —PRIMARY

Hosts

Cuterebriasis is a type of primary myiasis, in which the insect requires a specific living host for the larvae to feed on. It occurs primarily in rabbits and rodents housed outdoors or allowed access to the outdoors. Incidental hosts include humans and other animals. At least 10–70% of wild cottontail rabbits (*Sylvilagus* spp) are infected depending on geographic location and season.

Etiology

In North America, cuterebriasis is caused by larvae of bot flies, *Cuterebra* spp, found commonly in lagomorphs and rodents. The three larval stages are pathogenic, whereas the adult, whose short life span is dedicated mainly to breeding, is seen rarely. After hatching, bot fly larvae become buried subcutaneously, each with a breathing pore, after migrating randomly from their point of entry. Not only do the larvae cause lesions in different organs and tissues but they create conditions favorable for secondary bacterial infections and adverse immunologic reactions. In cases wherein larvae wander aberrantly to a sensitive tissue such as the brain, they may cause the death of an animal.

Predisposing Factors

Rabbits that are housed outdoors or allowed to roam freely in yards and fields are more likely to be exposed to bot flies and larvae. Because juvenile mammals tend to be more exploratory in nature and because their immunity is not yet developed fully, they are more likely to acquire cuterebriasis with adverse reactions. Marginal husbandry and management practices, such as neglecting wet, dirty, and diseased animals with gaping wounds or open sores, predispose the animal to attract flies, especially in the summer months.

Transmission

Cuterebra spp are obligate myiasis flies that deposit their ova in nests, logs, and burrows frequented by wild lagomorphs and rodents. The ova hatch into first-stage larvae and wait for susceptible animals to pass by. The larvae then cling to the passing host or are mechanically passed to other contact hosts. The life cycle is complex and occurs primarily in the definitive host.

Clinical Signs

Depending on the number, location, and developmental stages of the parasites, as well as the health and age of the host, the clinical signs of cuterebriasis may vary from inapparent infection to severe toxic shock. The relatively large larvae are generally found in subcutaneous sites on the back or rump area, front shoulder, neck or throat area, and ventral abdomen. Juvenile animals with greater than 9–10 bot flies may succumb with toxic signs. Clinical laboratory tests of infected hosts revealed anemia, alterations of CBC, WBC, and plasma proteins, as well as reduced fertility. Aberrantly migrating larvae have been reported intranasally, intraocularly, intraorally, and intracranially, where they may cause severe CNS signs that should be differentiated from the clinical signs of rabies. Crushing the *Cuterebra* spp larva in the subcutis may result in a fatal shock reaction. Additionally, death may ensue due to progressive debility resulting from chronic infection. If the animal survives, it loses considerable body condition and becomes a prime candidate for secondary bacterial infections and other complications, including predation.

Necropsy Signs

Gross lesions of *Cuterebra* spp are found mainly in the subcutis where they are associated with dead or live larvae and their breathing pores. In cases of aberrant migration, larvae may be found almost anywhere, especially in the brain, middle ear, or nasal passages. Because death may occur as a result of the toxins produced by the larvae, gross lesions in other areas of the body may be absent. Animals that die from chronic infection may be grossly emaciated with apparent splenomegaly, lymph-node enlargement, and cachexia.

Histologically, the severity of the infection is difficult to assess; however, marked inflammatory reactions and fibroblast proliferation are usually associated with aberrant migration of the larvae in certain organs.

Diagnosis

Diagnosis of cuterebriasis depends on finding boil-like or furuncular lesions associated with a fly larva. Furthermore, the larva is located by a 1–3 cm cone-shaped swelling with an apical pore. Careful dissection of the pore may reveal a *Cuterebra* spp larva in the first, second, or third stage of development. The larva is club-shaped with tapered ends and has a segmented body with circumferential rows of caudally projecting, spine-like denticles used for orientation. The mouth contains a pair of hooks, whereas the tail end contains the stigmatic plates used for breathing through the subcutaneous pores.

Treatment

Treatment may involve shaving the hair and surgical preparation of the affected skin. The *Cuterebra* spp larva is killed with alcohol, the pore is opened surgically, and the larva is removed carefully and intact. The resulting wound is kept dry and clean to facilitate rapid healing. Ivermectin has been used experimentally in cases of aberrant migration, but reaction to the dead larva is potentially fatal, necessitating concurrent use of corticosteroids.

Prevention

Prevention of myiasis in rabbits is accomplished with effective fly control measures such as proper disposal of manure, screened windows, fly traps, and use of safe insecticides and fly repellents. In addition, pet rabbits may be groomed prophylactically to remove fly ova, and access to the outdoors should be restricted during fly season. Dead and infected rabbits should be disposed of immediately and properly to prevent *Cuterebra* spp larvae from migrating to other rabbits.

Public Health Significance

Rabbit bot flies occasionally infect humans, especially children and the elderly. Cases of humans with intranasal, intracranial, and intraocular larval migration have been reported.

MYIASIS (FLY STRIKE) —SECONDARY

Hosts

Secondary myiasis occurs when flies that normally feed on decomposing organic matter or carrion develop in wounded, soiled, or immobilized animals. Flies causing secondary myiasis are opportunistic and will lay eggs indiscriminately. Fly strike occurs primarily in injured or debilitated rabbits or rodents housed outdoors but may also occur in indoor pets.

Etiology

Secondary myiasis is caused by Calliphorid flies, also called blow flies, which have characteristic metallic blue or green bodies. Common names also include "bluebottle" and "greenbottle" flies. These flies feed and lay ova on urine- or feces-stained fur and decaying flesh in exposed, untreated wounds or sores. The ova hatch and larvae, which are called maggots, are found locally and superficially. Marginal husbandry and management practices, such as neglecting wet, dirty, and diseased animals with gaping wounds, open sores, or soiled perineal areas, predispose the animal to attract flies, especially in the summer months when these animals are housed outdoors.

Predisposing Factors

Animals housed outdoors with blood, purulent or necrotic debris, feces, or urine on their fur will attract flies. Diseased and moribund animals that are nonambulatory with decubital ulcers become an easy target for flies to lay ova that hatch and become maggots. Accumulation of urine and fecal material around the perineum occurs in long-haired or obese rabbits, or those with hind end paralysis following spinal trauma. Animals that are neglected or handled rarely are more likely to develop conditions favorable to fly strike.

Transmission

Blow flies are opportunistic and will lay large numbers of eggs in any suitable location. Adult female blow flies deposit approximately 250 eggs at a time, which hatch into first-stage maggots within 24 hours. They feed and then molt into second-stage maggots, which feed for approximately 24 hours, and then molt into third-stage maggots. After more feeding, the third-stage maggots move away from the body and metamorphose into adult flies.

Clinical Signs

Clinical signs of fly strike are varied depending on the precipitating condition. General signs include depression, hunched appearance, reluctance to move, and unkempt hair coat. Maggots are not always readily visible, especially if they are covered by a mat of soiled hair, and owners are not always aware of the extent of the infestation.

Diagnosis

Maggots are usually associated with wounds, open sores, or wet folds of skin not readily accessible to the host when grooming. They are easy to see once hair mats and debris are cleared away. As in cuterebriasis, an overwhelming number of maggots on a rabbit may lead to terminal toxic shock.

Treatment

Rabbits should be stabilized with fluids, nutrition, and antibiotics if necessary, prior to maggot removal. Maggots and eggs should be removed, and the area washed with a generous amount of a mild disinfectant solution. The hair should be clipped around the affected area and an appropriate topical antibiotic applied several times daily until the wound heals completely. The animal should be confined indoors in clean, dry quarters during treatment. Any predisposing conditions, such as diarrhea, open wounds, or obesity, should be addressed to prevent recurrence.

Prevention

Prevention of myiasis in rabbits is accomplished with effective fly control measures such as regular disposal of uneaten greens and manure, screened windows, fly traps, and use of safe insecticides and fly repellents. Pet rabbits and rodents housed outdoors in the summer should be handled daily to detect any wounds, injuries, or diarrhea and may be groomed prophylactically to remove fly ova and soiled fur. Access to the outdoors should be restricted during fly season. Dead rabbits should be disposed of immediately to avoid attracting flies to the hutch.

Public Health Significance

Blow flies are opportunistic and may parasitize humans under the right circumstances.

References

Anderson GS, Huitson NR. Myiasis in pet animals in British Columbia: the potential of forensic entomology for determining duration of possible neglect. Can Vet J. 2004, 45:993–998.

Baird CR. Biology of Cuterebra lepusculi townsend (Diptera: Cuterebridae) in cottontail rabbits in Idaho. J Wildl Dis. 1983, 19:214–218.

Baird JK, Baird CR, Sabrosky CW. North American cuterebrid myiasis. Report of seventeen new infections of human beings and review of the disease. J Am Acad Dermatol. 1989, 21:763–772.

Bowman DD. Georgis' Parasitology for Veterinarians, 9th ed. Philadelphia: Elsevier Health Sciences, 2008; 22.

Cousquer, G. Veterinary care of rabbits with myiasis. In Pract. 2006, 28:342–349.

Doxanas MT, Waicher JR, Ludwig RA. Ophthalmomyiasis externa: a case report. Md Med J. 1992, 41:989–991.

Harriman, M. Fly strike. House Rabbit J. 1993, 2(12):8–9.

Hendrix CM, et al. Aberrant intracranial myiasis caused by larval Cuterebra infection. Comp Cont Educ Pract Vet. 1989, 11(5):550–562.

Hoppman E, Barron HW. Ferret and rabbit dermatology. J Exot Pet Med. 2007, 16:225–237.

Jacobson HA, McGinnes BS, Catts EP. Bot fly myiasis of the cottontail rabbit, Sylvilagus floridanus mallurus in Virginia with some biology of the parasite, Cuterebra buccata. J Wildl Dis. 1978, 14:56–66.

Lepitzki DA, Woolf A, Bunn BM. Parasites of cottontail rabbits of southern Illinois. J Parasitol. 1992, 78:1080–1083.

MYXOMATOSIS

Hosts

Myxomatosis is a viral disease of wild (*Sylvilagus*) and domestic (*Oryctolagus*) rabbits. Wild rabbits are the natural reservoir host in North and South America. The virus causes localized firm skin tumors (fibromas) in wild lagomorphs.

Etiology

The disease is caused by several strains of myxoma poxviruses on the more virulent end of the myxoma-fibroma spectrum of viruses. The highly virulent variant that occurs in western California and Oregon is, appropriately named, the California strain. The virus is endemic in the *Sylvilagus* population in California. A variety of other strains exist in South America, Australia, and Europe. Substantial variations exist between strains of myxoma virus from different parts of North and South America, based on serologic and biologic comparisons.

Transmission

The highly virulent virus is transmitted mechanically from wild reservoir hosts primarily by arthropod vectors, mosquitoes, and flies. The extent of viral transmission varies with seasonal changes in populations of mosquitoes, mites, and fleas feeding on rabbits. Other arthropods can act as mechanical vectors, as might birds, plants, and fomites. In the United States, an annual increase in myxomatosis is seen from August to November.

Clinical Signs

The first clinical signs after infection with the California strain of virus include a "sleepy-eyed" rabbit with mild lethargy, red eyes, swollen eyelids, fever, and a watery ocular discharge. If the rabbit survives the acute stage, the reddening and swelling extend to the lips, face, ears, and anogenital areas. Death follows in a large percentage of rabbits. When rabbits survive, they develop cutaneous hemorrhages. Affected rabbits in the terminal stages of disease are anorectic and dehydrated. Some will survive and the lesions regress over 1–3 months. In subacute to chronic cases, the disease is often complicated by pasteurellosis, which causes additional deaths.

Unlike the more severe signs in *Oryctolagus cuniculus*, only localized tumors are produced by the virus in the reservoir host, *Sylvilagus bachmani*, in California. Lesions in animals with the European and South American disease forms include the development of skin tumors, which may eventually rupture and ooze.

Necropsy

Gross necropsy signs after infection of European rabbits with the California strain of virus are subcutaneous edema and widespread visceral hemorrhage. Microscopically, there is extensive epithelial proliferation with ballooning of cells in the stratum granulosum and hyperkeratinization in the overlying epithelium. Large, eosinophilic, intracytoplasmic inclusion bodies are seen in the stratum germinativum. Lymphocytic depletion occurs in the spleen, and necrosis of lymphatic tissue occurs in several organs. Mucinous skin tumors and capillary and venule endothelial proliferation develop in rabbits in Europe.

Diagnosis

Diagnosis is based on clinical signs, necropsy findings, and the characteristic histopathologic appearance of the lesions. Intracutaneous inoculation of suspect tissue into young susceptible rabbits will result in lesions at the inoculation site within a week.

Treatment

A treatment for myxomatosis does not exist. Results from a therapeutic trial with acyclovir were inconclusive.

Prevention

Vector control through spraying, screening to exclude mosquitoes, avoidance of wild rabbits, quarantine of new arrivals, and vaccination with live attenuated vaccines in the face of an outbreak are methods of preventing myxomatosis. Owners of pet rabbits in Australia are not permitted to vaccinate their pets against myxomatosis virus.

Public Health Significance

Myxomatosis virus does not affect humans.

References

Bartrip PW. Myxomatosis in 1950s Britain. 20 Century Br Hist. 2008, 19(1):83–105.

Fenner F. Poxviruses of laboratory animals. Lab Anim Sci. 1990, 40:469–480.

Fenner F, Marshall ID. A comparison of the virulence for European rabbits (Oryctolagus cuniculus) of strains of myxoma virus recovered in the field in Australia, Europe and America. J Hyg (Camb.). 1957, 55:149–191.

Fenner F, Woodroofe GM. The pathogenesis of infectious myxomatosis: the mechanism of infection and the immunological response in the European rabbit (Oryctolagus cuniculus). Br J Exp Pathol. 1953, 34:400–411.

Grodhaus G, Regnery DC, Marshall ID. Studies in the epidemiology of myxomatosis in California. II. The experimental transmission of myxomatosis in brush rabbits (Sylvilagus bachmani) by several species of mosquitoes. Am J Hyg. 1963, 77:205–212.

Gumbrell RC. Myxomatosis and rabbit control in New Zealand. NZ Vet J. 1986, 34:54–55.

Marshall ID, Regnery DC. Myxomatosis in a California brush rabbit (Sylvilagus bachmani). Nature. 1960, 188:73–74.

McKercher DG, Saito JK. An attenuated live virus vaccine for myxomatosis. Nature. 1964, 202:933–934.

Patton NM, Holmes HT. Myxomatosis in domestic rabbits in Oregon. J Am Vet Med Assoc. 1977, 171:560–562.

Ross J, Sanders MF. The development of genetic resistance to myxomatosis in wild rabbits in Britain. J Hyg (Camb.). 1984, 97:255–261.

Saito JK, McKercher DG, Castrucci G. Attenuation of the myxoma virus and use of the living attenuated virus as an immunizing agent for myxomatosis. J Infect Dis. 1964, 114:417–428.

NASAL DERMATITIS (SORE NOSE) IN GERBILS

Hosts

"Sore nose," "rednose," or nasal or facial dermatitis occurs frequently in Mongolian gerbils (*Meriones unguiculatus*).

Etiology

Nasal dermatitis of gerbils is associated frequently with staphylococcal infections, but the primary cause may be the irritating nature of porphyrin-rich secretions from the Harderian glands that accumulate around the external nares, which are normally groomed onto the face and fur. *Staphylococcus* spp are usually isolated from gerbils with nasal dermatitis, thus implicating this bacterium in the pathogenesis. In a breeding colony of Mongolian gerbils, *S. xylosus* was the predominant isolate obtained from sporadic cases of nasal dermatitis and was the primary *Staphylococcus* spp cultured. The organism was considered an opportunistic pathogen.

Predisposing Factors

Gerbils are arid desert creatures and require an environment with low humidity for optimal skin health. In captivity, stressors such as changes in the cage, loss of or separation from cagemates, incompatible cagemates, and overcrowding result in increased chromodacryorrhea or "red tears" due to excess porphyrin-rich Harderian gland secretions. These secretions are removed normally by grooming with the forepaws over the pelage; however, accumulation of excessive amounts is irritating to the skin and may initiate "sore nose."

Illness and depression or management conditions, for example, applying Elizabethan collars that reduce and prevent removal of porphyrin secretions by natural grooming behavior, may also predispose animals to this condition. Overcrowding stress in gerbils results in greatly increased activity, especially burrowing, or pressing the nose through cage wires, which aggravates facial irritation. Although the sore nose lesion may be initiated by the irritating effects of porphyrin secretions and aggravated by cutaneous abrasions incurred while burrowing, subsequent *S. aureus* or *S. xylosus* infection may perpetuate a chronic dermatitis.

Clinical Signs

Nasal or facial dermatitis in gerbils is seen as a red-brown hairless area on the snout surrounding and below the external nares. If spontaneous recovery does not occur, normal grooming behavior may cause the lesion to progress into a chronic moist dermatitis involving the face and the inner aspects of the forepaws. With severe signs, the gerbil may lose condition, become anorectic, and, uncommonly, may die. The prognosis is good with treatment.

Diagnosis

Clinical signs, predisposing factors, culture, and isolation of *S. xylosus* or *S. aureus* from the nasal lesions provide information to make a diagnosis.

Treatment

The condition may be alleviated by removing stressors, cleaning the face, using clay or corncob bedding products instead of wood shavings or chips, and by applying appropriate ophthalmic ointments. Antibiotic sensitivity testing may be useful to effect more precise therapeutic measures for treating chronic ulcerative nasal dermatitis. Chloramphenicol palmitate and gentamicin have both been used effectively to treat sore nose. Streptomycins should be avoided in gerbils because of toxicity.

Prevention

Chromodacryorrhea and nasal dermatitis may be controlled by adherence to good husbandry and management practices. Elimination of environmental and social stressors, such as overcrowding, fighting, and disease, is important. Provision of dust baths or absorbent, fine bedding material such as clay will help to ameliorate the disease by reducing the amount of porphyrin accumulation on the face. In one study, surgical adenectomy of the Harderian glands prevented the occurrence of sore nose by eliminating the source of porphyrin in collared animals.

References

Bresnahan JF, et al. Nasal dermatitis in the Mongolian gerbil. Lab Anim Sci. 1983, 33:258–263.

Farrar PL, et al. Experimental nasal dermatitis in the Mongolian gerbil: effect of bilateral Harderian gland adenectomy on development of facial lesions. Lab Anim Sci. 1988, 38:72–76.

Hoppmann E, Wilson Barron H. Rodent dermatology. J Exot Pet Med. 2007, 16(4):238–255.

Solomon HF, Dixon DM, Pouch W. A survey of staphylococci isolated from the laboratory gerbil. Lab Anim Sci. 1990, 40:316–318.

Thiessen DD, Pendergrass M. Harderian gland involvement in facial lesions in the Mongolian gerbil. J Am Vet Med Assoc. 1982, 181:1375–1377.

NEOPLASIA

General Discussion

Although literature surveys of the incidence of neoplasia in rabbits and rodents contain lengthy lists of tumor types, each species, if not each strain, possesses a limited number of common tumors. Therefore, although a limited number of tumors is described in this section, individual animals may develop one or more of a variety of neoplasms.

General References on Neoplasia

Greenacre CB. Spontaneous tumors of small mammals. Vet Clin North Am Exot Anim Pract. 2004, 7(3):627–651.

Heydari AR, Unnikrishnan A, Lucente LV, et al. Caloric restriction and genomic stability. Nucleic Acids Res. 2007, 35(22):7485–7496.

Jones SR, et al. Naturally Occurring Neoplastic Diseases. In: Handbook of Laboratory Animal Science, vol. III. Melby EC, Jr, Altman NH (eds.). Cleveland, OH: CRC Press, Inc., 1976; 221–381.

Percy DH, Barthold SW. Pathology of Laboratory Rodents and Rabbits, 3rd ed. Ames, IA: Wiley-Blackwell, 2007.

Pour P, Ii Y, Althoff J. Comparative studies on spontaneous tumor incidence based on systematic histologic examination of rat and hamster strains of the same colony. Prog Exp Tumor Res. 1979, 24:199–206.

Prejean JD, et al. Spontaneous tumours in Sprague-Dawley rats and Swiss mice. Cancer Res. 1973, 33:2768–2773.

Squire RA, et al. Tumors. In: Pathology of Laboratory Animals, vol. II. Benirschke K, Garner FM, Jones TC (eds.). New York: Springer-Verlag, 1978; 2:1051–1283.

Stinson SF, Schuller HM, Reznik G (eds.). Atlas of Tumor Pathology of the Fischer Rat. Boca Raton, FL: CRC Press, 1990.

Neoplasia in the Rabbit

Adenocarcinoma of the uterine endometrium is the most common spontaneously occurring tumor of rabbits. Its occurrence is influenced by genetic background, age, and endocrinologic factors. Tumors are rarely seen in commercial rabbitries and research institutions because of the young age of the rabbits in these populations.

Uterine adenocarcinoma has been reported more often in tan, French silver, Havana, and Dutch breeds and less often (in descending order) in the Marten, English, chinchilla, Beveran, sable, Himalayan, and Polish breeds. The tumor was not found in the Belgian and rex breeds. Rabbits of the higher-incidence breeds younger than 3 years have an incidence of approximately 4%, whereas rabbits older than 3 years have an incidence of uterine adenocarcinoma approaching 50–80%.

The association of uterine adenocarcinoma with pregnancy toxemia, pseudopregnancy, and hyperestrogenism remains controversial. The dose of estrogen and its carcinogenic effects may be important factors that influence the development of uterine cancer. Because rabbits are induced ovulators, a nongravid doe is under estrogenic influences for most of the estrous cycle, which may play a factor in disease development. Further, a direct correlation exists between the incidence of uterine tumors and mammary carcinomas.

Senile atrophy of the endometrium may also predispose to tumor development. With increasing age, the endometrial cells, beginning deep in the glandular crypts, become less specialized, and the connective tissue stroma becomes less cellular and more collagenous. These progressive senile changes may underlie the transition to adenomatous, papillary, and cystic endometrial hyperplasia and then carcinoma. The hyperplastic stage lasts approximately 3 months, the carcinoma in situ 7 months, and the metastatic stage 10 or 12 months. The tumors are usually ovoid, firm, and hemorrhagic and are spaced regularly along the mesometrial junction. The neoplasm may invade the myometrium and seed the peritoneal cavity before hematogenous metastasis to the lungs and other organs occurs. Multiple uterine tumors may be of different sizes, but they are usually at the same stage of differentiation.

Clinical signs associated with uterine neoplasia in the rabbit include altered reproductive performance and eventually death over a period of 5–20 months after the tumor is first noted. During the subclinical period, affected does become less fertile, have smaller litters, abort or resorb fetuses, deliver stillborn kits, retain fetuses past term, and may have a bloody vulvar discharge or bloody urine. Typically, the multiple neoplastic nodules, which may be approximately 1 cm in diameter when first noticed, will grow to 5 cm by 6 months and can be palpated through the abdominal and uterine walls. The incidence or proportion of uterine tumors may decrease in SPF rabbits.

Lymphosarcoma is the most common tumor of juvenile and young adult domestic rabbits and is the second most common tumor of rabbits. Lymphosarcomas are characterized by pale, nodular enlargements in the renal cortices, hepatomegaly, splenomegaly, and intestinal lymphadenopathy. Cutaneous forms (epitheliotropic lymphoma) also occur.

A homozygous autosomal recessive gene may be necessary for development of lymphosarcoma. Lymphomas may be of either T or B cell origin.

Embryonal nephroma (Wilms' tumor) and bile duct adenomas rank third and fourth in tumor frequency in rabbits. It is tempting to speculate that bile duct tumors are a sequela of chronic *Eimeria stieae* infection. Squamous cell carcinoma is the second most common skin tumor after epitheliotropic lymphoma. Less frequently reported spontaneous neoplasms of the rabbit include testicular seminoma, thymoma, basal cell tumor, papilloma, squamous cell carcinoma, and osteogenic sarcoma with subcutaneous involvement.

The myxofibroma group of poxvirus-induced tumors occur as fibromas in *Sylvilagus* (cottontail) rabbits in both the eastern and western United States and in Europe, South America, and Australia. These antigenically related viruses are transmitted mechanically by mosquitoes and biting insects from cottontails to domestic rabbits, in which disease processes range from peracute, fatal myxomatosis to transitory single fibromas.

Myxomatosis, described elsewhere in this chapter, induces a generalized proliferation of reticuloendothelial cells and their mucin, which, with some strains of virus, results in the formation of irregular, subcutaneous, gelatinous tumors. These tumors, however, are not characteristic of the California disease.

A related poxvirus, endemic in Eastern cottontails (*S. floridanus*) causes self-limiting, subcutaneous fibromas in adult, domestic rabbits. In young *Oryctolagus*, the disease may become a disseminated fibromatosis. Prevention of the myxofibromatous diseases involves the exclusion of biting insects from the rabbitry and vaccination during an epidemic.

References

Baba N, von Haam E. Animal model: spontaneous adenocarcinoma in aged rabbits. Am J Pathol. 1972, 68:653–656.

Brown PJ, Stafford RA. A testicular seminoma in a rabbit. J Comp Pathol. 1989, 100:353–355.

Flatt RE, Weisbroth SH. Interstitial cell tumor of the testicle in rabbits: a report of two cases. Lab Anim Sci. 1974, 24:682–685.

Fox RR, et al. Lymphosarcoma in the rabbit: genetics and pathology. J Nat Cancer Inst. 1970, 45:719–729.

Heatley JJ, Smith AN. Spontaneous neoplasms of lagomorphs. Vet Clin Exot Anim. 2004, 7:561–577.

Hoover JP, et al. Osteogenic sarcoma with subcutaneous involvement in a rabbit. J Am Vet Med Assoc. 1986, 189:1156–1158.

Joiner GN, Jardine JH, Gleiser CA. An epizootic of Shope fibromatosis in a commercial rabbitry. J Am Vet Med Assoc. 1971, 159:1583–1587.

Kinkler RJ, Jepsen PL. Ependymoma in a rabbit. Lab Anim Sci. 1979, 29:255–256.

Kostolich M, Panciera RJ. Thymoma in a domestic rabbit. Cornell Vet. 1992, 82:125–129.

Li X, Schlafer DH. A spontaneous skin basal cell tumor in a black French minilop rabbit. Lab Anim Sci. 1992, 42:94–95.

Mews AR, et al. Detection of oral papillomatosis in a British rabbit colony. Lab Anim. 1972, 6:141–145.

Toth LA, et al. Lymphocytic leukemia and lymphosarcoma in a rabbit. J Am Vet Med Assoc. 1990, 197:627–629.

Weisbroth SH. Neoplastic Diseases. In: The Biology of the Laboratory Rabbit, 2nd ed. Manning PJ, Ringler DH, Newcomer CE (eds.). San Diego: Academic Press, 1994, 259–292.

Weisbroth SH, Scher S. Spontaneous oral papillomatosis in rabbits. J Am Vet Med Assoc. 1970, 157:1940–1944.

Neoplasia in the Guinea Pig

Rhabdomyomatosis, an accumulation of glycogen-bearing myocardial cells and not a neoplasm, is visible grossly as pale foci on the mural and valvular endocardial surfaces of the atria and ventricles. Another nonneoplastic proliferation in the guinea pig is the embryonic placentoma, a multilayered transitory growth of parthenogenic origin that occurs within the ovary of the young female. The placentoma is resolved by fibrosis and may be related to the neoplastic ovarian teratoma.

True neoplastic processes are rare in guinea pigs, but an age-related increase in incidence has been noted. Estimates of the incidence of neoplasia in guinea pigs over 3 years of age range up to 30%. Pulmonary neoplasia, usually bronchogenic papillary adenoma, is the most common category of tumor in the guinea pig, comprising 35% of the total. Tumors of the reproductive tract, the mammary glands, and the hematopoietic system comprise the remainder of the more commonly seen guinea pig tumors. Mammary gland tumors may occur in both male and female guinea pigs, of which approximately 30% are locally invasive adenocarcinomas.

Skin tumors affect up to 15% of aged guinea pigs, particularly trichofolliculoma, a benign form of basal cell tumor that is readily removed under anesthesia.

Leiomyomas were the most common reproductive tract tumors in a colony of aged (average 48 months) female guinea pigs and were seen frequently in conjunction with cystic rete ovarii. There is likely a relationship between the estrogen-secreting cysts and development of leiomyomas (similar to estrogen-dependent growth of fibroids in premenopausal women).

Spontaneous lymphocytic leukemia is a commonly reported acute, virally induced (c-type RNA virus) malignancy with a rapid course, which is often fatal within 2–5 weeks of onset. Strain 2 inbred guinea pigs are uniquely susceptible. The hair coat of the affected animal becomes rough, the mucus membranes are pale (anemia), and the liver and lymph nodes are enlarged. The white blood cell count may reach 250,000/mm^3, and typical 18–40 um leukemia cells are seen on blood smears. The disease responds favorably to chemotherapy.

References

Ediger RD, Rabstein MM. Spontaneous leukemia in a Hartley strain guinea pig. J Am Vet Med Assoc. 1968, 153:954–956.

Field KJ, Griffith JW, Lang CM. Spontaneous reproductive tract leiomyomas in aged guinea-pigs. J Comp Pathol. 1989, 101:287–294.

Frisk CS, Wagner, JE, Doyle, RE. An ovarian teratoma in a guinea pig. Lab Anim Sci. 1978, 28:199–201.

Greenacre CB. Spontaneous tumors of small mammals. Vet Clin Exot Anim Pract. 2004, 7(3):627–651.

Hong CC, Liu PL, Poon KC. Naturally occurring lymphoblastic leukemia in guinea pigs. Lab Anim Sci. 1980, 30:222–226.

Kaplow, LS, Nadel, E. Acute lymphoblastic leukemia. Animal model: transplantable guinea pig L2C leukemia. Am J Pathol. 1979, 95:273–276.

Kitchen DN, Canton WW, Bickford AA. A report of fourteen spontaneous tumors of the guinea pig. Lab Anim Sci. 1975, 25:92–102.

Vink HH. Rhabdomyomatosis (nodular glycogenic infiltration) of the heart in guinea-pigs. J Pathol. 1969, 97:331–334.

Zwart P, et al. Cutaneous tumours in the guinea pig. Lab Anim. 1981, 15:375–377.

Neoplasia in the Chinchilla

There is a paucity of information available regarding tumors of chinchillas. In the past, the majority of chinchillas were raised for fur production and did not survive long enough to develop tumors. Despite the fact that chinchillas live to be 20 years old or more, tumors are rarely seen in practice. Uterine leiomyosarcoma, lymphoma, osteosarcomas, and pulmonary tumors have been reported.

References

Greenacre CB. Spontaneous tumors of small mammals. Vet Clin North Am Exot Anim Pract. 2004, 7(3):627–651.

Simova-Curd S, Nitzl D, Pospischil A, Hatt JM. Lumbar osteosarcoma in a chinchilla (Chinchilla laniger). J Small Anim Pract. 2008, 49(9):483–485.

Neoplasia in the Hamster

The incidence of spontaneous neoplasia in the Syrian golden hamster is reportedly low. Variations depend on the source of the survey and the ages of the animals described. Reports vary from 4% as an overall population incidence up to 50% or more in select groups of hamsters over 2 years of age. Though the incidence of tumors is low, the variety of tumors in aged hamsters is large. Endocrine tumors of the adrenal cortex comprise the largest reported group. Next are tumors of the lymphoreticular system (predominantly lymphomas), tumors of the skin and subcutis, and tumors of the gastrointestinal tract (polyps, papillomas, and adenocarcinomas). Incidence varies substantially from colony to colony. Most tumors are benign. Benign follicular thyroid tumors are seen occasionally, especially if there is an iodine deficiency.

One of the most frequent sites for spontaneous neoplasms is the hematopoietic system. Reported tumors include malignant lymphomas with peripheral lymph node enlargement and lymphosarcomas. This is related to a hamster polyoma virus infection. Cutaneous lymphomas, resembling mycosis fungoides of humans, have also been reported in aging pet Syrian hamsters. Clinical signs included friable skin, hair loss, foul odor, erythroderma, dermal plaques with surface ulceration and crusting, papules, and lymphadenopathy, in addition to lethargy, anorexia, emaciation, and neuromuscular involvement. Progression of the disease was rapid, and systemic involvement was apparent at necropsy. A cutaneous hemangiosarcoma was reported in a 2-year-old female hamster with an ulcerated mass on its flank. The mass was removed surgically and did not recur.

Reproductive system tumors are infrequent and include thecomas and granulosa cell tumors of the ovaries, leiomyomas, and endometrial polyps of the uterus. Male reproductive tumors are rare, as are tumors of the central nervous system.

Tumors of the gastrointestinal system vary considerably between studies. In one report, polyps of the cecum and colon and gastric squamous papillomas were found. Cholangiomas (bile duct tumors) are common in some colonies, while cirrhosis is reported in others. Urinary system tumors are uncommon in hamsters. A wide variety of skin tumors have been seen. They include melanomas as the most common, followed by basal cell tumors, keratoacanthomas, squamous papillomas, Harderian gland adenomas, and warts. Hemangioendotheliomas of the vascular system are reported occasionally.

Hamsters are also susceptible to a range of experimentally induced tumors. The hamster's evertible cheek pouch is an easily accessed, immunologically protected site that was historically used for tumor transplantation. Immunodeficient mice have supplanted the use of the hamster cheek pouch for this purpose.

References

Deamond SF, et al. Longevity and age-related pathology of LVG outbred golden Syrian hamsters (Mesocricetus auratus). Exp Geron. 1990, 25:433–446.

Foster AP, Brown PJ, Jandrig B, et al. Polyomavirus infection in hamsters and trichoepitheliomas/cutaneous adnexal tumours. Vet Rec. 2002, 151(1):13–17.

Homburger F. Background data for tumor incidence in control animals (Syrian hamsters). Prog Exp Tumor Res. 1983, 26:259–265.

Kirkman H, Algard FT. Spontaneous and Nonviral-Induced Neoplasms. In: The Golden Hamster—Its Biology and Use in Medical Research. Hoffman RA, Robinson PF, Magalhaes H (eds.). Ames, IA: Iowa State University Press, 1968; 227–240.

Kondo H, Onuma M, Shibuya H, et al. Spontaneous tumors in domestic hamsters. Vet Pathol. 2008, 45:674–680.

Pour P, et al. Spontaneous tumors and common disease in three types of hamsters. J Nat Cancer Inst. 1979, 63:797–811.

Rich GA. Cutaneous lymphosarcoma in a Syrian hamster. J Small Exot Anim Med. 1992, 1:113–114.

Rosenthal K. Hemangiosarcoma in a hamster. J Small Exot Anim Med. 1991, 1:15.

Saunders GK, Scott DW. Cutaneous lymphoma resembling mycosis fungoides in the Syrian hamster (Mesocricetus auratus). Lab Anim Sci. 1988, 38:616–617.

Scherneck S, Ulrich R, Feunteun J. The hamster polyomavirus—a brief review of recent knowledge. Virus Genes. 2001, 22(1):93–101.

Strandberg JD. Neoplastic Diseases. In: Laboratory Hamsters. Van Hoosier GL, Jr, McPherson CW (eds.). Orlando: Academic Press, 1987; 157–178.

Turusov VS, et al. (eds.). Pathology of Tumours in Laboratory Animals. III. Tumours of the Hamster. Lyon, France: International Agency for Research on Cancer, 1982.

Van Hoosier GL, Jr, Trentin JJ. Naturally occurring tumors of the Syrian hamster. Prog Exp Tumor Res. 1979, 23:1–12.

Neoplasia in the Gerbil

The incidence of spontaneous neoplasia in gerbils older than 2 years is high. Neoplasms in gerbils cover a range of types, with tumors of the female reproductive system perhaps being the most common. Granulosa, thecal and lutein cell tumors, dysgerminomas, and teratomas have been reported in the ovary. Adenocarcinoma of the oviduct, uterine adenocarcinoma, and leiomyoma have also been reported. A few tumors of the male genital system have been reported: seminoma, teratoma, and prostatic adenomas. Adrenocortical adenomas and adenocarcinomas are also common tumors of gerbils. Neoplasms of the skin, which include those of the ventral scent gland, include basal cell carcinomas, melanomas, sebaceous adenomas, fibrosarcomas, squamous cell carcinomas, and cholesteatomas. Neoplasms have been reported in several other tissues. These include pancreatic islet cell adenomas, hepatic lymphangiomas, cecal adenocarcinomas, thymomas, splenic hemangiomas, Hodgkin's-like lymphoma, urinary hemangiomas, and osteosarcomas. Pseudoadenomatous structures of the skin, cystic ovaries, and periovarian cysts, which can cause infertility, are common, nonneoplastic processes that occur in the gerbil.

References

Benitz KF, KrAm AW Jr. Spontaneous tumors in the Mongolian gerbil. Lab Anim Care. 1965, 15:281–294.

Meckley PE, Zwicker GM. Naturally-occurring neoplasms in the Mongolian gerbil, Meriones unguiculatus. Lab Anim. 1979, 13:203–206.

Ringler DH, Lay DM, Abrams GD. Spontaneous neoplasms in aging Gerbillinae. Lab Anim Sci. 1972, 22:407–414.

Shumaker RC, Paik SK, Houser WD. Tumors in Gerbillinae: a literature review and a report of a case. Lab Anim Sci. 1974, 24:688–690.

Toft JD, II. Commonly observed spontaneous neoplasms in rabbits, rats, guinea pigs, hamsters and gerbils. Sem Av Exot Pet Med. 1992, 1:80–92.

Vincent AL, Ash LR. Further observations on spontaneous neoplasms in the Mongolian gerbil, Meriones unguiculatus. Lab Anim Sci. 1978, 28:297–300.

Vincent AL, Rodrick GE, Sodeman WA, Jr. The pathology of the Mongolian gerbil (Meriones unguiculatus): a review. Lab Anim Sci. 1979, 29:645–651.

Neoplasia in the Mouse

Neoplasia in mice is one of the most extensively investigated disease processes of rodents. Volumes have been written about the causation, pathogenesis, structure, and resolution of murine tumors. With the development of inbred strains and selection for tumor susceptibility and resistance, the pattern of tumor incidence in the laboratory mouse has become different from the pattern in its ancestor, the wild house mouse, or in the outbred white mouse. Neoplasia may be manifested clinically as weight gain or loss; cutaneous, subcutaneous, or abdominal swellings; infertility; paleness due to anemia from external or internal bleeding; increased susceptibility to infection; and death.

Adult, wild or random-bred, female breeder mice have the following approximate tumor incidences: pulmonary tumors, 28%; hemangioendotheliomas, 8%; ovarian tumors, 6%; mammary tumors, 6%; hepatomas, 4%; leukemias, 2%; reticulum cell sarcomas, 2%; and subcutaneous sarcomas, 2%. Fibrosarcomas are also common in pet mice. A thorough discussion of representative inbred strains and their approximate tumor incidences may be found in *The Mouse in Biomedical Research,* 2nd ed., vol 2: *Diseases,* 2007 (Brayton C).

Mammary tumors and lymphosarcomas are among the most common tumors of inbred strains. Some representative inbred strains and their associated neoplasms are mammary tumors in C3H mice, plasma cell tumors in BALB/c mice, type B reticulum cell sarcomas in SJL mice, and leukemias in AKR mice. More than 90% of AKR mice will develop leukemia by 1 year of age. Tumor incidence varies with sex, age, parity, diet, caloric intake, and substrain. Common experimental predisposing factors include radiation exposure and chemical carcinogens.

Mice develop a variety of spontaneous malignancies of the hematopoietic system, particularly of lymphopoietic origin. The incidence varies widely, depending on the strain of mouse, from 0 to virtually 100%. Similarly, environmental factors may also play a role in tumor development. Up to a 10-fold difference in the incidence of neoplasms may occur in the same strain maintained in different laboratories or under different environmental conditions. Thymic lymphoma is the most common malignancy of the hematopoietic system in the mouse. Histologically, the mediastinal mass is composed of lymphoblastic cells with numerous mitoses. Varying stages of differentiation may be observed. These tumors are of T cell origin. Committed T cells may originate in the bone marrow, then migrate to the thymus, where a thymic tumor develops. Thymic lymphomas are relatively common in SCID mice. Up to 20% of old *scid/scid* mice die with thymic lymphomas. Spontaneous thymic tumors are associated with endogenous retroviral infection and may be induced experimentally by chemical carcinogens (e.g., alkylnitrosamines).

Lymphopoietic tumors of B cell origin commonly affect spleen and lymph nodes with no thymic involvement. There may be infiltration of transformed lymphocytes into other tissues including liver, kidney, myocardium, leptomeninges, and so forth. Neoplastic cells often have large vesicular nuclei; prominent nucleoli, and abundant, poorly delineated cytoplasm, but tumors composed of relatively well-differentiated lymphocytes also occur. Cell type classification is similar to that used in other mammals.

Virtually all laboratory mice are contaminated with retroviruses. Unlike cells transformed by an oncogenic DNA virus, retrovirus-transformed cells may also produce infectious viral particles. Mice normally harbor endogenous retroviruses in a variety of types of cells, which are readily transmitted in germ cells to their progeny. Exogenous retroviruses also exist and are transmitted horizontally like conventional viruses but have largely been eliminated from laboratory mice. Retroviruses can also be transmitted horizontally via virus-containing urine, feces, milk, or saliva. There does not appear to be a good correlation between production of endogenous virus and spontaneous hematopoietic neoplasms. Frequently it appears that a chemical or physical carcinogen may be acting in concert with endogenous retrovirus to produce hematopoietic tumors. The two primary retroviruses that infect domesticated mice are murine leukemia virus (MuLV) and murine mammary tumor virus (MMTV).

Unlike the rat mammary tumor, which is removed easily, the mouse mammary adenocarcinoma is soft, fleshy, highly vascularized, and infiltrative. It cannot be removed without extensive tissue damage and hemorrhage.

Primary tumors of the lung are relatively common in the mouse, particularly in certain strains (e.g., BALB/c and C3H). These tumors do not appear to normally be virally induced but can be produced experimentally in mice by carcinogen administration. Thymectomized mice are more sensitive to induction of lung tumors than intact mice.

Although polyoma virus may infect cell lines and produce tumors in inoculated mice, hamsters, and guinea pigs, its occurrence as a natural infection is unlikely.

References

Bittner JJ. Some possible effects of nursing on the mammary gland tumor incidence in mice. Science. 1936, 84:162.

Brayton C. Spontaneous Diseases in Commonly Used Mouse Strains. In: The Mouse in Biomedical Research, 2d ed. Diseases. Fox JG, Barthold SW, Davisson MT, Newcomer CE, Quimby FW, Smith AL (eds.). Burlington, MA: Academic Press, 2007, 623–717.

Ceccarelli AV, et al. Outbreak of hindlimb paralysis in young CFW Swiss Webster mice. Comp Med. 2002, 52:171–175.

Crispens CG. Handbook on the Laboratory Mouse. Springfield, IL: Charles C. Thomas, 1975.

Dunn TB. Morphology of Mammary Tumors in Mice. In: Pathophysiology of Cancer. Homburger F (ed.). New York: Harper (Hoeber), 1959.

———. Normal and pathologic anatomy of the reticular tissue of laboratory mice, with a classification and discussion of neoplasms. J Nat Cancer Inst. 1954, 19:1281–1433.

Frith CH. Histiocytic Sarcoma, Mouse. In: Monographs on Pathology of Laboratory Animals: Hematopoietic System. Jones TC, Ward JM, Mohr U, Hunt RD (eds.). New York: Springer-Verlag, 1990; 58–65.

Frith CH, Ward JM. Color Atlas of Neoplastic and Non-Neoplastic Lesions in Aging Mice. New York: Elsevier, 1988.

———. A morphologic classification of proliferative and neoplastic hepatic lesions in mice. J Environ Pathol Toxicol. 1980, 3:329–351.

Frith CH, Ward JM, Chandra M. The morphologic, immunohistochemistry, and incidence of hematopoietic neoplasms in mice and rats. Toxicol Pathol. 1993, 21:206–218.

Hoger H, Gialamas J, Jelinek F. Multiple osteomas in mice. Vet Pathol. 1994, 31:429–434.

Krueger GRF. Lymphoblastic Lymphoma, Mouse. In: Monographs on Pathology of Laboratory Animals: Hematopoietic System. Jones TC, Ward JM, Mohr U, Hunt RD (eds.). New York: Springer-Verlag, 1990; 264–275.

Maronpot RR (ed.). Pathology of the Mouse. Vienna, IL: Cache River Press, 1999.

Riley V. Mouse mammary tumors: alteration of incidence as apparent function of stress. Science. 1975, 189:465–467.

Sundberg JP, et al. Myoepitheliomas in inbred laboratory mice. Vet Pathol. 1991, 28:313–323.

Neoplasia in the Rat

As with the mouse and other rodents, the incidence of spontaneous neoplasia in the rat varies with the age, sex, strain, diet, caloric intake, endocrine factors, and environmental circumstances of the population surveyed. Incidence of neoplasia in rats is up to 87% in select rat populations older than 2 years of age. The most common tumor in the rat is the mammary fibroadenoma, followed by pituitary adenomas and testicular interstitial cell adenomas (Leydig cell tumors). Tumors reported less often include uterine endometrial polyps, malignant lymphomas, mononuclear cell leukemias, histiocytic sarcomas, fibrosarcomas, Zymbal's gland tumor, thyroid adenomas, and hemangiosarcomas. Polyoma virus infections do not occur naturally in rats. Fischer rat large granular leukemia is a major cause of death in aging inbred F344 rats. Clinical signs include weight loss, anemia, jaundice, and depression. The liver and spleen are markedly enlarged at necropsy. This strain is also highly susceptible to mesothelioma and interstitial cell tumors.

Mammary neoplasms are most often benign fibroadenomas and are common in female Sprague-Dawley rats. Adenocarcinomas comprise less than 10% of mammary tumors in the aged female rat. Benign mammary tumors, seen occasionally in males, are usually single and may grow to 8 or 10 cm in diameter. Mammary fibroadenomas are well demarcated, ovoid or discoid, firm, and nodular. Size, growth rate, color, and consistency vary. Larger mammary tumors of rats may become ulcerated, hemorrhagic, and necrotic. The tumor is well tolerated by the host until the mass hinders locomotion or a septicemia or toxemia results from the ulceration and necrosis. Rats with large tumors will eventually lose weight and die. The encapsulated tumors may be removed surgically, but they recur frequently in another mammary gland. Care should be taken to ligate the large vessels entering the mass. Because mammary tissue is distributed widely in the subcutis of murine rodents, mammary tumors may be found behind the shoulders, on the neck, on the ventral abdomen and flank, or around the tail base. Spaying female rats will reduce the incidence of tumor development. The tumors are prolactin-responsive and may develop in the presence of a pituitary adenoma.

Pituitary gland neoplasms occur frequently in older female rats, particularly those on diets high in protein or calories. Chromophobe adenomas, the most common type of pituitary tumors, are soft, nonsecreting, and well circumscribed with irregular surfaces. Compression of brain tissue from chromophobe adenomas may cause hydrocephalus, head tilt, depression, and a variety of other clinical signs.

Lymphosarcoma and histiocytic sarcoma are seen with high frequency in aged animals. Lymphosarcomas tend to be multicentric, involving the mesenteric lymph nodes and spleen with terminal leukemia and neoplastic seeding of the hepatic parenchyma.

Other types of tumors occur spontaneously but are sporadic in nature.

References

Boorman SL, et al. (eds.). Pathology of the Fischer Rat: Reference and Atlas. San Diego: Academic Press, 1990.

Bresnahan JF, Wagner JE. Nephroblastoma with associated aortic rupture in a rat. Lab Anim Sci. 1982, 32:169–170.

Canton WW, Gries CL. Adenoma and Carcinoma, Pars Distalis, Rat. In: Monographs on Pathology of Laboratory Animals, Endocrine System. Jones TC, Mohr U, Hunt RD (eds.). New York: Springer-Verlag, 1986; 134–145.

———. Adenoma, Pars Intermedia, Anterior Pituitary, Rat. In: Monographs on Pathology of Laboratory Animals: Endocrine System. Jones TC, Mohr U, Hunt RD (eds.). New York: Springer-Verlag, 1986; 145–149.

Coleman GL, et al. Pathological changes during aging in barrier-reared Fischer 344 male rats. J Gerontol. 1977, 32:258–278.

Goodman DG, et al. Neoplastic and nonneoplastic lesions in aging F344 rats. Toxicol Appl Pharmacol. 1979, 48:237–248.

———. Neoplastic and nonneoplastic lesions in aging Osborne-Mendel rats. Toxicol Appl Pharmacol. 1980, 55:433–447.

Kaspareit-Rittinghausen J, Deerberg F. Spontaneous tumours of the spinal cord in laboratory rats. J Comp Pathol. 1989, 100:209–215.

MacKenzie WF, Garner FM. Comparison of neoplasms in six sources of rats. J Nat Cancer Inst. 1973, 50:1243–1257.

Pickering RG, Pickering CE. The effect of diet on the incidence of pituitary tumours in female Wistar rats. Lab Anim. 1984, 18:298–314.

Pollard M, Luckert PH. Spontaneous liver tumors in aged germfree Wistar rats. Lab Anim Sci. 1979, 29:74–77.

Rosol TJ, Stromberg PC. Effects of large granular lymphocytic leukemia on bone in F344 rats. Vet Pathol. 1990, 27:391–396.

Russo J, et al. Classification of Neoplastic and Nonneoplastic Lesions of the Rat Mammary Gland. In: Monographs on Pathology of Laboratory Animals: Integument and Mammary Glands. Jones TC, Mohr U, Hunt RD (eds.). New York: Springer-Verlag, 1989; 275–304.

Stromberg PC, et al. Behaviour of transplanted large granular lymphocytic leukemia in Fischer 344 rats. Lab Invest. 1985, 53:200–207.

———. Spleen cell population changes and hemolytic anemia in F344 rats with large granular lymphocytic leukemia. Vet Pathol. 1990, 27:397–403.

Troyer H, et al. Leydig cell tumor induced hypercalcemia in the Fischer rat. Am J Pathol. 1982, 108:284–290.

Turusov VS, et al. (eds.). Pathology of Tumours in Laboratory Animals, vol. 1, part 2. Tumours of the Rat. Lyon, France: International Agency for Research on Cancer, 1976.

Ward JM, Reynolds CW. Large granular lymphatic leukemia. A heterogeneous lymphocytic leukemia in F344 rats. Am J Pathol. 1983, 111:1–10.

NEPHROSIS

Hosts

Chronic progressive renal disease is an important cause of morbidity and is common in most small mammal species. The incidence may approach 25% or more. The disease may be quite variable clinically and the most common presentations are described below.

Etiology

The specific etiologies of the chronic renal diseases in these species have not been determined fully and the causes likely differ by species. When evaluating azotemia in these species, it is important to determine whether the origin is prerenal, renal, or postrenal in nature, prior to planning a therapeutic course of action. Primary renal disease is seen more frequently in aged males and the severity is often strain-dependent. Inappropriate diet, ad libitum feeding practices with secondary obesity, excessive protein content, mineral imbalances, high-carbohydrate diets, and infectious processes such as bacterial pyelonephritis have all been suggested as factors in the pathogenesis of the disease. Microscopically, lesions suggestive of renal degeneration can be seen as early as 8 weeks of age in some strains of rats and mice. In many small mammals with renal disease, the clinical signs are inapparent until the renal disease is quite advanced. Polyuria and polydipsia are often present but may be difficult to detect in an individual if animals are group-housed or deeply bedded.

The earliest detectable serum chemistry change in rats with primary renal disease is hypoalbuminemia. Blood urea nitrogen and creatinine levels may remain near normal until kidney failure is imminent. Histologically, it is reported that tubular basophilia indicative of proliferation is seen prior to glomerular changes, suggesting that the condition in rats has both a degenerative and regenerative aspect. Both diet-induced and spontaneous nephrocalcinosis is also seen in rats and consists of calcium phosphate deposits within the interstitium and tubules. Hydronephrosis, pyelonephritis, neoplasia, and obstructive nephropathy due to the presence of calculi or protein plugs in the urethra of male rats have all been reported as potential underlying causes of renal failure in rats.

A large percentage of aging Syrian hamsters demonstrate amyloid deposition within the glomerular basement membranes, in addition to other tissues. The condition is more severe in females. Hamsters may also develop polycystic disease, neoplasia, and a glomerulonephropathy similar to rats.

Urolithiasis is a common cause of renal disease in guinea pigs and chinchillas. Like rabbits, the calculi can be found anywhere within the renal system, including the renal pelvis. Clinical signs are dependent upon the location of the urolith, and animals may show lethargy, anorexia, hunched posture, and bruxism. Metastatic calcification, often iatrogenic in origin from feeding rabbit chow or inappropriate vitamin supplementation, is a common cause of renal failure in guinea pigs. Similarly, segmental nephrosclerosis, amyloidosis, or pyelonephritis may underlie kidney problems in this species. Bacterial cystitis is more common in female guinea pigs, likely because of the shorter urethra.

Interstitial nephritis and glomerulonephropathies are common renal lesions in various strains of aging mice. Amyloid deposition may also be seen in the kidneys and may be either primary (familial) or secondary (related to chronic inflammatory lesions). Amyloid is an insoluble protein and deposition leads to progressive disease and renal failure. Glomeruli are irreversibly damaged by amyloid deposition, leading to decreased filtration and chronic renal disease. Certain strains of mice such as the MRL, New Zealand black, and New Zealand white strains and their hybrids may commonly develop an autoimmune renal failure.

Renal disease also occurs in rabbits. In younger animals, infectious causes are more commonly diagnosed, for example, coliform- or *Pasteurella*-induced pyelonephritis, whereas in older animals the condition has a more degenerative appearance, with fibrosis and mineralization noted. Calcium-predominant uroliths may be found within the renal pelvises as well as within the lower urinary tract, and in severe cases, may induce obstruction.

Transmission

These diseases are not contagious.

Predisposing Factors

Laboratory rats on conventional laboratory diets have a high incidence of chronic renal disease. Nephrosis in conventionally housed rats is evident at 3–6 months of age. Renal changes are delayed and reduced in germ-free rats. Predisposing factors include advancing age; male sex; strain (e.g., a higher incidence is seen in Sprague-Dawley rats); diets high in certain proteins, carbohydrates, and calories or low in potassium; and immunologic characteristics of the strain.

Some strains of hamsters are more susceptible to amyloidosis than are others, and age and female sex are major predisposing factors in this species.

Clinical Signs

Chronic renal disease is usually subclinical and often is only detected at necropsy. In severe cases, usually in older animals, it is a major life-limiting disease. Affected animals progressively lose weight, become inactive, and die. A pronounced proteinuria (mostly albumin) appears in affected rats. Polyuria may appear in hamsters, guinea pigs, chinchillas, rabbits, and mice. Mice with autoimmune nephrosis may also have anemia and generalized edema.

Necropsy Signs

Chronic renal disease is by definition a bilateral nephrosis in which the kidneys may be enlarged in the earlier stages, small in more advanced stages; discolored, brown to pale tan to yellow; nodular with a granular or pitted surface; and have radial, pale striations on cut sections. The capsule may be difficult to peel back from the cortical surface because of multifocal cortical adhesions.

Histologic changes include tubular dilatation with proteinaceous or mineralized casts within the lumen, thickening of the mesangium by protein deposition with synechial formation between the glomerular tufts and Bowman's capsule, interstitial fibrosis with leukocytic infiltrate, and tubular atrophy and regeneration. Glomeruli may become sclerosed and shrunken in advanced disease. In hamsters, guinea pigs, and mice, amyloid is deposited on basement membranes and in the glomerular mesangium. Amyloid may be demonstrated with a differential stain (Congo red) and polarized light (apple green birefringence).

Diagnosis

Diagnosis of nephrosis is based on gross and microscopic lesions as described and on clinical signs. Clinical chemistry (BUN, creatinine) may not be useful in the early stages of the disease. Urinalysis may demonstrate an isosthenuric specific gravity and marked proteinuria.

Treatment

There is no treatment for this condition beyond palliative care. Animals should be provided with supplemental fluids and the diet should be modified. Potassium binding agents and low-protein/low-potassium diets may offer palliative support, and iron supplementation should be provided if anemia is present. Any underlying disease processes, for example, urolithaiasis or infections, should be treated, as appropriate.

Prevention

Ensuring a species-appropriate diet is fed and that the amount of diet fed is not excessive are important preventatives. Ad libitum access to potable water is important for these species, to prevent dehydration.

Rabbit and rodent salt wheels can be provided to encourage water consumption.

References

Alt JM, et al. Proteinuria in rats in relation to age-dependent renal changes. Lab Anim. 1980, 14:95–101.

Bras G. Age-associated kidney lesions in the rat. J Infect Dis. 1969, 120:131–135.

Fisher PG. Exotic mammal renal disease: causes and clinical presentation. Vet Clin Exot Anim. 2006, 9:33–67.

Gleiser CA, et al. Amyloidosis and renal paramyloid in a closed hamster colony. Lab Anim Sci. 1971, 21:197–202.

Hard GC, Khan KN. A contemporary overview of chronic progressive nephropathy in the laboratory rat, and its significance for human risk assessment. Toxicol Pathol. 2004, 32:171–180.

Hinton, M. Kidney disease in the rabbit: a histological survey. Lab Anim. 1981, 15:263–265.

Hubbard GB, Schmidt RE. Noninfectious Diseases. In: Laboratory Hamsters. Van Hoosier GL, Jr, McPherson CW (eds.). Orlando: Academic Press, 1987; 169–178.

Murphy JC, Fox JG, Niemi SH. Nephrotic syndrome associated with renal amyloidosis in a colony of Syrian hamsters. J Am Vet Med Assoc. 1984, 185:1359–1362.

Van Marck EAE, et al. Spontaneous glomerular basement membrane changes in the golden Syrian hamster (Mesocricetus auratus): a light and electron microscope study. Lab Anim. 1978, 12:207–211.

Weaver RN, Gray JE, Schultz JR. Urinary proteins in Sprague-Dawley rats with chronic progressive nephrosis. Lab Anim Sci. 1975, 25:705–710.

OXYURIASIS (PINWORMS)

Hosts

Pinworms, host-specific oxyurid nematodes that inhabit the intestinal tract, are common among vertebrate hosts, including several small mammal species. They have not been reported in guinea pigs or chinchillas.

Etiology

Passalurus ambiguus occurs in rabbits, cottontails, and hares. *Syphacia obvelata* occurs in mice and other rodents, including hamsters. *Syphacia muris* occurs in rats and other rodents. *Syphacia mesocriceti* occurs in hamsters. *Aspiculuris tetraptera* occurs in mice and other rodents. *Dentostomella translucida* occurs in gerbils.

Pinworms are commensal, mildly or nonpathogenic, ubiquitous, bacteria-feeding roundworms often seen by the dozens in the lower intestinal tract of rabbits and rodents. Pinworms have a direct life cycle. *Syphacia* spp have a prepatent period (duration of time from ingestion of ova to the appearance of ova in the feces) of 8–15 days, whereas *Aspiculuris* spp require approximately 23 days.

Transmission

Hosts are infected by ingesting embryonated ova in feces; fecal-contaminated feed, water, or debris; or through ingestion of ova adhering to the perianal skin (*Syphacia* spp only). *Aspiculuris* spp and *Passalurus* spp ova are passed in the feces; embryonation of *Aspiculuris* spp ova requires 6 days outside of the host. *Syphacia* spp ova on the perianal skin embryonate within a few hours of deposition, and retrograde infection may occur. Pinworm ova are light and are aerosolized easily. Typical sentinel monitoring programs detect only heavy ova burdens, and infections may remain undetected within a colony.

Predisposing Factors

Animals with diminished resistance are more susceptible to pinworm infections. Intestinal pinworm populations vary with the host's age and sex. In enzootically infected colonies, *Syphacia* spp numbers plateau in 5- to 6-week-old animals and then diminish as the host ages and develops immunity. *Aspiculuris* spp populations increase to a plateau when the host reaches approximately 10 weeks of age. Male hosts are generally more heavily parasitized by pinworms than are females, and worm populations vary with the composition of the intestinal microflora and among inbred strains. For example, DBA/2 mice are highly susceptible, whereas C3H mice are more resistant.

Clinical Signs

Clinical signs related directly to oxyuriasis are observed uncommonly even in hosts harboring dozens to hundreds of worms. Reported signs include diminished weight gains, decreased activity, rectal prolapse, and self-mutilation of the tail base from rectal irritation associated with severe *Syphacia* spp infections. Impaction, intussusception, increased stickiness of fecal pellets, and reproductive depression have also been reported. *Passalurus* spp nematodes are nonpathogenic for rabbits.

Necropsy Signs

Necropsy signs of pinworm infection are rare and are limited to intussusception and catarrhal enteritis. The small, adult worms are visible in the intestinal contents at the site of gastrointestinal infestation and eggs are typically seen in close association with the mucosa; *Syphacia* spp in the cecum and colon; *Aspiculuris* spp and *Passalurus* spp in the anterior colon and cecum; and *Dentostomella* spp in the small intestine. Larval forms (Figure 5.12) of mouse pinworms are frequently found at the base of mucosal glands near the rectum. Pinworms are confined to the intestinal lumen except for rare reported cases of penetration through the intestinal epithelium by *Aspiculuris* spp larvae. Histologically, there may be mild colonic inflammation. Characteristic profiles of the nematodes are seen commonly in the lumen of the cecum or colon when sections of these organs are examined microscopically.

Diagnosis

Diagnosis of oxyuriasis depends on finding the adult nematodes in the small intestine, cecum, or colon; finding ova in the feces; or, in the case of *Syphacia* spp, finding eggs or adult worms on cellophane tape pressed to the perianal skin. *Aspiculuris* spp and *Passalurus* spp do not deposit ova around the anus.

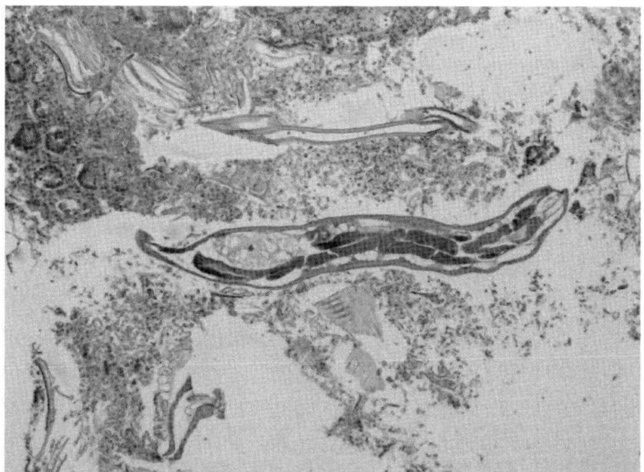

FIGURE 5.12. Photomicrograph of a pinworm larva within the cecum of a rat.

Adult worms range in length from 1 to 1.5 mm for *Syphacia* spp males to 11 mm for *Passalurus* spp females. Females are much longer than males for all species. Most are between 2 and 4 mm long with a tapered shape and pointed ends, thus the common name "pinworms." *Syphacia obvelata* ova are ellipsoidal (banana-shaped), approximately 120–150 um × 35–50 um, and somewhat flattened on one side. *Aspiculuris* spp ova are symmetrical and football-shaped. Adult worms and ova can be seen in fecal smears, but this method has limitations because worms in the cecum and large intestine lay ova in boluses and then die. Ova may be seen in cecal floation, cecal concentration preparations, fecal flotation, and fecal concentration preparations, as well as in histologic section. Perianal impressions on cellophane tape may be used for *Syphacia* spp detection. All methods are equally useful for detection of pinworms, although histology may be a more sensitive technique following pinworm eradication.

Treatment

Although numerous treatment regimens have been reported, treatment alone usually results in only a transient elimination of the intestinal nematodes. It is imperative that treatment of the environment occur concurrently. All chemicals used to treat pinworm infections may induce altered behavioral effects, may alter reproduction, or may induce toxicity in new strains of genetically engineered animals, particularly those with blood-brain barrier defects. For new colonies, it may be prudent to first test these drugs on a small number of animals to ensure safety.

Fenbendazole has been used with success to eliminate pinworms from rabbits and rodents. Diets containing fenbendazole may be irradiated but should not be autoclaved, as the compound is not heat stable. For rabbits, fenbendazole in the feed for 5 days at either 25 ppm or 50 ppm eliminated internal parasite infestation and was well tolerated by the animals. The addition of fenbendazole may alter feeding intake in rats.

In mice and rats, fenbendazole at 150 ppm in the food has continued to be a successful treatment to eradicate pinworms. This chemical is generally used in a "week on–week off" rotation for at least 3 cycles (i.e., minimum 6-week treatment plan).

Topical administration of ivermectin in a 0.01% spray solution misted over the animals is reported to be effective at eliminating pinworm infections in mice. No more than 1 mL of this dilute spray should be administered to each animal, and this treatment is not suitable for suckling mice. Topical selamectin at 0.6 or 6.0 mg/kg was reported to be ineffective against pinworm infections in mice and rats.

Piperazine as a 34% solution administered in the water is effective at eliminating pinworms. Animals are treated on a "week on–week off" basis for at least 3 cycles.

Prevention

Prevention and eradication of pinworm infection in rabbits and rodents can be extremely difficult. Bedding dusts and wild rodents should be reduced and eliminated. Filter tops should be used, and cages, rooms, and air ducts should be cleaned frequently. Quarantine should be initiated for animals with unknown health histories. Higher fiber diets are reported to reduce worm populations. Two percent peracetic acid or formaldehyde vapor treatments may not kill all pinworm ova in the environment, whereas hydrogen peroxide vapor may be effective at killing some egg forms.

The ovicidal effects of heat and a variety of chemical disinfectants were tested on ova of *Syphacia muris*. Seventy percent ethanol and heating at 80 °C for 30 minutes were the two most effective treatments for killing ova.

Impact on Research

Rats infected with pinworms may weigh 11–12% less than uninfected rats and may not be suitable for nutrition studies because infected rats do not have the growth potential of animals free of parasites. Studies that use organ weight relative to body weight data may introduce systematic error in calculations when infected animals are used. Although they are generally suspected to be largely nonpathogenic, pinworms may induce myelopoiesis or erythropoiesis and alter other cytokine and immune functions.

Public Health Significance

Humans are a dead-end host for these parasites.

References

Bugarski D, Jovcic G, Katic-Radivojevic S, et al. Hematopoietic changes and altered reactivity to IL-17 in Syphacia obvelata-infected mice. Parasitol Int. 2006, 55(2):91–97.

Coghian LG, et al. Practical and effective eradication of pinworms (Syphacia muris) in rats by use of fenbendazole. Lab Anim Sci. 1993, 43:481–487.

Dick TA, Quentin JC, Freeman RS. Redescription of Syphacia mesocriceti (Nematodai oxyuroidea) parasite of the golden hamster. J Parasitol. 1973, 59:256–259.

Duwel D, Brech K. Control of oxyuriasis in rabbits by fenbendazole. Lab Anim. 1981, 15:101–105.

Effler JC, Hickman-Davis JM, Erwin JG, et al. Comparison of methods for detection of pinworms in mice and rats. Lab Anim. 2008, 37(5):210–215.

Flynn BM, et al. Treatment of Syphacia obvelata in mice using ivermectin. Lab Anim Sci. 1989, 39:461–463.

Habermann RT, Williams FP, Jr. Treatment of female mice and their litters with piperazine adipate in the drinking water. Lab Anim Care. 1963, 13:41–45.

HamLen HJ, Kargas SA, Blum JR. Ivermectin overdose in a group of laboratory mice. Contemp Top Lab Anim Sci. 1994, 33:49–51.

Hill WA, Randolph MM, Lokey SJ, et al. Efficacy and safety of topical selamectin to eradicate pinworm (Syphacia spp.) infections in rats (Rattus norvegicus) and mice (Mus musculus). J Amer Assoc Lab Anim Sci. 2006, 45(3):23–26.

Huerkamp MJ. Ivermectin eradication of pinworms from rats kept in ventilated cages. Lab Anim Sci. 1993, 43:86–90.

Kerrick GP, Hoskins DE, Ringler DH. Eradication of pinworms from rats by using ivermectin in the drinking water. Contemp Top Lab Anim Sci. 1995, 34(2):78–79.

LeBlanc SA, Faith RE, Montgomery CA. Use of topical ivermectin treatment for Syphacia obvelata in mice. Lab Anim Sci. 1993, 43:526–528.

McNair DM, Timmons EH. Effects of Aspiculuris tetraptera and Syphacia obvelata on exploratory behavior of an inbred mouse strain. Lab Anim Sci. 1977, 27:38–42.

Miyaji S, Kamiya M, Shikata J. Ovicidal effect of heat and disinfectants on Syphacia muris estimated by in vitro hatching. Exp Anim. 1988, 37:399–404.

Mohn G, Phillip E-M. Effects of Syphacia muris and the anthelmintic fenbendazole on the microsomal

monooxygenase system in mouse liver. Lab Anim. 1981, 15:89–95.
Mullink, JWMA. Pathological effects of oxyuriasis in the laboratory mouse. Lab Anim. 1970, 4:197–201.
Owen D, Turton JA. Eradication of the pinworm Syphacia obvelata from an animal unit by anthelmintic therapy. Lab Anim. 1979, 13:115–118.
Pritchett KR, Johnston NA. A review of treatments for the eradication of pinworm infections from laboratory rodent colonies. Contemp Top Lab Anim Sci. 2002, 41(2):36–46.
Ross CR, et al. Experimental transmission of Syphacia muris among rats, mice, hamsters, and gerbils. Lab Anim Sci. 1980, 30:35–37.
Sueta T, Miyoshi I, Okamura T, et al. Experimental eradication of pinworms (Syphacia obvelata and Aspiculuris tetraptera) from mice colonies using ivermectin. Exp Anim. 2002, 51(4):367–373.
Taylor DM. Eradication of pinworms (Syphacia obvelata) from Syrian hamsters in quarantine. Lab Anim Sci. 1992, 42:413–414.
Vento PJ, Swartz ME, Martin LBE, et al. Food intake in laboratory rats provided standard and fenbendazole-supplemented diets. J Amer Assoc Lab Anim Sci. 2008, 47:46–50.
Villar D, et al. Biologic effects of fenbendazole in rats and mice: a review. J Amer Assoc Lab Anim Sci. 2007, 46:8–15.
Wagner M. The effect of infection with the pinworm (Syphacia muris) on rat growth. Lab Anim Sci. 1988, 38:476–478.
Wescott RB, Malczewski A, Van Hoosier, GL. The influence of filter top caging on the transmission of pinworm infections in mice. Lab Anim Sci. 1976, 26:742–745.

PARVOVIRUS INFECTIONS

Hosts

Parvoviruses have been identified in mice, rats, hamsters, and rabbits.

Etiology

Parvoviruses are small, nonenveloped, single-stranded DNA viruses that only replicate in rapidly dividing cell populations, such as those found in gut, skin, and lymphoid tissue. Compared with other domestic animals such as dogs and cats, parvoviral infections of rodents spare the gastrointestinal tract, and the disease is generally subclinical. In rabbits, a very mild enteritis has been produced following experimental infection, and the infection is likely subclinical under natural conditions. Therefore, this virus is not clinically important in pet practice.

Laboratory mice are frequently infected with parvoviruses of two closely related serotypes, mouse minute virus (MMV) and mouse parvovirus (MPV), each representing a family of distinct viral strains. The prime target tissues for viral receptors for both virus types are the small intestine, endothelial cells, and lymphoid tissue. MMV is transmissible to other rodents, particularly hamsters. Infant mice are more permissive hosts to MMV infection than adult mice.

Similarly, numerous strains of rat parvoviruses have been identified to date, including RV, H-1 virus, RPV-1a, minute virus (RMV-1a, -1b, -1c), and so forth. Only RV infection has been associated with clinical signs in rats, whereas the other viruses produce subclinical infections.

Parvoviruses have been identified and characterized in rabbits and hamsters, although this has not been an area of active research in recent years. Based on PCR evaluation, the hamster parvovirus is closely related to the mouse parvovirus MPV-1.

Transmission

Parvoviruses are thought to be transmitted by oral or nasal exposure. Recent studies evaluating MPV infectivity when transferring embryos, gametes (sperm and oocytes), and ovarian tissue from infected mice demonstrate a high rate of MPV infectivity (up to 68%) in pups following transfer. The viruses can also be transmitted via virus-contaminated mouse tissues, tumor lines, and various biologics.

Predisposing Factors

Parvoviruses are capable of infecting both juvenile and adult animals and immune competency is not a factor in terms of susceptibility to viral infection, although it may be important in viral clearance.

Clinical Signs

In mice, infection with MPV or MMV is generally subclinical even in immunodeficient animals, but immunomodulatory effects may occur that can interfere with the research objectives. The virus requires mitotically active cells and targets specific tissues by means of viral receptors. Experimental inoculation of newborn mice with MMV resulted in runting and cerebellar hypoplasia. MMV tends to cause a self-limiting infection in which the virus is cleared within approximately 1 month postinfection, whereas MPV may induce a chronic persistent infection. Both MMV and MPV may affect immune function in adult mice, and MPV replicates equally effectively in adult mice.

RV infection of rats can cause fetal resorption in pregnant animals, neonatal cerebellar hypoplasia with ataxia, hepatitis, steatorrhea, and jaundice. Hemorrhagic diathesis may be seen in adults, with cerebral and peritesticular hemorrhage; however, clinical signs are usually absent. Dental deformities and mortality have occurred in young hamsters post-exposure to Toolan's H-1 virus. Newborn hamsters inoculated with MMV displayed craniofacial lesions, periodontal disease, and death. Dental deformities, domed calvaria, cerebral mineralization, and testicular atrophy have been noted in hamsters exposed to hamster parvovirus, but the disease was confined to suckling and weanling animals.

Necropsy Signs

In mice, MMV infection may induce hemorrhagic lesions following virus-associated damage to endothelium as well as thrombocytopenia. Hepatitis and splenitis have been reported following experimental inoculation of animals with intranuclear inclusion bodies in hepatocytes. RV infection of rats may cause focal hepatitis, periorchitis, and cerebellar hypoplasia with loss of the external granular cell layer.

Diagnosis

Early serologic tests for MPV were based on hemagglutination inhibition assays, which detect antibodies to structural antigens (e.g., capsid proteins). Because the structural antigens for MPV and MMV are markedly different, MPV was not detected by these assays. When immunofluorescence assays were developed for viral identification, which use antigens to nonstructural proteins, MPV was subsequently detected, because the nonstructural proteins are almost identical between MPV and MMV. Antibody typically forms against the structural proteins, and thus humoral immunity to one virus is likely not cross-protective to other strains. MPV may not be detectable from all strains of mice (e.g., DBA). PCR of fecal pellets and mesenteric lymph nodes identifies mice with active infections. Males may be more sensitive for use in sentinel monitoring. As with MPV, RPV does not share structural antigens with RV, H-1, or RMV.

Serology and PCR or immunohistochemistry of mesenteric lymph nodes are sensitive means to detect active parvoviral infections. Detection is difficult in cryptic infections. These infections occur when the virus infects a nonactively dividing cell. The virus remains dormant until the cell begins to divide, allowing the virus to be propagated. Seroconversion to rat parvovirus (RV) and Toolan's H-1 virus has been observed in hamsters.

Treatment

There is no treatment for parvovirus infections. MMV and RV infections are generally short-lived and the viruses are cleared from the system, if the animal survives infection. RV may cause persistent infections in young animals born to nonimmune dams. MPV often causes chronic, latent infections.

Because they are nonenveloped, parvoviruses can survive temperature extremes and can only be destroyed in the environment following lengthy exposure to caustic viricides, bleach solutions, and ultraviolet radiation.

Prevention

Routine use of dirty bedding sentinel systems for virus detection is not an efficient means of detecting parvoviruses in mouse and rat colonies, as viral shedding may be low in infected animals. Despite this, the technique remains the most common method for evaluation of infections with low prevalence. Care must be used when designing these programs to ensure that sensitive strains of animals are used as sentinels, that they are an appropriate age for infection, and that bedding exposure programs are set at optimal intervals to maximize detection. Biologics and cell lines must be screened for microbiologic contamination prior to use in vivo.

Impact on Research

Parvoviruses induce immunomodulatory effects and thus potentially may interfere with many research models, e.g., diabetes, multiple sclerosis, cancer, neurodegenerative disease, infectious disease, and immunologic studies. MMV may suppress bone marrow progenitor cells with chronic infection.

References

Agka Y, et al. Detection of mouse parvovirus in Mus musculus gametes, embryos and ovarian tissue by polymerase chain reaction assay. Comp Med. 2007, 57:51–56.

Besselsen DG, Besch-Williford CL, Pintel DG, et al. Detection of newly recognized rodent parvoviruses by PCR. J Clin Microbiol. 1995, 33:2859–2863.

Besselsen, DG, et al. Effect of mouse strain and age on detection of mouse parvovirus 1 by use of serologic testing and polymerase chain reaction analysis. Comp Med. 2000, 50(5):498–502.

———. Transmission probabilities of mouse parvovirus 1 to sentinel mice chronically exposed to serial dilutions of contaminated bedding. Comp Med. 2008, 58:140–144.

Coleman GL, et al. Naturally occurring lethal parvovirus infection of juvenile and young adult rats. Vet Pathol. 1983, 20:49–56.

Gaertner, DJ, et al. Persistent rat virus infection in juvenile athymic rats and its modulation by immune serum. Lab Anim Sci. 1995, 45:249–253.

Hansen GM, Paturzo FX, Smith AL. Humoral immunity and protection of mice challenged with homotypic or heterotypic parvovirus. Lab Anim Sci. 1999, 49:380–384.

Jacoby RO, et al. Prevalence of rat virus infection in progeny of acutely or persistently infected pregnant rats. Comp Med. 2001, 51:38–42.

———. Special topic overview: rodent parvovirus infections. Lab Anim Sci. 1996, 46:370–380.

Kilham L, Margolis G. Fetal infections of hamsters, rats and mice induced with minute virus of mice (MVM). Teratol. 1971, 4:43–62.

Matsunaga Y, Chino F. Experimental infection of young rabbits with rabbit parvovirus. Arch Virol. 1981, 68:257–264.

Matsunaga Y, Matsuno S, Mukoyama J. Isolation and characterization of a parvovirus of rabbits. Infect Immun. 1977, 18(2):495–500.

McKisic MD, et al. Mouse parvovirus infection potentiates rejection of tumor allografts and modulates T cell effector functions. Transplant. 1996, 61:292–299.

Redig AJ, Besselsen DG. Detection of rodent parvoviruses by fluorogenic nuclease polymerase chain reaction. Comp Med. 2001, 51:326–331.

Segovia JC, et al. Parvovirus infection suppresses longterm repopulation of hematopoietic stem cells. J Virol. 2003, 77:8495–8503.

———. Severe leukopenia and dysregulated erythropoiesis in SCID mice persistently infected with parvovirus minute virus of mice. J Virol. 1999, 73:1774–1784.

Smith P, et al. Reliability for soiled bedding transfer for detection of mouse parvovirus and mouse hepatitis virus. Comp Med. 2007, 57:90–96.

Thomas ML, et al. Gender influences infectivity of C57BL/6 mice exposed to mouse minute virus. Comp Med. 2007, 57:74–81.

Wan C-H, et al. Molecular characterization of three newly recognized rat parvoviruses. J Gen Virol. 2002, 83:2075–2083.

PASTEURELLA MULTOCIDA INFECTIONS

Hosts

Pasteurella multocida induces significant disease in rabbits, but rodents, birds, and farm animals may also be infected by this common animal pathogen. In commercial operations, pasteurellosis may account for mortalities of up to 15–20% in young fryers.

Etiology

Pasteurella multocida is a small, Gram-negative, bipolar staining, coccobacillus bacterium. Colonies on blood agar vary substantially and are considered mucoid, smooth, or rough. Several somatic:capsular serotypes occur in rabbits, with types 3:A, 12:A, and 12:D among the more common. Capsular type A bacteria produce a necrolytic and osteolytic toxin that induces atrophic rhinitis in swine and rabbits. Within rabbitries and colonies, *Pasteurella multocida* isolates are uniform, but between colonies isolates vary.

Significant differences exist in the virulence of various *P. multocida* isolates from rabbits. Some strains predictably cause fatal septicemia, whereas others induce chronic forms of rabbit pasteurellosis such as snuffles.

Transmission

The bacterium is transmitted by direct contact between cagemates, a chronically infected doe and her litter, or between breeding pairs. In breeding operations, the primary means of transmission is between the doe and her kits. Neonates may be infected in the vaginal passage, during nursing, and from contaminated sipper tubes. Maternal antibodies to *P. multocida* persist in young to 6 weeks of age but are not protective. Transmission by respiratory aerosol occurs over short distances, but noninfected rabbits housed in cages adjacent to *Pasteurella* spp shedders but without direct contact require weeks to months to develop culture-positive nasal infections.

Asymptomatic carriers of *P. multocida* are common, although rabbits used in biomedical research in North America are typically free of *P. multocida*. The organism resides in the nares, paranasal sinuses, tympanic bullae, conjunctiva, vagina, and lungs, where it elicits a minimal inflammatory response.

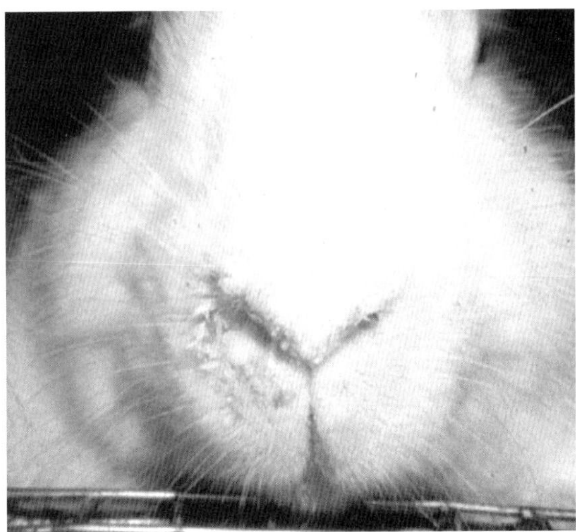

FIGURE 5.13. Pasteurellosis infection in a rabbit characterized by a mucopurulent rhinitis.

Predisposing Factors

The ubiquity of asymptomatic carriers and chronically diseased adult rabbits, the ease of transmission to the young by contact, the virulence of the organisms, and preexisting bacterial infections, such as *Bordetella bronchiseptica*, are factors that predispose to pasteurellosis. Environmental factors such as increased ammonia level, temperature fluctuations, drafts, and poor sanitation all contribute to the development of clinical pasteurellosis, as do the stresses of reproduction and older age.

Breed of rabbit and strain of the organism may affect predisposition to infection as well as severity of disease. The pathogenicity of *P. multocida* A:3 was compared in Flemish giant and New Zealand white rabbits. Flemish giants were much more severely affected than were New Zealand white rabbits, and the score of pneumonia and pleuritis was three times higher in Flemish giants. The pathogenesis of this difference was speculated to be due to greater depression of local immunity in Flemish giants in response to *P. multocida* infections.

Clinical Signs

Clinical signs of *P. multocida* infection range from inapparent, in carrier animals, to peracute death. Septicemia, chronic abscessation, and suppuration in adult rabbits are other signs of the disease. The primary locus of the infection can occur in almost any tissue or organ and spread by the blood to any other tissue or organ, although the nasopharnx and oropharynx are considered the most common primary sites. Abscessation in the liver is rarely caused by *P. multocida*.

Signs exhibited depend on the site of infection and may include nasal discharge (Figure 5.13), snuffling, runny eyes, torticollis or "wry neck" (head tilt), cutaneous ulceration, subcutaneous swelling, enlarged testes (abscesses), vaginal discharge, infertility, weight loss, and sudden or lingering death. Pneumonia has few clinical signs in rabbits.

Acute enzootic pneumonia is the most common clinical syndrome in young rabbits with *P. multocida* infections, whereas abscesses and suppuration occur more commonly in older animals. Neonates may die from a septicemia. Pulmonary impairment may cause cyanosis of the iris in albino breeds and a short, terminal period of dyspnea.

Necropsy Signs

Gross lesions of *P. multocida* infection may involve one or more of the following: generalized visceral congestion, sanguineous nasal discharge, and focal hemorrhages resulting from septicemia; well-demarcated reddish-gray foci of bronchopneumonia; diffuse fibrinopurulent pleuritis and pneumonia (Figure 5.14), and fibrinopurulent or mucopurulent

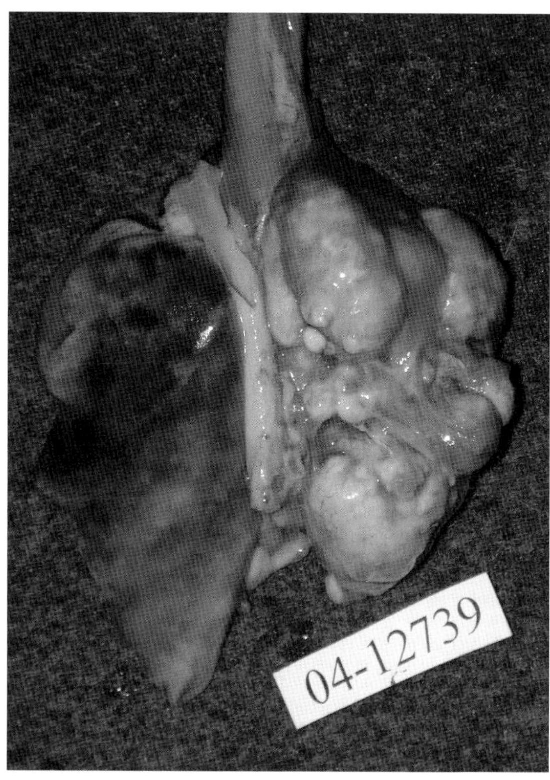

FIGURE 5.14. Lungs from an apparently normal rabbit that died acutely during anesthetic induction. This animal was harboring a subclinical *Pasteurella*-induced bronchopneumonia. Courtesy of Emily Martin.

reactions and abscesses in the meninges and brain (Figure 5.15), middle and inner ear, thoracic and abdominal viscera, nasal passages, subcutaneous tissues, bones, or the reproductive organs. Rabbit pus in a *P. multocida* abscess is characteristically creamy-white and thick.

Turbinate atrophy occurs in rabbits. It has been associated with both A and D types of *Pasteurella multocida* but not *B. bronchiseptica* infection.

Diagnosis

Diagnosis of *P. multocida* infection is based on the observation of clinical signs and on the isolation of the causative organism from blood or affected tissues. Nasal swab cultures can be somewhat unreliable as indicators of infection because some carrier animals may be culture-negative and carry the infection at a site other than the nares, such as the middle ears. In any case, a deep nasal culture taken 2–4 cm

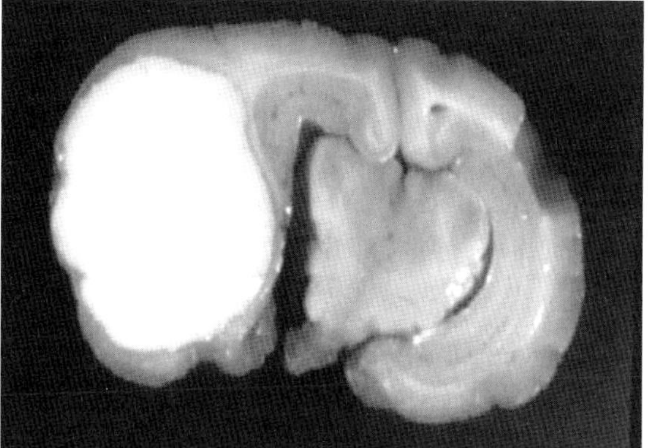

FIGURE 5.15. Brain abscess in a rabbit secondary to *Pasteurella multocida* infection.

into the median aspect of the nares is necessary to detect a nasal or pharyngeal infection. Rabbits may require sedation for this procedure. Finding two sequential negative IgG determinations in sera collected a month apart is useful to confirm a *Pasteurella*-free status in isolated rabbits. Serologic tests may not detect acute infections, whereas culture methods may not detect chronic infections. Both approaches are needed when determining the status of a colony.

Culture of large numbers of animals and culture of sites in addition to the nasal cavities and the oropharynx will help to confirm a carrier state. Purulent processes in rabbits are usually due to *P. multocida* or *Staphylococcus aureus*. Both grow on blood agar. *Pasteurella multocida* is nonhemolytic and produces large, translucent, smooth or mucoid colonies up to 3–4 mm in diameter. *Staphylococcus* colonies are smaller, dry, opaque, and often hemolytic. Gram staining will provide a final diagnosis. *Pasteurella multocida* should also be differentiated from *Pasteurella pneumotropica* and *Bordetella bronchiseptica* infections through the use of indole, glucose, and urea cultures.

ELISA tests are also available for serologic monitoring of bacterial status. Skull radiographs are very helpful when trying to determine the extent of disease in chronic infections, such as atrophic rhinitis and otitis media.

Treatment

Although aggressive antibiotic treatment may eliminate the bacterium in acute infections, it is important to be aware that treatment of chronically infected pet rabbits is likely to be palliative. Antibiotics have poor penetration into abscessed lesions, and owners should be warned that treatment will be symptomatic, intermittent, and lifelong.

Antibiotic therapy should be based on culture and sensitivity findings. Enrofloxacin, ciprofloxacin, parenteral procaine pencillin, chloramphenicol, gentamicin, and trimethoprim-sulfa have all been used with good effect to suppress clinical signs of the disease following a 14- to 21-day course of treatment. Quinolone antibiotics should not be used in young animals, as they may induce arthropathies and they can be irritating when given by SC routes. Owners should always be cautioned to watch for changes in activity, appetite, and fecal output whenever antibiotics are administered to rabbits. It is important to note that there are no vaccines or drugs currently approved for specifically treating pasteurellosis in meat-type rabbits. Segregated-medicated early weaning methods can be used to eliminate the bacterium from commercial operations, as have been used effectively in swine production facilities.

Removal of environmental irritants such as dusty bedding and moldy hay or straw, provision of a nutritious and appropriate diet, and general attention to routine husbandry and management of animals will go a long way toward minimizing clinical signs of the disease and keeping animals comfortable.

Conjunctivitis can be treated with an appropriate ophthalmic ointment or drop containing gentamicin, ciprofloxacin, chloramphicol, or tetracycline. If there is discharge, the nasolacrimal ducts should be flushed with warm saline following administration of a topical anesthetic and using a 21-gauge teflon IV catheter. Ophthalmic ointment can be instilled as a final flush. Careful and gentle cleaning of matted fur surrounding the eye will add to rabbit comfort.

Prevention

Rabbit pasteurellosis is enzootic in most rabbitries and pet rabbits and is difficult to eradicate. Selection of *Pasteurella*-free or *Pasteurella*-resistant stock, repeated culture surveys of rabbits in the colony with culling of affected individuals, and provision for a 3-week entry quarantine with culture or serologic screening are methods of preventing entry and eliminating the organism from a rabbitry.

High husbandry standards, elimination of ammonia, and stabilization of the environment preclude the development of the more severe forms of the disease in adults. As the young are susceptible to pulmonary infection, chronically infected does should be culled. Weaning the young at 4 or 5 weeks reduces exposure to the infected mother. More frequent manure removal and good ventilation reduce accumulation of ammonia.

The prophylactic use of sulfaquinoxaline-supplemented water (0.05%) may reduce the incidence of enzootic pneumonia in exposed young until they can be isolated at weaning. Antibiotic eradication schemes have many shortcomings, including the generation of diarrhea, and are no substitute for culling, cleaning, and repopulation with *P. multocida*-free or *P. multocida*-resistant rabbits.

Public Health Significance

Although transmission of a rabbit infection to humans is unlikely, *P. multocida* can cause skin infections, arthritis, meningitis, peritonitis, pneumonia, and septicemia in susceptible humans. Identical serotypes of *Pasteurella multocida* can be cultured in poultry, cattle, rabbits, and cats, making cross-species transmission of the bacterium likely in extensive operations where two or more of these species co-exist.

References

Anderson LC, Rush HG, Glorioso JC. Strain differences in the susceptibility and resistance of Pasteurella multocida to phagocytosis and killing by rabbit polymorphonuclear neutrophils. Amer J Vet Res. 1984, 45:1193–1198.

Brogden KA. Physiological and serological characteristics of 48 Pasteurella multocida cultures from rabbits. J Clin Microbiol. 1980, 11:646–649.

Broome RL, Brooks DL. Efficacy of enrofloxacin in the treatment of respiratory pasteurellosis in rabbits. Lab Anim Sci. 1991, 41:572–576.

DeLong D, et al. Colonization of rabbits by Pasteurella multocida: serum IgG responses following intranasal challenge with serologically distinct isolates. Lab Anim Sci. 1992, 42:13–18.

DiGiacomo RF, Allen V, Hinton MH. Naturally acquired Pasteurella multocida subsp. multocida infection in a closed colony of rabbits: characteristics of isolates. Lab Anim. 1991, 25:236–241.

DiGiacomo RF, et al. Atrophic rhinitis in New Zealand white rabbits infected with Pasteurella multocida. Amer J Vet Res. 1989, 50:1460–1465.
DiGiacomo RF, et al. Naturally acquired Pasteurella multocida infection in rabbits: immunological aspects. Lab Anim Sci. 1990, 40:289–292.
DiGiacomo RF, et al. Toxin production by Pasteurella multocida isolated from rabbits with atrophic rhinitis. Amer J Vet Res. 1993, 54:1280–1286.
DiGiacomo RF, Garlinghouse LE, Jr, Van Hoosier GL, Jr. Natural history of infection with Pasteurella multocida in rabbits. J Am Vet Med Assoc. 1983, 183:1172–1175.
DiGiacomo RF, Jones CDR, Wathes CM. Transmission of Pasteurella multocida in rabbits. Lab Anim Sci. 1987, 37:621–623.
Dillehay DL, et al. Pathogenicity of Pasteurella multocida A:3 in Flemish Giant and New Zealand white rabbits. Lab Anim. 1991, 25:337–341.
Furie RA, et al. Pasteurella multocida infection: report in urban setting and review of spectrum of human disease. NY State J Med. 1980, 80:1597–1602.
Gaertner DJ. Comparison of penicillin and gentamicin for treatment of pasteurellosis in rabbits. Lab Anim Sci. 1991, 41:78–80.
Garlinghouse LE, Jr., et al. Selective media for Pasteurella multocida and Bordetella bronchiseptica. Lab Anim Sci. 1981, 31:39–42.
Holmes HT, et al. A method for culturing the nasopharyngeal area of rabbits. Lab Anim. 1987, 21:353–355.
———. Serologic methods for detection of Pasteurella multocida infections in nasal-culture-negative rabbits. Lab Anim Sci. 1986, 36:650–654.
Kumar AA, et al. Prevalent serotypes of Pasteurella multocida isolated from different animal and avian species in India. Vet Res Commun. 2004, 28:657–667.
Lu YS, Ringler DH, Park JS. Characterization of Pasteurella multocida isolates from the nares of healthy rabbits and rabbits with pneumonia. Lab Anim Sci. 1978, 28:691–697.
Manning PJ. Serology in Pasteurella multocida in laboratory rabbits: a review. Lab Anim Sci. 1982, 32:666–671.
RimLer RB. Presumptive identification of Pasteurella multocida subgroups A, D and F by capsule depolymerization with mucopolysaccharides. Vet Rec. 1994, 134:191–192.
Rush HG, et al. Resistance of Pasteurella multocida to rabbit neutrophil phagocytosis and killing. Amer J Vet Res. 1981, 42:1760–1768.
Sharpnack DD, et al. Quinolone arthropathy in juvenile New Zealand white rabbits. Lab Anim Sci. 1994, 44:436–442.

PASTEURELLA PNEUMOTROPICA INFECTIONS

Hosts

Mice and rats are susceptible to infections and clinical disease caused by *Pasteurella pneumotropica*, which is distributed worldwide in conventional and barrier colonies. *Pasteurella pneumotropica* has been isolated from a variety of hosts, including Syrian hamsters and guinea pigs, but infections in these species are typically incidental and nonclinical and they are not discussed further. This is generally not a disease of major concern in pet rodents.

Etiology

Pasteurella pneumotropica is a Gram-negative, nonmotile, 1–2 um long, pleomorphic coccobacillus that is a weakly pathogenic, opportunistic invader. The prevalence of infection is high in wild rodents.

Transmission

Pasteurella pneumotropica often exists in a latent, carrier state in the upper respiratory tract and uterus and is considered part of the normal gut flora of rodents. It may be disseminated by respiratory aerosol or fecal contamination, biting, licking, and intrauterine contamination. Typically, in enzootically infected colonies, nasopharyngeal colonization of laboratory rodents occurs around the time of weaning.

Predisposing Factors

With the proliferation and increased use of immunocompromised and genetically engineered mice, opportunistic infections with bacteria such as *P. pneumotropica* have emerged as significant problems in some research facilities. Because *P. pneumotropica* is an opportunistic pathogen, circumstances that decrease the host's resistance, particularly other infections, may precipitate clinical disease. *Pasteurella pneumotropica* in conjunction with Sendai virus infection of mice results in fatal pneumonia, and *P. pneumotropica* may complicate

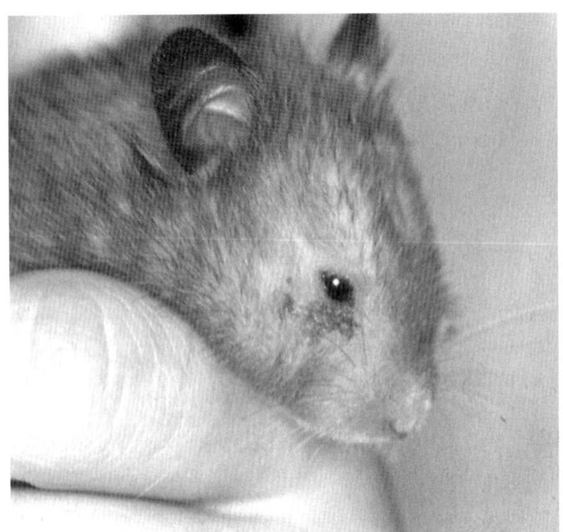

FIGURE 5.16. Conjunctivitis in a hamster. This condition may be seen with *Pasteurella pneumotropica* infection.

Mycoplasma pulmonis infection or other infections in rats and mice.

Clinical Signs

Characteristically, morbidity and mortality are low. *Pasteurella pneumotropica* is widespread as a latent infection, but the bacterium causes clinical disease only sporadically. Signs associated with *P. pneumotropica* infection include chattering, labored respiration, weight loss, skin abscesses, head tilt, Harderian gland abscesses, conjunctivitis (Figure 5.16), panophthalmitis, mastitis, infertility, bulbourethral gland infections, abortions, internal and subcutaneous abscesses, and death.

Necropsy Signs

The manifestations of infection and the target organs vary, but chronic suppurative bronchopneumonia (frequently as a co-pathogen), chronic endometritis, otitis media, chronic suppurative mastitis, preputial gland abscesses, and conjunctivitis are commonly seen. The muscles of mastication may be infected with the bacterium in young pups, leading to anorexia and death. Lesions are especially common in athymic nude mice and infection may lead to chronic wasting in these animals.

Rats may have a severe, multifocal to coalescing, acute to subacute, necrotizing to fibrinous bronchopneumonia, which must be differentiated from pneumonias caused by *Streptococcus* spp and *Corynebacterium* spp.

Diagnosis

A definitive diagnosis of *P. pneumotropica* infection is established through recovery of the organism on culture. After 24 hours of aerobic incubation at 37 °C on blood agar, the colonies are small (1 mm), circular, convex, smooth, and surrounded by a zone of slight greenish discoloration. An ELISA diagnostic test using *P. pneumotropica* lipooligosaccharide antigen has been helpful in detecting *P. pneumotropica* infections in mice.

Treatment

Enrofloxacin given subcutaneously or in the drinking water was superior to tetracycline in attempts to eliminate *P. pneumotropica* from oropharyngeal and gastrointestinal sites in mice. Large-scale embryo transfer rederivation may be necessary for breeding colonies of mice with associated bacterial problems.

Prevention

Elimination of murine respiratory infection from a colony requires a known disease-free stock placed into a clean and barrier-sustained colony. Newly arrived animals should be quarantined until their microbial status has been determined. Caesarean derivation should be done with the knowledge that *P. pneumotropica* is a common uterine inhabitant, as is *M. pulmonis*. The bacterium is most efficiently transmitted by direct contact, and dirty bedding sentinel systems may not be sensitive enough in all cases to detect this bacterium.

Public Health Significance

Pasteurella pneumotropica can infect humans, but rodent-to-human transmission is rarely reported. In one recent report, *Pasteurella pneumotropica* was transmitted by a hamster bite to a child undergoing dialysis, inducing peritonitis. Humans may be inadvertent sources of infection for barrier-sustained rodents.

References

Artwohl JE, et al. Outbreak of Pasteurella pneumotropica in a closed colony of stock Cd^{tm1Mak} mice. Contemp Top Lab Anim Sci. 2000, 39:39–41.

Barbier Frebourg N, et al. Septicemia due to Pasteurella pneumotropica: 16S rRNA sequencing for diagnosis confirmation. J Clin Microbiol. 2002, 40:687–689.

Blackmore DK, Casillo S. Experimental investigation of uterine infections of mice due to Pasteurella pneumotropica. J Comp Pathol. 1972, 82:471–475.

Boot R, et al. Colonization and antibody response in mice and rats experimentally infected with Pasteurellaceae from different rodent species. Lab Anim. 1994, 28:130–137.

Campos A, Taylor AH, Campbell M. Hamster bite peritonitis: Pasteueralla pneumotropica peritonitis in a dialysis patient. Pediatr Nephrol. 2000, 15:31–32.

Carthew P, Gannon J. Secondary infection of rat lungs with Pasteurella pneumotropica after Kilham rat virus infection. Lab Anim. 1981, 15:219–221.

Hong CC, Ediger RD. Chronic necrotizing mastitis in rats caused by Pasteurella pneumotropica. Lab Anim Sci. 1978, 28:317–320.

Lescher RJ, Jeszenka EV, Swan ME. Enteritis caused by Pasteurella pneumotropica infection in hamsters. J Clin Microbiol. 1985, 22:448.

Macy JD, et al. Dual infection with Pneumocystis carinii and Pasteurella pneumotropica in B cell–deficient mice. Comp Med. 2000, 50:49–55.

Manning PJ, et al. An enzyme-linked immunosorbent assay for detection of chronic subclinical Pasteurella pneumotropica infection in mice. Lab Anim Sci. 1991, 41:162–165.

Moore TD, Allen AM, Ganaway JR. Latent Pasteurella pneumotropica infection of the gnotobiotic and barrier-held rats. Lab Anim Sci. 1973, 23:657–661.

Scharmann W, Heller A. Survival and transmissibility of Pasteurella pneumotropica. Lab Anim. 2001, 35(2):163–166.

Sebesteny A. Abscesses of the bulbourethral glands of mice due to Pasteurella pneumotropica. Lab Anim. 1973, 7:315–317.

Ueno Y, et al. Elimination of Pasteurella pneumotropica from a contaminated mouse colony by oral administration of enrofloxacin. Exp Anim. 2002, 51(4):401–405.

Ward GE, Moffatt R, Olfert E. Abortion in mice associated with Pasteurella pneumotropica. J Clin Microbiol. 1978, 8:177–180.

PEDICULOSIS

Hosts

Lice as a whole have a wide host range, but individual species are host-specific. Mites and lice sometimes occur together on the same host.

Etiology

Lice are flattened insects, with six legs and no wings. *Polyplax* spp and *Haemodipsus* spp are of the suborder Anoplura—sucking lice. *Haemodipsus ventricosis*, the rabbit louse, has a life cycle of 30 days and its ova hatch 7 days after being laid. *Polyplax serrata*, the house mouse louse, is a blood-sucking louse and has a life cycle of 13 days. *Polyplax spinulosa*, the spined rat louse, is common in wild rats, has a life cycle of approximately 26 days, and is also a blood-sucking louse. Its ova hatch 6 days after being laid.

Gliricola spp and *Gyropus* spp are of the suborder Mallophaga—biting lice. *Gliricola porcelli*, the slender guinea pig louse, and *Gyropus ovalis*, the oval guinea pig louse, abrade the skin to obtain fluid. Of the species listed, *Gliricola* spp and *Polyplax* spp are relatively common, while *Gyropus* spp and *Haemodipsus* spp are relatively uncommon.

Transmission

All life cycle phases occur on the host. Ova (nits) are cemented to hair. Transmission of lice is by direct contact with an infected host or bedding. Lice seldom leave a living host.

Predisposing Factors

Animals with decreased resistance or young animals housed in unsanitary conditions may experience more severe infections and clinical consequences than do normal animals.

Clinical Signs

Infection by the rabbit louse, *Haemodipsus ventricosis*, may cause pruritus, alopecia, weakness, and anemia. The rabbit louse affects dorsolateral areas of the trunk more often than other areas of the body.

Infections with *Gliricola* spp and *Gyropus* spp, the guinea pig lice, are usually benign but can cause scratching, partial alopecia, and scabs, usually around the ears.

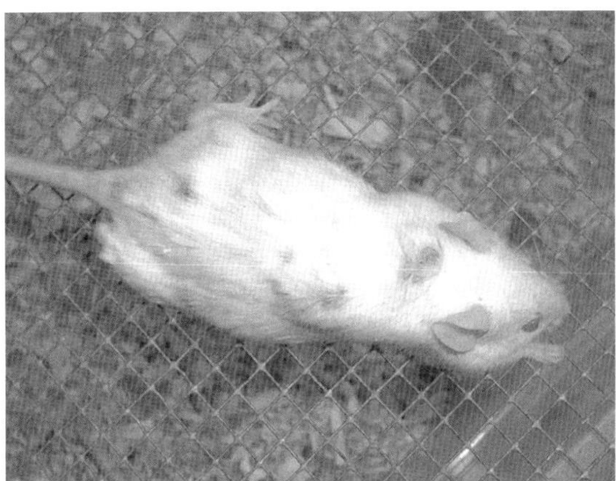

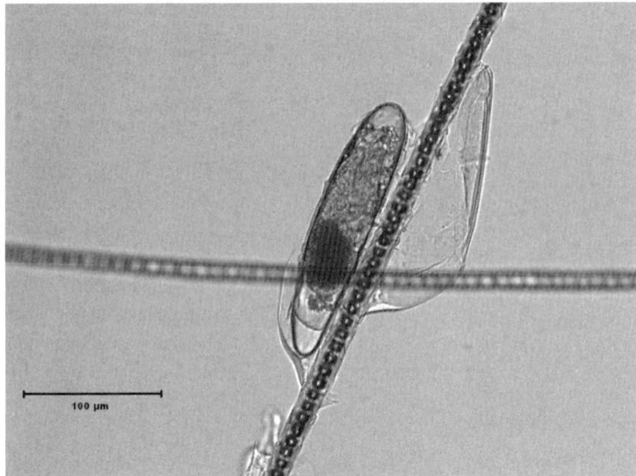

FIGURE 5.17. Multifocal ulcerations and swellings in a mouse infested by *Polyplax serrata* (left). Nits were demonstrated on the pelage of many mice in the affected colony (right).

Polyplax spp, mouse and rat lice, are found on the neck and body. They may cause debilitation, anemia, scratching, numerous small, scabbed wounds over the side and back, and death (Figure 5.17). *Polyplax serrata* of mice transmits the blood-borne protozoal agent of murine eperythrozoonosis, and *P. spinulosa* of rats transmits the blood-borne protozoan agent of murine haemobartonellosis. Animals without a history of louse infection and no history of receiving a parenteral inoculation of contaminated biological materials should be free of these protozoal infections.

Diagnosis

A hand lens or dissecting microscope is used to observe the pelt for adult or immature ectoparasites, especially the margin of lesions and the nape of the neck. Nits are readily visible on hair shafts. If the animal is dead, direct observation for lice is easier if the pelt is cooled in the refrigerator for 30 minutes, removed for 10 minutes, and then examined with a lens. The parasites migrate from the cool skin toward the warmer hair tips. Placing the suspect pelt on a dark paper within a frame of double-gummed cellophane tape or petroleum jelly will trap the lice and facilitate detection. *Haemodipsus* spp are 1.2–2.5 mm long and have an oval abdomen. *Polyplax* spp are slender and are 0.6–1.5 mm long. *Gliricola* spp have a narrow head and body approximately 1.0–1.5 mm long. *Gyropus* spp have a wide head and oval abdomen and are 1.0–1.2 mm long.

Treatment

Lice may be killed with the treatments described in the section on acariasis. Elimination of ectoparasites from a room requires treatment, removal of the animals from the room, thorough mechanical scrubbing of equipment and surfaces, and formaldehyde fumigation of equipment and premises. Self-grooming by the rodent host helps in the control of the louse population.

Prevention

Pediculosis is prevented by installing parasite-free stock in a parasite-free facility. Examination for lice during and after quarantine and barrier housing will protect a colony. If lice are a problem elsewhere in a facility, the animals should be quarantined and treated, and the equipment should be cleaned and disinfected. Wild rodents and lagomorphs may have pediculosis and should be excluded from colonies of domestic animals.

Public Health Significance

Haemodipsus ventricosis is a vector for the transmission of *Francisella tularensis* (tularemia) from rabbits to humans. *Gliricola* spp and *Gyropus* spp do not affect humans. *Polyplax* spp may serve as vectors for rickettsial organisms. Because of their high host specificity, humans are unlikely to acquire pediculosis from laboratory rabbits and rodents.

References

Berkenkamp SD, Wescott RB. Arthropod transmission of Eperythrozoon coccoides in mice. Lab Anim Sci. 1988, 38(4):398–401.

Hofing GL, Kraus AL. Arthropod and Helminth Parasites. In: The Biology of the Laboratory Rabbit, 2nd ed. Manning PJ, Ringler DH, Newcomer CE (eds.). San Diego: Academic Press, 1994, 231–257.

Kim SH, Jun HK, Yoo MJ, et al. Use of a formulation containing imidacloprid and moxidectin in the treatment of lice infestation in guinea pigs. Vet Dermatol. 2008, 19(3):187–188.

Murray MD. The ecology of the louse Polyplax serrata (Burn.) on the mouse Mus musculus. Aust J Zool. 1961, 9:1–13.

PNEUMOCYSTOSIS

Hosts

Pneumocystosis is usually a subclinical pulmonary condition that occurs widely in mammalian species including domestic rodents and domestic rabbits, primates, ungulates, carnivores, and numerous other animal species, including humans. The most relevant clinical disease occurs in immunodeficient mice.

Etiology

Pneumocystis spp are unicellular fungal organisms that are ubiquitous in the environment. Four basic stages of the organism—trophozoites, precysts, cysts, and intracystic bodies—inhabit the alveoli of infected animals. The cyst forms are 4–6 um in diameter and contain eight crescent-shaped sporozoites. Trophozoites are polymorphic with a single nucleus and are 1–5 um in diameter. They adhere tightly to the alveolar wall.

Mouse (*P. murina*) and rat (*P. carinii*) derived isolates are distinct species and infections are host-specific.

Transmission

The organism is transmitted by the respiratory route or as an aerosol. Because of the ubiquitous nature of this organism, conventional rodents should be envisioned as living in a cloud of *Pneumocystis* spp spores. They are typically infected as 3- to 4-week-old juveniles. Immunity to the organism develops rapidly, and young animals are initially protected by colostrum antibodies. Virtually all rodents in the 4- to 12-week-old age groups should be considered to be infected and shedding. The organism doesn't cross the placenta, thus Caesarean-section rederivation will eliminate the organism.

Predisposing Factors

Subclinical infections with *Pneumocystis* spp are relatively common in mice and rats. Immunocompetent animals develop a mild subclinical infection that resolves in 5–6 weeks, whereas immunodeficient animals (either natural or acquired) are unable to clear the organism from their respiratory tree and develop a chronic infection. Thymectomy is not a predisposing factor.

Clinical Signs

Continuous antibiotic therapy, genetic factors, and concurrent viral or bacterial infections frequently play an important role in the incidence of clinical disease. Hunched posture, dyspnea, and wasting have been observed in infected mice.

Necropsy Signs

At necropsy, the lungs appear edematous, are pale, and fail to collapse. Diffuse alveolitis, mobilization of alveolar macrophages, and the presence of vacuolated eosinophilic proteinaceous material within alveoli are characteristic microscopic findings. Typical spherical cyst forms may be demonstrated by PAS reactions or silver stains on fixed specimens. Lesions are particularly severe in severe combined immunodeficient (SCID) or athymic nude mice. The organism is thought to be species-specific, thus interspecies transmission is unlikely to occur.

Other conditions may result in accumulations of foamy or proteinaceous material in the lungs of mice, and because of the long-term implications for colony management, it is important to confirm the diagnosis.

Diagnosis

Examination of methenamine-silver-stained paraffin-embedded sections for trophozoites and cysts and PCR techniques are sensitive means of detecting the organism. Electron microscopy is no more sensitive than histology in detecting clinical infections.

Serology is only useful for monitoring immune competent animals.

Treatment

It is important to note that antibiotic treatment controls disease signs but does not eradicate the infection. Trimethoprim-sulfa suspensions (40 mg trimethoprim/200 mg sulfamethoxazole per mL) administered via drinking water is a convenient means to treat affected colonies. The suspension is added at a rate of 15.6 mL per 500 mL water bottle. The drug will settle out of solution and the water bottle must be shaken daily to resuspend the agent. Treatment may be either continuous or following a "3 days on–4 days off" pattern with regular water being supplied in the off treatment days. Treatment should be considered to be palliative only.

Prevention

Prevention of pneumocystosis is achieved by purchasing stock known to be free of *Pneumocystis* spp. Once established in a colony, it is difficult to eliminate.

Public Health Significance

Isolates for animals are distinct from human isolates.

References

An C-L, et al. Exposure of immunocompetent adult mice to Pneumocystis carinii f.sp. muris by cohousing: growth of Pneumocystis carinii f.sp. muris and immune responses. Infect Immun. 2003, 71:2065–2070.

Barton EG, Jr, Campbell WG, Jr. Pneumocystis carinii in lungs of rats treated with cortisone acetate. Am J Pathol. 1969, 54:209–236.

Cushion MT, Ruffolo JJ, Walzer PD. Analysis of the developmental stages of Pneumocystis carinii, in vitro. Lab Invest. 1988, 58:324–331.

Frenkel JK, Good JT, Shultz JA. Latent pneumocystis infection of rats; relapse, and chemotherapy. Lab Invest. 1966, 15:1559–1577.

Furuta R, et al. Cellular and humoral immune responses of mice subclinically infected with Pneumocystis carinii. Infect Immun. 1985, 47:544–548.

Keeley SP, et al. Phylogenetic identification of Pneumocystis murina sp nov, a new species in laboratory mice. Microbiol. 2004, 150:1153–1165.

Pintozzi RL, Blecka LJ, Nanos S. The morphologic identification of Pneumocystis carinii. Acta Cytol. 1979, 23:35–39.

Pohlmeyer G, Deerberg G. Nude rats as a model of natural Pneumocystis carinii pneumonia: sequential morphological study of lung lesions. J Comp Pathol. 1993, 109:217–230.

Ruffolo JJ, Cushion MT, Waizer PD. Techniques for examining Pneumocystis carinii in fresh specimens. J Clin Microbiol. 1986, 23:17–21.

Sundberg JP, et al. Identification of Pneumocystis carinii in immunodeficient mice. Lab Anim Sci. 1989, 39:213–218.

Walzer PD, et al. Outbreaks of Pneumocystis carinii pneumonia in colonies of immunodeficient mice. Infect Immun. 1989, 57:62–70.

Weir EC, Brownstein DG, Barthold SW. Spontaneous wasting disease in nude mice associated with Pneumocystis carinii infection. Lab Anim Sci. 1986, 36:140–144.

PODODERMATITIS

Hosts

Ulcerative pododermatitis in rabbits, a common condition known as "sore hocks," occurs unilaterally or bilaterally on the plantar metatarsal surfaces (footpads of the rear feet) or, less often, on the palmar metacarpal surfaces. A variation of this condition known as "bumblefoot" affects guinea pigs, chinchillas, and rats but less frequently than rabbits.

Etiology

The condition is thought to be caused by pressure necrosis of the epidermis, primarily on the plantar metatarsal surfaces of large rabbits housed on hard or wet floors and in large guinea pigs, chinchillas, and rats housed on wire floors or on coarse woodchip bedding. Poor hygiene leading to wet cage conditions and contamination of the open wound with urine and feces increases the severity of the lesions, as does obesity.

Predisposing Factors

Factors that predispose to pododermatitis in rabbits include increased body weight as seen in heavy breeds such as the rex, Flemish giant, or checkered giant; reduced plantar fur pad thickness; bruising;

obesity, restraint, inanition, or lack of movement in a small cage; and abrasions caused by irregular cage flooring and coarse and irritating bedding. Affected animals should be culled and not used as breeders. The incidence of pododermatitis increases with age and weight (more than 3 kg) and is seen more during hot humid weather, especially in males. It is doubtful that ulcerative pododermatitis is caused or exacerbated by thumping in excessively excitable animals. Rabbits with heavily furred feet, immature animals, or light-weight breeds are affected less frequently.

In rodents, the condition predominantly arises from housing animals on wire-bottom floors with oversized grids or metal irregularities leading to abrasions; in unsanitary conditions leading to localized infections; or secondary to coarse bedding. Some softwood chip beddings release oils that are irritating to the unhaired footpad of these species.

Clinical Signs

The lesion consists of unilateral or bilateral rounded, focal, scab-covered, often hemorrhagic, cutaneous ulcers on the plantar metatarsal surfaces (Figure 5.18). When secondary infection is present, *Staphylococcus aureus* is often cultured. In addition to these signs, cellulitis, abscessation, and osteomyelitis may be seen in severe cases. Animals may be reluctant to move and may show signs of variable depression, anorexia, refusal to breed, loss of body condition, and even death.

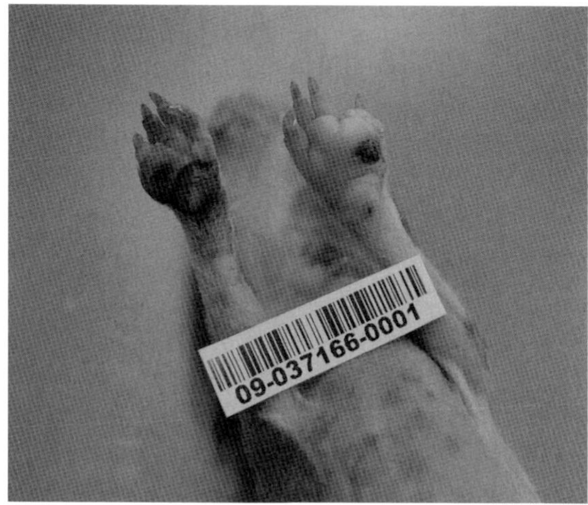

FIGURE 5.18. Bilateral pododermatitis of the metatarsals of a guinea pig. Courtesy of Marina Brash.

Diagnosis

Clinical signs and predisposing factors provide the diagnosis. The animal should be firmly restrained in a towel wrap during examination of the plantar metatarsal surfaces to avoid further trauma to the animal and injury to the handler. Chemical restraint is usually not necessary.

Treatment

Treatment includes cleansing, toenail trimming, and application of a topical antiseptic or protective cover. Frequently, healing is prolonged and complicated by secondary bacterial infection. The prognosis may be poor for complete recovery in animals with intractable pododermatitis, as chronic infection and ulceration may lead to osteomyelitis.

In addition to providing soft, dry, clean bedding and a solid cage surface, the affected foot can be soaked in warm Epsom salt solutions to promote healing. In general, bandaging of the extremities is poorly tolerated; however, a light protective dressing in conjunction with a thin layer of antibiotic ointment may be useful. Systemic antibiotics for severe cases, resting boards, and application of topical over-the-counter ointments such as Bag Balm® or Preparation H® have been described.

Prevention

Pododermatitis occurs in rabbits housed on both solid and wire floors and in almost any type of cage or confinement device. Prevention is achieved by housing rabbits in clean cages on soft, clean, dry bedding. Selection of breeders with thick plantar metatarsal fur pads may also help. Eliminating stressful conditions in the environment, providing adequate nutrition and exercise, and guarding against obesity through limited feeding are measures that may help prevent sore hocks. Excessively warm and moist environments may result in a thinner fur coat and a less dense plantar metatarsal hair covering, leaving the foot more susceptible to ulcers and infections.

Rats housed continuously on wire typically do not develop foot lesions until they are at least 6 months of age. Despite this propensity, rats show a strong preference for solid-bottom flooring and the use of wire-bottom cages should be avoided in rodents, whenever possible.

References

Brown C, Donnelly TM. Treatment of pododermatitis in the guinea pig. Lab Anim. 2008, 37(4):156–157.

Hoppmann E, Wilson Barron H. Ferret and rabbit dermatology. J Exot Pet Med. 2007, 16:225–237.

———. Rodent dermatology. J Exot Pet Med. 2007, 16:238–255.

Manser CE, Elliot H, Morris TH, et al. The use of a novel operant test to determine the strength of preference for flooring in laboratory rats. Lab Anim. 1996, 30(1):1–6.

Manser CE, Morris TH, Broom DM. An investigation into the effects of solid or grid cage flooring on the welfare of laboratory rats. Lab Anim. 1995, 29(4):353–363.

Peace TA, Singer AW, Niemuth NA, et al. Effects of caging type and animal source on the development of foot lesions in Sprague Dawley rats (Rattus norvegicus). Contemp Top Lab Anim Sci. 2001, 40(5):17–21.

PREGNANCY TOXEMIA

Hosts

This group of clinically similar diseases occurs in female cattle, rabbits, guinea pigs, hamsters, sheep, goats, nonhuman primates, and humans. Among small mammal species, the disease occurs most frequently in guinea pigs and to a lesser extent in rabbits. Toxemia secondary to hepatic lipidosis and obesity may also be seen in male guinea pigs and rabbits but is obviously not related to pregnancy in these instances.

Etiology

In guinea pigs, the clinical signs are similar, but there are two distinctly different patterns of disease that are seen, a metabolic form and a circulatory form. Both forms occur in sows in advanced pregnancy, and because both syndromes result in similar endpoints, the syndromes may be indistinguishable clinically.

The metabolic form (pregnancy ketosis) of the disease is most common in obese sows carrying 4 or more fetuses. Adverse stress factors such as poor environment, dietary changes, and low-roughage diets can predispose animals to this condition. The disease can be reproduced experimentally by fasting pregnant (or nonpregnant) guinea pigs, and it can also occur in obese boars and bucks and obese, pregnant does.

The circulatory form (preeclampsia) is seen in very large sows in advanced pregnancy. The uterine content of guinea pigs in late gestation may represent up to 50% of the body weight of the nonpregnant dam. In this condition, uteroplacental ischemia occurs due to compression of the aorta caudal to the renal vessels by the gravid uterus. This leads to up to a 30% reduction of blood flow to the uterus, infarction of the placenta, and terminal disseminated intravascular coagulation. This syndrome is very similar to preeclampsia in women. Toxemia has been produced experimentally in guinea pigs by banding the uterine arteries. Hypertension, proteinuria, and elevated creatinine levels were observed.

Predisposing Factors

Factors that predispose a guinea pig or rabbit to pregnancy toxemia are multiple. Specific influences include obesity, heredity, change in diet, change in feeding routine, anorexia, large fetal load that may either compress or overextend the vascular supply to the uterus, hypoplasia of vessels supplying the uterus or failure of those vessels to enlarge adequately to supply the primigravid uterus, lack of exercise, and nonspecific environmental stressors. A tendency for more cases to occur during the winter has been noted. Obese boars also develop the metabolic form of the syndrome, though much less frequently than pregnant sows.

Obesity and fasting are also predisposing factors in ketosis in rabbits. The Dutch, Polish, and English breeds have a predisposition to toxemia, as do pregnant, pseudopregnant, and postparturient does, although obese nonpregnant does and bucks may succumb also.

Clinical Signs

The condition usually occurs during the last week of gestation in rabbits and during the last 2–3 weeks of gestation or the first postpartum week in guinea pigs. The condition may be asymptomatic, rapidly fatal, or involve weakness, depression, reluctance to move, incoordination, anorexia, abortion, dyspnea, convulsions, coma, and death over a 4- to 6-day period. The urine becomes clear (acidic), and proteinuria, ketonuria, and hyperkalemia may develop. This condition is responsible for high fetal wastage in many production guinea pig colonies.

General statements regarding serum calcium, phosphorus, and glucose levels are misleading because of considerable variation among species and stages of the disease within a single species.

Necropsy Signs

Necropsy signs of pregnancy toxemia, when evident, include reduced gastric content, abundant body fat, dead and decomposed fetuses, uterine and placental hemorrhage, adrenal enlargement and hemorrhage, and an enlarged tan liver that is greasy on cut section.

Histologically, hepatic lipidosis, fatty changes in the kidneys and adrenal glands, and the presence of lipids within vessels are typical microscopic findings. Uterine ischemia may be seen in cases of the circulatory form of the disease. Diagnosis is based on clinical, necropsy, and microscopic signs.

Treatment

If toxemia is detected in progress, several unproven treatments can be tried, including administration of lactated Ringer's solution, calcium gluconate, propylene glycol, 5% glucose, and corticosteroids. Use of magnesium sulfate solution to dilate arteries has been attempted in small animals, but results are inconclusive. Guinea pigs under treatment for ketosis frequently die from acute enteritis due, in part, to stress and dysbiosis from inanition and bacterial overgrowth.

Prevention

A critical consideration in preventing toxemia is to avoid fasting animals and to supply fresh water and a nutritious diet. Pregnant guinea pigs should not be subjected to dietary changes or stressors such as transport or drastic changes in environment. Breeding animals should not be permitted to become obese, and weight reduction strategies should be gradual. For this reason, anorexia should always be treated as a serious clinical sign.

References

Abitbol MM, et al. Production of experimental toxemia in the pregnant rabbit. Am J Obstet Gynecol. 1976, 124:460–470.

Bruce NW. The effect of ligating a uterine artery on fetal and placental development in the rat. Biol Reprod. 1976, 14:246–247.

Ganaway JR, Allen AM. Obesity predisposes to pregnancy toxemia (ketosis) of guinea pigs. Lab Anim Sci. 1971, 21:40–44.

Golden JG, Hughes HC, Lang CM. Experimental toxemia in the pregnant guinea pig (Cavia porcellus). Lab Anim Sci. 1980, 30:174–179.

Leland SE, Brownstein DG, Weir EC. Pancreatitis and pregnancy toxemia in a New Zealand white rabbit. Contemp Top Lab Anim Sci. 1995, 34(6):84–85.

Percy DH, Barthold SW. Guinea Pig. In: Pathology of Laboratory Rodents and Rabbits, 3rd ed. Ames, IA: Wiley-Blackwell, 2007.

Richter AG, Lausen NC, Lage, AL. Pregnancy toxemia (eclampsia) in Syrian golden hamsters. J Am Vet Med Assoc, 1984, 185:1357–1358.

Seidl DC, et al. True pregnancy toxemia (preeclampsia) in the guinea pig (Cavia porcellus). Lab Anim Sci. 1979, 29:472–478.

RABIES VIRUS INFECTION

Hosts

Most veterinarians practicing in North America are keenly aware of the potential risk of occurrence of rabies in cats and dogs. Small mammal species such as rabbits and rodents appear to be naturally more resistant to development of rabies infections; however, the disease may occur rarely in these species, particularly if housed outdoors, or in small mammal species adopted from the wild. There are no vaccines approved for use in these species. No human has ever been reported to have developed rabies following a rodent or lagomorph bite. Clients who allow animals to graze outdoors or who shelter their animals outside should be cautioned to protect their animals from feral animal exposures.

References

Eidson E, et al. Rabies virus infection in a pet guinea pig and seven pet rabbits. J Am Vet Med Assoc. 2005, 227:932–935.

Karp BE, et al. Rabies in two privately owned domestic rabbits. J Am Vet Med Assoc. 1999, 215:1824–1827.

RINGTAIL

Hosts

Tail necrosis or "ringtail" can occur in any rodent species with a glabrous (nonhaired) tail. It is seen in infant mice and rats between 7 and 15 days of age as well as other rodent species, such as juvenile *Mystromys albicaudatus* (white-tailed mice).

Etiology

The disease has been classified as primarily an environmental disorder with the pathogenesis attributed to low humidity and either low or high temperatures, which may result in an aberrant response of the temperature-regulating vessels in the tail of the suckling rodents. Other potential causes cited include a deficiency in essential fatty acids and dehydration.

Predisposing Factors

Age and strain are determining factors in the development of ringtail. The incidence in suckling animals is greater than in adults. Long-Evans and Sherman rats are less susceptible than are Wistar and Sprague-Dawley rats. Additionally, conditions that cause lower ambient humidity such as occurs with wire cages, hygroscopic bedding, and excessive air flow rates predispose animals to ringtail. In the Northern Hemisphere, ringtail is seen most often between November and April, when facilities are artificially heated and interior humidity drops. Nutrient deficiencies, including lack of essential fatty acids in the diet of lactating dams, may predispose infants to ringtail, which can be further exacerbated by low ambient humidity.

Clinical Signs

Animals with mild clinical signs have hyperemic tails with few if any annulations and they usually recover uneventfully. In moderately affected cases, the animals are left with permanent annular constrictions on their tails. In severe cases, the tails become dry and necrotic and slough. The stumps will heal without complications. Affected rats usually have no other apparent clinical or metabolic abnormalities or signs of discomfort.

Diagnosis

Recognition of clinical signs and knowledge of husbandry practices and experimental protocol are helpful in making a diagnosis. Ringtail lesions present as edema, inflammation, and possibly necrosis. These can cause the tail distal to the lesion to slough, leaving a stubby, short tail.

Treatment

Specific treatment for ringtail is usually not necessary as long as all possible predisposing factors are corrected and the animals are housed with clean bedding and fed a balanced diet. Lanolin has been used as a topical ointment to prevent progression of ringtail in rat pups diagnosed early in the course of the condition. Preventing other diseases and environmental stresses from compromising the overall health and immune status of the animal is an important measure in promoting healing and an uneventful recovery.

Prevention

In some instances, ringtail can be prevented by providing a solid-bottom plastic cage with both adequate bedding and nesting material. Use of microisolator caging tops will increase local cage humidity by 5–10% compared with room humidity and may help to prevent the condition. In most cases prevention depends on maintaining the relative humidity of the room at approximately 50% or higher. Nutritional requirements, including essential fatty acid levels, should be met.

References

Crippa L, et al. Ringtail in suckling Munich Wistar Fromter rats: a histopathologic study. Comp Med. 2001, 50:536–539.

Ellison GTH, Westlin-van Aarde LM. Ringtail in the pouched mouse (Saccostomus campestris). Lab Anim. 1990, 24:205–206.

Stuhlman RA, Wagner JE. Ringtail in Mystromys albicaudatus: a case report. Lab Anim Sci. 1971, 21:585–587.

Taylor DK, Rogers MM, Hankenson FC. Lanolin as a treatment option for ringtail in transgenic rats. J Amer Assoc Lab Anim Sci. 2006, 45(1):83–87.

Weichbrod RH, et al. Diagnostic exercise: tail sloughing in mice. Lab Anim Sci. 1987, 37:644–645.

ROTAVIRUS INFECTIONS

Hosts

Rotaviruses are species-specific enveloped RNA viruses that produce significant intestinal disease in a variety of young hosts, including mice (epizootic diarrhea of infant mice [EDIM]), rats (infectious diarrhea of infant rats [IDIR]), rabbits, calves, and humans. EDIM occurs worldwide in conventional mouse colonies. IDIR in rats is similar to EDIM of mice.

Etiology

Rotaviruses are 60–80 nm in diameter, contain double-stranded RNA, are nonenveloped, and have capsomers on the surface. Rotaviruses are placed in lettered groups (A, B, C, D, etc.) based on genetic relatedness. Group A rotaviruses cause EDIM, diarrhea in rabbits, and acute gastroenteritis in human infants during the winter months. One of the group B viruses causes diarrhea in infant rats. The viruses cause an inhibition of the intestinal absorptive mechanism through epithelial damage and transport system blocking. Concurrent infection with EDIM and MHV produces a disease that resembles what was once described as lethal intestinal viral infection of mice (LIVIM). Similarly, concurrent infection with enterotoxigenic *E. coli* increases the severity of rotaviral disease.

Postexposure, the virus may replicate in enterocytes throughout the intestinal tract and may escape the intestine to infect extraintestinal tissues. Manifestations of the disease are most common in the small intestine, but histologic evidence of infection has been noted on occasion in other tissues in rats.

Previous infection by EDIM may affect response of mice to human rotavirus challenges during vaccine efficacy testing.

Transmission

The viruses of EDIM and IDIR are transmitted predominantly by oral-fecal contamination. In all species, the disease is highly contagious. Animals surviving the clinical disease shed the virus for weeks. The filter cover concept was introduced initially to prevent transmission of the EDIM agent among susceptible mice. Mouse rotaviruses are not infectious for rats. Little is known about the transmission of rotavirus infection in rabbits.

Predisposing Factors

Clinically apparent diarrheal disease is seen in mice and rats up to 12 or 13 days of age, and it is more severe in mice born to primiparous females. Older animals may be susceptible to rotaviral infections and may shed the virus in large quantities following infection, but they rarely exhibit evidence of clinical disease. The increased susceptibility of neonatal animals to clinical disease appears to be due in part to the reduced kinetic rate of enterocyte turnover in very young animals. Neonatal animals are unable to replace these epithelial cells fast enough, resulting in collapse of villi and diarrhea.

Clinical Signs

EDIM and IDIR are diarrheal diseases of high morbidity and low mortality. Affected suckling mice and rats have watery, yellow diarrhea and steatorrhea due to malabsorption, but infants continue to nurse and have a milk-filled stomach that is visible through the ventral abdominal wall (milk spot). Sometimes constipation is seen during the convalescent stages.

In rats, diarrhea is usually seen in 8- to 12-day-old pups. The diarrhea persists for 5–6 days and may be associated with erythema, cracking, and bleeding of the perianal skin. Although affected rodents continue to eat, they do not grow normally, and stunted growth is a common sequela. Weaning percentage (percentage of young weaned compared with litter size at birth) may be slightly reduced. When weaned, the young are somewhat underweight for their age. Primary rotaviral infections rarely produce diarrhea in rabbits, but they may play a role in the enteritis complex in this species.

Necropsy Signs

The stomach of the affected mouse is usually filled with milk, unlike sucklings with MHV infection. The gastrointestinal tract of the affected mouse, rabbit, or rat may appear normal or be distended with gas and watery, yellow feces.

In the small intestine, rotaviruses replicate selectively in enterocytes lining the distal tips of villi. In suckling mice, villous atrophy and vacuolation of enterocytes occur during the course of the disease but without the syncytial giant cell formation seen frequently in coronaviral enteritides.

Rats, like pigs with rotaviral infections, develop villous epithelial syncytial cell formations, particularly in the distal one-third of the small intestine. Numerous viral particles can be seen with electron microscopy in syncytial cells.

Serologic surveys of commercial rabbitries suggest that the virus is endemic in conventional animals. Histologic alterations following infection may be seen in rabbits as old as 11 months.

Diagnosis

A diagnosis of rotaviral infection is usually made on the basis of clinical signs, case history, and histologic findings. Electron microscopy of negatively stained specimens prepared from diarrheic feces has been used to diagnose rotaviral infections. ELISA and immunofluorescence assays are also available commercially.

Treatment

Little can be done to treat EDIM or IDIR; however, supportive treatment of rabbits and rodents with diarrhea may be indicated.

Prevention

Selection of disease-free stock and the use of cage filter covers will reduce or prevent outbreaks of EDIM. Barrier housing will markedly reduce chances of new infections.

Public Health Significance

Mouse rotaviruses are not thought to affect humans. Rat rotaviruses may be zoonotic and neonatal rats are susceptible to human rotavirus infection.

References

Barthold SW. Murine Rotavirus Infection, Mouse. In: Monographs on Pathology of Laboratory Animals: Digestive System. Jones, TC, et al (eds.). New York: Springer-Verlag, 1997; 384–389.

Choi AH, et al. Intranasal or oral immunization of inbred and outbred mice with murine or human rotavirus VP6 proteins protects against viral shedding after challenge with murine rotaviruses. Vacc. 2002, 20:3310–3321.

Ciarlet M, et al. Rotavirus disease, but not infection and development of intestinal histopathological lesions, is age restricted in rabbits. Virol. 1998, 251:343–360.

Coelho KIR, et al. Pathology of rotavirus infection in suckling mice: a study by conventional biology, immunofluorescence, ultra thin sections, and scanning electron microscopy. Ultrastruct Pathol. 1981, 7:59–80.

Crawford SE et al. Rotavirus viremia and extraintestinal viral infection in the neonatal rat model. J Virol. 2006, 80:4820–4832.

De Castro L. Serological evidence of rotavirus infection in a guinea pig colony. Mem Inst Oswaldo Cruz. 1988, 83(4):411–413.

DiGiacomo RF, Thouless ME. Age-related antibodies to rotavirus in New Zealand rabbits. J Clin Microbiol. 1984, 19:710–711.

———. Epidemiology of naturally occurring rotavirus infection in rabbits. Lab Anim Sci. 1986, 36:153–156.

Eiden J, Vonderfecht S, Yolken RH. Evidence that a novel rotavirus-like agent of rats can cause gastroenteritis in man. Lancet. 1985, ii:8–11.

Femer WT, et al. Comparison of methods for detection of serum antibody to murine rotavirus. J Clin Microbiol. 1987, 25:1364–1369.

Gastrucci G. Isolation and characterization of cytopathic strains of rotavirus from rabbits. Arch Virol. 1985, 83:99–104.

Huber, AC, et al. Pathology of infectious diarrhea of infant rats (IDIR) induced by an antigenically distinct rotavirus. Vet Pathol. 1989, 26:376–385.

McNeal MM, et al. Discovery of a new strain of murine rotavirus that is consistently shed in large quantities after oral inoculation of adult mice. Virol. 2004, 320:1–11.

Peeters JE, Charlier G, van Opdenbosch E. Rotavirus in commercial suckling rabbits: some preliminary observations. Vet Bull. 1982, 52:724.

Schoeb TR, et al. Rotavirus-associated diarrhea in a commercial rabbitry. Lab Anim Sci. 1986, 36:149–152.

Shirane K, Nakagomi O. Interspecies transmission of animal rotaviruses to humans as evidenced by phylogenetic analysis of the hypervariable region of the VP4 protein. Microbiol Immunol. 1994, 38:823–826.

Smith AL, et al. Detection of antibody to epizootic diarrhea of infant mice (EDIM) virus. Lab Anim Sci. 33:442–445, 1983.

Thouless ME, et al. The effect of combined rotavirus and Escherichia coli infections in rabbits. Lab Anim Sci. 1996, 46:381–385.

SPECIFIC DISEASES AND CONDITIONS

———. Pathogenicity of rotavirus in rabbits. J Clin Microbiol. 1988, 26:943–947.

Vonderfecht SL, et al. Infectious diarrhea of infant rats produced by a rotavirus-like agent. J Virol. 1984, 52:94–98.

SALMONELLOSIS

Hosts

Salmonella spp are widespread in nature and affect a broad range of vertebrates. The agent is not common in pet rabbits and rodents and is rare in research colonies, but may commonly be found in colonies of feeder mice. Guinea pigs are highly susceptible and develop severe clinical disease; mice are also susceptible and may carry subclinical infections for long periods. Rabbits, chinchillas, hamsters, rats, and gerbils are infected less often, but severe outbreaks have occurred in each species.

Etiology

Salmonella typhimurium and *S. enteritidis* are the pathogenic species most often isolated from laboratory animals, but many other species of *Salmonella* spp of equal or lesser pathogenicity have been cultured and typed.

Transmission

Transmission is by the fecal-oral route through ingestion of feces, feces-contaminated feed, or bedding. The conjunctiva is a portal of entry in guinea pigs and probably other species. *Salmonella* spp frequently exist in a subclinical carrier state in the intestinal tract and are continually shed into the environment, making elimination of infection difficult. Control is made even more difficult because of the ability of *Salmonella* spp to survive in the environment. Because of good hygienic management and barrier housing, *Salmonella* spp infections are seen rarely in research facilities.

An outbreak of *Salmonella typhimurium* infections was reported in a commercial rabbitry in New South Wales that resulted in serious economic loss. The source of infection was believed to be local farm hay of poor quality that was used in nest boxes of kindling does. Commercial rabbits and chinchillas are frequently exposed to *Salmonella* spp in the feed. In another study, a *Salmonella* Group D infection was thought to have spread from cockroaches to gerbils via mosquitoes and a contaminated filarial inoculum.

Predisposing Factors

Among predisposing factors increasing susceptibility to salmonellosis are youth or old age, stress of pregnancy, nutritional deficiencies, concomitant diseases, genetic predisposition, serotype of organism involved, and environmental and experimental stresses. Guinea pigs are highly susceptible in the winter at parturition and at weaning. C57BL/6, DBA/1, and BALB/c mice are considered among the more susceptible strains.

Clinical Signs

Salmonellosis in laboratory animals is an enteric and systemic infection that may be enzootic or epizootic. Sporadic outbreaks with high mortality are the rule in guinea pig and chinchilla colonies and rabbitries, but in smaller rodents clinical signs are usually inapparent.

Specific signs, when present, include anorexia, rapid deterioration, rough hair coat, pyrexia, weight loss, light-colored soft feces, conjunctivitis, ocular discharge, small litters, lethargy, dyspnea, abortions, and sporadic deaths, particularly of pregnant dams in the late stages of pregnancy. Rats in one infected colony had no sign other than soft feces.

Necropsy Signs

Lesions of acute salmonellosis include enlargement, congestion, and focal necrosis of the liver, spleen, lymphoid tissues, and intestine. The gut may contain decreased contents and increased amounts of gas and fluid. Pregnant animals may have necrotic metritis.

In subacute or chronic cases the spleen may be enlarged, the liver and gut may be hyperemic, and necrotic foci may be prominent in the viscera. Enlarged and prominent Peyer's patches may be seen throughout the ileal subserosa.

Microscopically, vasculitis and thrombosis are seen in hamsters. Foci of necrosis surrounded by mononuclear cell infiltrates occur in the viscera along with a suppurative lymphadenitis.

Diagnosis

Although necropsy signs may be suggestive of salmonellosis, cultures of the mesenteric lymph nodes, conjunctiva, feces, cecum, or freshly aborted material (if available) are methods of choice for confirming an outbreak or a carrier state of this condition. The agents do not hydrolyze urea and usually do not use lactose. Media may include Gram-negative, selenite, or tetrathionate brilliant green broth to enhance growth of *Salmonella* spp from fecal samples. A battery of additional biochemical tests can be used to identify further suspect colonies in culture. Suspected *Salmonella* spp isolates must be confirmed by serotyping because several nonpathogenic enteric bacteria may have similar biochemical reactions. A final determination of serotype is usually performed in a reference laboratory.

Treatment

Treatment of salmonellosis may suppress an epizootic to an enzootic infection, but elimination of carriers is difficult. Because of the major public health concern, colonies infected with *Salmonella* spp usually should be eliminated, premises sanitized, and proven clean animals used for restocking. Infection of valuable rodents by minimally pathogenic strains of *Salmonella* spp may be controlled or eliminated by intense culture, isolation, and treatment. *Salmonella* spp serovars of low virulence may disappear spontaneously without treatment from colonies or other populations. This is more likely to occur in well-maintained barrier facilities.

A therapeutic regimen that has been followed with some success is the addition of oxytetracycline to the drinking water at 10 g/L for 10 days or 250 mg/kg body weight per day. Treated mice were isolated, the remainder of the colony euthantized, the room disinfected, and first litters monitored for *Salmonella* spp.

Prevention

Rigid, high husbandry standards and screening of new arrivals and resident populations of other species, especially dogs, nonhuman primates, and animal care personnel, will reduce the possibility of outbreaks. Birds, wild rodents, and contaminated feed must be excluded from the facility. Elimination of infection from conventional colonies by treatment is extremely difficult; euthanizing affected animals, disinfecting, and restocking may be more practical.

Public Health Significance

Salmonellosis occurs in humans and can be contracted from, or given to, pet and laboratory animals. Clients and staff should be instructed in proper hygiene when handling small mammal pets or research animals, including rigid posthandling handwashing practices. Within breeding, pet store, and distribution operations, *Salmonella* spp can be cultured from cages, food, and bedding, emphasizing the need for environmental control if the bacteria are found and strict hygiene control measures to minimize the spread of infection to other susceptible species (e.g., reptiles, dogs, and cats). Routine culturing of pet feces is not warranted but may be advisable in households with immunocompromised individuals or whenever *Salmonella* spp is cultured from a symptomatic client family member. Several outbreaks of salmonellosis have also been linked to consumption of undercooked rabbit meat contaminated with *Salmonella* spp bacteria. Rabbit meat must be thoroughly cooked to avoid foodborne disease outbreaks.

References

Casebolt DB, Schoeb TR. An outbreak in mice of salmonellosis caused by Salmonella enteritidis serotype enteritidis. Lab Anim Sci. 1988, 38:190–192.

Clark JD, et al. Salmonellosis in gerbils induced by nonrelated experimental procedure. Lab Anim Sci. 1992, 42:161–163.

Corazzola S, Zanin B, Bersani G. Food poisoning in man following an outbreak of salmonellosis in rabbits. Vet Ital. 1971, 22:370–373.

Harwood DG. Salmonella typhimurium infection in a commercial rabbitry. Vet Rec. 1989, 125:554–555.

Holmberg SD, et al. Drug-resistant Salmonella from animals fed antimicrobials. N Eng J Med. 1984, 311:617–622.

Kirchner BK, et al. Recovery and pathogenicity of several Salmonella species isolated from mice. Lab Anim Sci. 1982, 32:506–508.

Naglki T, et al. Outbreak of Salmonella enteritidis and isolation of Salmonella sofia in chinchillas (Chinchilla laniger). Vet Rec. 2003, 152:719–720.

Okewole PA, et al. Uterine involvement in guinea pig salmonellosis. Lab Anim. 1989, 23:275–277.

Olfert ED, Ward GE, Stevenson D. Salmonella typhimurium infection in guinea pigs: observations on monitoring and control. Lab Anim Sci. 1976, 26:78–80.

Olson GA, Shields RP, Gaskin JM. Salmonellosis in a gerbil colony. J Am Vet Med Assoc. 1977, 171:970–972.

Seepersadsingh N, Adesiyun AA. Prevalence and antimicrobial resistance of Salmonella spp. in pet mammals, reptiles, fish aquarium water, and birds in Trinidad. J Vet Med. 2003, B50:488–493.

Seps SL, et al. Investigations of the pathogenicity of Salmonella enteritidis serotype Amsterdam following a naturally occurring infection in rats. Lab Anim Sci. 1987, 37:326–330.

Shimi A, Keyhani M, Hedayati K. Studies on salmonellosis in the house mouse, Mus musculus. Lab Anim. 1979, 13:33–34.

Simmons DJC, Simpson W. Salmonella montevideo salmonellosis in laboratory mice: successful treatment of the disease by oral oxytetracycline. Lab Anim. 1980, 14:217–219.

Smith K, et al. Outbreak of multidrug-resistant Salmonella typhimurium associated with rodents purchased at retail pet stores. Morbid Mort Weekly Rep. 2005, 54:429–433.

Swanson SJ, et al. Multidrug-resistant Salmonella enterica serotype typhimurium associated with pet rodents. N Eng J Med. 2007, 356:21–28.

SENDAI VIRUS INFECTIONS

Hosts

Mice, rats, hamsters, guinea pigs, and swine are hosts for Sendai virus infection. Chinchillas can be infected experimentally with the virus, while gerbils appear to be resistant. Suckling and weanling mice are most commonly and seriously affected. Although viral multiplication is largely limited to the nasal epithelium, laboratory rabbits are also susceptible to Sendai virus infection. Historically in North America, Sendai virus infections caused some of the most significant diseases of laboratory rodents. The disease remains enzootic in research mice in many parts of the world.

Etiology

Sendai virus, an RNA virus of the family Paramyxoviridae, genus *Paramyxovirus*, is also known as parainfluenza type 1. Many viruses in the paramyxovirus-parainfluenza group share common antigens. Clinical disease due to Sendai virus is often complicated by mycoplasmal and bacterial infections.

Following aerosol exposure, Sendai virus replicates in respiratory epithelial cells of the nasal passages, trachea, and bronchi, and, depending on various factors (including strain of mice), virus may also replicate in type II pneumocytes. In nude mice, Sendai virus replicates in both type I and type II pneumocytes. Intranuclear inclusions have been observed in bronchial epithelium of infected nude mice.

Transmission

Natural infection occurs via respiratory transmission, and passage may be by direct contact, contaminated fomites or tissues, or respiratory aerosol. The disease is extremely contagious. Acutely infected weanling mice (4–6 weeks of age) provide the principal reservoir for transmission in enzootically infected colonies. Disease-free or specific pathogen free animals are highly susceptible to infection.

Predisposing Factors

Some inbred mouse strains (129/J and DBA/2) are very susceptible to Sendai virus infection, but other strains (C57BL/6 and SJL) and random-bred mice are moderately resistant. DBA/2 mice are immunocompetent but have a delayed immune response following infection, which permits the virus to become established in the lower respiratory tract. A subsequent vigorous immune response induces significant host tissue damage.

Concurrent *Pasteurella pneumotropica*, *Corynebacterium kutscheri*, and *Mycoplasma pulmonis* infections greatly increase morbidity and mortality. In susceptible colonies, the disease is overt and epizootic especially if concurrent diseases produce a synergism. An inapparent enzootic form of disease is seen when most dams have been infected and pass maternal antibodies to their young.

Clinical Signs

In enzootically infected colonies, newborn mice are passively protected by maternal antibody until they are 4–6 weeks of age, at which time they become infected and develop an acquired immunity that is probably lifelong. Because adults in enzootically infected colonies have acquired immunity, they rarely show disease. Frequently, the disease is subclinical in weanling mice. Sendai virus infections are nearly always subclinical in rats, hamsters, guinea pigs, and rabbits. Clinical signs of an acute infection in susceptible animals include rough hair coat, chattering, weight loss, dyspnea, decreased breeding efficiency, and variable mortality.

Epizootic disease occurs when animals in an uninfected colony encounter Sendai virus infection. In this case, any and all animals may show clinical signs. There may be high mortality with many sick animals among sucklings. After several weeks of epizootic disease, an enzootic pattern ensues and persists as long as susceptible animals are present; usually weanlings or newly introduced naive or nonimmune mice are susceptible. Athymic mice and other immunodeficient mouse strains are highly susceptible and develop a persistent infection with wasting.

Necropsy Signs

In many animals, rhinitis will be the only visible sign of infection. Acute bronchopneumonia is grossly evident as plum-colored lungs with anteroventral consolidation.

The virus preferentially targets airways and necrotizing bronchiolitis is a classic lesion. Proliferation with or without destruction of bronchiolar epithelium, increased cellularity of alveolar septa, proteinaceous exudation, and the presence of alveolar macrophages and neutrophils in bronchioles and alveoli are frequent findings during the acute phase of the disease. The sloughing of virus-infected bronchiolar epithelial cells corresponds with the appearance of detectable antibody. During the regenerative phase, there is hyperplasia of type II pneumocytes lining airways, with fibrosis, thickening, and mononuclear cell infiltration in alveolar septa. Lesions in airways and alveoli are particularly extensive in athymic and SCID mice.

Diagnosis

Consideration of the species, strain, and age of animals involved and of the clinical, necropsy, and characteristic histologic lesions permits a provisional diagnosis of Sendai virus infection.

Sendai virus can usually be recovered from the lower respiratory tract from 6 to 8 days postinoculation. The elimination of the virus normally coincides with the appearance of detectable Sendai virus antibody in the peripheral blood. Serologic tests are not useful for many immune-deficient mouse strains.

Antigens shared among parainfluenza viruses confuse diagnostic serology efforts. Parainfluenza virus 3 (PI-3) may infect guinea pigs giving false positive results in ELISA serologic tests for Sendai virus (PI-1).

Animals vaccinated with live attenuated or killed vaccines develop titers that may be impossible to distinguish from titers associated with the naturally occurring disease. Inoculation of suspect materials into cell cultures can be used to diagnose Sendai virus infection before antibodies appear and suppress active infection.

Prevention

Prevention of the highly contagious but usually subclinical Sendai virus infection involves selection of rodents from a Sendai-free source and continual seromonitoring of the colony. Because young, recently weaned hamsters, mice, rats, rabbits, and guinea pigs constitute a reservoir population in which the infection maintains itself, the elimination of such young and the exclusion of additional young for 1–2 months may stop an outbreak. Commercial producers successfully use this method to eliminate Sendai virus from breeding colonies.

Previously, a killed vaccine of duck embryo origin was available commercially. The vaccine was prepared in 50-dose vials, and 0.1 mL of the vaccine given intraperitoneally provided approximately 7 months of protection. Others have successfully vaccinated with a temperature-sensitive mutant. Embryo transfer successfully eliminated Sendai virus from infected colonies. There is no evidence of transplacental infection with Sendai virus.

Effect on Research

Researchers should be apprised that a variety of physiologic functions are altered by concurrent Sendai virus infection, for example, depression of cell-mediated immunity, blast cell transformation, phagocytosis, and decreased intrapulmonary antibacterial activity. The disease generally has a major impact on animals used in immunologic research, transplantation, and pulmonary carcinogenesis studies.

In animal facilities where the virus is enzootic, it is advisable to purchase vaccinated or older animals, that is, 6 weeks old versus 3 weeks old, when possible. Older animals of susceptible strains have lower mortality and clinical disease is milder.

Public Health Significance

Sendai virus is antigenically related to human parainfluenza virus-1. Although the virus replicates productively in the upper and lower respiratory tracts of several nonhuman primate species, it has not been demonstrated to infect humans spontaneously.

References

Artwohl JE, et al. The efficacy of a dirty bedding sentinel system for detecting Sendai virus infection in mice: a comparison of clinical signs and seroconversion. Lab Anim Sci. 1994, 44:73–75.

Brownstein D. Genetics of natural resistance to Sendai virus infection in mice. Infect Immun. 1983, 41:308–312.

Carthew P, Sparrow S. A comparison in germfree mice of the pathogenesis of Sendai virus and mouse pneumonia virus infections. J Pathol. 1980, 130:153–158.

Castleman WL, Owens SB, Brundage-Anguish, LJ. Acute and persistent alterations in pulmonary inflammatory cells and airway mast cells induced by Sendai virus infection in neonatal rats. Vet Pathol. 1989, 26:18–25.

Dillehay DL, Lehner NDM, Huerkamp MJ. The effectiveness of a microisolator cage system and sentinel mice for controlling and detecting MHV and Sendai virus infections. Lab Anim Sci. 1990, 40:367–370.

Iwata H, et al. Aerosol vaccination with a Sendai virus temperature-sensitive mutant (HVJ-pb) derived from persistently infected cells. J Infect Dis. 1989, 162:402–407.

Jakab GJ. Interactions between Sendai virus and bacterial pathogens in the murine lung: a review. Lab Anim Sci. 1981, 31:170–177.

Machii K, et al. Infection of rabbits with Sendai virus. Lab Anim Sci. 1989, 39:334–337.

Makino S, et al. An epizootic of Sendai virus infection in a rat colony. Exp Anim. 1973, 22:275–280.

Okamoto M, Matsushita S, Matsumoto T. Cleaning of sendai virus-infected mice by embryo transfer technique. Exp Anim. 1990, 39:601–603.

Parker JC, Whiteman MD, Richter CB. Susceptibility of inbred and outbred mouse strains to Sendai virus and prevalence of infection in laboratory rodents. Infect Immun. 1978, 19:123–130.

Porter WP, Kudlacz EM. Effects of parainfluenza virus infection in guinea pigs. Lab Anim. 1992, 26:45–49.

Rottinghaus AA, Gibson SV, Wagner JE. Comparison of serologic tests for detection of antibodies to Sendai virus in rats. Lab Anim Sci. 1986, 36:496–498.

Skiadopoulos MH, et al. Sendai virus, a murine parainfluenza virus type 1, replicates to a level similar to human PIV1 in the upper and lower respiratory tract of African green monkeys and chimpanzees. Virol. 2002, 297(1):153–160.

Tsukui M, et al. Protective effect of inactivated virus vaccine on Sendai virus infection in rats. Lab Anim Sci. 1982, 32:143–146.

SPIRONUCLEOSIS

Hosts

The enteric flagellate *Spironucleus muris* infects mice, rats, hamsters, and wild rodents. Clinical disease is seen only in weanling, stressed, immune-suppressed, or inbred mice.

Etiology

Spironucleus muris is an opportunistic pathogen of laboratory mice, and occasionally outbreaks of diarrhea with weight loss occur. Co-infection with organisms such as *Giardia* spp or intestinal viruses or dietary changes may precipitate diarrhea, particularly in young animals. *Spironucleus* trophozoites reside primarily in the intervillar spaces and crypts of the upper small intestine. When associated with disease, blunting of villi, hyperplasia of crypt epithelium, and hypercellularity in the lamina propria, mononuclear cells predominating, are typical pathologic findings. In a morphologic study of kinetics of mucosal turnover of the small intestine in mice chronically infected with *Giardia muris* and *Spironucleus muris*, the enterocyte turnover was twice the rate in infected compared with uninfected mice.

The torpedo-shaped trophozoites (2–3 um × 20–25 um, flagella included) have two anterior nuclei and eight flagella (two posterior and six anterior). Small, oval cysts (5 um) have a banded "Easter egg" appearance. The direct life cycle is incompletely known. Resistant cysts survive stomach passage. The prepatent period is 2–3 days. *Spironucleus* spp feeds on bacteria, probably lactobacilli. It has been proposed that *Spironucleus* spp can be divided into two main groups. One group is infective for mice and golden hamsters, while the second group is exclusively infective for rats. This conclusion was based on interspecies cyst transfer studies.

Transmission

The environmentally resistant cyst of *S. muris* facilitates transmission by the fecal-oral route. Young and athymic nude mice pass larger numbers of cysts than do adults and other strains of mice.

Predisposing Factors

Susceptibility to *S. muris* infection varies with factors that raise or lower resistance. Co-infection with enterotropic strains of mouse hepatitis virus is common. Inbred strains such as C3H, NZW, and DBA/2 and the athymic nude mouse are very susceptible. Mice of both sexes between 3 and 8 weeks of age have the highest levels of clinical infection. Specific stressors include irradiation, steroid administration, crowding, nutrition, surgery, and chilling. A mild increase in the ambient temperature to 75–80 °F (27 °C) has reduced mortality. *Spironucleus muris* inhibits macrophage activity and may act synergistically with bacteria to cause disease.

Clinical Signs

Spironucleosis is an acute, chronic, or latent disease, depending on predisposing factors and duration of infection. The acute disease is characterized by a hunched posture, depression, dehydration, a rough, dull hair coat, distended abdomen, and often a soft, sticky stool. Death at the peak of an outbreak occurs 1–4 days following the onset of clinical signs, and mortality rates may approach 50%. Older mice have a marked variation in signs. Many have no clinical signs. Some may show progressive wasting, listlessness, and sporadic death.

Necropsy Signs

The common necropsy finding is an anterior small intestine grossly distended with a bubbly froth, giving the appearance of postmortem autolysis. The froth may be variably colored but rarely contains blood. The duodenum and anterior jejunum are affected grossly. Other findings may include diarrhea, an enlargement and thickening of the wall of the duodenum, enlarged mesenteric lymph nodes, ascites, and splenic and thymic atrophy.

Histopathologic signs are those of acute catarrhal enteritis or chronic mucosal hyperplasia with minimal mononuclear cell infiltration. Reduction in height of villi, epithelial desquamation, lymphocytic infiltration, villous edema, and the presence of organisms deep in the crypts between villi are common microscopic findings.

Diagnosis

Sprionucleus spp infections may not be detected with dirty bedding sentinel systems. Cysts and trophozoites may be seen on microscopic examination of direct smears of duodenal contents or in fixed and stained sections; however, histology may be more sensitive for detection than direct examination of smears because the trophozoites autolyze rapidly in unfixed preparations. Trophozoites can be seen in hematoxylin and eosin-stained or PAS-reaction sections distending the lumen of the crypts of Lieberkuhn in the duodenum (mice and hamsters) and in the pylorus (rats). Alternatively, PCR tests may be used to detect the organism in tissues. Cysts, which may be quantitated, are better seen with iodine staining or phase contrast optics. In direct smears diluted in an isotonic saline solution, the trophozoites of *S. muris* have a fast, forward, erratic movement, whereas the larger *Giardia* spp trophozoites are spoon- or half-moon-shaped and have a rolling motion in a liquid environment.

Treatment

When the antiprotozoal agent dimetridazole was given in the drinking water (0.04–0.1%), mortality was reduced but *Spironucleus* spp was not eliminated from infected animals. Subsequently, the entire class of 5-hydroxyimidazole compounds has been removed from the U.S. market because of potential carcinogenicity concerns.

Prevention

Prevention is based on good colony management, which includes proper sanitation of caging and isolation, testing, and quarantine procedures. Cysts are resistant to commonly used disinfectants. Cysts of *S. muris* are sensitive to temperatures above 45 °C (113 °F) for 30 minutes or 60 °C (140 °F) for 1 minute, 70% ethanol, and 4% formalin. They survive cold, low pH, and desiccation. Caesarean derivation and cross-fostering onto clean dams can be used to rederive infected animals.

Public Health Significance

Spironucleus muris is not pathogenic for humans.

References

Boorman GA, et al. Synergistic role of intestinal flagellates and normal intestinal bacteria in a post-weaning mortality of mice. Lab Anim Sci. 1973, 23:187–193.

Fain MA, Karjala Z, Perdue KA, et al. Detection of Spironucleus muris in unpreserved mouse tissue and fecal samples by using a PCR assay. J Amer Assoc Lab Anim Sci. 2008, 47(5):39–43.

Flatt RE, Halvorsen JA, Kemp RL. Hexamitiasis in a laboratory mouse colony. Lab Anim Sci. 1978, 28:62–65.

Keast D, Chesterman FC. Changes in macrophage metabolism in mice heavily infected with Hexamita muris. Lab Anim. 1972, 6:33–39.

Kunstyr I. Infectious form of Spironucleus (Hexamita) muris: banded cysts. Lab Anim. 1977, 11:185–188.

Kunstyr I, Ammerpohl E. Resistance of faecal cysts of Spironucleus muris to some physical factors and chemical substances. Lab Anim. 1978, 12:95–97.

Lussier G, Loew FM. An outbreak of hexamitiasis in laboratory mice. Can J Comp Med. 1970, 34:350–353.

Perdue KA, Copeland MK, Karjala Z, et al. Suboptimal ability of dirty-bedding sentinels to detect Spironucleus muris in a colony of mice with genetic manipulations of the adaptive immune system. J Amer Assoc Lab Anim Sci. 2008, 47(5):10–17.

Schagemann G, et al. Host specificity of cloned Spironucleus muris in laboratory rodents. Lab Anim. 1990, 24:234–239.

Sebesteny A. Transmission of Spironucleus and Giardia spp. and some nonpathogenic intestinal protozoa from infested hamsters to mice. Lab Anim. 1979, 13:189–191.

Wagner JE, et al. Hexamitiasis in laboratory mice, hamsters, and rats. Lab Anim Sci. 1974, 24:349–354.

SPLAYLEG IN RABBITS

Hosts

Congenital or acquired abnormalities of the hip and shoulder have been described in rabbits, dogs, calves, and humans.

Etiology

Splayleg is a descriptive term applied to a variety of inherited or acquired developmental abnormalities in which the rabbit in ventral recumbency is unable to adduct (to bring together toward the median axis) one or more limbs and rise to a standing position. These abnormalities include improper development of the spine, pelvis, coxofemoral junction, or long bones. The muscles of the affected limbs may remain functional or become partially or totally paralyzed. Unlike paralysis associated with vertebral fracture or luxation, splayleg usually has a familial inheritance pattern.

Splayleg has also developed in rabbits raised on smooth floor surfaces.

Predisposing Factors

Genetic predisposition to splayleg occurs in a variety of rabbit breeds and in both sexes with similar frequencies. In an early study on splayleg in rabbits, it was concluded that its manifestation is the result of a mutant autosomal gene that is inherited in a simple autosomal recessive pattern. The disease is not primarily an arthritis or osteochondritis.

In one study evaluating the impact of floor surface on acquired splayleg, rabbits housed on Plexiglas® or waxed cardboard surfaces had a significantly higher incidence of acquired hip dysplasia than animals housed on a textured surface. Affected animals had splaying of one or both hind limbs, flattening and reduction of the femoral head, subluxation of the hip, and patellar luxation.

Clinical Signs

Splayleg may be seen initially at birth, a few days after birth, after the rabbit leaves the nest, or after several months. The affected rabbit is usually alert and responsive, although its growth may be stunted slightly. With adequate nursing care, rabbits can be sustained for months until adverse clinical sequelae develop. If the rabbit is maintained long enough, joint disease, specifically, chronic traumatic osteoarthritis, subluxation, or dislocation, may result in a false joint.

Necropsy Signs

Besides the obvious postural and conformational abnormality, gross pathologic changes are strictly confined to bony structures of the femoral neck and the subtrochanter region. Surrounding structures such as the femoral head or the acetabulum and other soft tissues are usually normal except as a sequela to a chronic condition. Histopathologic changes are an uncommon feature of the congenital abnormality.

Diagnosis

Clinical signs consistent with radiographic findings and a history of onset at a young age supported by a genetic predisposition, such as a history of siblings with a similar affliction, are confirmatory factors in making the diagnosis. Other conditions leading to weakness of rear limbs such as ataxia, trauma, malnutrition, severe *Sarcocystis* spp infection, and toxoplasmosis should be included in the differential diagnosis.

Treatment

There is no known satisfactory treatment for splayleg. The affected rabbit, because of limited mobility, is prone to predation, starvation (if unable to access food), and secondary skin disease because of frequent exposure to urine, trauma, and abrasions. Hence, such animals should be euthanatized.

Prevention

Animals with congenital splayleg should be eliminated from the colony and their dams and sires removed from breeding stock. Acquired splayleg may be prevented by ensuring that growing animals are housed on surfaces with firm footing.

References

Arendar GM, Much RA. Splayleg, a recessively inherited form of femoral neck anteversion, femoral shaft torsion and subluxation of the hip in the laboratory lop rabbit. Clin Orthop. 1966, 44:221–229.

Cosgrove M, Wiggins JP, Rothenbacher H. Sarcocystis spp. in the Eastern cottontail (Sylvilagus floridanus). J Wildl Dis. 1982, 18:37–40.

Joosten HF. Splayleg: a spontaneous limb defect in rabbits. Genetics, gross anatomy, and microscopy. Teratol. 1981, 24(1):87–104.

Lindsey JR, Fox RR. Inherited Diseases and Variations. In: The Biology of the Laboratory Rabbit, 2nd ed. Manning PJ, Ringler DH, Newcomer CE (eds.). San Diego: Academic Press, 1994, 293–319.

Owiny JR, Vandewoude S, Painter JT, et al. Hip dysplasia in rabbits: association with nest box flooring. Comp Med. 2001, 51(1):85–88.

STAPHYLOCOCCOSIS

Hosts

Staphylococcus aureus infections occur commonly in a variety of animals, including humans. The organism is an opportunistic agent and is commonly carried subclinically in the nasopharynx and on the skin of rabbits and rodents. Staphylococcal abscesses are common in some colonies of immunocompromised mice, and staphylococcal dermatitis occurs from time to time in rats and other rodent species, possibly secondary to undetermined genetic, autoimmune, and other inciting causes.

Etiology

Staphylococcus aureus is an aerobic, nonsporeforming, variably alpha- and beta-hemolytic, catalase-positive, Gram-positive coccus. Although several human phage types have been recovered from animals, animals usually have species-specific staphylococcal serotypes or biotypes.

Transmission

Two important considerations in the transmission and persistence of *S. aureus* are human carriers and the resistance of the organism to drying and environmental factors. The organism may spread by direct contact between animals and man or by contaminated food, feces, cages, and bedding. Aerosol spread is possible also, as is invasion through traumatized skin or open umbilical stumps.

Predisposing Factors

Staphylococci are common microflora of the skin, mucous membranes, and upper respiratory tract. Initiation of clinical disease usually involves a cutaneous wound, constant skin wetting, or a stressor, such as crowding, dietary changes, fighting, low dietary protein, or high environmental temperatures. Contact with infected caretakers has been implicated as a predisposing factor.

Clinical Signs

Clinical signs of *S. aureus* infection, other than sudden death from pneumonia, septicemia, or toxemia, include fever, anorexia, depression, urinary tract infections, moist dermatitis, conjunctivitis (Figure 5.19), foot swelling, subcutaneous lumps, enlarged mammary glands, or a purulent discharge. Pruritic skin lesions may elicit self-mutilation or the animals may develop scabs and heal spontaneously. Dermatitis is often exacerbated by scratching. Infections caused by infectious agents such as *Staphylococcus* spp may alter sleep patterns.

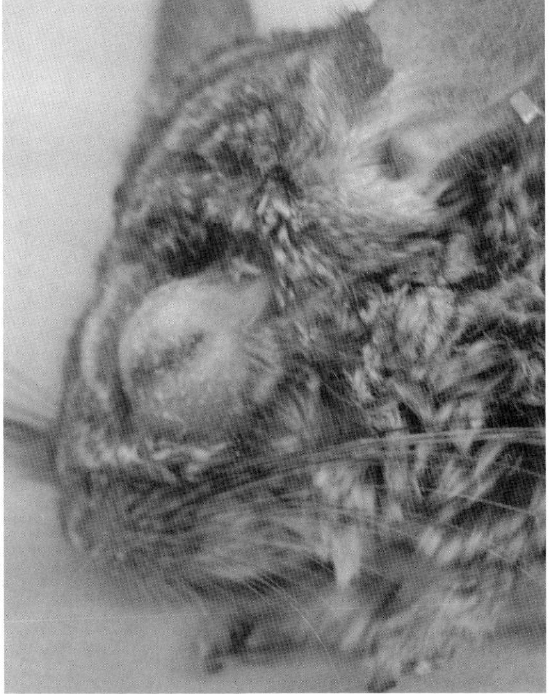

FIGURE 5.19. Severe staphylococcal conjunctivitis in a chinchilla.

Among the staphylococcal dermatopathies, which range from alopecia and reddening to extensive ulceration, are cheilitis and exfoliative dermatitis in guinea pigs; ulcerative to gangrenous pododermatitis of rabbits, chinchillas, guinea pigs, and rats; pustular and ulcerative dermatitis in rats and mice; ulcerative dermatitis and "sore nose" in gerbils; conjunctivitis in rabbits; mastitis and subcutaneous abscesses in chinchillas and rabbits; and moist dermatitis due to ear tag irritation in mice.

Internal staphylococcal lesions, which may have specific (purulent discharge) or nonspecific signs, include acute to chronic rhinitis, gingivitis, pneumonia, and cystitis. Abscessation or suppuration can occur in any tissue, including the tympanic bullae, preputial glands, brain, heart, urogenital system, lymph nodes, and spleen. Death following *S. aureus* infection may be peracute, likely related to exotoxin elaboration. Staphylococcal mastitis in rabbits, originating from scratches, bites, or nest box wounds, results in a variation of the "young doe syndrome." The resulting toxemia involves swollen glands, fever, anorexia, and death in nursing does. The young may also die.

Necropsy Signs

Lesions of staphylococcal infection vary with host, site, and duration, but characteristics range from diffuse cellulitis to suppuration with abscessation, necrosis, and granuloma formation. Clumps of large Gram-positive cocci are readily seen on impression smears or in lesions examined microscopically.

Diagnosis

Recovery of *S. aureus* on culture does not confirm a diagnosis, although it does confirm the presence of the organism at the site. Other bacteria, including *Pasteurella* spp, *Salmonella* spp, *Pseudomonas* spp, and *Streptococcus* spp, produce dermatitis or abscessation in rabbits and rodents. Trimming toenails may be useful to reduce self-mutilation.

Treatment

Treatment of staphylococcal infections, if indicated, includes cleaning, drainage, or excision of the lesion; removal of the cause of traumatic insult, if any; and selection of topical and parenteral antibiotics based on culture, sensitivity testing, and host idiosyncrasies.

Rodents are active groomers and quickly remove and consume materials applied topically. Topical agents, such as zinc ointment, should be applied in a thin coat, and often over-the-counter medications can provide soothing relief without upsetting gastrointestinal flora. Elizabethan collars, properly constructed and applied, may be useful in preventing animals from removing topical preparations.

Antibiotics that have been used to treat staphylococcal infections include gentamicin, kanamycin, procaine penicillin G (20,000–40,000 units/kg for 3 days), nitrofuran topical ointments, oxytetracycline (55 mg/kg fresh daily in water for 4 days), and tetracycline hydrochloride (0.3 g/100 mL water for 14 days). Penicillins and cephalosporins are generally well tolerated in mice and rats but may induce fatal dysbiosis when used in rabbits and other rodent species.

Prevention

The spread of *S. aureus* or the initiation of clinical disease in carrier animals is reduced or prevented by good sanitation, elimination of sharp or abrasive surfaces, use of clean feed and bedding, reduction of stress, and monitoring of caretakers and animals. Elimination of carriers by treatment is difficult.

Public Health Significance

Strains of methicillin-resistant *Staphylococcus aureus* (MRSA) have been cultured from clinically normal rabbits, guinea pigs, and chinchillas. Appropriate hand-washing practices should always be used after handling small rodents and rabbits.

References

Blackmore DK, Francis RA. The apparent transmission of staphylococci of human origin to laboratory animals. J Comp Pathol. 1970, 80:645–651.

Bradfield JF, Wagner JE, Boivin GP. Epizootic fatal dermatitis in athymic nude mice due to Staphylococcus xylosus. Lab Anim Sci. 1993, 43:111–113.

Carolan MG. Staphylococcosis in rabbits. Vet Rec. 1986, 119:412.

Chew BP, Zamora CS, Luedecke LO. Effect of vitamin A deficiency on mammary gland development and susceptibility to mastitis through intramammary infusion with Staphylococcus aureus in mice. Amer J Vet Res. 1985, 46:287–293.

Clarke MC, et al. The occurrence in mice of facial and mandibular abscesses associated with Staphylococcus aureus. Lab Anim. 1978, 12:121–123.

Cover CE, Keenan CM, Bettinger GE. Ear tag induced Staphylococcus infection in mice. Lab Anim. 1989, 23:229–233.

Donnelly RM, Stark DM. Susceptibility of laboratory rats, hamsters, and mice to wound infection with Staphylococcus aureus. Amer J Vet Res. 1985, 46:2634–2638.

Holliman A, Girvan GA. Staphylococcosis in a commercial rabbitry. Lab Anim Sci. 1986, 36:187.

Millichamp NJ, Collins BR. Blepharoconjunctivitis associated with Staphylococcus aureus in a rabbit. J Am Vet Med Assoc. 1986, 189:1153–1154.

Morgan M. Methicillin-resistant Staphylococcus aureus and animals: zoonosis or humanosis? J Antimicrob Chemother. 2008, 62(6):1181–1187.

Peckham JC, et al. Staphylococcal dermatitis in Mongolian gerbils (Meriones unguiculatus). Lab Anim Sci. 1974, 24:43–47.

Toth LA, Krueger JM. Alteration of sleep in rabbits by Staphylococcus aureus infection. Infect Immun. 1988, 56:1785–1791.

Walther B, et al. Methicillin-resistant Staphylococcus aureus (MRSA) isolated from small and exotic animals at a university hospital during routine microbiological examinations. Vet Microbiol. 2008, 127(1–2):171–178.

STREPTOCOCCUS PNEUMONIAE INFECTIONS IN RODENTS

Hosts

Streptococcus pneumoniae affects a wide range of animals, but the guinea pig and rat are particularly susceptible. Rabbits, mice, and other small rodent species are less susceptible.

Etiology

Streptococcus pneumoniae infections in the guinea pig are caused by serotypes III, IV, and XIX. Serotypes reported in rats include II, III, VIII, XVI, and XIX. *Streptococcus pneumoniae* are Gram-positive, oval or lanciform, capsulated cocci that often occur in distinct pairs or short chains. Genus

SPECIFIC DISEASES AND CONDITIONS

synonyms are *Diplococcus* spp and *Pneumococcus* spp. Infections in rodent colonies tend to be monotypic.

Transmission

Transmission of *S. pneumoniae* is by respiratory aerosol or direct contact. Clinically normal guinea pigs and rats may carry the organism in the upper respiratory passages. Depending on the season of the year, 40–70% of human populations carry *S. pneumoniae* in the respiratory passages and may be the source of the infection in animals.

Predisposing Factors

Losses from *S. pneumoniae* are greater during the winter, after shipment, and in animals on marginal diets, especially in guinea pigs with hypovitaminosis C. Carrier animals frequently succumb when stressed by dietary deficiencies, concurrent diseases such as mycoplasmosis and Sendai virus infection in rats, pregnancy in guinea pigs, experimental procedures, shipment, and poor husbandry. Inbred strains of guinea pigs are more susceptible than are random or outbred stocks. Infected animals should not be used in research.

Clinical Signs

Carrier animals may have upper respiratory infections without clinical signs. Acute episodes or prolonged epizootics with variable morbidity and mortality may both occur. In guinea pigs, clinical signs include sneezing, nasal and ocular discharges, anorexia, weight loss, coughing, dyspnea, depression, torticollis if the inner ear or brain is affected, and death. Abortions are associated with both general and uterine infections.

Similar signs, along with hematuria, are seen in affected rats. Carrier rats and guinea pigs, after experimental manipulations, are prone to clinical disease due to *S. pneumoniae*, for example, peritonitis after intraperitoneal injections, encephalitis after placement of intracranial implants, and pleuritis after cardiac puncture.

Necropsy Signs

Gross lesions of *S. pneumoniae* infection include seropurulent and fibrinopurulent polyserositis, including pleuritis, pericarditis, epicarditis, peritonitis, orchitis, meningitis, otitis media and interna, metritis, and bronchopneumonia.

Diagnosis

Diagnosis is established by observation of the Gram-positive, oval or lanciform, coccal bacteria in pairs or short chains on a stained, direct smear of the inflammatory exudate. Cultures for routine monitoring can be collected from the nasal passages with a small swab or by nasal lavage. Histologically, unlike with many bacterial diseases, large numbers of organisms can be seen in smears and tissue sections. Recovery of *S. pneumoniae* on blood agar culture in the presence of 5–10% CO_2 confirms the diagnosis. An ELISA is available for serodiagnosis of pneumococcal infections.

Treatment

Treatment in most cases is impractical because the condition may be advanced at the time of detection. Antibiotic therapy likely will not eliminate the agent from infected colonies. Oxytetracycline at 0.1 mg/mL in the drinking water for 7 days has controlled an epizootic but not eliminated the carrier state. Such treatment assumes that the animal will drink the liquid and tolerate changes in intestinal flora, and that the antibiotic will reach the organisms. *Streptococcus pneumoniae* organisms are generally sensitive to benzathine-based penicillins, ampicillin, bacitracin, chloramphenicol, erythromycin, lincomycin, and methicillin, but most of these antibiotics may produce fatal reactions in guinea pigs. Broad-spectrum antibiotics such as chloramphenicol and trimethoprim-sulfa may be useful in guinea pigs. For rats, 150 units/g body weight of benzathine penicillin has been recommended.

Prevention

Good husbandry, closed-colony maintenance, elimination of carriers, and reduction of environmental stress reduce the possibility and severity of outbreaks. Ordinary disinfectants readily kill pneumococci. A vaccine that contains capsular polysaccharides from multiple serotypes is used to prevent human infections. To minimize shedding and bacterial transmission, human caregivers with streptococcal infections should not handle rabbits or rodents.

Public Health Significance

Streptococcus pneumoniae can cause respiratory and meningeal disease in humans, especially in elderly people, and in people who lack spleens. In some cases, the serotypes that affect animals may also affect humans.

References

Borkowski FL, Griffith J. Diagnostic exercise: pneumonia and pleuritis in a rat. Lab Anim Sci. 1990, 40:323–325.

Fallon MT, et al. Inapparent Streptococcus pneumoniae type 35 infection in commercial rats and mice. Lab Anim Sci. 1988, 38:129–132.

Matsubara J, et al. Serodiagnosis of Streptococcus pneumoniae infection in guinea-pigs by an enzyme-linked immunosorbent assay. Lab Anim. 1988, 22:304–308.

Witt WM, Hubbard GB, Fanton, J. Streptococcus pneumoniae arthritis and osteomyelitis with vitamin C deficiency in guinea pigs. Lab Anim Sci. 1988, 38:192–194.

STREPTOCOCCUS ZOOEPIDEMICUS INFECTIONS IN GUINEA PIGS

Hosts

Streptococcal organisms are found in a variety of hosts, but among small rodents the guinea pig is most often affected clinically with *Streptococcus zooepidemicus*.

Etiology

A beta-hemolytic, Gram-positive, encapsulated, Lancefield's Group C *Streptococcus*, *S. zooepidemicus*, is involved occasionally in clinical disease in conventionally housed pet and laboratory origin guinea pigs. The cervical lymphadenitis caused by this agent closely resembles a less common disease caused by *Streptobacillus moniliformis*.

Transmission

Transmission of *S. zooepidemicus* occurs through cutaneous wounds, via aerosol into the respiratory tract, or by the genital route. In many cases, the agent likely enters the host through small abrasions in the oral cavity. The oral cavity abrasions may be caused by sharp or coarse plant feeds, such as hay and oats. After penetration, the agent is transported via the lymphatics to the draining regional cervical lymph nodes, where it proliferates. The conjunctiva and nasal mucosa represent excellent sites for entry of *S. zooepidemicus* infections that result in cervical lymphadenitis in young guinea pigs.

Predisposing Factors

Poor husbandry and general stress factors predispose to streptococcal infections. Biting facilitates transmission, as does the traumatic effect of overgrown teeth and coarse dietary roughage. Dietary deficiencies, especially vitamin C deficiency in guinea pigs, must be resolved, as they may predispose the animals to infection.

Clinical Signs

In its chronic or enzootic form, *S. zooepidemicus* causes cervical lymphadenitis, a sporadic, pyogenic infection with abscessation and, in many cases, external drainage of the ventral cervical lymph nodes. Abscesses caused by this agent may occur in almost any organ, but cervical and other lymph nodes are by far the most common site. This lymphadenopathy is sometimes referred to as "lumps." Septicemias and acute pneumonias with high mortality occur in the epizootic form.

Torticollis or "wry neck" results from streptococcal infection of the middle ear with variable extension to the inner ear. Respiratory involvement is manifested clinically by nasal and ocular discharge and by signs of acute pneumonia, including dyspnea and cyanosis. Chronic infection can progress to septicemia if the host is stressed or an abscess ruptures spontaneously or is opened surgically. Abortions, stillbirths, hematuria, and hemoglobinuria have been associated with septicemias. Reproductive patterns also may be disturbed by the numerous small uterine abscesses seen in some *S. zooepidemicus* infections.

Necropsy Signs

Infection with *S. zooepidemicus* ranges from an acute, fatal septicemia to a chronic, suppurative process in the lymph nodes, especially the cervical nodes, thoracic and abdominal viscera, uterus, and middle and inner ears. Extensive pulmonary consolidation, focal hepatic necrosis, and fibrinous pleuritis are additional signs.

Diagnosis

A presumptive diagnosis can be made when cervical abscesses are palpated or observed. Chains of Gram-positive cocci may be seen in stained direct smears of material from abscesses. Confirmatory diagnosis depends on in vitro culture from abscesses, heart blood, or affected lungs in the case of acute disease. At 24 hours on blood agar, beta-hemolytic colonies of streptococci are mucoid, 2–3 mm in diameter, and are surrounded by a clear zone of hemolysis.

Treatment

Concerns in therapy include the number of infected and contact animals, distribution of abscesses, presence of fistulous tracts, potential for septicemia if the abscess is opened, and the antibiotic sensitivity of the organism. Abscesses should be removed intact from anesthetized animals, whenever possible, to minimize environmental contamination and transmission to other guinea pigs in the household or colony. With or without surgical treatment, a systemic antibiotic, such as chloramphenicol, enrofloxacin or ciprofloxacin (10 mg/kg IM or PO every 12 hr), or trimethoprim-sulfa is given. Chloramphenicol palmitate, one of the few antibiotics safe to use in guinea pigs, is given at 50 mg/kg orally for 5–7 days.

Prevention

Epizootics with high mortality usually follow introduction of affected stock into a formerly infection-free colony or mixing susceptible stock with resistant carrier animals. Good husbandry practices, general preventive measures, and routine palpation for enlarged cervical lymph nodes reduce the possibility of streptococcal infection in guinea pigs. Affected guinea pigs are removed from the colony or treated until the abscesses have drained and healed. In cases of epizootic *S. zooepidemicus* infection with widespread pneumonia, septicemias, and abscesses, the entire colony may have to be eliminated.

Killed bacterins have not been effective in preventing this disease, but scratch injections into the oral cavity with American Type Culture Collection strain 12960 of a group C *Streptococcus* has stimulated immunity. The organism is grown for 24 hours in trypticase soy broth and 0.1 mL is scratched into the oral mucosa.

Public Health Significance

Beta-hemolytic streptococci (not *S. zooepidemicus*) are recovered frequently from human infections, but *S. zooepidemicus* is strictly an animal pathogen.

References

Ahem PF, Archer RK, Sparrow S. An infection in rats caused by Beta-haemolytic streptococci of group C. Vet Rec. 1979, 104:507–508.

Fleming MP. Streptobacillus moniliformis isolations from cervical abscesses of guinea pigs. Vet Rec. 1976, 99:256.

Henderson JD, Jr. Cervical lymphadenitis in the guinea pig. Vet Med Small Anim Clin. 1976, 71:462–463.

Mayora J, Soave O, Doak R. Prevention of cervical lymphadenitis in guinea pigs by vaccination. Lab Anim Sci. 1978, 28:686–690.

Murphy JC, et al. Cervical lymphadenitis in guinea pigs: infection via intact ocular and nasal mucosa by Streptococcus zooepidemicus. Lab Anim Sci. 1991, 41:251–254.

Olson LD, et al. Experimental induction of cervical lymphadenitis in guinea-pigs with group C streptococci. Lab Anim. 1976, 10:223–231.

TRANSMISSIBLE COLONIC HYPERPLASIA IN MICE

Hosts

Transmissible murine colonic hyperplasia caused by *Citrobacter rodentium* is a naturally occurring disease seen predominantly in mice; however, infections have also been reported in guinea pigs and gerbils.

Etiology

The causative agent of transmissible colonic hyperplasia is a Gram-negative bacillus, formerly designated as *Citrobacter freundii* 4280 and more recently as *C. rodentium*. Transmissible murine colonic hyperplasia is a naturally occurring infectious disease of mice characterized by mucosal hyperplasia of the distal colon. *C. rodentium* is related to *E. coli* strains and induces attaching and effacing lesions. Following oral inoculation, the organism initially colonizes the small intestine and then selectively colonizes the descending colon, attaching to the mucosa and displacing other aerobic bacteria and inducing an intense mucosal hyperplasia.

There are isolated reports of *C. rodentium*–associated enteric disease in gerbils and guinea pigs.

Transmission

Transmission of the causative bacterium is by the fecal-oral route. Fomites may be involved in cage-to-cage spread. Outbreaks in a colony are often prolonged over weeks or months, although the duration of infection in any individual animal is likely short. The source of infection for mouse colonies frequently remains unknown. Humans are suspected carriers.

Predisposing Factors

Dietary changes, diet composition, age, genetic background, stress, and virulence of the *C. rodentium* strain affect susceptibility to clinical disease. Newly weaned mice have a higher mortality and more obvious clinical signs than do older mice. C3H mice have more severe clinical signs than do NIH Swiss, C57BL/6, and DBA/2 mice.

Clinical Signs

Clinical signs include ruffled hair coat, stunting, passage of dark, sticky feces, and occasionally rectal prolapse. Moderate mortality occurs in mice infected at around 2–6 weeks of age, and mortality rates are low to nil in mice infected as adults. There is a great variation in strain susceptibility to the clinical disease, and diet may also influence susceptibility. After the acute phase, colonic hyperplasia regresses.

Necropsy Signs

The outstanding sign at necropsy of affected mice is a grossly detectable thickening (to 0.5 cm diameter) and turgidity of the rectum and terminal 1–3 cm of the descending colon. The thickening is due to hyperplasia of enterocytes, a reaction in both young and adult mice. Inflammation accompanies the hyperplasia in young mice.

Microscopically, mucosal hyperplasia is seen in the descending colon. There is a marked increase in the height of the affected mucosa (crypt height may be up to 3 times normal), increased mitotic index, erosions of affected epithelium, presence of bacterial colonies in crypts and lamina propria, leukocytic infiltration, and goblet cell hyperplasia.

In gerbils, the clinical signs and pathology are similar to those seen in laboratory mice.

Diagnosis

Diagnosis is based on recovery of *Citrobacter rodentium* from affected mice and on the characteristic colonic hyperplasia. *C. rodentium* is normally recoverable on culture only during the early stages of the disease. When present, the agent is readily cultured in vitro and has a characteristic biochemical reaction profile. Most isolates are lactose positive and use citrate as a sole source of carbon.

Nonpathogenic *Citrobacter* biotypes are commonly isolated from the intestines and feces of rodents; thus, microbiologists working with rodent samples must be aware of in vitro tests necessary to distinguish the pathogenic *Citrobacter rodentium* biotypes from other nonpathogenic biotypes. Other enteric diseases of mice that should be considered in the differential diagnosis include enzootic diarrhea of infant mice, mouse hepatitis virus infection, giardiasis, reovirus and rotavirus infections, colibacillosis, salmonellosis, spironucleosis, *Helicobacter* spp infection, pinworm infestation, and *Clostridium piliforme* infection (Tyzzer's disease).

Transmission to sentinel animals via dirty bedding transfer is inefficient, and this method may not detect the presence of the bacterium.

Treatment

Ingestion of 0.1% solution of sodium sulfamethazine in the drinking water for 60 days has reduced clinical signs of experimental *Citrobacter* spp infection in a mouse colony. Tetracycline at 450 mg/L of drinking water or neomycin sulfate at 2 mg/mL is reported to suppress the disease and eliminate the bacteria in mice.

Prevention

Good husbandry and sanitation will reduce opportunities for entry of the bacterium into a colony. *Citrobacter rodentium* is occasionally isolated from the intestinal tracts of clinically normal mammals, including laboratory rodents and man, a finding that raises concerns about sources of contamination.

Public Health Significance

Citrobacter rodentium variants have been found in human feces, but the potential pathogenicity of these and other *Citrobacter* spp for humans is unknown. *Citrobacter rodentium*–infected mice are commonly used as a model for enteropathogenic *E. coli* infections of humans.

References

Barthold SW. The microbiology of transmissible murine colonic hyperplasia. Lab Anim Sci. 1980, 30:167–173.

Barthold SW, et al. Transmissible murine colonic hyperplasia. Vet Pathol. 1978, 15:223–236.

Borenshtein D, et al. Development of fatal colitis in FVB mice infected with Citrobacter rodentium. Infect Immun. 2007, 75(7):3271–3281.

De La Puente-Redondo VA, et al. Epidemic infection caused by Citrobacter rodentium in a gerbil colony. Vet Rec. 1999, 145:400–403.

Maggio-Price L, et al. Diminished reproduction, failure to thrive, and altered immunologic function in a colony of T-cell receptor-deficient transgenic mice. Lab Anim Sci. 1998, 48:145–155.

Mundy R, et al. Citrobacter rodentium of mice and men. Cell Microbiol. 2005, 7:1697–1706.

Schnaur DB, et al. Genetic and biochemical characterization of Citrobacter rodentium sp. nov. J Clin Microbiol. 1995, 33:2064–2068.

Silverman J, et al. A natural outbreak of transmissible murine colonic hyperplasia in AU. mice. Lab Anim Sci. 1979, 29:209–213.

TULAREMIA

Hosts

Tularemia is a common, often fatal septicemic disease of over a hundred species of wild animals, especially rodents, wild lagomorphs, and certain gallinaceous birds (pheasants and quail). Tularemia has a broad host spectrum, and rodents and lagomorphs are highly susceptible and have been involved in many epizootics. Tularemia is rare in domestic rabbits and rodents, although animals raised outdoors and exposed to ticks are much more likely to contract infections than are similar animals kept indoors in a home or laboratory animal resource facility.

Etiology

Francisella tularensis is an aerobic nonmotile, Gram-negative, pleomorphic, bipolar coccobacillus. The agent is particularly prevalent in the south central United States and has been classified by U.S. Centers for Disease Control and Prevention as a "select agent," requiring strict containment and documentation for experimental studies.

Transmission

Transmission is direct, via bites, inhalation, or ingestion of bacilli, and has not been documented to occur from human to human. Only a few (5–10) organisms are required for infection by the respiratory route, while many times more are required if ingested (10^6–10^8). Blood-sucking arthropods, especially ticks, biting flies, and mosquitoes, are an important means of bacterial transmission. The tissues, blood, and feces of infected animals harbor the organism.

Predisposing Factors

The tularemia bacterium is highly infectious and affects otherwise healthy animals. The disease is more common in the fall and winter when carrier animals concentrate in buildings and other enclosed spaces to obtain protection from the cold.

Clinical Signs

The disease has a range of signs in mammals depending upon bacterial type, dose, and route of exposure. Symptoms include fever, lethargy, lymphadenopathy, pneumonic disease, septicemia, and death. Affected animals may initially demonstrate a roughened hair coat, depression, tendency to huddle, anorexia, ataxia, and death. The course of the disease in cottontail rabbits (*Sylvilagus* spp) lasts approximately 1 week. Asymptomatic infections are common in wildlife based on the high prevalence of serum antibody.

Necropsy Signs

Signs of septicemia include pulmonary congestion and consolidation, subpleural petechial hemorrhage, numerous pinpoint, small, and bright white hepatic foci, and congestion and enlargement of the liver and spleen. The miliary white spots on the dark background of the congested liver and spleen have been described as resembling the Milky Way galaxy. Lymph nodes are enlarged and the bacteria are distributed widely in blood vessels.

Diagnosis

Diagnosis is based on necropsy findings of a septicemic bacterial disease. Stained impression smears of affected tissues or fluids may contain small Gram-negative coccobacilli among debris and within cells and can aid in making a tentative diagnosis at necropsy.

In vitro recovery of *F. tularensis* requires special attention. Special enriched media such as blood-glucose-cysteine agar grow colonies that are minute and translucent. The agent is highly hazardous to man and must be handled with extreme caution in the laboratory. Intraperitoneal injection of potentially contaminated blood into a guinea pig produces lymphoid necrosis, serofibrinous peritonitis, septicemia, and death in 8–10 days.

Treatment

Treatment is not indicated for animals. Tetracyclines and streptomycin are among the antibiotics used to treat human infections.

Prevention

Avoid or minimize contact with animals that may have been exposed to *Francisella tularensis*. Exclusion of wild mammals and insect vectors from the colony are preventive measures. Hunters should avoid "lazy" cottontail rabbits and wear gloves when skinning game.

Public Health Significance

Up to 90% of human cases of tularemia are linked to wild lagomorph exposure. Humans are very susceptible and tularemia is a reportable disease in the United States. Because contamination of inapparent skin lesions results in human infections, persons handling suspect tissues should always wear gloves. Laboratory culture should be attempted only where adequate biohazard culture facilities are available. Cutaneous lesions, septicemias, and meningitis occur in cases of human tularemia. Bites of two and three host ticks are particularly dangerous, as ticks transmit the bacterium.

Recent cases in humans in Canada and the United States have been associated with pet hamster bites, the hamsters often dying of mysterious illnesses before a diagnosis is determined. In all cases, the infected animals have been traced back to large rodent breeders or distribution centers. Human cases have also occurred after well-meaning individuals have picked up and attempted to treat feral squirrels and rabbits that appeared sick. If these animals are taken into clinics for evaluation, it is important to ensure that appropriate hygiene and personal safety measures are in place to minimize the risk of potential disease transmission.

References

Hoff GL, et al. Tularemia in Florida: Sylvilagus palustris as a source of human infection. J Wildl Dis. 1975, 11:560–561.

Lepitzki DA, Woolf A, Cooper M. Serological prevalence of tularemia in cottontail rabbits of southern Illinois. J Wildl Dis. 1990, 26:279–282.

Moe JB, et al. Pathogenesis of tularemia in immune and nonimmune rats. Amer J Vet Res. 1975, 36:1505–1510.

Pape J, et al. Brief report: tularemia associated with a hamster bite. Morbid Mort Weekly Rep. 2005, 53:1202–1203.

Rohrbach BW. Tularemia. J Am Vet Med Assoc. 1988, 193:428–432.

TYZZER'S DISEASE

Hosts

The number of species known to be susceptible to Tyzzer's disease, an infection caused by *Clostridium piliforme*, continues to increase. The spectrum includes mice, rats, hamsters, gerbils, rabbits, guinea pigs, chinchillas, horses, cattle, rhesus monkeys, marmosets, cats, dogs, several wildlife species, and others. A single case of Tyzzer's disease has been reported in an HIV-infected patient. Tyzzer's disease is a common disease of gerbils and is found occasionally in rats, rabbits, and other rodents. Many rat colonies have a high incidence of seropositive animals without evidence of clinical disease. Rat, hamster, and mouse colonies (barrier- and nonbarrier-sustained) may have clinically inapparent infections.

Etiology

Clostridium piliforme is a spore-forming, motile, narrow, rod-shaped, PAS-positive, nonacid-fast, obligate, Gram-negative intracellular organism. Each species of animal seems to have a specific substrain of *C. piliforme*, but within some animal species there may be multiple substrains of the bacterium. The organism is a common benign intestinal inhabitant that persists for years in spore form outside the host. *Clostridium piliforme* has been grown in tissue culture of 3T3 cells, and it can be propagated in embryonated hen eggs.

Transmission

Transmission is thought to be by the fecal-oral route. Infectious spores survive for years in bedding, soil, or contaminated feed. The vegetative form is extremely labile.

Predisposing Factors

Poor environmental sanitation, shipping stress, and immunosuppressive therapy such as radiation, corticosteroids, concurrent disease, thymectomy, and crowding contribute to the development of clinical disease. The acute, highly fatal disease is seen most often in weanling animals, but adults may be affected also. Use of sulfaquinoxaline to prevent coccidiosis and pneumonia in rabbits has been associated with an epidemic of Tyzzer's disease.

Clinical Signs

The most common form of infection is probably subclinical, with sporadic outbreaks of clinical disease when spores in the environment are ingested. Tyzzer's disease in weanling or stressed animals is a peracute to acute enzootic disease causing rough hair coat, lethargy, and death within 48–72 hours. Watery diarrhea and perineal fecal staining may or may not accompany the disease. More chronically infected animals, in which hepatic lesions may be more pronounced, exhibit weight loss, rough hair coat, and eventually death.

Necropsy Signs

The classical lesions of *C. piliforme* infection consist of a triad typically involving the gut, liver, and heart. The liver may be enlarged with few to numerous necrotic foci, 1–2 mm in diameter. The liver is not necessarily involved, and the intestine or heart may be the only organs affected. The absence of liver lesions does not rule out Tyzzer's disease. In more acute cases, there may be edema, congestion, hemorrhage, and focal ulceration of the intestine, particularly around the ileocecal-colonic junction. The gut is often atonic and filled with a yellowish fluid. Mesenteric lymph nodes may be enlarged. The abdomen and small intestine of affected rats may be distended grossly due to megaloileitis. Five-week-old SD rats from seropositive colonies had a low incidence of megaloileitis, while seronegative colonies had no megaloileitis. A proteinaceous exudate may be found in the abdominal cavity of infected guinea pigs and gerbils.

Pale myocardial foci have been noted in rabbits, rats, mice, and hamsters with Tyzzer's disease. There are no reports of splenic lesions.

The hepatic, intestinal, and myocardial foci that variably characterize this disease are areas of necrosis surrounded initially by a scant, mixed inflammatory cell population. These foci probably arise via an embolic shower of organisms from a primary infection in the intestine. The filamentous organisms may be visualized in tissue sections within the cytoplasm of cells adjacent to the necrotic area using a Steiner or Warthin-Starry silver stain, often in a "bundle of sticks" arrangement.

Diagnosis

Necropsy signs and tissue sections stained with silver, Giemsa, or PAS stains demonstrate the intracellular, filamentous *C. piliforme* organisms in hepatocytes, enterocytes, or other tissues, providing a definitive diagnosis of Tyzzer's disease. Indirect fluorescent antibody tests are also a diagnostic aid.

The diagnosis of Tyzzer's disease may be difficult to establish. Even with special stains, organisms in tissues may be difficult to find because of their paucity. Feces from suspect animals inoculated per os into known *C. piliforme*–free weanling gerbils (which are highly susceptible) is a valuable aid for detecting the presence of the Tyzzer's disease agent in a suspect colony. Little is known about the incidence of Tyzzer's disease among animals in commercial and private stock colonies because colonies are not screened regularly for

Tyzzer's disease, in part because of the absence of a good screening test.

Treatment

The peracute to acute (1- to 4-day) course of the disease and the intracellular location of the organism reduce the effectiveness of treatment. Oxytetracycline in the drinking water at 0.1 g/L for 30 days has suppressed an outbreak. Tetracycline at 10 mg/kg body weight for 5 days "on-off-on" or at 400 mg/L for 10 days has also been used. The agent of Tyzzer's disease is also sensitive to penicillin, cephalosporins, chloramphenicol, and erythromycin. Sulfonamides, streptomycin, and kanamycin apparently do not affect the agent.

Prevention

Purchase of stock from a reputable vendor, preferably one using Caesarean derivations and barrier-rearing techniques, and good husbandry practices are the best preventive measures. Antibiotics may suppress infections, but carriers may develop. Spores survive freeze-thaw cycles but are killed if heated at 56°C (133°F) for 1 hour or 80°C (176°F) for 30 minutes. Spores are resistant to ethanol and quaternary ammonia compounds and may persist in the environment. A 0.5% sodium hypochlorite solution and peracetic acid are effective in spore inactivation. Filter cage covers aid in reducing transmission. Traditional rederivation methods have successfully eliminated Tyzzer's disease from a large rat-breeding colony.

Public Health Significance

No public health significance is known, but the report of *C. piliforme* infection in a rhesus monkey and an immunosuppressed human should be noted. Antibodies to *C. piliforme* have been found in pregnant women. Because *C. piliforme* affects such a wide spectrum of animal species, humans are likely susceptible to clinical disease under certain circumstances, such as systemic immune deficiency.

References

Boivin GP, et al. Development of a monoclonal antibody-based competitive inhibition enzyme linked immunosorbent assay for detection of Bacillus piliformis isolate-specific antibodies in laboratory animals. Lab Anim Sci. 1994, 44:153–157.

Boot R, Walvoort HC. Vertical transmission of Bacillus piliformis infection (Tyzzer's disease) in a guinea pig: case report. Lab Anim. 1984, 18:195–199.

Dillehay DL, Lindsey JR. Diagnostic exercise: diarrhea in guinea pigs. Lab Anim Sci. 1988, 38:472–473.

Engelhardt JA. What's your diagnosis? Hepatic lesions in gerbils. Lab Anim. 1988, 17:11–12.

Franklin CL, et al. Tyzzer's infection: host specificity of Clostridium pilforme isolates. Lab Anim Sci. 1994, 44:568–572.

Fujiwara K, Nakayama M, Takahashi K. Serologic detection of inapparent Tyzzer's disease in rats. Jpn J Exp Med. 1981, 51:197–200.

Ganaway JR. Effect of heat and selected chemical disinfectants upon infectivity of spores of Bacillus piliformis (Tyzzer's disease). Lab Anim Sci. 1980, 30:192–196.

Ganaway JR, McReynolds RS, Allen AM. Tyzzer's disease in free-living cottontail rabbits (Sylvilagus floridanus) in Maryland. J Wildl Dis. 1976, 12:545–549.

Goto K, et al. A serological survey on Bacillus piliformis infection in laboratory rabbits in Japan. Exp Anim. 1991, 40:231–233.

Hansen AK, Dagnaes-Hansen F, Mollegaard Hansen KE. Correlation between megaloileitis and antibodies to Bacillus piliformis in laboratory rat colonies. Lab Anim Sci. 1992, 42:449–453.

Hansen AK, et al. Rederivation of rat colonies seropositive for Bacillus piliformis and the subsequent screening for antibodies. Lab Anim Sci. 1992, 42:444–448.

Hansen AK, Svendsen O, Mollegaard-Hansen KE. Epidemiological studies of Bacillus piliformis infection and Tyzzer's disease in laboratory rats. Z Versuchstierkd. 1990, 33:163–169.

Livingston RS, et al. A novel presentation of Clostridium piliforme infection (Tyzzer's disease) in nude mice. Lab Anim Sci. 1996, 46:21–25.

Motzel SL, Gibson SV. Tyzzer's disease in hamsters and gerbils from a pet store supplier. J Am Vet Med Assoc. 1990, 197:1176–1178.

Motzel SL, Riley LK. Subclinical infection and transmission of Tyzzer's disease in rats. Lab Anim Sci. 1992, 42:439–443.

Ononiwu JC, Julian RJ. An outbreak of Tyzzer's disease in an Ontario rabbitry. Can Vet J. 1978, 19:107–109.

Peeters JE, et al. Naturally occurring Tyzzer's disease (Bacillus piliformis infection) in commercial rabbits: a clinical and pathological study. Ann Rech Vet. 1985, 16:69–79.

Smith KJ, et al. Bacillus piliformis infection (Tyzzer's disease) in a patient infected with HIV-1: confirmation with 16S ribosomal RNA sequence analysis. J Am Acad Dermatol. 1996, 34:343–348.
Tsuchitani M, et al. Naturally occurring Tyzzer's disease in a clean mouse colony: high mortality with coincidental cardiac lesions. J Comp Pathol. 1983, 93:499–507.
Waggie KS, et al. A study of mouse strain susceptibility to Bacillus piliformis (Tyzzer's disease): The association of B-cell function and resistance. Lab Anim Sci. 1981, 31:139–142.
Waggie KS, et al. Lesions of experimentally induced Tyzzer's disease in Syrian hamsters, guinea pigs, mice and rats. Lab Anim. 1987, 21:155–160.
Yokoiyama S, Fujiwara K. Effect of antibiotics on Tyzzer's disease. Jpn J Exp Med. 1971, 41:49–57.

ULCERATIVE DERMATITIS (MOIST DERMATITIS)

Hosts

Ulcerative or moist dermatitis occurs sporadically in rabbits and rodents.

Etiology

Ulcerative dermatitis or moist eczema refers to a localized reddened exudative inflammatory skin lesion that can be caused by a variety of irritating infectious agents. Generally bacterial agents cannot become established unless the skin is traumatized or continually wetted. Noninfectious factors include scratching at an allergic reaction site, abrasions, cuts, puncture wounds, urine scald, and chemical or thermal burns. Bacteria involved may be *Staphylococcus* spp, *Treponema* spp, *Streptococcus* spp, *Fusobacterium* spp, *Corynebacterium* spp, and *Pseudomonas* spp, whose blue-green pigment causes "blue fur" disease. Specific or named conditions include "sore nose" in gerbils (discussed earlier in the chapter) and "wet dewlap," "slobbers," ptyalism, and "hutch bum" in rabbits.

In mice, the condition is considered multifactorial, and defining a specific etiologic cause has been elusive despite years of research by many laboratories. The syndrome has been variously associated with immune-mediated vasculitis, innate immune dysfunctions, and behavioral peculiarities of C57BL/6 and related strains. The condition may be associated with a non-H2 linked gene or combination of genes but has an epigenetic component, and the syndrome is exacerbated by the presence of mites or ectoparasites. A retrospective study found that 4.1% of C57BL/6 mice became affected with the condition during their lifetime, and it was more common in female mice that were 10–16 months of age.

Predisposing Factors

Conjunctivitis, drooling from malocclusion or other dental disease, use of water pans and crocks, leaking sipper tubes, chronic diarrhea, obesity, urinary incontinence, parasitisim, and damp cages predispose to moist dermatitis. Overcrowding, stress, fighting, and the use of abrasive or nonabsorbent bedding may exacerbate or aggravate moist dermatitis conditions. Reducing or eliminating these factors may result in alleviation of signs.

Clinical Signs

Ulcerative dermatopathies may range from superficial erythema with minimal exudation to suppuration and deep ulceration. Regional lymph nodes may be enlarged if the dermal reaction is extensive. The hair surrounding the lesion is usually moist and matted. Lesions occur most frequently on the face or ventral areas in contact with water. Frequently, *Staphylococcus* spp can be recovered from the inflamed or ulcerated areas. Pyocyanin, a pigment produced by some strains of *Pseudomonas aeruginosa*, sometimes imparts a blue-green color to affected fur. *Pseudomonas aeruginosa* also produces several toxins that cause dermal necrosis and may be lethal.

Ulcerative dermatitis of rats is seen more often in young males. The lesions, which usually begin on the neck, shoulders, or anterior trunk, first appear as an irregularity in the hair coat. This small focus of alopecia or ulceration then enlarges over the next several days to form small to extensive ulcerations. Some lesions scab and regress, and others are pruritic and stimulate scratching and self-mutilation, necessitating euthanasia.

Ulcerative dermatitis is a common disease of mice of C57BL/6 background. The condition presents with pruritus and can result in alopecia, ulceration, crusting, exudation with potential secondary bacterial infections, and skin necrosis. The lesions are most often observed on the back of the head, neck, and between the scapula but can extend into the axilla, ventrum, and inguinal areas.

Diagnosis

Diagnosis is aided by microbiologic culture and microscopic examinations of lesions.

Treatment

Ulcerative dermatitis is treated by clipping hair over and adjacent to the lesion, cleansing the area affected, administering topical or systemic antibiotics or applying an antiseptic, and removing the underlying cause.

In mice, treatment can be frustrating and animals must often be euthanized because of extensive ulceration of the skin. One study evaluated the consequences of treating the condition by dietary vitamin E supplementation (0.1 mL Derm Caps® PO once daily for 7–10 days) at the onset of clinical signs. Of 71 mice, 45% had complete reepithelialization of the skin with an average recovery time of 2–5 weeks following institution of therapy.

Other therapies attempted in mice and rats include topical triple antibiotic ointment applied once every other day, topical cyclosporine therapy (0.2% cyclosporine in 2% lidocaine supplemented with 50 ug/mL gentamicin) once or twice daily until resolved, and zinc oxide ointment applied topically every 1–2 days.

Prevention

Prevention includes using nonabrasive bedding that is maintained clean and dry in a nonabrasive, dry cage. Use of hopper feeders and sipper tube waterers instead of bowls and crocks reduces throat abrasion and wetting. Balls or stones placed in water crocks reduce wetting while drinking. Obesity is often associated with this syndrome, so proper nutrition and activity reduce risk of occurrence. The water supply is a frequent source of *P. aeruginosa* infections and the sanitation schedule for watering implements and the source should be checked for this bacterium if a clinical problem develops.

References

Andrews EJ. Muzzle trauma in the rat associated with the use of feeding cups. Lab Anim Sci. 1977, 27:278.

Hoppman E, Wilson Barron H. Ferret and rabbit dermatology. Sem Exot Pet Med. 2007, 16:225–237.

Kastenmayer RJ, Fain MA, Perdue KA. A retrospective study of idiopathic ulcerative dermatitis in mice with a C57BL/6 background. J Amer Assoc Lab Anim Sci. 2006, 45(6):8–12.

Lawson PT. Vitamin E as a treatment for ulcerative dermatitis in C57BL/6 mice and strains with a C57BL/6 background. Contemp Top Lab Anim Sci. 2005, 44(3):18–21.

Maronpot RR, Chavannes J-M. Dacryoadenitis, conjunctivitis, and facial dermatitis of the mouse. Lab Anim Sci. 1977, 27:277–278.

McDonald RA, Pinheiro AF. Water chlorination controls Pseudomonas aeruginosa in a rabbitry. J Am Vet Med Assoc. 1967, 115:863–864.

O'Donaghue PN, Whatley BF. Pseudomonas aeruginosa in rabbit fur. Lab Anim. 1971, 5:251–255.

Scharffetter-Kochanek K, Lu H, Norman K, et al. Spontaneous skin ulceration and defective T cell function in CD18 null mice. J Exp Med. 1998, 188(1):119–131.

Walther B, Wieler LH, Friedrich AW, et al. Methicillin-resistant Staphylococcus aureus (MRSA) isolated from small and exotic animals at a university hospital during routine microbiological examinations. Vet Microbiol. 2008, 127(1–2):171–178.

UROLITHIASIS

Hosts

Of rabbits and rodents, uroliths (stones in the urinary tract) are the most common in rabbits, rats, and guinea pigs. The predominant mineral in urinary concretions of rabbits and guinea pigs is calcium (calcium carbonate, calcium phosphate, and calcium oxalate) with much smaller amounts of magnesium and phosphorus (ammonium magnesium phosphate or struvite). In rats, struvite uroliths predominate.

Etiology and Predisposing Factors

Although the cause of urolith formation is obscure, predisposing factors include genetic predisposition, metabolic disorders, nutritional imbalances, inadequate water intake, nematode infestion (*Trichosomoides crassicauda* in rats), and bacterial infections. Typically, signs of urolithiasis are more common in males because their urethra is longer, narrower, and less distensible than in females, resulting in partial or complete urethral obstruction when stones are present.

The predisposition of rabbits to develop calcium-containing renal and urinary calculi may be related to peculiarities in the calcium metabolism of this species. Excessive calcium intake is regulated through greatly increased elimination by the kidneys, not by reduced absorption in the intestine, which increases the risk of precipitation of urinary solutes, especially if the urine pH becomes too alkaline. Normal rabbit urine pH is 8.2. At pH 8.5–9.5, crystals precipitate in the urine.

In a colony of 170 guinea pigs, aged females were more predisposed to cystitis and urolithiasis than were males and young guinea pigs. The cause may have been related to infection of the urinary tract with *E. coli* or *Staphylococcus* spp, irritation and trauma of the urinary bladder due to the cystic calculi, preexisting diabetes mellitus, and female guinea pig urogenital anatomy and function (shorter urethra and ease of bacterial retrograde movement).

In an outbreak of pneumonia and septicemia due to *Streptococcus pyogenes* in a breeding colony of 800 guinea pigs, 50% of the adult females had urolithiasis, which was believed to be a sequela of cystitis caused by the streptococcal infection.

Clinical Signs

Signs of urolithiasis in rabbits may be absent or may include anorexia, weight loss, listlessness, hunched posture, anuria or hematuria, and dense abdominal masses evident by palpation or on radiographs. Discrete urinary stones may be difficult to distinguish from calcium "sludge" that is common in rabbit urinary bladders. Affected rabbits may have an abnormal serum biochemical profile, although nonrenal factors may affect BUN levels, and serum creatinine levels do not generally increase until 75% or more of renal function is lost. Urine may be difficult to express because of calcium sludging or because of urethral or ureteral obstruction by calculi, in which case the urinary bladder may be quite turgid.

Perineal soiling and urine scald may be seen with pollakiuria and incontinence, further contributing to animal discomfort.

Necropsy Signs

On necropsy, fine sand or numerous irregularly shaped stones, all of about the same size, may be found in the renal pelvis, ureters, bladder, or urethra. Structures between the nephron and the concretion may be dilated and filled with fluid. Cystitis is a common sequela to urinary stasis.

Urethral proteinaceous obstructions occur in aged male guinea pigs, rats, and mice. These are composed primarily of congealed ejaculum that may become infected; a suppurative infection ensues. A variety of bacteria may be isolated from these infections, especially *Pseudomonas aeruginosa*, *Escherichia coli*, and *Proteus* spp.

Diagnosis

Diagnosis is based on clinical signs, palpation, radiography, urinalysis, culture, and a chronic hematuria refractory to antibiotic therapy.

Treatment

In general, diets to dissolve uroliths are ineffective in rabbits and rodents. Treatment for urolithiasis is surgical removal of calculi with a guarded prognosis for long-term cure, particularly in the case of renoliths, as recurrence of calculi is common. Postoperative management should include an appropriate course of antibiotics preferably based on urine culture and sensitivity testing (chloramphenicol, trimethoprim-sulfa, and enrofloxacin are all potential selections), a low-calcium diet that limits pellets and alfalfa intake, and follow-up radiographs.

T. crassicauda infection in rats may be treated with ivermectin at 3 mg/kg PO (0.4% w/v solution of ivermectin in propylene glycol) given with a 1 mL syringe and polyethylene tubing.

Prevention

Because of the uncommon occurrence and uncertain etiology of urolithiasis, specific preventive measures, other than good husbandry practices and a balanced diet, have not been described. A standard recommendation for preventing urolithiasis in nonbreeding pet rabbits is to reduce the dietary component of high-calcium pellets and to increase the amount of grass hay. Not feeding rabbits more calcium than is required, around 5 g/kg (maintenance) and approximately 8 g/kg (growth, lactation) and less than 25 ug (1000 I.U.) cholecalciferol/kg diet, has been recommended to control urinary stones, gravel, and calcium sludge.

There may be sufficient empirical justification for combining a grass hay of lower calcium content with a limited pelleted diet if plasma calcium levels exceed 16 mg/dL (4 mmol/L) or if there are signs of metastatic calcification or urolithiasis. Young, old, or lactating rabbits may not obtain sufficient energy from a higher fiber feed. Excessive vitamin D supplementation should be avoided in all species to minimize the risk of urolith development.

References

Bauck LAB, Hagan RI. Cystotomy for treatment of urolithiasis in a hamster. J Am Vet Med Assoc. 1984, 184:99–100.

Boll RA, Suckow MA, Hawkins EC. Bilateral ureteral calculi in a guinea pig. J Small Exotic Anim Med. 1991, 1:60–63.

Fisher PG. Exotic mammal renal disease: diagnosis and treatment. Vet Clin Exot Anim. 2006, 9:69–96.

Garibaldi BA, Goad MEP. Hypercalcemia with secondary nephrolithiasis in a rabbit. Lab Anim Sci. 1988, 38:331–333.

Gilmore MM. Urolithiasis in a gerbil. Vet Rec. 1978, 103:102.

Huerkamp MJ, Dillehay DL. Struvite uroliths in a male mouse. Lab Anim Sci. 1991, 41:642–643.

Kamphues J. Macrominerals and urine pH: calcium metabolism of rabbits as an etiological factor for urolithiasis. J Nutr. 1991, 121:595–596.

Okewole PA, et al. An outbreak of Streptococcus pyogenes infection associated with calcium oxalate urolithiasis in guinea pigs (Cavia porcellus). Lab Anim. 1991, 25:184–186.

Summa MEL, et al. Efficacy of oral ivermectin against Trichosomoides crassicauda in naturally infected laboratory rats. Lab Anim Sci. 1992, 42:620–622.

Wahry WT, Peper RL. Calcium carbonate urolithiasis in a rabbit. Lab Anim Sci. 1994, 44:534–536.

Zimmerman TE, et al. Soft tissue mineralization in rabbits fed a diet containing excess vitamin D. Lab Anim Sci. 1990, 40:212–215.

VENEREAL SPIROCHETOSIS (TREPONEMATOSIS)

Hosts

Domestic rabbits, wild lagomorphs, and hares are susceptible to venereal spirochetosis. The disease is also known as treponematosis, rabbit syphilis, and vent disease.

Etiology

Treponema paraluiscuniculi is a slender, spiral-shaped bacterium between 10 and 30 um in length. Antibodies to *T. paraluiscuniculi* cross-react with antigens of *T. pallidum*, the agent of human syphilis.

Transmission

The spirochete is transmitted by direct contact, especially during mating. Exchange of bucks among breeders promotes dissemination of the organism. Infection of kits may occur at birth or during the nursing period, but infection is uncommon in virgin rabbits. The disease is uncommon in most well-managed rabbit colonies but may be seen occasionally in pet rabbits and commercial operations.

Predisposing Factors

Rabbits in cold environments are predisposed to the clinical disease. Susceptibility, extent, and severity of lesions vary among rabbit breeds. Breeding animals are at higher risk than individual or laboratory animals.

Clinical Signs

Serologically positive rabbits are often encountered, but clinical, epizootic disease is uncommon. Whereas more attention has been paid to the disease in males because they have more obvious clinical signs, females may also contract the infection. Females may develop metritis, retained placentas, and abortions, possibly unnoticed, which occur at 12–22 days of gestation. The herd may have a history of low conception rates and a high incidence of nest box fatalities in young less than 9 days of age. Clinical signs, when they appear, begin with vesicular swelling and reddening followed by dry scaliness of the swollen prepuce and vulva. This early stage is followed by the development of macules, papules, erosions, ulcers, and crusts on the external genitalia, perineal areas, nose, eyelids, and lips.

A case has been described of venereal spirochetosis in an adult buck that had a firm, slightly raised, nonpruritic, scab-covered mass on the right nasal margin. The scab was removed easily and revealed a red, ulcerated surface. A modified silver stain was used to visualize spirochetes in the superficial dermis and epidermis.

Affected rabbits remain alert, and the condition regresses after several weeks. If the prepuce is affected severely, apparent and transient infertility may result. Preputial and scrotal scars are indicative of healed lesions.

Necropsy Signs

In most cases, there are no internal gross lesions. The perineal and genital skin and the mucous membranes of the external genitalia are the tissues most often affected, although some cases only involve the external nares. Inguinal lymph nodes may be enlarged. Histologically, the thickened epidermis may be hyperkeratotic, and the dermis infiltrated by monomorphonuclear inflammatory cells, primarily plasma cells.

Diagnosis

The gross lesions of venereal spirochetosis in rabbits resemble those caused by trauma, dermatophytes, or pasteurellosis (facial crusting). The use of the cardiolipin antigen Wassermann-type test or the rapid plasma reagin (RPR) card test will provide evidence of a *T. paraluiscuniculi* infection. Absence of clinical disease in the absence of concurrent treatment with antibiotics and two negative RPR tests 30 days apart are suggested as evidence of noninfection.

A fluorescent antibody test has also been used in diagnosis. The spirochetes may be demonstrated using darkfield microscopy in wet preparations of tissue fluids expressed from active lesions in the epidermis, dermis, uterus, or lymph nodes. One can also obtain a diagnosis by staining sections of fixed tissue or smears with silver salts. *Treponema paraluiscuniculi* should be considered in the differential diagnosis of unexpected inflammatory skin lesions in rabbits, especially those around the nose, anus, and genitals.

Treatment

Penicillin given intramuscularly at 40,000 units/kg per day for 3–5 days provides a cure, although penicillin exposure may precipitate an enterotoxemia. Alternately, long-acting penicillin (benzathine penicillin G) can be given intramuscularly at 84,000 units/kg three times at weekly intervals. Owners should carefully monitor animals for signs of enterotoxemia and discontinue antibiotics if animals go off feed or develop diarrhea.

Prevention

Routine serologic screening provides an indication of exposure. Periodic examination of breeding does and bucks for cutaneous lesions followed by treatment or culling will eliminate clinical carriers. Infected animals should not be bred. It may be possible to eliminate the infection from small herds by treating all animals simultaneously. In young animals or fryers bred for meat production, there may be restrictions on the use of certain antimicrobial agents or specific withdrawal times for meat, which must be followed. Maintaining a closed breeding herd prevents introduction of venereal spirochetosis. If new animals must be introduced, they should be clinically and serologically free of disease. It may be advisable to quarantine and treat all new arrivals intended for breeding.

Public Health Significance

Although rhesus monkeys and a chimpanzee have been infected experimentally, humans are not believed to be susceptible to *T. paraluiscuniculi* infection.

References

Cunliffe-Beamer TL, Fox RR. Venereal spirochetosis of rabbits: description and diagnosis. Lab Anim Sci. 1981, 31:366–371.

DiGiacomo R, et al. Clinical course and treatment of venereal spirochetosis in New Zealand white rabbits. Br J Vener Dis. 1984, 60:214–218.

———. Treponema paraluiscuniculi infection in a commercial rabbitry: epidemiology and serodiagnosis. Lab Anim Sci. 1983, 33:562–566.

Froberg MK, et al. Pathology of congenital syphilis in rabbits. Infect Immun. 1994, 61:4743–4749.
Gaertner DJ, Barthold SW. Diagnostic exercise: nasal mass in a rabbit. Lab Anim Sci. 1989, 39:440–441.

VIRAL HEMORRHAGIC DISEASE IN RABBITS

Hosts

Rabbit viral hemorrhagic disease (VHD) is a peracute infection of European rabbits (*Oryctolagus* spp), the only known host. Rodents appear not to be susceptible. A closely related virus causes a similar hemorrhagic disease syndrome known as the European brown hare syndrome (EBHS). Synonyms for this disease include rabbit plague, rabbit or viral hemorrhagic pneumonia, rabbit viral septicemia, rabbit viral sudden death, and others.

Epidemiology

Though first described in China in 1984, a similar disease, EBHS, was recorded among *Lepus europaeus* on an island near Sweden in 1980. It spread throughout the mainland of southern Sweden in 1981 and by 1982 became widespread in Denmark. The disease was subsequently reported in Korea in 1985 and in Italy in 1986. The disease emerged in France and Poland in 1988. An outbreak in Mexico started in December of 1988 but was eradicated successfully by 1992. Since that time, the disease has appeared on at least three separate occasions among commercial rabbit farms and exotic mammal exhibits, predominantly in the western United States.

Etiology

The causative agent is a calicivirus (RNA, single-stranded) that is closely related to the EBHS virus. Experimental inoculation studies indicate that the viruses are species-specific and genetically dissimilar. During the past few years, scientists in Australia have studied the potential of VHD virus as a means of biological control of the wild rabbit population in that country. Initial inoculation studies were performed on Wardang Island off the south coast of Australia. The virus subsequently escaped to the mainland and proved highly lethal initially to wild and pet rabbits.

Transmission

The highly contagious VHD virus is transmitted horizontally by direct contact with secretions or excretions from infected rabbits or indirectly via aerosol exposure to contaminated fomites, pelts, other rabbit byproducts, and frozen rabbit meat. The 1988–1990 outbreak of VHD in Mexico was traced to 18 tons of frozen rabbit meat imported from China. There is no evidence that it is transmitted by arthropod vectors; however, mechanical means of transmission via birds, rodents, and insects cannot be ruled out. Filtered liver homogenate from infected animals is used experimentally as a source of infectious material because the virus has been difficult to culture in vitro. The origin of the virus in recent U.S. outbreaks has not been determined.

Predisposing Factors

The virus is extremely virulent in rabbits older than 2 months. In endemic areas, carriers or serologically positive, unvaccinated young rabbits may expose naive adult animals to the disease, thus perpetuating the infection and resulting in eradication failures. Although rabbits younger than 1 month cannot be infected clinically, a small percentage of those between 1 and 2 months old are still susceptible to natural infection. Nutritional inadequacy and environmental stress may increase susceptibility to VHD. Resistance or natural immunity of young rabbits to experimental infections was not correlated with levels of maternal antibodies, and resistance declined with advancing age.

Clinical Signs

The hallmark of this disease is sudden death without premonitory signs. Morbidity and mortality may be as high as 80–100%. The virus has a short incubation period, from 16 hours to 3 days, followed by high fever (40.5–41 °C; 104.9–105.8 °F) and death within 24 hours. Other signs, not consistently seen, include depression, anorexia, dyspnea, hematuria, vaginal hemorrhage, convulsions, and epistaxis (bleeding from the nose). Because death is acute, affected animals are often in good body condition. The acute form is seen primarily in epizootic areas. Subacute cases with milder symptoms are seen in the later and enzootic stages of an outbreak. Although most

SPECIFIC DISEASES AND CONDITIONS

animals that survive are resistant to reinfection, some of those that are serologically positive may still carry the virus and shed the virus intermittently. Chronic nonclinical infection is rare because seroconversion usually affords complete protection, but when present, it is assumed to occur in suckling rabbits.

Clinical signs similar to those of VHD in rabbits have been described in wild hares stricken with the EBHS, which is caused by a related virus.

Necropsy Signs

Blood-tinged nasal discharge, hepatomegaly, splenomegaly, and serosal ecchymoses are typical findings at necropsy. Hepatic necrosis, cryptal necrosis, pulmonary edema and hemorrhage, and lympholysis have been described.

Histologically, there is multifocal to coalescing liver necrosis notable with little, if any, inflammation. Microscopic changes in the spleen include necrosis and microthrombi in small vessels. Microinfarctions due to disseminated intravascular coagulation may be seen scattered throughout the myocardium, kidneys, and other organs. Central nervous system changes, such as microthrombosis, may be found, but they are less common in the CNS than in the other organs.

Diagnosis

Diagnosis of VHD is based on the characteristic peracute clinical signs and high mortality; gross and histologic lesions, especially necrosis and hemorrhage of the liver and the respiratory system; and detection of virus neutralizing antibodies. Besides ELISA, hemagglutination assay, and PCR of tissue extracts, immunohistochemical staining of frozen and paraffin-embedded tissue sections may be used to demonstrate the disease and confirm the diagnosis.

Treatment

There is no treatment for rabbit VHD. A commercial vaccine is available but its use is prohibited in the United States and Canada. Nonpharmacologic support may be offered to diseased rabbits; however, the prognosis for recovery is grave.

Prevention

Selection of VHD-free stock, strict husbandry, quarantine, and serologic screenings are measures to exclude potential sources of infection. During an outbreak, complete depopulation and proper disposal of all infected animals and their fomites with thorough disinfecting of equipment and cages were effective in eliminating the disease and preventing recurrence in Mexico. The disease is reportable in the United States, and if the virus is suspected, a state and federal veterinarian should be contacted immediately and a quarantine should be put into effect.

Because VHD virus is stable, its elimination from the environment requires decontamination of floors, walls, and fomites using 10% bleach or 3% formalin followed by 2% sodium hydroxide. The premises should be kept empty of animals for 2 weeks during warm weather or 2 months in colder seasons.

Public Health Significance

The lack of evidence of disease in millions of people who have consumed infected rabbit meat and in the large number of farmers, veterinarians, and laboratory technicians who have been in contact with VHD virus indicates that humans are not susceptible to the virus.

References

Alexandrov M, et al. Immunohistochemical localization of the rabbit haemorrhagic disease viral antigen. Arch Virol. 1992, 127:355–363.

Campagnolo ER, et al. Outbreak of rabbit hemorrhagic disease in domestic lagomorphs. J Am Vet Med Assoc. 2003, 223:1151–1155.

Chasey D. Rabbit hemorrhagic disease: the new scourge of Oryctolagus cuniculus. Lab Anim. 1996, 31:33–44.

Cooke BD. Rabbit haemorrhagic disease: field epidemiology and the management of wild rabbit populations. Rev Sci Tech. 2002, 21(2):347–358.

Gavier-Widen D, Momer T. Descriptive epizootiological study of European brown hare syndrome in Sweden. J Wildl Dis. 1993, 29:15–20.

Krogstad AP, Simpson JE, Korte SW. Viral diseases of rabbits. Vet Clin Exot Anim. 2005, 8:123–138.

Lawson M. Rabbit virus threatens ecology after jumping the fence. Nature. 1995, 378:531.

Liebermann HT, et al. Some physicochemical properties of the virus of rabbit haemorrhagic disease. J Vet Med. 1992, 39B:317–326.

Mandelli G, et al. An approach to viral haemorrhagic disease (VHD): pathogenesis by histopathological and immunohistochemical assay. J Appl Rabbit Res. 1992, 15:1535–1543.

Meldrum KC. Viral haemorrhagic disease of rabbits. Vet Rec. 1992, 130:407.

Nauwynck P, et al. Susceptibility of hares and rabbits to a Belgian isolate of European brown hare syndrome (EBHS) virus. J Appl Rabbit Res. 1992, 15:1348–1354.

Pages Mante A, Artigas C. Advisable vaccinal programme against myxomatosis and rabbit haemorrhagic disease viruses on wild rabbits. J Appl Rabbit Res. 1992, 15:1448–1452.

Park JH, Ochiai K, Itakura C. Aetiology of rabbit haemorrhagic disease in China. Vet Rec. 1993, 133:67–69.

Parra F, Prieto M. Purification and characterization of a calicivirus as the causative agent of a lethal hemorrhagic disease in rabbits. J Virol. 1990, 64:4013–4015.

Smid B, et al. Rabbit haemorrhagic disease: an investigation of some properties of the virus and evaluation of an inactivated vaccine. Vet Microbiol. 1991, 26:77–85.

Yongkun, W., et al. Development of a vaccine protective against viral hemorrhagic disease. J Appl Rabbit Res. 1992, 15:1355–1359.

Chapter 6

Case Reports

The case reports described in this chapter were taken, with minor modifications, from the files of the diagnostic laboratories at Colorado State University, University of Saskatchewan, University of Guelph, University of Missouri–Columbia, Pennsylvania State University, and Mississippi State University. These cases reveal the complexity of disease in rabbits and rodents and demonstrate how field cases may differ considerably from textbook descriptions. Students may find it helpful to consider how the case would be managed in a private practice versus a laboratory setting. Suggested short answers and selected references are supplied in the second section of the chapter.

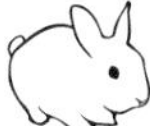

THE RABBIT

Case 1: Death in Rabbits Sharing a Lawn with Cats

A distraught laboratory employee consults with you about one of her five prized French lop show rabbits that became sick over the past 2 weeks and died, and a second one that is looking ill. The rabbits are housed in elevated wood and wire mesh hutches in her backyard. The diet consists primarily of commercial rabbit pellets supplemented with fresh vegetables and grass hay. Water is provided ad libitum in bowls. Occasionally, the rabbits are allowed to graze on the lawn. Dogs, cats, raccoons, and foxes are known to wander through the area on occasion.

The rabbits that died had developed varying clinical signs before death, including anorexia, ataxia, muscle tremor, posterior weakness, and paralysis, which lasted approximately 2 days and was followed by death. You are able to examine the second animal and note a mild head tilt to the left, weakness on the right, and decreased mentation.

a. *What are some differential diagnoses to consider when CNS signs are seen in a rabbit?*
b. *How would you diagnose an etiologic agent?*
c. *What is the most likely mode of transmission and source of protozoal or larval migrans disease in the rabbits?*
d. *What public health concerns do you have?*
e. *What therapy would you institute and what is the prognosis?*

Case 2: Reproductive Disorders in Rabbits

A large commercial rabbitry experienced the following reproductive abnormalities: (1) increased fetal and maternal mortality; (2) kindling rate reduced 25%; (3) increased perinatal and neonatal mortalities; and (4) reduction in average litter size. These problems occurred after feeding a newly formulated diet for 4 months. Postmortem evaluation of does with reproductive disorders (prolonged gestation or abortion) revealed moderate to severe suppurative metritis with the recovery of *Pasteurella multocida* from some rabbits. Of the 32 aborted or stillborn fetuses and neonates examined, 3 aborted fetuses had hydrocephalus and cleft palate. The brains of the affected fetuses had cortical atrophy. All other organs appeared normal. The clinical syndrome involved was suggestive of toxicity or a dietary deficiency manifested by fetal resorption, abortion, stillbirths, and hydrocephalus in the fetuses and neonates.

a. *Which vitamins should be implicated as a cause of reproductive abnormalities? Which tissue samples should be submitted for analysis?*
b. *What are potential causes of a vitamin deficiency or excess? How would you confirm your suspicion?*
c. *What are other clinical signs of hypervitaminosis A? What are some differential diagnoses of*

reproductive disorders in the rabbit? What is the potential role of P. multocida *in this case?*
d. What is the diagnosis?

Case 3: Bloody Urine in a Rabbit

An adult gray chinchilla rabbit doe frequently dribbled several milliliters of bloody urine and reportedly had not eaten for at least 3 days. The student owner brought the rabbit to your clinic for examination.

The perineum was stained with blood, and palpation of the lower abdomen revealed a firm, distended bladder. Radiography revealed an irregularly shaped, opaque mass in the lower abdomen.

a. What is the probable diagnosis? What is the cause?
b. How would you proceed with treatment?
c. What dietary recommendations would you make to the client?

Case 4: Growth Around a Rabbit's Cornea

A 4-month-old pet Florida white rabbit developed a thin fold of tissue surrounding and growing over the upper half of the left cornea. The owner indicated that the growth had been present for approximately 5 weeks, and the rabbit seemed normal otherwise.

You sedate and examine the rabbit and are able with gentle pressure to lift the conjunctival fold off the eyeball. The abnormal skin is thin and avascular, and there is no evidence of suppurative inflammation.

a. What is the most likely diagnosis?
b. What is the treatment for this condition?
c. What is the prognosis?

Case 5: Ataxia in Dwarf Rabbits

A colony of dwarf rabbits has experienced sporadic deaths among the young. The closed colony is housed indoors in suspended wire cages equipped with crocks for feed and water. Affected rabbits were first evident at 3–4 weeks of age, when runting, weakness, and ataxia were seen in one animal in approximately 40% of the litters. The runted animals weighed half that of their normal siblings and invariably died at 10–12 weeks. Necropsy revealed no gross lesions or obvious congenital abnormalities.

a. Which specific conditions in rabbits could produce ataxia?
b. Which common infectious disease of rabbits might produce abnormal neurologic signs?
c. Which tissues should be collected and examined for histologic signs of this disease? Which tissue stains would be used?

Case 6: Pot-Bellied Rabbit

A weanling rabbit was brought to a veterinary clinic for examination. The rabbit had a firm but distended upper abdomen and was cachetic. There were no abnormal intestinal sounds or diarrhea.

a. What diagnostic procedures would contribute to making an accurate diagnosis?
*b. Eventual necropsy examination of the rabbit revealed an enlarged liver that contained numerous raised pale yellow foci. How could you differentiate hepatic coccidiosis from cysticercosis (*Taenia pisiformis*) and tularemia?*
c. What is the causative organism of hepatic coccidiosis?

Case 7: Maternal Neglect by a Doe

A primiparous (first litter) doe had a long, difficult delivery. Shortly after the kindling process she partially cannibalized several kits, abandoned some, and nursed a few.

a. What causes cannibalism of newborn rabbits?
b. How can such behavior be prevented?
c. What may cause a doe to abandon her young?

Case 8: Death of a Pregnant Doe

An obese, 3-year-old, pregnant (27 days) doe that had died suddenly was submitted for necropsy examination. The rabbit had been fed table scraps and cow's milk. Gross lesions included multifocal, small (1–2 mm) pits on the renal surface, 10 dead fetuses, a light tan liver, and mineralized arteries.

a. What agent is the probable cause of the renal pitting? How is this agent transmitted? Did this agent contribute to the animal's death?
b. What is the probable cause of death and what is the pathogenesis of this condition? What husbandry steps might prevent or reduce the incidence of this disease in a rabbitry?
c. How long is the rabbit's gestation period?

Case 9: Foul-Smelling Diarrhea in Does

An owner of a herd of 60 does reported the death of 17 does within a 12-hour period. Affected adult and weanling animals developed dull, watery eyes, weakness, and incoordination, but the most prominent sign was a fulminating, smelly diarrhea. Body temperatures in terminal cases were between 40 and 41 °C.

a. *Which conditions are probable differential diagnoses in this case?*
b. *What diagnostic procedures would you use to determine the cause of enteropathies in the does?*
c. *What would you do to prevent further devastation of this valuable breeding herd?*

Case 10: Multiple Skin Ulcers in a Pet Rabbit

A pet rabbit has an ulcerated area on his nose that constantly exudes serous fluid. As the fluid dries, the lesion becomes crusted, and after a week the crust looked like a small horn. The crust can be removed, but a raw, moist, ulcerated surface remains. The rabbit also has several small scabs and crusts on the penis and scrotal pouches and several small crusted nodules on the lips. Treating with chlorhexidine, topical steroids, and triple antibiotic ointment was not effective. Culture of plucked hairs from the edge of the lesions did not result in growth on D.T.M. media, and scrapings examined for mites were negative.

a. *Which diseases should be considered in the differential diagnosis and what further diagnostics should be performed?*
b. *What should be done to establish a definitive diagnosis?*
c. *What treatment do you recommend?*

Case 11: Aggression in Male Rabbits

A woman brought three intact adult male rabbits into the veterinary clinic. All three rabbits were cagemates and had recently started chewing on their fur and biting one another over the back and around the scrotum. Examination of stool specimens revealed an absence of internal parasites. The animals were destined for adoption as pet animals.

a. *What dietary deficiencies may induce fur chewing?*
b. *Is the housing situation a factor in the chewing and biting?*
c. *What surgical procedures would you recommend?*

Case 12: Facial Problems in a Buck

An adult male rabbit was submitted for necropsy examination. The animal had a purulent conjunctivitis, rhinitis, and a wet chin and dewlap with sticky, matted fur.

a. *What are the causes of wet dewlap? How is this condition prevented and treated?*
b. *How would a* Pasteurella multocida *organism reach the orbit from the nasal passage?*
c. *How would you treat the conjunctivitis?*

Case 13: Posterior Paresis in a Doe

A 2-month-old doe was submitted with a feces-soiled perineum. The attending clinician noted that the animal was dragging the rear limbs.

a. *What is the differential diagnosis for the paresis? How would you proceed to a definitive diagnosis?*
b. *What is the probable explanation for the fecal staining of the perineum?*
c. *In cases of spinal luxation, what factors determine a recommendation of cage rest or euthanasia?*

Case 14: Unthrifty Rabbit

A 7-year-old, intact, male New Zealand white rabbit presented to a veterinary clinic with a 2-month history of weight loss and a 2-week history of being off feed. The owner indicated that the animal had been seen previously by another veterinarian for chronic respiratory disease for which it had been treated with tetracycline in the water for the past 2 years.

On physical examination, the animal was lethargic and depressed with sticky mucous membranes, flaccid muscle tone, and a poor hair coat.

A CBC and clinical chemistry panel reveal the following profile for this animal (normal reference range values for parameters are indicated in parentheses):

PCV	19%	(33–50%)
TP	74 g/dL	(54–83 g/dL)
Ca	3.0 mM	(1.4–3.1 mM)
P	3.4 mM	(1.3–2.2 mM)
Gluc	5.6 mM	(4.2–8.7 mM)
Creat	689.5 uM	(131–155 uM)
BUN	191 mg/dL	(3.6–6.9 mg/dL)
Na	151 mM	(131–155 mM)
K	6.4 mM	(3.6–6.9 mM)
ALT	63 U/L	(48–80 U/L)
Urine SG	1.010	(1.003–1.036)

a. What is your tentative diagnosis for this case? Is the condition acute or chronic? What evidence do you have from the profile?
b. What are your plans for treating this animal?
c. What is the prognosis for this animal?

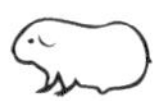

THE GUINEA PIG

Case 15: Abdominal Pain in a Guinea Pig

A 3-year-old male guinea pig is presented because it is hunched and appears to be in pain. Radiographs are obtained (see Figures 6.1 and 6.2).

a. What is your radiographic diagnosis?
b. What is the most likely cause of this condition?
c. What is the treatment of choice?
d. What is the prognosis?

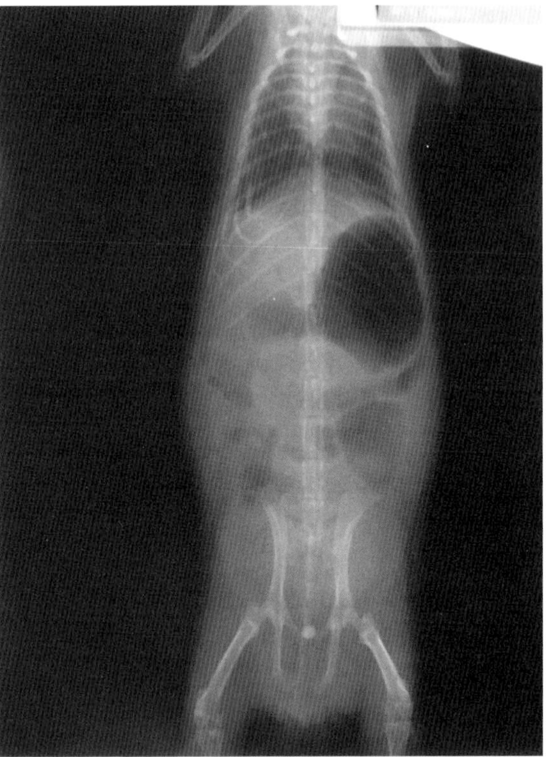

FIGURE 6.1. Ventrodorsal view of a guinea pig.

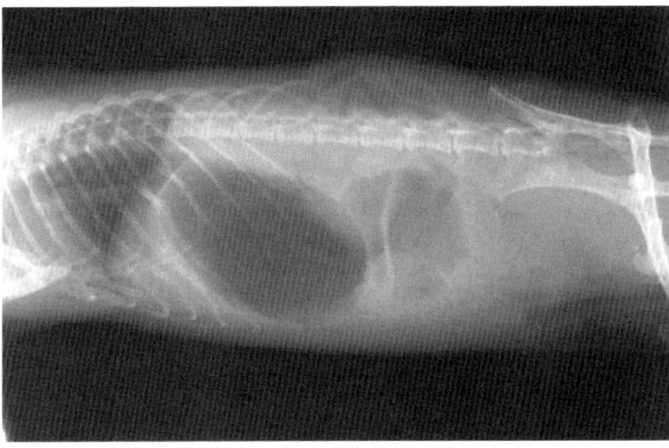

FIGURE 6.2. Lateral view of a guinea pig.

Case 16: Soft Stool in Guinea Pigs

A young male guinea pig had a 3-week history of persistent soft stool and lethargy. The animal remained thin despite the owner's attempts to improve the diet and enhance growth. After 3 weeks, the guinea pig died and was submitted to a veterinary clinic for evaluation. Necropsy revealed mucosal reddening within the ileum, cecum, and colon and a brown, watery content with no evidence of blood. Histopathologically, there was moderate villous blunting and fusion in the distal small intestine; however, no Tyzzer's bacilli were observed.

a. What diseases should be considered in the differential diagnosis of cases involving soft feces in young guinea pigs?
b. Cryptosporidium *spp oocysts were found in the guinea pig's feces. What does* Cryptosporidium *spp look like? Describe the technique for finding this organism in the feces.*
c. How is Cryptosporidium *spp transmitted? Is it a zoonotic disease?*

Case 17: Fatal Pneumonia in Guinea Pigs

A local pet store received a shipment of 30 2-year-old, mixed-sex guinea pigs. Within 3 days of delivery, two animals developed respiratory distress, crusty eyelids, rough hair coat, depression, and anorexia, and died 4 days later. Necropsy examination revealed pulmonary consolidation and purulent exudates in the upper and lower airways.

a. What bacteria should be considered as possible etiologic agents for this disease outbreak? What are predisposing factors?
b. How could this outbreak have been prevented?
c. What therapy should be administered for the remaining animals? What is the prognosis for these animals?

Case 18: Mistreatment of Scurvy

A pet guinea pig was brought to a veterinary clinic. The animal exhibited joint swelling and had a history characteristic of an animal with scurvy, including vocalization when being picked up and food refusal. The veterinarian dispensed vitamin drops containing vitamin C adequate to eliminate hypovitaminosis C. After 2 weeks, the guinea pig was returned to the clinic with new problems. Despite a good appetite, the animal had become very thin and had lost most of its hair, although the obvious signs of scurvy had receded.

a. Which vitamin product might the veterinarian have prescribed or the client mistakenly purchased?
b. When is supplemental (in addition to that in the feed) vitamin C recommended for guinea pigs? How much is given daily?

Case 19: Guinea Pigs with "Lumps"

Sporadic deaths occurred in 25 of 40 animals participating in an exhibition at a county fair. The clinical signs reported by the various owners included submandibular swellings in several animals and dyspnea in many. Necropsy signs included conjunctivitis, enlarged cervical lymph nodes, pneumonia, pleuritis, otitis media, and metritis.

a. Which pathogenic bacterium is probably involved?
b. This agent caused abortions in contact animals. What other factors may produce abortions or stillbirths in guinea pigs?

Case 20: Septicemia in a Guinea Pig

A student submitted a 600-g female guinea pig with a recent history of anorexia and peracute death. Gross necropsy examination revealed atelectasis and consolidation of the entire left lung and congestion and focal abscessation of the right lung. The spleen was enlarged and had several white foci on the capsular surface. Bilaterally, multifocal white foci were present on the capsular surface of the kidneys.

a. The lesions in this guinea pig indicate a septicemia. The enlarged spleen with the necrotic foci is suggestive of which diseases?
b. Is diarrhea a frequent finding in acute salmonellosis in small mammal pets?
c. What prognosis can be given for colonies with endemic salmonellosis?

Case 21: Incomplete History and Physical Examination

An adult female guinea pig was submitted for necropsy examination. A diagnosis of scurvy had been given by the veterinarian. A superficial gross necropsy examination of external structures and the thoracic and abdominal cavities revealed no ectoparasites or gross lesions. The animal weighed 365 g.

a. Is this an appropriate weight for an adult female guinea pig?
b. Anorexia and emaciation are common in guinea pigs. Suggest several causes for this problem in pet guinea pigs besides the presumptive diagnosis made by the clinician.
c. What can be done to reverse anorexia in a guinea pig?

Case 22: Swollen Feet in a Guinea Pig

A guinea pig with marked painful swelling, ulceration, and crusting of the plantar surface of the right hind foot was noted in a breeding colony. The animal was brought to a veterinary clinic, anesthetized with isoflurane in oxygen, and the foot lesion was evaluated and incised with a sterile scalpel. Several attempts to locate an abscess were unsuccessful. The foot was subsequently bandaged and the animal was held 2 days for observation, during which time it went off feed and developed ketosis. The animal did not bear weight on the limb postoperatively and the lower portion of the affected limb was later amputated, following which the animal was returned to the colony.

a. What factors predispose to pododermatitis in guinea pigs?
b. If the inflammatory response in pododermatitis is a chronic arthritis and not abscess formation, what treatment would you recommend?
c. Why might this guinea pig have become ketotic during the observation period?

Case 23: Consequences of Mastitis

A 620-g guinea pig sow, which had delivered two pups 5 days previously, was submitted for clinical examination. The right mammary gland was swollen and discolored but the animal was otherwise bright and alert. The referring veterinarian treated the guinea pig with an injection of amoxicillin and the animal was sent home.

a. What are the likely causes of mastitis in guinea pigs? How should this condition be treated in sows?
b. The guinea pig died 3 days after the amoxicillin injection. What was the probable cause of death?
c. What provisions should be made for the orphaned 8-day-old pups?

Case 24: Stillbirths and Mortality in a Guinea Pig Breeding Colony

Ten guinea pigs were presented for evaluation from a colony with a recent history of increased mortality in near-term sows, stillbirths, and perinatal mortality in neonates. No significant gross lesions were seen at necropsy. Histologic evaluation revealed numerous intranuclear eosinophilic inclusions in mandibular salivary gland ductular epithelial cells of two of the sows.

a. What virus produces these characteristic inclusions in the mandibular salivary gland ductular epithelium of guinea pigs? What are other potential rule-outs for this case?
b. What clinical signs are usually associated with this viral infection in guinea pigs?
c. Is this a zoonotic infection?

CASE REPORTS

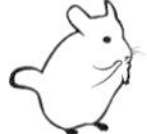

THE CHINCHILLA

Case 25: Head Tilt in a Chinchilla

An 11-year-old pet chinchilla was brought to a veterinary clinic because the owner had noticed the head was tilted to the right. The veterinarian also noted the right ear and lip were droopy. The chinchilla had been normal until a couple of days before and usually spent a lot of time outside of its cage, enjoying jumping on furniture and banking off walls. Skull radiographs were obtained (Figure 6.3).

a. What abnormalities are visible on the skull radiograph?
b. What is the likely cause of the abnormalities seen on clinical examination and radiographs?
c. What are the differential diagnoses for head tilt in a chinchilla?

Case 26: Hair Loss in a Chinchilla

A 7-year-old chinchilla has several patches of hair loss on its face and neck. A child in the household has also developed a sore on the arm.

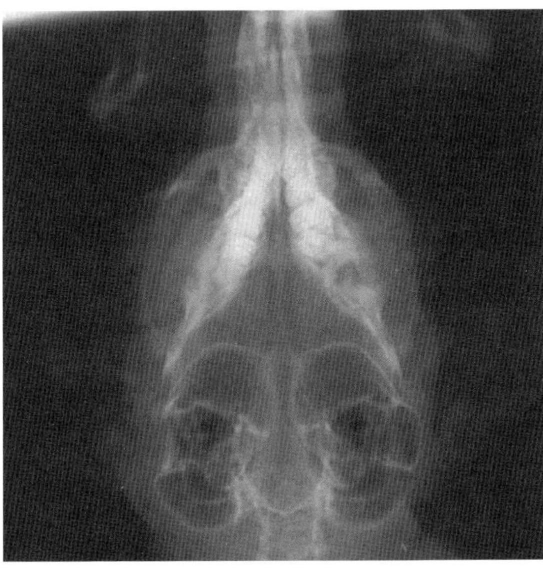

FIGURE 6.3. Ventrodorsal view of a chinchilla skull.

a. What is the most likely diagnosis and etiologic agent?
b. What treatment options are available?
c. What was the most likely source of infection in the chinchilla?

Case 27: Enteritis in a Chinchilla

A 3-year-old neutered male chinchilla was seen by a veterinarian for anorexia and diarrhea. The chinchilla had been taken to an emergency clinic 2 days previously for treatment of a cat bite and had received fluids, pain medication, and antibiotics, which the owner had been continuing at home. The chinchilla was now depressed, hunched, and had developed diarrhea. The chinchilla was normally fed a good-quality pellet, grass hay, and the occasional piece of apple or raisin as a treat; however, the owner reported that it had not been interested in eating for at least a day. The veterinarian also noted dehydration and pain on abdominal palpation.

a. What additional history might be important in determining the cause of the chinchilla's problem?
b. What is the treatment for this condition?
c. What is the prognosis?

Case 28: Abortion and Death in Chinchillas

A chinchilla rancher requested postmortem examination of two chinchillas, both of which had aborted before death. Of 64 females, 34 had died, many experiencing abortions prior to death. No clinical signs of disease other than loss of appetite were observed before death. The animals were fed a high-quality pelleted ration and were occasionally given raisins as treats. On postmortem examination, the animals were cachectic, anemic, and had multifocal, pinpoint white foci on the liver capsule and mesenteric lymph nodes, and on the serosa of the colon.

a. What are the differential diagnoses for this finding?
b. What other clinical signs could result from infection with this agent?
c. What is the most likely source of infection?
d. What management advice could be given to the owner?

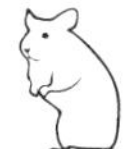

THE HAMSTER

Case 29: Dermatitis in a Hamster

A 19-month-old male Syrian hamster owned by a 12-year-old developed alopecia and scabs over the back and rear limbs. The hairless area was pruritic and the hamster was observed to bite the affected area.

a. What are rule-outs for the condition described in this animal?
b. What diagnostics should be performed?
c. How would this case be treated?

Case 30: Hamster Alopecia

A 1-year-old pet golden hamster was reported to be losing hair for 2 weeks but was otherwise normal. The owner recently bought a new, larger cage for the hamster.

a. What are the differential diagnoses for non-pruritic alopecia in the golden hamster?
b. What diagnostic procedures should be undertaken to determine the cause of the hair loss?

Case 31: Fatal Enteritis in Hamsters

A pet store supplier is experiencing high mortality in his teddy bear hamster stocks. Seven of 25 animals have been found dead with no premonitory signs, and 3 have diarrhea and are huddling. Rats and mice housed in the same area are not demonstrating clinical signs. The animals are fed standard rodent blocks and reared in fish tanks with wire lids at the back of the store. Tanks are cleaned out weekly. Animals are obtained from other local suppliers and breeders approximately monthly. The owner agrees to bring in the three sick animals for examination. You are presented with one weanling and one adult hamster that are hunched, dehydrated, and have unkempt hair coats. Two of the hamsters have perineal fecal staining and are moribund. You anesthetize one animal, collect blood via a cardiac puncture, and perform a complete necropsy. Gross examination reveals a thickened ileum and multifocal white spots on the liver.

a. What additional tests would you recommend?
b. What is your provisional diagnosis and what therapy would you recommend?
c. What is the prognosis?

Case 32: Swollen Hamsters

Two laboratory hamsters from a group of five that are control animals in an infectious disease study present within 2 weeks of each other with severe subcutaneous edema (anasarca). The animals are 18-month-old SPF females that have been provided with routine husbandry. The other three animals look normal. The hamsters have been housed individually to avoid fighting.

a. What rule-outs will you consider and what diagnostics do you recommend? Are any therapeutics indicated?
b. What are common nonneoplastic, noninfectious diseases seen in aged hamsters?

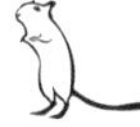

THE GERBIL

Case 33: Skin Mass and Head Tilt in Gerbils

Two 4-year-old gerbils were brought to a veterinary clinic for examination. One gerbil had a soft, subcutaneous mass (1×2 cm) on the midventral abdomen posterior to the xiphoid process. An abscess was detected by aspiration. The abscess was drained and flushed, and the gerbil was given trimethoprim/sulfa in a cherry-flavored syrup and sent home. One month later the gerbil returned to the clinic with a firm mass in the same area. The second gerbil had developed a mild but fixed head tilt. This animal was treated successfully with corticosteroids and systemic antibiotics.

a. For the first gerbil, the abscess was a secondary problem. What primary disorder might be suspected?
b. Chloramphenicol and dexamethasone successfully stopped the progression of the torticollis in the second animal. What are potential differential diagnoses for head tilt in a gerbil? What is the therapeutic function of the steroid?

CASE REPORTS

Case 34: Death of Young Gerbils

Two 17-day-old gerbils were presented to a veterinary clinic for necropsy examination. The gerbils were found to be cachetic and dehydrated, and the stomach of both animals had multifocal hemorrhages on the mucosal surface, consistent with acute ulceration. The dam and 2 other littermates were reportedly in good health. The diet provided was a high-quality, pelleted chow, and water was provided via a bottle with a sipper tube attached to the side of the cage.

a. At what age are gerbils weaned?
b. What husbandry conditions might have resulted in the death of the 2 littermates?

Case 35: Rough Hair in Gerbils

A family purchased a pair of 6-week-old gerbils. The family was hoping to breed the animals and requested general information about breeding gerbils from a veterinarian. The clients were also concerned about the gerbils' rough hair coats.

a. What causes gerbils to have rough hair coats?
b. How do you verify that the gerbils are a breeding pair?
c. What type of cage, feed, bedding, feeding and watering devices, and nesting boxes should the practitioner recommend?

Case 36: Sudden Death in Gerbils

A young adult female gerbil and several weanlings died suddenly with no other clinical signs. The ileocecal-colonic junction was hyperemic, and the liver surface was seen to have multifocal pale white foci on the surface.

a. What common enteric condition of rabbits and rodents also causes focal hepatic necrosis?
b. How is the causative agent transmitted? Does it persist in the cage environment?
c. How would one obtain a specific diagnosis in this case?

Case 37: Ocular and Nasal Discharge in Gerbils

One animal of a pair of male gerbils developed a copious, red-brown purulent discharge from the left eye and nares. Adjacent skin and nose were hairless, moist, and erythematous. The swollen lids and pus covered the intact eyeball. *Staphylococcus aureus* was isolated in pure culture from the purulent material.

a. What is the most likely etiology of this condition?
b. What is the source or cause of the reddish-brown pigment in the pus?
c. How should this gerbil be treated?

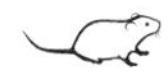 THE MOUSE

Case 38: Paresis in a Male Mouse

A male mouse developed a slowly progressive posterior paresis, diarrhea, and perineal swelling. This pet mouse had been taken from a cage containing another male mouse.

a. What is the probable cause of the clinical signs seen in this mouse?
b. What recommendations might be made to the owner to avoid this condition in pair- or group-housed male mice in the future?

Case 39: Fatal Disease in a Colony of Mice

Inbred C3H female mice were inoculated with mouse serum obtained from a commercial supplier as part of an immunization protocol. Over the next 3 weeks, all recipient mice died. Clinical signs, when they occurred, included a rough hair coat, facial swelling, conjunctivitis, and death.

a. What fatal diseases of mice should be considered in this outbreak?
b. What precautions should be taken to reduce the possibility of the spread of an infectious disease from this colony?
c. How could the disease be diagnosed?

Case 40: Prolapsed Rectums in Mice

Six young male mice, four alive and two dead, were emaciated and had soft, bloody feces around the anus. All mice had evidence of either catarrhal or hemorrhagic enteropathy and had grossly thickened colons. The livers of the animals were pale, and the spleens were enlarged. Two animals had prolapsed rectums. Culture of the colonic contents resulted in a heavy growth of *Proteus* spp and coliform-like organisms.

a. Why did the mice have pale viscera?
b. What pathologic processes might account for the thickened colon?
c. What etiologic agents might be suspected in this case?
d. How would you contain an outbreak of enteritis in a large mouse colony?

Case 41: Diarrhea in Neonatal Mice

Ten 5- to 7-g 2-week-old mice with stunted growth, rough, fecal-stained hair coats, focal alopecia, and watery diarrhea were submitted for necropsy examination. The large intestine contained fluid feces. Several other litters in the room had died recently.

a. What viral conditions cause diarrhea in weanling mice? How would you differentiate these conditions?
b. What agents or processes might cause focal alopecia in mice?
c. What murine viruses are carried subclinically in the mouse gut?
d. Define morbidity. Define mortality.

Case 42: Itchy Mice

A client presents several mice from a colony that he raises in his basement to provide food for his snakes. He has noted hair loss, bleeding, and itching on most of the animals in the colony. On physical exam, you noted scabs and exudative dermatitis around the face and head. Animals were noticeably pruritic. The client has not noted any unusual deaths and both males and females of various ages were affected.

a. Given this history, what is the most likely diagnosis?
b. If animals were nonpruritic, males had scabs, and females had areas of alopecia without dermatitis, what conditions would you suspect?
c. What diagnostic tests would you perform? How do these exams differ from similar procedures in the dog or cat?

d. Assume you are able to diagnose your top rule-out. What would you use to treat the animals? What would you tell the client when he asks whether he can feed the sick animals or those under treatment to his snakes?

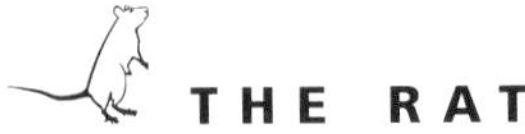

THE RAT

Case 43: Respiratory Disease in Rats

A client presents a 2-year-old male rat that has lost weight recently and become less active. Upon examination you note an unkempt hair coat, labored respiration, and red discharge from the eyes and nose. The rat weighs 300 g.

a. What is the normal weight range of an adult male rat?
b. What is the likely cause of the red discharge?
c. What diagnostic procedures are available to differentiate among the several organisms that might be involved in this case?
d. What is the most likely diagnosis, an appropriate therapy, and long-term prognosis?
e. What noninfectious diseases might be present in an animal with this signalment?

Case 44: Moveable Masses in Rats

A young girl brings two adult, female pet rats to the clinic. Both rats have single, 2-cm, firm, moveable, subcutaneous masses in the axillary region. Fibrous connective tissue cells are seen by fine needle aspirates taken from the masses.

a. What is the probable origin of the masses?
b. What histologic type of neoplasm occurs most often in the mammary gland of the rat?
c. What is an appropriate treatment for this condition?
d. Are the masses likely to reoccur if they are removed?

Case 45: Sore Eyes in Rats

A colony of 40 Long-Evans rats housed in open-top caging experienced an outbreak of "squinting" eyes and sneezing associated with a serous conjunctivitis. The eyelids were swollen, and exudate matted the surrounding fur. After a week the outbreak subsided, although several rats had clouded corneas. Histopathologic examination of the Harderian glands revealed acute edematous inflammation, necrosis, and squamous metaplasia of the glandular epithelium. *Staphylococcus aureus* was recovered in pure culture from the conjunctival sac of three rats. No organisms were cultured from the conjunctiva of several other affected animals.

a. What is the hair color pattern of the Long-Evans rat?
b. What is the probable classification of the etiologic agent? How could it be definitively diagnosed?
c. Why would corneal damage occur?
d. What management practices could be instituted to prevent spread of the disease?

Case 46: Dermatitis in Rats

A rat that had been presented for spay returned to the clinic postprocedure because of reddening of the dorsal skin along the length of the body. The animal had been anesthetized with isoflurane in oxygen during the procedure and had been warmed using a heating pad set on the low setting.

a. What is the most probable cause of the lesions?
b. How could the lesions be prevented?

Case 47: Rats with White Streaks in the Urinary Bladder

A feeder colony of rats is maintained for a small private zoo. The owners have noticed some sneezing among the rats and submitted several animals for necropsy evaluation. Following gross and histological examination, the only lesions noted are small thread-like white worms in the wall of the urinary bladder and parasitic larval forms with associated leukocytic infiltrates in the lungs.

a. What one parasite could cause both the respiratory and urinary tract abnormalities?
b. What laboratory tests can be conducted to provide confirming diagnostic evidence?
c. How can the condition be treated and eliminated from the colony?
d. Discuss the life cycle of this parasite.

CASE REPORTS

SUGGESTED SOLUTIONS

The following answers to questions posed in the clinical cases are intended to emphasize the main points for each case and are not meant to include detailed discussions of each case or problem.

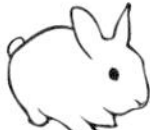

RABBITS

Case 1

a. Bacterial encephalitis, poisoning, enterotoxemia, rabies, nutritional deficiencies, heat stroke, encephalitozoonosis, toxoplasmosis, and nematode migration (*Baylisascaris procyonis*) in the brain should be included among the differential diagnoses.
b. Definitive ante mortem diagnosis is difficult. Serology can be used to help rule out *Encephalitozoon* spp, and an MRI or CT scan can help to differentiate the pathologies caused by each agent. Culture and isolation and special stains of affected tissues can be used to search for a specific cause postmortem. Encephalopathies due to *E. cuniculi* should be ruled in or out by examining histologic sections of the brain and kidney.
c. Rabbits may be infected with *Toxoplasma gondii* by ingesting grass contaminated with cat feces containing oocysts shed by feral cats. Only cats have been recognized to support all life phases of *Toxoplasma gondii.* The organism can be transmitted transplacentally in rabbits and other animal species. *Encephalitozoon cuniculi* is usually transmitted in early life from dam to offspring. *Baylisascaris* spp larval migrans results when rabbits graze in areas that are contaminated with fecal oocytes shed by raccoons or skunks. Oocytes are shed in very high numbers by these species and are highly resistant to dessication in the environment (Figure 6.4).

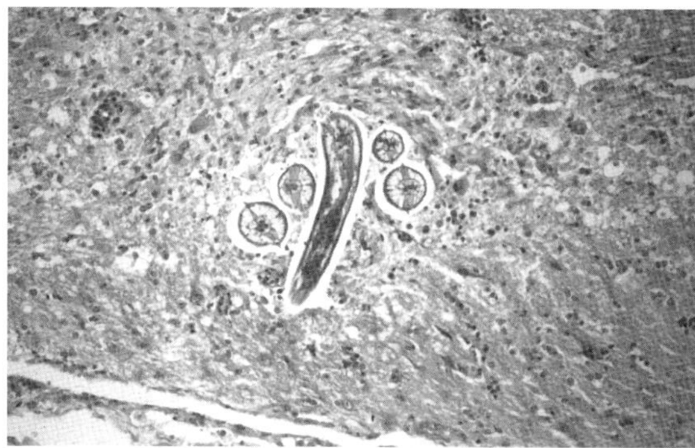

FIGURE 6.4. Photomicrograph of brain from a rabbit with cerebral larval migrans due to *Baylisascaris procyonis*. Several sections of the larva can be seen.

d. Pregnant women and individuals with a compromised immune system should be apprised of the high zoonotic potential of toxoplasmosis when oocysts are shed into the environment by cats. Humans are also susceptible to *Baylisascaris* spp larval migrans. The condition is most common in children, who may ingest dirt or play in areas in which cats, raccoons, and other species may defecate. Both toxoplasmosis and *Baylisascaris* spp infection require ingestion of oocyts in the environment. Although rabbits do not shed oocysts when infected by *T. gondii*, infection can also be transmitted when undercooked rabbit meat containing cysts is consumed. A thorough history and clinical evaluation are very important in confirming the diagnosis and in the execution of preventive measures.
e. Without a specific diagnosis, symptomatic therapy can be instituted. This would include hand feeding and watering, consideration of steroid therapy and broad spectrum antibiotics, and albendazole for treatment of potential parasitic disease. The prognosis is guarded.

References

Deeb BJ, DiGiacomo RF. Cerebral larva migrans caused by Baylisascaris sp. in pet rabbits. J Am Vet Med Assoc. 1994, 205(12):1744–1747.

Dubey JP, et al. Fatal toxoplasmosis in domestic rabbits in the USA. Vet Parasitol. 1992, 44:305–309.

Furuoka H, Sato H, Kubo M, et al. Neuropathological observation of rabbits (Oryctolagus cuniculus) affected with raccoon roundworm (Baylisascaris procyonis) larva migrans in Japan. J Vet Med Sci. 2003, 65(6):695–699.

Harcourt-Brown FM, Holloway HK. Encephalitozoon in pet rabbits. Vet Rec. 2003, 152(14):427–431.

Leland MM, Hubbard GB, Dubey JP. Clinical toxoplasmosis in domestic rabbits. Lab Anim Sci. 1992, 42:318–319.

Case 2

a. Vitamin A deficiency or excess can provoke release of hydrolases as a result of compromised structural and functional integrity of cellular lysosomes. In particular, excess vitamin A promotes decreased plasma and liver vitamin E levels, which can contribute to reproductive problems. Vitamin E is an essential dietary substance that protects cellular membranes and organelles from endogenous peroxidation. Kidney, plasma, and liver samples may be analyzed for vitamins A and E levels.
b. Deficiency of vitamin A or other nutrients can result from general malnutrition or anorexia stemming from illness. Infrequently, deficiency and excess of vitamin A is the result of an improperly formulated ration, as in this case. To confirm this diagnosis, analysis of feed should be conducted in conjunction with consideration of response to management changes and therapeutic supplementation or reduction of the vitamin in question.
c. Hypervitaminosis A can lead to follicular hyperkeratosis, anemia, increased susceptibility to infection and cancer, and night blindness. Toxicities involving arsanilic acid, DDT, nitrates, various mycotoxins such as zearalenone and aflatoxin, infections such as listeriosis, salmonellosis, aspergillosis, chlamydiosis, and other less well-defined conditions such as systemic disease and colony overcrowding should be included in the differential diagnoses of reproductive disorders in rabbits. The recovered *P. multocida* is probably an opportunistic invader responding to the retained and dead fetuses along with the uterine pathology associated with the vitamin imbalance.
d. The most likely diagnosis is hypervitaminosis A or, less likely, hypovitaminosis E.

References

DiGiacomo RF, Deeb BJ, Anderson RJ. Hypervitaminosis A and reproductive disorders in rabbits. Lab Anim Sci. 1992, 42:250–254.

Hafez AH, Gomma A, Mousa SA, et al. Aflatoxin and aflatoxicosis. IV. The effect of dietary aflatoxins on adult fertile male and female rabbits at various reproductive conditions. Mycopathol. 1983, 83:183–186.

Ismail AM, et al. Hypervitaminosis A in rabbits. I. Dose response. J Appl Rabbit Res. 1992, 15:985–994.

Yamini B, Stein S. Abortion, stillbirth, neonatal death, and nutritional myodegeneration in a rabbit breeding colony. J Am Vet Med Assoc. 1989, 194:561–562.

Case 3

a. The probable cause is urinary tract obstruction by a urolith and an associated hemorrhagic cystitis. The cause of urolithiasis in rabbits is not known, but it may be associated with chronically elevated plasma calcium levels, excessive vitamin D intake, and almost certainly other factors. Other rule-outs in this case would include uterine adenocarcinoma, ruptured endometrial aneurysms, and mummified fetuses. Porphyruria, or accumulation of porphyrin pigments in the urine, should also be considered.
b. Treatment involves a cystotomy and removal of the urolith, or uropropulsion in the case of "bladder sludge," follow-up antibiotic therapy (e.g., trimethoprim/sulfa), dietary adjustments, and resolution of postoperative dehydration and anorexia. Acidification of rabbit diets to prevent recurrence of stones should not be attempted because rabbits are herbivores, and consequently, their urine is normally basic; considerable acidification would be required to achieve an aciduria.
c. Dietary recommendations include providing a lower calcium diet by feeding fewer pellets that are typically high in calcium and more grass hays that are usually lower in calcium. Water should be provided at all times.

References

Garibaldi BA, Pecquet-Goad ME. Hypercalcemia with secondary nephrolithiasis in a rabbit. Lab Anim Sci. 1988, 38:331–333.

White RN. Management of calcium ureterolithiasis in a French lop rabbit. J Small Anim Pract. 2001, 42(12):595–598.

Case 4

a. Conjunctival overgrowth or hyperplasia. This is an unusual abnormality unique to the rabbit, in which conjunctival tissue grows across the sclera onto the cornea. It has also been called pseudopterygium, aberrant conjunctival stricture, conjunctival centripetalization, precorneal or epicorneal membranous occlusion, and circumferential conjunctival hyperplasia.

b. Treatment involves making several incisions into the overgrowing conjunctiva from the free edge to the limbus followed by transpalpebral fixation to restore the conjunctival fornix.
c. The prognosis is good if the conjunctival tissue is sutured as described above. Prognosis is guarded if the tissue is simply trimmed away, as recurrence is common.

References

Allgoewer I, et al. Abberant conjunctival stricture and overgrowth in the rabbit. Vet Ophth. 2008, 11:18–22.

Katsuta O, et al. Pseudopterygium: unique conjunctival stricture observed in Japanese White Rabbit. J Toxicol Pathol. 2008, 21:239–241.

Case 5

a. Traumatic spinal or limb injury, inherited defects, infectious diseases, toxin effect, metabolic upset, and neuromuscular disease can cause ataxia.
b. A common cerebral disease of rabbits is encephalitozoonosis, but clinical signs are rare. Cerebral nematodiasis also can cause incoordination.
c. The brain and kidneys are tissues to be examined. A Gram stain will be positive for *Encephalitozoon cuniculi*, while a PAS reaction is less predictive for rabbit strains of the organism.

Reference

Pakes SP, Gerrity LW. Protozoal Diseases. In: The Biology of the Laboratory Rabbit, 2nd ed. Manning PJ, Ringler DH, Newcomer CE (eds.). San Diego: Academic Press, 1994; 205–209.

Case 6

a. Diagnostic procedures to determine the cause of a distended abdomen, diarrhea, and cachexia in the rabbit would involve palpation, radiography, or ultrasonography for intestinal distention, hepatomegaly, and a gastric hair ball. The oral cavity should be examined for malocclusion and the feces for coccidial oocysts.
b. In hepatic coccidiosis, the lesions are linear and irregular (they follow the bile ducts) with indistinct margins. A smear of a cut section of the liver or gallbladder would reveal oocysts on microscopic examination. *Taenia* cysticercus lesions are usually rounded and have distinct margins. Larval cysts may be present in the peritoneal cavity. The miliary white foci of necrosis caused by *Francisella tularensis* will occur throughout the abdominal parenchyma and not just the liver. Tularemia is rare in domestic rabbits but more common in wild rabbits, especially in tick-infested areas.
c. *Eimeria stiedae* is the causative organism of hepatic coccidiosis in rabbits.

Reference

Pakes SP, Gerrity LW. Protozoal Diseases. In: The Biology of the Laboratory Rabbit, 2nd ed. Manning PJ, Ringler DH, Newcomer CE (eds.). San Diego: Academic Press, 1994; 205–209.

Case 7

a. Cannibalism of neonate rabbits has been associated with prolonged delivery, poor nest building, chilling of young, hereditary nervousness, consumption of placentas, disturbance of the doe, presence of abnormal or dead young, water deprivation, improper nest box design, low caloric diets, and a myriad of other factors difficult to define.
b. Correct any of the previously listed deficiencies. Keep the doe calm at kindling time. Place the hutch and nesting box away from loud or unusual noises, strangers, and predators (snakes, opossums, raccoons, foxes, coyotes, dogs, cats, and other feral animals). Fresh drinking water and a sufficient amount of food should be provided. Mortality may decrease if the doe-kit contact is restricted to one 15- to 30-minute daily nursing session. Does that cannibalize successive litters should be culled.
c. If a rabbit nest is split or if one or more young is out of the nest, the doe may not retrieve and combine the young. Some stimuli—for example, low body temperature of the neonate, odor, or a behavioral or physical abnormality—may cause rejection.

References

González-Redondoa P, Zamora-Lozano N. Neonatal cannibalism in cage-bred wild rabbits (Oryctolagus cuniculus). Arch Med Vet. 2008, 40:281–287.

Rödel HG, Starkloff A, Bautista A. Infanticide and maternal offspring defence in European rabbits under natural breeding conditions. Ethol. 2008, 114:22–31.

Rödel HG, von Holst D, Kraus C. Family legacies: short- and long-term fitness consequences of early-life conditions in female European rabbits. J Anim Ecol. 2009 Mar 9. [Epub ahead of print]

Case 8

a. The renal lesion may be a manifestation of interstitial nephritis caused by *Encephalitozoon cuniculi* (passed in the urine). Infection with this agent is usually asymptomatic, though CNS symptoms can occur.
b. Pregnancy toxemia (acidosis) is the probable cause of death and is related to mobilization of fats during times of high-energy demand. Obese animals and those on poor diets are at higher risk. Some causes of pregnancy toxemia or ketosis are prevented by eliminating obesity in breeding does through reduced food intake or feeding high-fiber feed. The underlying defect may be inadequate nutrients reaching the fetuses because of damaged uterine vessels.
c. The rabbit's gestation period is between 28 and 34 days.

Reference

Brower M. Practitioner's guide to pocket pet and rabbit theriogenology. Theriogenol. 2006, 66(3):618–623.

Case 9

a. Clostridial enterotoxemia is a probable diagnosis. Rotavirus infection, Tyzzer's disease, colibacillosis, or coccidiosis should be considered also.
b. Clinical history, a fecal examination for coccidial oocysts, necropsy examination, determination of enterotoxin or centrifugation of cecal content for cytological evaluation of *Clostridium spiroforme* and culture might provide a diagnosis. A specific diagnosis is usually difficult to determine.
c. The prognosis is poor. Higher fiber feed should be provided, along with fluid therapy, but the fatal event is probably an enterotoxemia. Symptomatic therapy may save a few animals. Prevention of recurrence includes strict sanitation, reduction of stress, provision of higher fiber feed, selection of *Clostridium*-free breeding rabbits, and cessation of practices that effect rapid changes in the quantity of feed consumed. Pregnant does on restricted feeding should gradually be introduced to full feed with high-energy feeds after kindling.

Reference

Perkins SE, Fox JG, Taylor NS, et al. Detection of Clostridium difficile toxins from the small intestine and cecum of rabbits with naturally acquired enterotoxemia. Lab Anim Sci. 1995, 45(4):379–384.

Case 10

a. Differential diagnoses should include rabbit syphilis, caused by *T. pallidum,* myxomatosis, bacterial dermatitis, and neoplasia (Shope fibroma, papilloma, or squamous cell carcinoma). The last three rule-outs should be considered but are less consistent with the clinical presentation. Dermatophytosis and ectoparasitism cannot be entirely ruled out even though initial diagnostics were negative.
b. These are classic lesions of rabbit syphilis and further testing may be unnecessary. Biopsy and histopathologic examination, impression smear evaluation for spirochetes, and serologic tests for syphilis could be conducted.
c. Penicillin, 50,000–200,000 IU per 4.5 kg BW, administered intramuscularly for 3 days, is recommended and works well, although penicillin administered orally may cause fatal enterotoxemias. Amoxicillin and ampicillin should never be used orally or parenterally in rabbits.

Reference

Treponematosis. The Merck Veterinary Manual Online. http://www.merckvetmanual.com/mvm/index.jsp?cfile=htm/bc/171321.htm. Accessed April 14, 2009.

Case 11

a. Fur chewing may indicate a fiber deficiency or a stress response. Selectively altering protein, salt, fiber (hay), or MgO (5 lb per ton of feed) in the diet and making certain that potable drinking water is available may eliminate the fur-chewing problem. Rabbits and other species may ingest fur or other high-fiber materials to decrease pain from acute enteritis.

b. Housing sexually mature male rabbits in separate cages will reduce or eliminate fur-chewing behavior and will eliminate biting and fighting. Alternatively, providing hiding places and escape routes for group-housed rabbits will permit more subordinate animals to escape the unwanted attentions of dominant rabbits.
c. These rabbits should be neutered to improve behavioral attributes as pets and to decrease incidence of reproductive diseases as they age.

Reference

Bradley T. Rabbit care and husbandry. Vet Clin North Am Exot Anim Pract. 2004, 7(2):299–313, vi.

Case 12

a. Drooling or ptyalism in rabbits may be caused by malocclusion, or the dewlap may become wet and abraded if the rabbit feeds or drinks from crocks. Obese females are predisposed to this condition. A wet dewlap, often associated with a moist, bacterial dermatitis, may be prevented by correcting malocclusion or by feeding from hopper feeders and watering through sipper tubes rather than crocks or bowls. Superficial, moist dermatitis is treated by shaving the hair over the lesion, cleansing the skin with an antiseptic soap, rinsing, and applying a topical antibiotic powder or ointment.
b. *Pasteurella multocida* may reach the conjunctival sac from the nasal cavity via the nasolacrimal duct or by transmission on the forepaws from the nares.
c. Conjunctivitis in rabbits may be treated with an ophthalmic ointment containing an antibiotic or by systemic antibiotics. Treatment of the conjunctival infection does not necessarily eliminate the organism in the nasal passage. Flushing of the nasolacrimal duct with saline and then an antibiotic solution will reduce bacterial numbers and allow conjunctival exudate to drain to the nasal area and thus reduce matting of hair around the eye. Underlying causes of the conjunctivitis, including tooth root abscesses, should be investigated.

Reference

Rougier S, Galland D, Boucher S, et al. Epidemiology and susceptibility of pathogenic bacteria responsible for upper respiratory tract infections in pet rabbits. Vet Microbiol. 2006, 115(1–3):192–198.

Case 13

a. A congenital abnormality involving the spine, coxofemoral junction, or rear limb bones may exhibit a familial inheritance pattern, or the condition may be associated with flooring with poor traction during limb development. A traumatic injury would have a history of sudden onset and an association with a fall, improper restraint, or other traumatic event in most cases. Rabbits with hypovitaminosis E may not be able to use their rear limbs because of dystrophic muscles. A definitive diagnosis would be established by thorough history and physical examination, including neurologic examination and imaging studies.
b. Neurologic control of defecation and urination is often impaired following traumatic lumbosacral dislocation or luxation due to damage to the spinal cord. Increased soiling also occurs if animals are dragging their rear legs due to neurological impairment.
c. The prognosis of posterior paresis in the rabbit depends on the extent of the damage to the vertebral column, spinal cord, and nerve trunks. If the lesion is due to focal spinal cord edema and inflammation, cage rest for 7–10 days and use of drugs to reduce edema and inflammation (i.e., corticosteroids) may restore motor function. If the vertebrae are fractured with displaced fragments or the spinal cord or nerves are severed or severely injured, recovery will not occur. Food and water should be placed so that the animal can readily access it, urinary bladder expression may be required, frequent cleaning of the perineal area is required to prevent urine scalding and fecal soiling, and increased cage cleaning should be performed.

References

Keeble E. Common neurological and musculoskeletal problems in rabbits. In Pract. 2006, 28:212–218.

Owiny JR, VandeWoude S, Painter JT, et al. Hip dysplasia in rabbits: association with nest box flooring. Comp Med. 2001, 51(1): 85–88.

Case 14

a. The tentative diagnosis is chronic renal failure (BUN, CREAT, urine S.G.). The condition is likely chronic because of the low PCV resulting from reduced erythropoietin expression.
b. Plans might include giving a balanced electrolyte solution IV immediately to correct the hydration status and then teaching the client to administer SC fluids subsequently. Potassium levels of the patient would have to be monitored and adjusted by supplementation in the fluids, as needed. The anemia could be treated by ferrous sulphate and B complex vitamins could be added. The animal may require oral gavage or nasogastric tube feeding of a high-quality food, such as a herbivore-specific critical care diet to treat anorexia. The urine should be cultured to determine whether a urinary tract infection is present, as this is common with chronic renal disease.
c. The treatment is palliative only and the owner should be counselled that the condition is chronic and degenerative. Quality of life may determine further clinical decisions pursued.

Reference

Fisher PG. Exotic mammal renal disease: diagnosis and treatment. Vet Clin North Am Exot Anim Pract. 2006, 9(1):69–96.

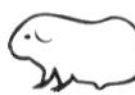

GUINEA PIGS

Case 15

a. There is a round, radiodense structure present in the pelvis, which is likely a urolith present at the neck of the bladder or in the urethra.
b. The cause of urolithiasis in guinea pigs is not known. Predisposing factors may include genetic predisposition, metabolic disorders, nutritional imbalances, inadequate water intake, and bacterial cystitis.
c. Treatment of choice is surgical removal after stabilization. Urethral calculi are more difficult to remove surgically. Catheterizing the urethra and back-flushing may retropulse the urolith into the bladder. Culture of the urine, stone, and bladder wall should be performed.
d. The prognosis is poor, as recurrence is common. Dietary manipulations are generally not successful, and urinary acidifiers are not indicated in guinea pigs as they have difficulty removing acid excess.

Reference

Fisher PG. Exotic mammal renal disease: diagnosis and treatment. Vet Clin North Am Exot Anim Pract. 2006, 9(1):69–96.

Case 16

a. Tyzzer's disease, salmonellosis, coccidiosis, and cryptosporidiosis should be considered in cases involving chronic diarrhea in guinea pigs.
b. Cryptosporidial oocysts are 3–6 um in diameter and are morphologically similar to yeasts. Diagnosis of cryptosporidial infection can be made from microscopic examination of concentrated fecal flotation samples or from acid-fast stains of fresh or formalin-fixed fecal smears or tissue sections.
c. *Cryptosporidium* spp is highly infectious and may be transmitted by the fecal-oral route from various animal species to humans. It is a common cause of disease in immunodeficient humans.

Reference

Chrisp CE, Reid WC, Rush HG, et al. Cryptosporidiosis in guinea pigs: an animal model. Infect Immun. 1990, 58(3):674–679.

Case 17

a. This scenario is highly suggestive of bacterial infection exacerbated by stress. *Bordetella bronchiseptica* and *Streptococcus pneumoniae* should be considered and can be confirmed by culture. A likely scenario is that highly susceptible uninfected guinea pigs came in contact with asymptomatic carrier animals and that the stress associated with shipment resulted in the disease presentation.
b. The use of an autogenous bacterin or canine bacterium might have prevented a clinical outbreak of *Bordetella* infection, but this is not a common practice. Good husbandry, elimination of carriers, and stress reduction diminish the impact of streptococcal infections.

c. A broad-spectrum antibiotic, such as enrofloxacin, should be administered to any animals that demonstrate respiratory signs or decreased activity or appetite. Nebulization can be considered for any animals that have respiratory involvement. Appropriate diet and husbandry and a low-stress environment should be provided, and these animals should be separated from other guinea pigs in the facility. Strains of *Bordetella bronchiseptica* and *Streptococcus pneumoniae* can be carried by several species of animals, including rabbits, guinea pigs, cats, dogs, rats, and wild rodents, as well as humans.

Reference

Sparrow S. Diseases of pet rodents. J Small Anim Pract. 2008, 21:1–16.

Case 18

a. If a multivitamin product was used in this guinea pig, other vitamins, especially vitamins D and A, may have been administered in excessive amounts.
b. Supplemental vitamin C should be provided whenever the vitamin C content of the feed is suspected to be inadequate. Excess vitamin C will be excreted in the urine as long as the animal is well hydrated and has functional kidneys. Many commercially available feeds for pets do not provide adequate levels of vitamin C and should routinely be supplemented. Heat, length of storage, improper formulation, and dampness contribute to breakdown of the vitamin. Treatment dosages are between 25 and 50 mg/kg per day for animals with clinical disease.

Reference

Hickman DL, Wasson K, Ehrhart EJ. Morbidity and mortality in a group of young guinea pigs. Subclinical hypovitaminosis C. Lab Anim. 2003, 32(9):23–25.

Case 19

a. *Streptococcus zooepidemicus* is the probable etiologic agent.
b. Dystocia, large fetal loads, salmonellosis, streptococcal infections, cytomegalovirus infections, miscellaneous infections, nutritional deficiencies, stress, and ketoacidosis may cause abortion or stillbirths in guinea pigs.

Reference

Murphy JC, Ackerman JI, Marini RP, et al. Cervical lymphadenitis in guinea pigs: infection via intact ocular and nasal mucosa by Streptococcus zooepidemicus. Lab Anim Sci. 1991, 41(3):251–254.

Case 20

a. Salmonellosis in guinea pigs may cause generalized visceral congestion and focal necrosis of the spleen and liver.
b. Diarrhea may occur with *Salmonella* spp infections, but this sign is an inconsistent finding. Affected animals may have a soft, discolored stool or may present with other nonspecific signs of illness.
c. Because of the epizootic and fatal consequences of a *Salmonella* spp outbreak in a colony of animals, the persistence of the disease in a carrier state, and the public health significance, infected animals are generally euthanized.

Reference

Singh BR, Alam J, Hansda D. Alopecia induced by salmonellosis in guinea pigs. Vet Rec. 2005, 156(16):516–518.

Case 21

a. A typical adult female guinea pig should weigh between 700 and 900 g. This animal was clearly emaciated.
b. Emaciation in guinea pigs is often caused by malocclusion of the cheek teeth. Other causes of weight loss in pet guinea pigs include metastatic calcification, vitamin C deficiency, ectoparasitism, chronic renal disease, pain, and anorexia induced by changes in the taste or composition of the feed or changes in the feeding and watering devices.
c. Anorexia in guinea pigs is life-threatening and must be reversed or overcome within a few days of onset. Any primary causes for anorexia should be specifically treated. If a variety of fruits and vegetables are offered and not eaten, the animal must be force-fed a high caloric food mixed, perhaps, with mashed pellets. Yogurt and other food combinations are used also. In all cases, fluids and vitamin C should be given PO or SC.

References

Jekl V, Hauptman K, Knotek Z. Quantitative and qualitative assessments of intraoral lesions in 180 small herbivorous mammals. Vet Rec. 2008, 162(14):442–449.

Legendre LF. Malocclusions in guinea pigs, chinchillas and rabbits. Can Vet J. 2002, 43(5):385–390.

Case 22

a. Pododermatitis in guinea pigs is most often encountered in heavy older animals raised on a rough or abrasive floor, such as wire.

b. Treatment of pododermatitis is difficult because the inflammation is chronic, diffuse, and relatively isolated from the vascular system. Staphylococci are frequently isolated from such lesions. Topical antibiotics given with DMSO, softening of the skin of the foot, and surgical debridement may be attempted, but the prognosis for recovery is poor.

c. Ketosis in guinea pigs is a common sequelae to anorexia. This animal may have been painful in the postoperative period, leading to anorexia. Pain needs to be managed with close attention to avoid prolonged periods of fasting, which may lead to irreversible ketosis and death.

Reference

Brown C, Donnelly TM. Treatment of pododermatitis in the guinea pig. Lab Anim. 2008, 37(4):156–157.

Case 23

a. Mastitis in guinea pigs is commonly caused by *Streptococcus zooepidemicus* infections; however, other potential etiologic agents include staphylococcal, *Pasteurella* spp, and coliform organisms. Pups should be removed from the dam and sows should be treated with parenteral broad-spectrum antibiotics (e.g., fluorquinolone antibiotics), analgesics, and hot packing of the affected glands. Affected animals may go off feed and become dehydrated. Sows should be tempted to eat with tasty food supplements and given access to fresh water.

b. Penicillin, and most other antibiotics, used in the guinea pig or hamster may induce an alteration of the intestinal flora that results in fatal enteritis or enterotoxemia.

c. Orphaned guinea pigs or those from dams with agalactia can be bottle-fed with KMR diluted two or three to one with water. By 5–7 days, the young pups will begin to eat softened pelleted feed and can be weaned from milk by the third week. Guinea pig pups that are less than 55 g at birth rarely survive.

Reference

Kinkler RJ, Jr, et al. Bacterial mastitis in guinea pigs. Lab Anim Sci. 1976, 26:214–217.

Case 24

a. Cytomegalovirus (CMV) infection produces eosinophilic intranuclear inclusions in submandibular salivary gland ductular epithelial cells. The ductal epithelial cells are markedly enlarged in infected guinea pigs. Smaller intranuclear inclusions may be found in renal tubular epithelial cells and occasionally in other tissues. Other potential infectious rule-outs for this clinical case include acute adenoviral infection or acute bacterial infection with a range of agents such as *Bordetella bronchiseptica*, *Streptococcus* spp, *E. coli*, and *Salmonella* spp.

b. Cytomegalovirus infections are usually subclinical in guinea pigs. The prevalence of infection in conventionally housed and managed animals is usually high.

c. Although the guinea pig is an animal model for cytomegalovirus infections of humans, there is no evidence that the guinea pig virus can be transmitted between guinea pigs and humans. In fact, attempts to transmit guinea pig CMV to other species have failed.

References

Griffith BP, Hsiung GD. Cytomegalovirus infection in guinea pigs. IV. Maternal infection at different stages of gestation. J Infect Dis. 1980, 141:787–793.

Griffith BP, et al. Enhancement of cytomegalovirus infection during pregnancy in guinea pigs. J Infect Dis. 1983, 147:990–998.

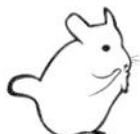

CHINCHILLAS

Case 25

a. Indentation or collapse of the lateral mid-portion of the right bulla and lucency in the caudal portion of left mandibular body are visible (Figure 6.5).
b. Head tilt is due to damage to the vestibulocochlear nerve secondary to trauma, infection, inflammation, neoplasia. Droopy right ear and lip is likely caused by damage to the facial nerve secondary to trauma, infection, inflammation, neoplasia. Indentation or collapse of the lateral mid-portion of the right bulla was likely caused by fracture secondary to trauma. The bulla wall is very thin and chinchillas are very agile and enjoy running and jumping, and the animal may have hit its head against the wall. Lucency in the caudal portion of the left mandibular body is interpreted as a chronic finding likely due to a tooth root abscess and possibly osteomyelitis of the surrounding bone.
c. Differential diagnoses for head tilt in a chinchilla include trauma, infections (otitis media/interna), parasites, neoplasia, central vestibular disease, and cerebrospinal nematodiasis.

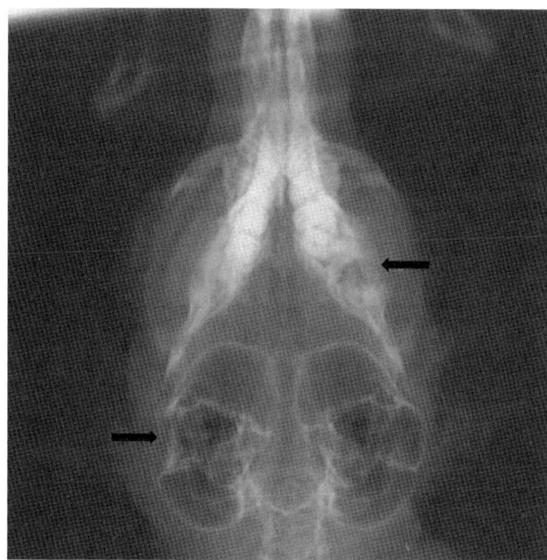

FIGURE 6.5. Ventrodorsal view of a chinchilla skull showing indentation of right bulla and lucency in left mandibular body (arrows).

Reference

Wideman WL. Pseudomonas aeruginosa otitis media and interna in a chinchilla ranch. Can Vet J. 2006, 47(8):799–800.

Case 26

a. Dermatophytosis is most likely, as it is zoonotic and can be transmitted to people. In chinchillas, *Trichophyton mentagrophytes* is most commonly isolated, although *Microsporum canis* and *M. gypseum* may also occur.
b. Treatment options include topical or systemic antifungals, or a combination of both. Topical treatment removes spores from the hair shaft. Systemic treatment acts at the hair follicle. Topical treatment includes 2% chlorhexidine/2% miconazole shampoo, 0.2% enilconazole rinse, lime sulphur dips once weekly for 6 weeks, or orthocaptan fungal powder added to dust (1 tsp per 2 cups of dust). Note that orthocaptan may be carcinogenic and hands should be washed carefully after handling treated animals. Systemic treatment includes griseofulvin (25 mg/kg PO q24h × 30–60 d), ketoconazole (10–15 mg/kg PO q24h), itraconazole (5–10 mg/kg q24h), and terbinafine (8–20 mg/kg PO q24h).
c. The chinchilla likely acquired the infection from another chinchilla and may have been carrying the organism asymptomatically until now.

References

Donnelly TM. Disease Problems of Chinchillas. In: Ferrets, Rabbits, and Rodents: Clinical Medicine and Surgery, 2nd ed. Quesenberry KE, Carpenter JW (eds.). St. Louis: Saunders, 2004; 255–265.

Marshall KL. Fungal diseases in small mammals: therapeutic trends and zoonotic considerations. Vet Clin Exot Anim. 2003, 6:415–427.

Case 27

a. It is important to know what type of antibiotics the chinchilla is being given. Inappropriate antibiotic use can result in intestinal dysbiosis, which favors overgrowth of *Clostridium* spp, elaboration of toxins, and fatal enterotoxemia. Antibiotics implicated in enterotoxemia of chinchillas include penicillins (including ampicillin and amoxicillin), cephalosporins, clindamycin, erythromycin, and lincomycin.

b. Treatment for antibiotic-associated enterotoxemia is supportive. The suspect antibiotic should be immediately discontinued. Provision of fluids warmed to body temperature are important to replace losses and maintain blood pressure. Intravenous or intraosseous administration is most helpful. Subcutaneous fluids may not be absorbed quickly enough to be effective. Analgesics are also indicated to minimize abdominal discomfort. Syringe-feeding a palatable, high-fiber diet will help prevent ileus and provide nutritional support. Pediatric simethicone may help reduce gas. The chinchilla should be kept warm but not overheated.

c. Antibiotic-associated enterotoxemia is a life-threatening condition and the prognosis is poor.

Reference

Donnelly TM, Brown CJ. Guinea pig and chinchilla care and husbandry. Vet Clin Exot Anim. 2004, 7:351–373.

Case 28

a. Differentials include any bacteria that could result in septicemia, with *Listeria* spp being the most likely, due to the epizootic nature of the infection. Toxoplasmosis may also cause abortions and pinpoint liver lesions.

b. *Listeria monocytogenes* may also cause sudden death, encephalitis with neurological signs, weight loss, depression, hunched appearance, droopy ears, diarrhea or constipation with rectal prolapse, abdominal pain (stretching or rolling), bruxism, and vocalization.

c. The source is usually contamination of feed and/or water with rodent droppings.

d. Recommendations include improved sanitation of cages, water bottles and dust baths, minimizing stress, storeage of food in rodent-proof containers, and purchasing food from reputable suppliers.

Reference

Sabocanec R, et al. Incidence of listeriosis in farm chinchillas (Chinchilla laniger) in Croatia. Veterinarski Arhiv. 2000, 70:159–167.

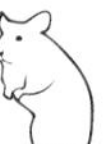

HAMSTERS

Case 29

a. Dermatophytosis, bite wounds from another hamster, cutaneous lymphoma, allergic or bacterial dermatopathies, and acariasis (*Demodex* spp) might cause lesions similar to those seen in this animal.

b. A thorough history should be performed to determine the type of bedding used and any other recent changes (weight or appetite loss, other hamster introductions in particular). A skin scraping, DTM culture, and possibly a biopsy or bacterial culture should be performed. Because this animal is owned by a child, it is important to rule out dermatophytes.

c. Prior to identification of the underlying cause, the animal should be cleansed with an antibacterial/antifungal agent such as chlorhexidine. Any husbandry-related recommendations (i.e., change bedding from cedar to hardwood, remove other hamsters that might be inflicting trauma) should be instituted. The cause of the problem should be determined and an appropriate treatment used, such as ivermectin for demodicosis, systemic or local antifungals for dermatophytes, or systemic antibiotics for bacterial infections. Care should be exercised in administration of therapies with potential side effects.

Reference

Tani K, Iwanaga T, Sonoda K, et al. Ivermectin treatment of demodicosis in 56 hamsters. J Vet Med Sci. 2001, 63(11):1245–1247.

Case 30

a. Pheochromocytomas, adrenocortical adenomas, and adenocarcinomas have been reported in golden hamsters and all may result in alopecia. They are relatively common among the neoplasms of hamsters. Cage trauma and demodecosis should also be considered. Neoplasia may predispose animals to demodecosis.

b. A scraping from the margin of the skin lesion should be examined for *Demodex* spp and dermatophytes, although dermatophytosis is rare in the golden hamster. Alopecia in hamsters is also commonly associated with endocrinologic disease. Affected animals are generally over 14 months old, and while alopecia with or without comedones and hyperpigmentation may be the initial presenting sign, animals will develop polyuria, polydipsia, and skin fragility with time. There is no diagnostic test currently available for hamsters and diagnosis is usually a process of elimination. Similarly, there is no treatment other than supportive care for the condition.

Reference

Collins B. Endocrine diseases of rodents. Vet Clin Exot Anim. 2008, 11(1):153–162.

Case 31

a. Histopathology with silver stains of the liver and ileum are recommended to rule out Tyzzer's disease (*C. piliforme*) and transmissible ileal hyperplasia ("wet tail") caused by *Lawsonia intracellularis*. In addition, a fecal evaluation should be performed for parasites, and fecal culture may also be indicated. It is important to consider that multiple etiologies may be involved and are likely related to husbandry factors, such as poor diet, inappropriate environmental conditions, transportation, and so forth.
b. Both transmissible ileal hyperplasia and Tyzzer's disease seem likely as they are common in pet store animals and present with symptoms similar to those described. Provision of appropriate husbandry is key to controlling further disease in the colony. Treatment includes supportive fluids (oral or parenteral electrolytes or lactated Ringer's solution) for dehydration, an antidiarrheal agent, such as bismuth subsalicylate, and appropriate antibiotics, such as tetracycline, enrofloxacin, metronidazole, or trimethoprim/sulfa, which can be administered orally or via the drinking water. Rats and mice in the facility may be carriers for Tyzzer's disease and should be housed in separate areas.
c. The prognosis is guarded for any animals that develop symptoms, as animals often do not respond to therapy.

References

Motzel SL, Gibson SV. Tyzzer's disease in hamsters and gerbils from a pet store supplier. J Am Vet Med Assoc. 1990, 197:1176–1178.

Motzel SL, Riley LK. Subclinical infection and transmission of Tyzzer's disease in rats. Lab Anim Sci. 1992, 42:439–443.

Shauer DB, et al. Proliferative enterocolitis associated with a dual infection with enteropathogenic Escherichia coli and Lawsonia intracellularis in rabbits. J Clin Microbiol. 1998, 36:1700–1703.

Case 32

a. Renal disease with subsequent hypoproteinemia as well as cardiomyopathy with subsequent heart failure and poor peripheral circulation should be considered in these animals. A thorough history should also investigate other experimental factors that might have contributed to disease. A urinalysis could reveal urine specific gravity and protein content and an ultrasound might be performed to assess cardiac function if the appropriate transducers are available. Whole-body radiographs might also reveal cardiac or renal abnormalities. If the investigator decides to euthanize the animals, a necropsy should be performed. Diuretics can be initiated if this will not interfere with the experimental study.
b. Amyloidosis of the kidneys and other organs, cardiomyopathy, and renal disease are all common metabolic diseases of aged hamsters. Anasarca has been reported in cases of cardiomyopathy and amyloidosis.

References

Murphy JC, Fox JG, Neimi SM. Nephrotic syndrome associated with renal amyloidosis in a colony of Syrian hamsters. J Am Vet Med Assoc. 1984, 185(11):1359–1362.

Ottenweller JE, Tapp WN, Natelson BH. The effect of chronic digitalis therapy on the course of heart failure and on endocrine function in cardiomyopathic hamsters. Res Commun Chem Pathol Phamarcol. 1987, 58(3):413–416.

GERBILS

Case 33

a. Cutaneous neoplasms have been associated with the ventral midline sebaceous scent gland in the gerbil. These neoplasms are usually benign but are occasionally malignant. In either case, resection of the mass is generally curative.

b. Torticollis indicates an inflammation of the inner ear or brain and may be secondary to otitis media/interna, a brain abscess or tumor, aural cholesteatoma, or trauma. If an inflammatory process damages the vestibular apparatus of the inner ear, the animal may never regain a normal posture. Administration of a steroid may reduce inflammation. If the torticollis is not severe, an affected animal may compensate and continue to eat and drink despite the head tilt. Alternately, head tilt can also result from pressure on the tympanic membrane due to the accumulation of keratin plugs produced by aural cholesteatomas in the external auditory canal.

References

Chole RA, et al. Cholesteatoma: spontaneous occurrence in the Mongolian gerbil, Meriones unguiculatus. Am J Otol. 1981, 2:204–210.

Henry KR, et al. Age-related increase of spontaneous aural cholesteatoma in the Mongolian gerbil. Arch Otolaryngol. 1983, 109:19–21.

Schiffer SP, Lukas VS, Chrisp CE. Diagnostic exercise: head tilt in a gerbil. Lab Anim Sci. 1986, 36(2):176–177.

Case 34

a. Gerbils are weaned between 20 and 26 days of age. The gerbils in this case were sucklings.

b. Death in 2 animals just prior to weaning could be due to congenital defects that impaired prehension, such as malocclusion or hydrocephalus. No clinical signs were evident on necropsy that supported these diagnoses. Husbandry considerations would be related to temperature, particularly hyperthermia (unlikely because the mother and 2 littermates were unaffected), or inability to eat or drink. This would be possible if the animals could not reach or chew the food pellets, or if the sipper tube was inaccessible due to cage height. Stomach content and hydration status at necropsy could help to ascertain these parameters. In the case of this diagnosis, the other 2 littermates would presumably still be nursing or might be larger and therefore able to reach and procure food and water more effectively.

Case 35

a. Rough hair coats in gerbils occur when the relative humidity is 50% or higher. Gerbils may also have rough hair coats if they are febrile, the water bottle leaks, or if the bedding is damp or contains resin. Gerbils can be provided with dust baths or bedding that is firmer and more abrasive than wood shavings (such as corncobs) to maintain high coat quality.

b. Gerbils are sexed by noting the anogenital distance, which in adults is about 5 mm for females and 10 mm for males. The female has a vulvar opening at the base of the urogenital papilla, whereas the male has a larger papilla. If the gerbils have identical arrangements of the anal and urogenital structures, they are not a male-female pair.

c. Gerbils should be provided with deep bedding and a concealed nesting and hiding place within the cage. Gerbils should be fed a quality, pelleted rodent feed from a hopper feeder and watered from a water bottle that is readily accessible. The water conservation mechanism of the gerbil is a mechanism for survival in the desert and should not be used as a rationale for excluding water from the pet or laboratory gerbil. Nesting boxes may be simple metal boxes, cans, or short pieces of plastic pipe or tubing.

Case 36

a. Tyzzer's disease often involves focal hepatic necrosis, but other enteric conditions, including coliform infections, can pass via the portal circulation to the liver.

b. *Clostridium piliforme* is transmitted primarily through the ingestion of contaminated feces. Infectious, spore-like bodies from the filamentous organism may remain viable in the environment for months or years.

c. The classic triad of gross necropsy signs—myocarditis, hepatic necrosis, and typhlitis—together with Warthin-Starry visualization of bacilli in histologic sections, are commonly used methods for identifying the disease and the intracellular organism.

References

Motzel SL, Gibson SV. Tyzzer's disease in hamsters and gerbils from a pet store supplier. J Am Vet Med Assoc. 1990, 197:1176–1178.

Veazey RS, Paulsen DB, Schaeffer DO. Encephalitis in gerbils due to naturally occurring infection with Bacillus piliformis (Tyzzer's disease). Lab Anim Sci. 1992, 42:516–518.

Case 37

a. The cause of this is likely an increase in secretion of porphyrin material from the Harderian gland, which is irritating to the skin. Various skin bacteria, such as *Staphylococcus* spp, then act opportunistically to produce dermatitis.
b. The reddish-brown pigment is likely porphyrin from the Harderian gland. Stressors, such as those resulting from overcrowding or high humidity, are thought to increase secretion.
c. Keeping the gerbil in a dry environment, minimizing stress, and providing a sand bath may help prevent this condition. Antibiotic eye ointment can be used in the eye and on the skin. Parenteral antibiotics, such as chloramphenicol or trimethoprim/sulfa, are indicated in severe infections. Trauma to the nose from chewing at the bars of a wire cage or from a roughened cage surface may exacerbate the condition.

Reference

Donnelly TM. Disease Problems of Small Rodents. In: Ferrets, Rabbits, and Rodents: Clinical Medicine and Surgery, 2nd ed. Quesenberry KE, Carpenter JW (eds.). St. Louis: Saunders, 2004; 299–315.

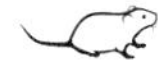

MICE

Case 38

a. Adult male mice housed in groups without adequate shelters or hiding places will often fight and bite one another. The fighting wounds, usually seen over the back, rump, and tailhead, include alopecia, scabbing, swelling, and ulceration. In some cases abscessation occurs. The social hierarchy existing within the group influences the relative severity of the lesions.
   This mouse had a staphylococcal abscess extending from beside the anus through the posterior abdomen and into the spinal cord and canal. Differential diagnoses include traumatic injury and neoplasia.
b. Adult male mice can be housed individually or given appropriate cage enrichment items to allow subordinate animals to escape unwanted attention from more dominant animals.

Case 39

a. Mousepox should be suspected in all cases of epizootic mortality in a mouse colony, especially when that mortality is high and when the introduction of biological products or mouse tissues precedes the outbreak. Salmonellosis or other peracute bacterial infections could cause sudden deaths in susceptible strains of mice and should also be considered.
b. Recommendations should include PCR testing of the tissue for mouse pathogens or inoculation of the tissue into test mice maintained under strict quarantine (MAP test), use of sentinel mice within the experimental room, necropsy and histopathology of tissues from affected animals, and repeated serologic testing.
c. Serologic testing, PCR testing, or virus inoculation of susceptible cell lines, mouse inoculation, and histopathologic examination are used to diagnose mousepox.

References

Lipman NS, Nguyen H, Perkins S. Mousepox: a threat to U.S. mouse colonies. Lab Anim Sci. 1999, 49(3):229.

Lipman NS, Perkins S, Nguyen H, et al. Mousepox resulting from use of ectromelia virus-contaminated, imported mouse serum. Comp Med. 2000, 50(4):426–435.

Case 40

a. Pale viscera are indicative of anemia. As some of these mice had hemorrhagic enteritis, this may account for the anemia.

b. Inflammation of the intestinal wall, with edema and inflammatory cell infiltration, will result in a thickened intestinal wall, as will hyperplasia of the intestinal epithelium seen typically with *Citrobacter rodentium* or *Lawsonia intracellularis* infection. The rectum of mice is predisposed to prolapse with straining and hyperplastic colitis.
c. Enteric organisms that may be involved in colitis in mice include *Helicobacter* spp, *E. coli*, *Citrobacter rodentium*, *Lawsonia intracellularis*, *Salmonella* spp, MHV, and heavy pinworm infestations.
d. A complete necropsy with histopathology, serology, and culture for relevant organisms should be performed. Rooms with affected mice should be isolated; the affected mice should be quarantined and treated or euthanized pending diagnosis. The facility should be thoroughly disinfected and restocked, if feasible. Use of microisolator caging will reduce the transmission of the highly infectious disease agents.

Reference

Percy DH, Barthold SW. Mouse. In: Pathology of Laboratory Rodents and Rabbits, 3rd ed. Ames, IA: Wiley-Blackwell, 2007.

Case 41

a. Diarrhea in infant mice may be caused by a wide variety of organisms, including rotavirus (epizootic diarrhea of infant mice [EDIM]), coronavirus (mouse hepatitis virus [MHV]), and reovirus 3. EDIM affects weanling mice under 21 days of age. Mortality remains low, and the feces may be pasty and yellow. Reovirus 3 infections are characterized by steatorrhea (oily diarrhea) in suckling mice. At necropsy, mice affected with reovirus 3 may have pale foci in the liver and other viscera. MHV, the most common of these three in research colonies, can result in high mortality, and the enteric form usually affects suckling animals. This case is most consistent with an outbreak of MHV. ELISA or indirect fluorescent antibody tests are serologic tests that may be used to establish a definitive diagnosis in exposed and recovered animals. PCR can also be used to diagnose active infections.
b. Dermatophytoses, excessive grooming or barbering by cagemates, biting, urine-fecal irritation, and abrasion on a cage surface will cause focal alopecia in mice.
c. Many murine viruses may be shed asymptomatically in the feces. More commonly shed viruses include TMEV, MHV, rotavirus, MPV, and MMV.
d. Morbidity refers to the number of animals affected or infected. Mortality refers to the number of animals that die.

Reference

Rehg JE, Blackman MA, Toth LA. Persistent transmission of mouse hepatitis virus by transgenic mice. Comp Med. 2001, 51(4):369–374.

Case 42: Itchy Mice

a. The most likely diagnosis for this syndrome, given the widespread nature of the condition and pruritus, is lice or mite infestation.
b. If the condition were confined to scabs and wounds in males, the likely diagnosis would be fighting. If females had areas of alopecia with no dermatitis, and were lacking whiskers, then barbering should be considered.
c. Skin scrape and DTM culture should be performed. Instead of performing a deep follicular scrape, which could cause significant trauma to the mouse, particularly if the wounds are around the eyes, shafts of hair around the affected lesions could be plucked and examined under mineral oil. DTM cultures are similar to those performed in dogs and cats. If one animal can be euthanized, histopathology and examination of the pelage for mites can be performed. Response to therapeutic trials with antiparasitics can also be used to assess infestation.
d. A variety of agents can be used to treat mouse lice. These include ivermectins, pyrethrins, and organophosphates. Ivermectins are highly effective and have a high therapeutic index, though some rare strains lack a complete blood-brain barrier and can suffer neurotoxicity following

exposure to ivermectin and its derivatives. Environmental decontamination should also be performed simultaneously. While feeding a snake a mouse that has recently been treated with ivermectin should be avoided, the drug is not toxic to reptiles.

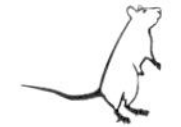

RATS

Case 43

a. An adult male rat typically weighs 450–520 g; this rat is in poor body condition.
b. The red discharge is likely chromodacryorrhea, or excessive porphyrin excretion in tears that is associated with stress.
c. Direct smear, gross and microscopic signs, culture, and serologic testing will provide a diagnosis.
d. Bacteria associated with pneumonia in rats include *Mycoplasma pulmonis*, cilia-associated respiratory bacillus (CARB), *Streptococcus pneumoniae*, *Corynebacterium kutscheri*, and *Pasteurella pneumotropica*. *Mycoplasma pulmonis* is a very common respiratory pathogen in rats that results in chronic pneumonia presenting as dyspnea in older rats. CARB and coronaviruses may also contribute to chronic respiratory disease of rats. Therapy for chronic respiratory disease includes provision of oxygen supplementation, if dyspnea is severe, and broad-spectrum antibiotics administered parenterally or via nebulization. Note that antibiotic therapy is palliative and not curative in chronic respiratory disease. Feeding moistened high-quality food will help support nutritional needs and hydration. The long-term prognosis is poor.
e. Older male rats are also predisposed to neoplasia, including testicular tumors (interstitial cell or Leydig tumors), chronic renal disease, and myocardial degeneration.

Reference

Percy DH, Barthold SW. Rat. Pathology of Laboratory Rodents and Rabbits, 3rd ed. Ames, IA: Wiley-Blackwell, 2007.

Case 44

a. Subcutaneous masses in rats are usually mammary neoplasms, although abscesses and fibrosarcomas should also be considered.
b. Mammary neoplasms in rats are most often benign fibroadenomas, although adenocarcinomas may also occur.
c. Surgical removal under general anesthetic is an appropriate treatment as masses are typically benign.
d. The masses are unlikely to reoccur following surgical excision, but other mammary tumors may grow from other sites. It is impractical to ablate all the mammary tissue in the mouse as it is extensive. Concurrent spay may reduce the incidence of tumor growth; however, prolactin-secreting pituitary adenomas may also induce mammary tumor growth in rats.

Reference

Hotchkiss CE. Effect of surgical removal of subcutaneous tumors on survival of rats. J Am Vet Med Assoc. 1995, 206(10):1575–1579.

Case 45

a. Long-Evans rats have dark hair over the head and dorsoanterior trunk and are often described as "hooded" rats.
b. The causative agent of sialodacryoadenitis in rats is a coronavirus. It could be definitively diagnosed by culture or PCR during active infection or serologic analysis after recovery.
c. Corneal damage would result from the decreased or absent lacrimal secretion and from trauma resulting from scratching the irritated area with the feet (self-traumatization).
d. Use of microisolator caging can slow the spread of disease, which is highly contagious. Strict hygiene including changing all clothing and autoclaving and complete sanitization of all bedding, cages, and implements that could serve as fomites should be instituted to prevent further spread of the disease.

Reference

Hajjar AM, DiGiacomo RF, Carpenter JK, et al. Chronic sialodacryoadenitis virus (SDAV) infection in athymic rats. Lab Anim Sci. 1991, 41(1):22–25.

Case 46

a. Judging by the location of the lesions on lesser-haired parts of the body and the histologic appearance, the lesions were probably thermal burns caused by heat from the heating pad. Heat lamps or hot water bottles may cause similar burns.

b. Anesthetized animals are susceptible to burns from hair dryers, heat lamps, or heating pads because animals cannot move away from the heat source and anesthesia suspends reflex vasoconstriction in response to heat. A circulating water blanket with a calibrated temperature setting should always be used in lieu of a heating pad.

Case 47

a. Findings are consistent with *Trichosomoides crassicauda* infection.

b. Examine urine for parasite ova by collecting urine (use of metabolism cages and 2% glucose in 0.09% saline for drinking water to cause diuresis), followed by filtration. Use a syringe to force the urine through a 22-mm diameter, coarse Millipore prefilter, which retains the eggs and examine the filter microscopically at 40×. The dark, brownish-yellow, bioperculate eggs are seen readily. Histologically, one may see profiles of adult parasites and eggs in the walls of the urinary bladder, ureter, or pelvis of the kidney, as well as migrating larval forms in the lungs.

c. Administration of a single 200 ug/kg SC dose of ivermectin and institution of an effective cage cleaning routine associated with repeated transfer of recently treated animals to clean cages represents an appropriate course of action. This will eliminate cages as fomites for transmission of eggs.

d. Adult female worms live partially embedded in the mucosa of the urinary tract and pass eggs intermittently in the urine. The small males reside inside the reproductive tract of female worms. Eggs ingested by a rat hatch in the stomach, and the resulting larvae migrate, via the lungs, to the kidneys and urinary bladder, where the worms mature.

Reference

Findon G, Miller TE. Treatment of Trichosomoides crassicauda in laboratory rats using ivermectin. Lab Anim Sci. 1987, 37:496–499.

INDEX

B

Prostatitis, rats, 244

Q

R